Sarcoidosis

Sarcoidosis

J. G. Scadding

MD, FRCP
Emeritus Professor of Medicine,
University of London.
Honorary Consulting Physician,
Brompton Hospital and Hammersmith Hospital

and

D. N. Mitchell

MD, MRCP
Consultant Physician,
MRC Tuberculosis and Chest Diseases Unit,
Brompton Hospital.
Honorary Consultant Physician,
Brompton Hospital and
Central Middlesex Hospital.
Honorary Senior Lecturer,
Cardiothoracic Institute,
University of London

SECOND EDITION

Springer-Science+Business Media, B.V.

First published 1985 by
Chapman and Hall Ltd
11 New Fetter Lane,
London EC4P 4EE

© 1985 Scadding and Mitchell
Originally published by Chapman and Hall in 1985.
Softcover reprint of the hardcover 2nd edition 1985

ISBN 978-0-412-21760-9   ISBN 978-1-4899-2971-6 (eBook)
DOI 10.1007/978-1-4899-2971-6

British Library Cataloguing in Publication Data

Scadding, J.G.
    Sarcoidosis.——2nd ed.
    1. Sarcoidosis
    I. Title   II. Mitchell, D.N.
    616.9   RC182.S14

Contents

Preface to the Second Edition

Since the first edition of this book in 1967, interest in sarcoidosis has increased world-wide, leading to increasing numbers of published clinical, epidemiological and laboratory studies, notably in immunology and in the pathogenesis of granulomatous inflammation. A series of international conferences which started as an informal gathering in London in 1958 has continued at approximately three-yearly intervals with increasing numbers of participants and more formal organisation, and the proceedings of all but the first have been published.

When the preparation of a second edition was suggested to me, I considered several questions. Is there still a place for a comprehensive, clinically-orientated book on sarcoidosis? Although the reports of the international conferences bring together research reports and some reviews of topics of contemporary interest, they are useful principally to specialists in the subject; and, like the original papers scattered through many journals, are not convenient sources of reference for clinicians. Continued enquiries about the availability of the first edition long after it had gone out of print suggested that it had provided such a source. I therefore concluded that a second edition should be prepared, and then had to consider whether, as a physician retired from academic and hospital appointments, I was the right person to undertake the major task of incorporating in it the still-relevant parts of the first edition, the considerable amount of new information that had accumulated since 1967, and a conspectus of current studies. To meet some of the difficulties implied by this question, I decided to seek the collaboration of a colleague still actively engaged in clinical and laboratory study of sarcoidosis as joint author, and was pleased when Donald Mitchell consented to join me.

J. G. S.

Having agreed to collaborate, we agreed also that our principal objective would continue to be to provide a comprehensive account of the complex clinico-pathological features of sarcoidosis which should be of value both to clinicians concerned with the problems of individual patients, especially those with unusual manifestations of the disease, and to investigators concerned with the unsolved problems of pathogenesis and aetiology. We have therefore maintained the general pattern of the first edition, in which pathology, incidence, and clinical manifestations were described, with illustrative case-reports where appropriate, before immunology and aetiology were discussed. The chapters dealing with these subjects retain only condensed summaries of those they replace, as more or less historical introductions to accounts of more recent work in these fields and of the position at the time of writing.

We are aware that our views on some controversial points are not shared by all; for instance on definition, on the propriety of adapting diagnostic criteria to differing clinical manifestations, on the use of corticosteroids in management, on the interpretations of the Kveim reaction, and on the need for complete open-mindedness about possible causal agents. Nevertheless, we have tried, as in the first edition, to keep clear the distinction between observations and interpretations, and to present the arguments on controversial matters fairly.

We thank Bridget Rogers and Verrall Lyle who have typed the manuscript and Neil Papworth for assistance in the reproduction of the chest radiographs and histological microphotographs. Our publishers have been extremely co-operative and we thank in particular Barry Shurlock and Peter Altman for all their help.

J. G. S.
D. N. M.

Ciba-Geigy Pharmaceuticals have made a generous donation to support the coloured illustrations in this book as a contribution to medical education, and we gratefully acknowledge this help.

Preface to the First Edition

In 1937, Professor I. Snapper, then Professor of Clinical Medicine at the University of Amsterdam, gave two University of London lectures on 'Pseudotuberculosis in Man'. The first of these summarised in masterly fashion what was then known of the disease now generally called sarcoidosis. My interest in this disease dates from my attendance at these lectures, and thus extends over more than a quarter of a century. During this time the importance of the disease has been increasingly recognised in many parts of the world, notably in Scandinavia, Holland, France, Germany and the United States. Its varied manifestations brought it to the notice first of dermatologists, then of physicians, ophthalmologists and radiologists; later specialists in many fields of clinical medicine and surgery found occasional examples of it; it has been found to have aspects of interest to biochemists and immunologists; it is now frequently discovered in mass radiographic surveys; and geographic variations in its incidence have attracted the attention of epidemiologists. Because of the wide interest which it has thus excited, much has been written about it in both general and specialist journals, and in many languages.

This book represents an attempt to provide a comprehensive account of sarcoidosis by correlating my personal experience and views with the published experience and views of others. Although my principal interest is in diseases of the respiratory system, colleagues have over the years referred to me patients with a variety of manifestations of sarcoidosis, and, of course, those patients presenting with intrathoracic manifestations frequently have extrathoracic changes also. Nevertheless, one individual can observe few examples of the rarer manifestations of a disease, so that in describing these I have had to rely largely on reviews of scattered accounts of a single or a few cases. Where my own experience has been more extensive, I have based my account primarily upon it, and have referred to the work of others principally to indicate differences both in objective experience and in subjective interpretation of that experience. In discussing the many controversial uncertainties, notably those relating to aetiology, I have tried to present observations and interpretations separately. Thus I hope that – in what is intended to be in the main a personal monograph – the reader will be able to distinguish between those parts which are based upon personal experience and those which are derivative, and to discern exactly what is the experience upon which personal opinions are based.

Many people have helped directly or indirectly in the production of this book. I am indebted to many physicians, both at the Brompton and Hammersmith Hospitals and in hospitals, clinics and practices throughout the country, who, knowing my interest in the disease, have referred patients with sarcoidosis to me; and to my registrars and house physicians who, over the years, have helped in the investigation and management of these patients. Among the latter, Dr K. M. Citron, now, happily, my colleague on the staff of the Brompton Hospital, must be mentioned specially for his collaboration over many years. My colleagues in Departments of Pathology, notably Dr K. F. W. Hinson, have been unfailingly helpful in allowing me access to their histological preparations and in discussion of problems of interpretation. My thanks are due similarly to my radiologist colleagues. Mr P. J. Bishop, Librarian of the Institute of Diseases of the Chest, has given me much valued bibliographical assistance and has been zealous in tracing references not readily available even in the great medical libraries of London. Most of the photomicrographs were made by Mr W. H. Brackenbury of the Photomicrographic Unit, Pathology Department, Postgraduate Medical School of London, the clinical photographs by Mr D. Kemp and Mr A. Curd of the Photographic Department, Institute of Diseases of the Chest, and the reproductions of many of the radiographs and some from colour transparencies by the Department of Medical Photography, Royal Marsden Hospital.

Finally, I owe a special debt of gratitude to my secretary, Miss Dorothy Hunt, for devoted and untiring help, not only in the preparation of the typescript but also in the tedious task of assembling case records, radiographs and other material.

J. G. S.

Chapter 1

Historical Survey

The earliest published reports of cases that can be accepted retrospectively into the diagnostic category now called sarcoidosis related to patients presenting with skin eruptions of several types. The concept of sarcoidosis as a systemic disease arose from recognition that these eruptions had a common histological pattern, and were accompanied by changes in internal organs showing a similar pattern; and later that changes of this sort may occur without skin involvement. Some of the names at first used for this systemic disease were derived from those used for the skin eruptions and others were eponyms, based upon claims for priority of description (Scadding, 1981a).

LUPUS PERNIO

In February 1889, Ernest Besnier, (Fig. 1.1), then the leading French dermatologist, showed a man aged 34 with lesions on the face and upper limbs 'of a type incompletely known and described' at a meeting at the Hôpital St Louis, Paris, and the case-report was subsequently published in *Annales de Dermatologie et de Syphiligraphie*. The patient was a cooper, working in the open air and exposed to the weather. His mother had died of pulmonary tuberculosis. The disease had started ten years earlier in the cold winter of 1879–80 with changes in the ears, which later ulcerated, though in this first report this ulceration is mentioned only briefly. After three years, a red swelling appeared on the nose, at first localized and gradually extending, and swellings attributed to synovitis of the tendon-sheaths of the fingers appeared on the backs of the hands. Both the patient and wax models of the earlier appearances were shown at the meeting. The nose was described as twice its normal volume, of purplish-red colour and shiny surface, with shallow erosions in front of the nostrils. The affected parts were not anal-

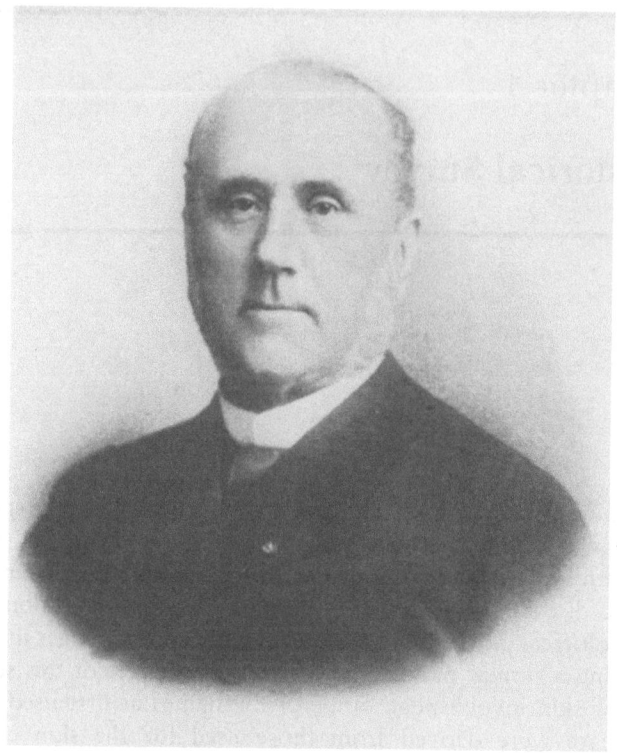

Figure 1.1   Ernest Besnier, 1831–1909.

gesic, and were not cold. In the hands there was, in addition to the swellings attributed to synovitis, purplish-red discolouration of several fingers, and dystrophic changes in the nails of the swollen little and ring fingers of the right hand. Epitrochlear lymph-nodes, but no others, were palpable, and no evidence of involvement of internal organs was found. Besnier described the eruption on the face as 'une variété de lupus erythèmateux à forme d'érythème pernio ou d'asphyxie locale', and proposed the name 'lupus pernio' for it. He regarded it as close to, but not identical with, the chilblain lupus ('lupus-engelure') of Hutchinson. These various combinations of 'lupus', which at that time would generally have been taken to refer to lupus vulgaris, with 'pernio', 'chilblain' and 'engelure' all meaning the same in different languages, are obviously liable to cause confusion. Case-reports by Hutchinson in his *Smaller Atlas of Illustrations of Clinical Surgery* (1895) show that he used the term 'chilblain lupus' for eruptions which he thought resulted from the combined effects of the factors causing lupus with those causing chilblains; he distinguished this from lupus erythematosus, which he illustrated separately.

Besnier made no histological studies; but the condition to which he gave the name lupus pernio presents a very distinctive clinical appearance, and in 1892 Tenneson reported a case which had been studied histologically. Quinquaud described the histology of this case as follows: 'an excessive predominance of epithelioid cells and a great rarity of giant cells . . . In summary, these lesions are those of a lupus, but a lupus with special histological characteristics, which can be defined anatomically: lupus of myxomatous and oedematous type'. He stated that a guinea-pig had been inoculated; at the time of the report, the animal was not yet dead, but its tuberculin reaction was positive. It is tantalizing that the fate of that guinea-pig does not seem to have been made generally known.

The published reports of Besnier's and Tenneson's cases were not illustrated; but wax models of the appearance of their patients were used to illustrate lupus pernio in an atlas of skin diseases, edited by Besnier and published in Paris in 1895–97, and translated into English and edited by Pringle (1897). Plate XXXV of this Atlas shows the appearance of the nose in Besnier's patient over a period of nine years, and of the hand at a single time. The ulceration of the ears mentioned briefly in the earlier report, is emphasized; it led to considerable loss of tissue, but unfortunately was not illustrated. In his commentary, Besnier expressed the opinion that lupus pernio is an infiltrating tuberculosis, and that 'in certain regions it invariably ulcerates'. It seems clear from this that Besnier regarded lupus pernio as a variant of lupus vulgaris. Plate XVIII evidently refers to Tenneson's 1892 case, which was that of a 46 year old woman with a purplish-red swelling over the nose and cheeks, similar eruptions on the arms, and swellings of the dorsal aspects of the hands and of some fingers, with trophic changes in nails. The description of the histology in this report differs somewhat from the 1892 account, omitting reference to 'myxomatous and oedematous' features: it refers only to 'common nodules of tuberculous lupus. Many of them have spontaneously developed into cicatricial tissue'. In an editorial commentary, Pringle stated that Hutchinson had expressed the view that these lesions were those of lupus vulgaris in tissues made vulnerable by weak peripheral circulation, though (rather unaccountably) different from those which he had described as chilblain lupus.

Both Besnier and Tenneson seem to have regarded the eruptions in their cases as unusual forms of the then very prevalent lupus vulgaris, and Besnier certainly labelled the changes in the hands tuberculous synovitis. In view of certain discordant features, notably the ulceration of the ears in Besnier's case, it is arguable whether the diagnosis of sarcoidosis can be regarded as established for either of them. But Besnier's description of lupus pernio certainly drew attention to a pattern of skin involvement subsequently shown to occur in the disease now called sarcoidosis. Neither Besnier nor Tenneson made any further observations contributing to knowledge of this disease.

'MORTIMER'S MALADY'

'Mortimer's malady' was described by Jonathan Hutchinson (Fig. 1.2) of London in 1898. He used this name for the disease because 'the first and as yet the most marked example' of it which he had observed was 'that of a very respectable elderly woman named Mortimer'. She was 65 years old, and her skin disease had been present about a year. It consisted of separate patches in groups on her cheeks and on the backs of the upper arms. The patches were symmetrical but rather larger and more abundant on the left cheek and right arm than on the opposite parts. They were raised and well defined, of dusky red colour and rather soft. There was no ulceration or pustulation, but some showed slight scaling. There was no scarring, though some of the patches had depressed centres. Six months later, the patches had increased in number and size. The lobule of the right ear was affected, and the nose 'was much swollen across the bridge, but without any implication of the skin, presenting a thick, soft tumour'. This description suggests that the eruption included elements resembling both Besnier's lupus pernio and the 'multiple sarcoids' described by Boeck in the following year; but unfortunately, no histological evidence was obtained. Hutchinson recorded that when biopsy was suggested, the patient did not return to see him for two years. In the same paper, Hutchinson described one other case in a man aged about 45 which he regarded as of the same disease, and two others about whose identity with Mortimer's malady he felt less certain. He thought that Mortimer's malady 'may not improbably be a tuberculous

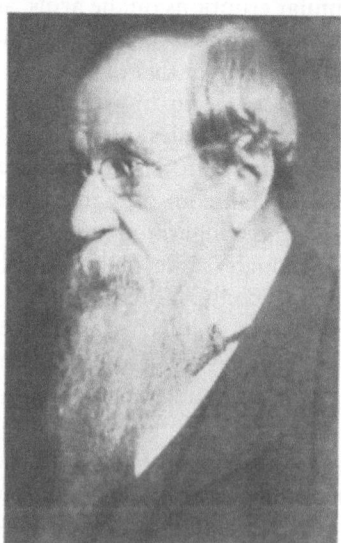

Figure 1.2   Jonathan Hutchinson, 1828–1913.

affection and one of the lupus family, but if so it differs widely from all other forms of lupus, both in its features and its course'. Because of this, he suggested the name 'lupus vulgaris multiplex non-ulcerans et non-serpigin-osus'. He later recorded that Mrs Mortimer died five years after the appearance of the eruption after a brief illness with abdominal pain and swelling, found at necropsy to be due to enlarged para-aortic and mesenteric lymph-nodes, histology of which showed only 'hyperplasia of normal gland-tissue'.

'MULTIPLE BENIGN SARKOIDS'

In 1899, Caesar Boeck (Fig. 1.3) of Christiania (Oslo) described the case of a policeman, aged 36, who had scattered spots and patches on the skin, appearing first on the brow and later spreading to affect the scalp, the face, the back of the trunk, the extensor surfaces of the arms, the back of one thigh and the lower legs. Over the right patella, there was irregular infiltra-tion in and around an old scar. The patches were slightly elevated and could be felt as well-defined nodules and infiltrations. The smaller ones were of a uniform yellow-brown colour, sometimes slightly scaling. Larger ones showed a slight central depression of bluish-red tint, so that in the largest

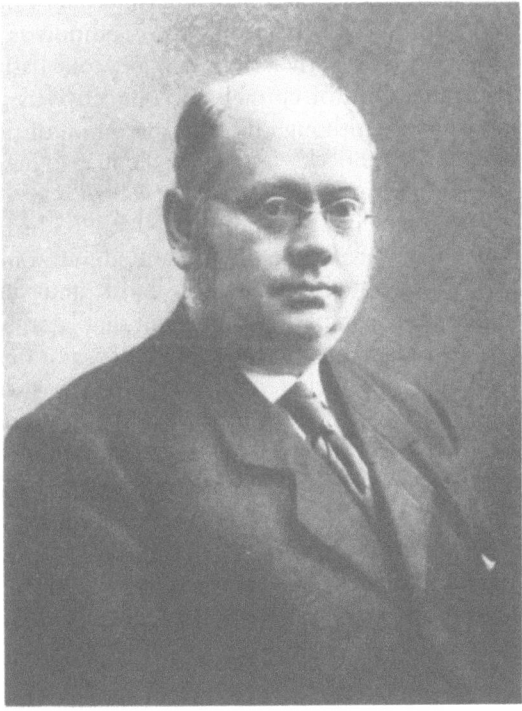

Figure 1.3 Caesar Boeck, 1845–1917.

the centre appeared atrophic with a network of dilated capillaries, surrounded by a narrow raised border. Plate II of Boeck's original paper shows the lesions on the back and trunk of his patient; the appearance is very similar to that of the skin of the patient shown in Fig. 7.3. Boeck noted in his patient that the cubital (epitrochlear) lymph-nodes were 'enormously swollen', the axillary nodes enlarged but not so much, the cervical nodes very little, and the femoral nodes 'so enlarged as to be visible when the patient stood upright'. He removed two skin nodules for histological examination, one recent, the other more advanced. He found 'through the whole depth of the corium from the papillary layer to the limits of the subcutaneous tissue, sharply circumscribed foci of a new growth', whose 'cells were of the type of epithelioid connective-tissue cells . . . The nuclei were sometimes multiple . . . In a few instances I found true giant cells of the sarcomatous type. Mitosis was scarcely anywhere to be detected'. He thought that most of these foci developed in the perivascular lymph spaces, but some from the corium, independent of the vessels. The outer epidermis and skin appendages were little affected. Boeck mentioned that he had seen one other similar case in Norway, and discussed the resemblance of his two cases to those previously described by Jonathan Hutchinson as Mortimer's malady. He proposed the name 'multiple benign sarkoid of the skin' for the disease observed in his two cases, regarding the condition as a new growth which 'might be described as perivascular sarcomatoid tissue built up by excessively rapid proliferation of epithelioid connective-tissue cells in the perivascular lymph spaces'. Although this interpretation of this histology is now known to be incorrect, Boeck was clearly the first to describe not only the skin lesion of the disease now generally called sarcoidosis and its histology, but also involvement of lymph-nodes. By 1905 he had revised his opinion both about the nature of the disease and about nomenclature. He explained that he had suggested the name sarcoid to indicate in a general way the connective-tissue origin of the lesions; but that later, on the strength of the discovery of acid-fast bacilli in the nasal mucosa of one patient, and of other evidence, he had concluded that the disease was 'a bacillary infectious disease, which is either identical with tuberculosis or closely related to it', and therefore preferred the term 'lupoid'. Because of the benign nature of the process and because the infiltration always developed in small distinct miliary foci, he proposed the name 'benign miliary lupoid'. By 1916 he had recognized the identity of Besnier's lupus pernio with benign miliary lupoid, and the occurrence of a very chronic affection of the lungs and of changes in bone and in conjunctiva, as well as of the previously mentioned manifestations in this disease.

Boeck's first patient with skin sarcoids died at the age of 80 from a hypernephroma with metastases; Danbolt (1947) published an account of the necropsy, at which no remaining evidence of sarcoidosis could be found.

'LIVID PAPILLARY PSORIASIS'

In a paper entitled 'Hutchinson-Boeck's disease', Hunter (1936) suggested that a case first seen by Hutchinson in 1869 and described in 1877 in his *Illustrations of Clinical Surgery* may have been one of the same condition as he subsequently described as Mortimer's malady, and most subsequent accounts of the history of sarcoidosis have accepted this as the first recorded case. Hutchinson headed his account of this case 'Anomalous Disease of Skin of Fingers, etc. (Papillary psoriasis?)', with the page heading 'Case of Livid Papillary Psoriasis'. The illustration shows the hand of a man aged 58, with large livid patches of induration on the middle finger, in the cleft between the middle and ring fingers and on the dorsum of the hand. These were raised and smooth – though with some dry scaling – of irregular shape, with abrupt margins, not tender and of purple colour. Similar patches but with less thickening were present on the front of the left tibia. The patient was otherwise in good health, apart from gout. Although the description seems compatible with the suggestion that this was a sarcoid infiltration of the skin, the illustration, about which Hutchinson remarked that the artist had not been very successful in representing the peculiarities described, would not immediately suggest this diagnosis. Hutchinson stated that in 1869 he had seen in the University Museum in Oslo a drawing showing a precisely similar condition on the hand of a Swedish sailor who was a patient of Professor Boeck. At first sight it might appear that this case may have been one of those later described by Caesar Boeck, but the Boeck whose clinic Hutchinson visited in 1869 must have been Carl William who died in 1875 and was uncle of Caesar. This incident therefore provides no connection between Hutchinson's case published in 1875 and Boeck's benign sarkoid. Hutchinson's patient had gout and died from kidney disease, and Hutchinson referred to him in a discussion of eruptions associated with gout, published in a paper which followed immediately that in which he described Mortimer's malady. It is thus clear that Hutchinson himself did not at any time identify this as a case of Mortimer's malady, and the grounds for making this identification retrospectively seem tenuous.

SUBCUTANEOUS SARCOIDS

In 1906, Darier and Roussy described the cases of five healthy middle-aged women with subcutaneous nodules, most frequently on the trunk, but sometimes on the limbs. In four of these, nodules were removed for biopsy, and a histological appearance similar to that of Boeck's sarcoids of the skin was found. Darier and Roussy therefore regarded the lesions in their cases as subcutaneous sarcoids.

INVOLVEMENT OF INTERNAL ORGANS

As noted above, Boeck early recognized that the lungs, lymph-nodes, nasal mucosa, eyes and other organs might show changes in patients with cutaneous sarcoids, and further evidence about these manifestations was soon published.

BONES

In 1904, Karl Kreibich, later Professor of Dermatology in Prague, but then working in Vienna, described cystic changes in the bones of the hands in connection with lupus pernio. His paper was based upon four cases, and is illustrated by an excellently reproduced radiograph of the hands of one of them; the histology of the skin was studied in another. In 1910, Rieder of Munich reported a condition which he interpreted as chronic osteomyelitis of several fingers in two cases of lupus pernio, and this paper also is illustrated by very clear radiographs. These bones changes were described again in two cases in 1920 by Jüngling, under the title 'ostitis tuberculosa multiplex cystica'. He thought the condition tuberculous; he mentioned Rieder's paper in a footnote, but seems to have been unaware of Kreibich's paper at this time. Later (1928) he recognized the close association of this condition with lupus pernio and Boeck's sarcoids, and described the histology and the detailed radiology. Jüngling's name has been rather widely associated with these changes in the bones of the hands and feet, but there is no doubt that Kreibich has priority. Not only was his paper published 14 years before Jüngling's first paper, but it was based upon twice as many cases, in one of which histological evidence was obtained and he clearly recognized the association with lupus pernio. Danbolt (1958) claimed priority for a case described by Kienböck in 1902; but this was in a paper on the radiology of syphilitic disease of the bones of the extremities, and although the published radiograph and the observations that the skin over the affected digits was red, tense and swollen and that a red swelling appeared over the bridge of the nose leave little doubt that this was indeed a case of lupus pernio with bone changes, Kienböck certainly thought that it was due to syphilis, on the basis of a history of infection five years earlier.

EYES

Although Boeck had mentioned involvement of the conjunctiva, and other early authors noted iritis accompanying sarcoids of the skin (Schumacher, 1909), the frequency of ocular involvement was not recognised for a long time. In 1909, Heerfordt of Copenhagen described under the title 'febris uveo-parotidea subchronica' a syndrome of enlargement of parotid and sometimes other salivary glands, chronic or subacute uveitis, and in many cases paresis of cerebral nerves, especially the facial. Heerfordt inclined to the view that this was a chronic form of mumps, but later the discovery of a tuberculoid histological pattern led to the suggestion that the disease should be named uveo-parotid tuberculosis or pseudo-tuberculosis. It was not until 1936 that Dutch and later French authors showed that this syndrome is a manifestation of sarcoidosis (Bruins Slot, 1936; Pautrier, 1937; Bruins Slot *et al.*, 1938). This conclusion was based on the finding of the typical histological pattern in the parotid glands and in other tissues and of clinically evident involvement of other organs, including the skin, lymph-nodes and lungs in patients with this syndrome. It is now generally recognized that while the full Heerfordt syndrome is rare, uveitis and other ocular changes are frequent in sarcoidosis (Chapter 8).

GENERALIZED GRANULOMATOSIS

In 1915, Kuznitsky and Bittorf of Breslau described the case of a man, aged 27, with Boeck's sarcoids on the legs and subcutaneous nodules on the arms, biopsy of lesions from both these sites showing the typical histology; he also had an enlarged spleen, enlargement of superficial lymph-nodes, slight albuminuria and cylindruria, and lung changes demonstrable both clinically and radiologically. He did not react to tuberculin, and no tubercle bacilli were found in the sputum. They considered that in this case the internal organs were involved by the same disease-process as was causing Boeck's sarcoid in the skin, and that this constituted a hitherto unrecognized disease of the internal organs, especially the lungs.

In 1914, Jörgen Schaumann (Fig. 1.4) of Stockholm wrote a prize essay on lupus pernio, in which he expressed the view that Besnier's lupus pernio and Boeck's multiple benign sarcoids or miliary benign lupoids were manifestations of the same disease; that this disease might involve also the lymph-nodes, the mucosa of the nose, the tonsils, the benes of the hands and the lungs; and that all these manifestations where characterized by a histological pattern which he summarized as 'a tuberculoid granulomatous process, presenting minimal phenomena of exudative type, and an exclusively proliferative character'. He suggested that since this disease appeared to involve predominantly the lymphatic system, it should be called lymphogranulomatosis benigna. In this essay, which does not appear to have been published until 1934, he described and illustrated, accompanying lupus pernio, radiographic changes in the bones of the toes and in the lungs, and typical histological changes in skin, lymph-nodes and tonsils. He pointed out that the skin changes should not be considered the cardinal and unique symptom of the disease, and that it was possible that the disease might sometimes affect only the lymph-nodes and internal organs, without causing

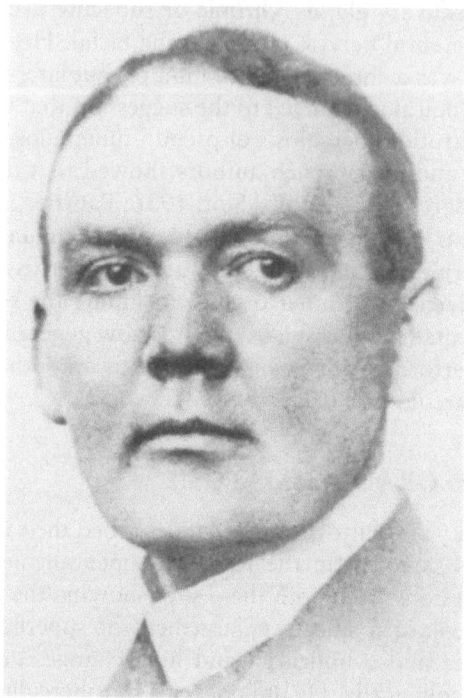

Figure 1.4 Jörgen Schaumann, 1879–1953.

any skin changes. In a long series of later papers, published from 1917 onwards, he produced clinical evidence in favour of these views. In 1936, he expressed the opinion that lymphogranulomatosis benigna is a generalized disease, without or with skin manifestations, in all probability of a tuberculous nature, that may cause death by destruction of the haemopoietic apparatus, by localization in vital organs or by the effect on the heart of the increased resistance to its work caused by the pulmonary lesions, but more often by the supervention of a classical tuberculosis.

LÖFGREN'S SYNDROME

About 1940, Scandinavian physicians noted that bilateral hilar lymph-node enlargement, with or without erythema nodosum, might be associated with sarcoidosis. In 1946, Sven Löfgren of Stockholm confirmed this association certainly for six and probably for nine more of a series of 212 cases of erythema nodosum; and in 1953 he showed clearly that the 'bilateral hilar lymphoma syndrome' represented an early stage of sarcoidosis (Chapter 5). This was a most important contribution, for the discovery of bilateral hilar lymph-node enlargement by routine radiography is now one of the most frequent ways in which sarcoidosis is discovered.

OTHER MANIFESTATIONS

In addition to the organs already mentioned, almost every tissue in the body has been reported to have been involved. The central nervous system and the heart are especially important though rare sites of localization, about which knowledge has accumulated largely through the publication of clinical and pathological case-reports. There are important changes in immunological reactivity, and in some cases in calcium metabolism, both of which have special characteristics. Interest in sarcoidosis has stimulated much investigation of the pathogenesis of granuloma formation, and many attempts have been made to isolate a causal agent from patients with sarcoidosis. In spite of these efforts, the aetiology of sarcoidosis remains obscure.

THE KVEIM REACTION

In 1941, Kveim, working in Danbolt's department of dermatology in Oslo, observed the development of slowly developing nodules having the histology of sarcoids at the site of intradermal injection of a suspension of tissue particles from a sarcoid lymph-node in patients with sarcoidosis. This reaction has been extensively investigated both as a possible diagnostic test, notably by Siltzbach of New York, and in relation to its implications for the pathogenesis of sarcoidosis (Chapter 21).

NOMENCLATURE

While ideas about sarcoidosis were developing, many names were suggested and used both for individual manifestations and syndromes and for the general disease of which they appeared to be partial expressions. Many of these have been eponymous, and in the past this has led, as is not unusual, to much pointless controversy about priority. The names of Besnier, Boeck, Schaumann, Hutchinson and Tenneson have been applied eponymously to the general disease, singly or in various combinations of two or three. Of these, only Boeck and Schaumann developed the concept of a systemic disease. Besnier was the first to describe one of the skin manifestations, lupus pernio, but did not describe the histology or anything beyond an affection of the skin. Tenneson was the first to report the histology of this condition. Hutchinson described the skin lesions later described by Boeck as multiple benign sarcoids, but made no histological studies. Boeck not only made histological studies, but continued his interest in the disease for many years, perceived the identity of skin sarcoids and lupus pernio, and recognized several of the non-cutaneous manifestations. Schaumann insisted upon the general character of the disease, and was the first to suggest that the skin changes might be an incidental and not a necessary event in its evolution; his prolonged studies of it added greatly to the understanding of its course and of its morbid anatomy.

Among non-eponymous names, Schaumann's 'lymphogranulomatosis benigna' has already been mentioned. He suggested this to indicate the general character of the disease, and its tendency to localize in the reticulo-endothelial system, and to contrast it with 'lymphogranulomatosis maligna' or Hodgkin's disease. The latter implication – that the disease is essentially one of the reticulo-endothelial system, having certain analogies with Hodgkin's disease but following a benign course – carries with it certain corollaries which are at least doubtful, and possibly for this reason the name was not generally adopted. It is perhaps ironic that 'sarcoid' has entered into general use. It was introduced by Boeck on a mistaken first impression from the histology that the skin lesion he described was a tumour of the connective tissue, and was later abandoned by him. But although the word sarcoidosis is reduced to nonsense by strict etymological examination (σαρξ-flesh), it might also be interpreted rather more freely as denoting a disease characterized by histological changes similar to those found in Boeck's benign sarcoids of the skin. Moreover, the impossibility of reading etymological sense into it may have a compensating advantage, in that it frees the word from unwanted aetiological implications.

The name 'sarcoidosis' is now used to refer to a systemic disease. Two sorts of observations led to the concept that a number of eponymous syndromes and affections of the skin and other organs, apparently unrelated at the time of their first description, should be regarded as manifestations of the same systemic disease. First, in clinical practice cases were found in which two or more of the syndromes were associated with each other, sometimes in incomplete forms. And second, a common histological pattern was found in all affected tissues, and even, when opportunity for more complete histological study presented itself, in some organs not presenting clinical symptoms or signs. In the next two chapters we shall therefore consider the pathology more fully, and then examine the problem of the definition of a disease in general and of sarcoidosis in particular.

Chapter 2

Pathology

The histological pattern that characterizes sarcoidosis can be described briefly as a non-caseating tuberculoid granulomatosis. Granulomatosis is here defined as a chronic inflammatory response in which cells of the mononuclear phagocyte series are prominent, usually forming focal aggregations (Williams and Williams, 1983). When these are well-marked, they are recognizable as tubercles. Knowledge of this sort of inflammation started from the study of the disease which owes its name, tuberculosis, to the recognition of the tubercle as its distinctive morbid-anatomical characteristic, but since Koch discovered its causal agent, it has been definable, and now is generally defined, aetiologically. In the following discussions, the word 'tubercle' is used in its original morbid-anatomical sense, without aetiological implications.

THE TUBERCLE

Early studies of the tubercle which develops in response to mycobacterial infection were reviewed by Rich (1951). It is composed characteristically of epithelioid cells, which are mononuclear phagocytes modified by enlargement both of cytoplasm and of nucleus, the latter becoming pale because its chromatin does not increase proportionately. A rather unconvincing resemblance of this modified macrophage to an epithelial cell gave rise to a generally used term 'epithelioid cell' to refer to it. A tubercle consists of a more or less well defined group of epithelioid cells, together with variable numbers of multinucleate giant cells. The typical giant cell of the tubercle is the Langhans type, with nuclei in an arc or a circle around a central granular zone, but the foreign-body type, with nuclei scattered through the cytoplasm, may also be seen. Variable numbers of lymphocytes may be found within the tubercle, especially at its periphery, and non-granulomatous chronic inflammatory cell infiltration of varying extent usually surrounds it. In mycobacterial tuberculosis the centre of a tubercle or of a coalescent group of tubercles may undergo necrosis without autolysis, resulting in caseation. In spite of much investigation, the factors determining the development of tubercles in response to mycobacterial infection remain incompletely known. While certain lipid fractions of mycobacteria stimulate their formation, the quantity required to produce this effect is far greater than that which would be contained in any number of bacilli likely to be present in the tissues. The development of tubercles does not depend upon the virulence of the bacilli, nor upon the susceptibility or hypersensitivity of the host. Studies of experimental granulomas, reviewed below (p. 28), and of the cellular immunology of granulomatous diseases (Chapter 20, p. 442) have thrown light upon the cellular processes leading to granuloma formation, but knowledge of the factors which underlie variability between individuals in cellular response to mycobacterial infection remains incomplete.

Tubercles occur most typically as the leading histopathological feature of tuberculosis and other diseases caused by mycobacteria, including leprosy; they also occur in a number of fungal diseases, including histoplasmosis, coccidioidomycosis, blastomycosis and cryptococcosis, as a less prominent feature in some other bacterial diseases, including brucellosis, tularaemia, syphilis and lymphogranuloma inguinale, and in some metazoal infestations, such as schistosomiasis. They may also be part of the histopathology of some diseases of unknown cause, such as Wegener's granulomatosis and related diseases, vasculitides, cryptogenic eosinophilic pneumonia, and primary biliary cirrhosis. But in these, granulomas are part only of a complex picture, rarely have the characteristics of a fully-formed tubercle, and may not be prominent. In sarcoidosis, however, epithelioid cell tubercles without caseation constitute the essential element of the histological pattern.

THE TUBERCULOID GRANULOMA OF SARCOIDOSIS

The distinction between the epithelioid-cell tubercles of sarcoidosis and those of mycobacterial tuberculosis and of the other diseases in which tubercles may occur consists in the different relative prominence of various features. The sarcoid tubercle (Fig. 2.1) is characterized by the well-defined appearance of the rounded collection of large epithelioid cells with pale-staining nuclei within the tissue in which it occurs, by the sparsity of lymphocytes at its centre though a variable number are present peripherally, and by the absence of caseation. None of these by itself is distinctive. In mycobacterial tuberculosis, tubercles at a distance from a caseating focus may show an identical appearance. Even the absence of caseation may reflect a difference of degree rather than an absolute criterion of differentia-

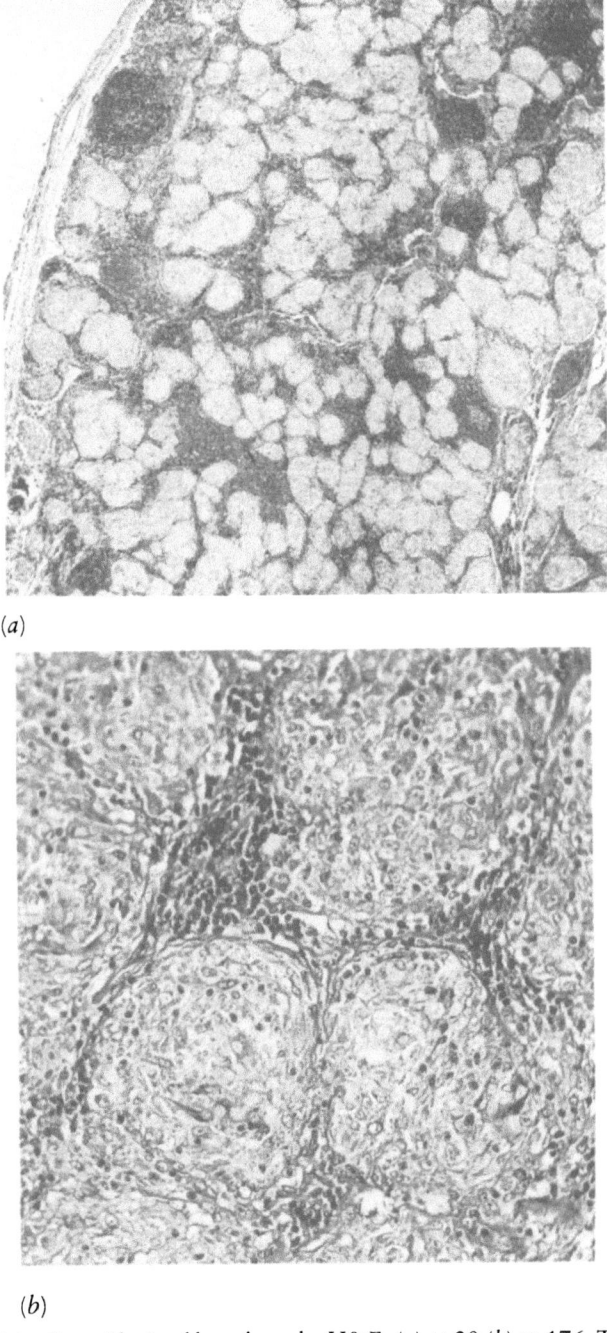

(a)

(b)

Figure 2.1 Sarcoidosis of lymph-node. H&E. (a) × 20 (b) × 176. This is the characteristic pattern of discrete non-caseating epitheloid cell tubercles.

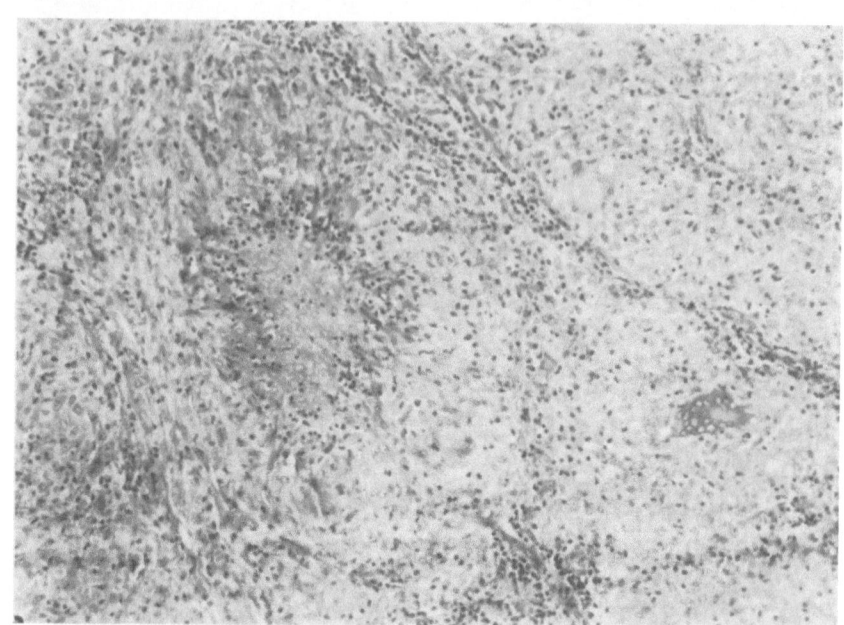

Figure 2.2 Central granular necrosis in sarcoidosis of lymph-node. Note also giant cells H&E. × 140.

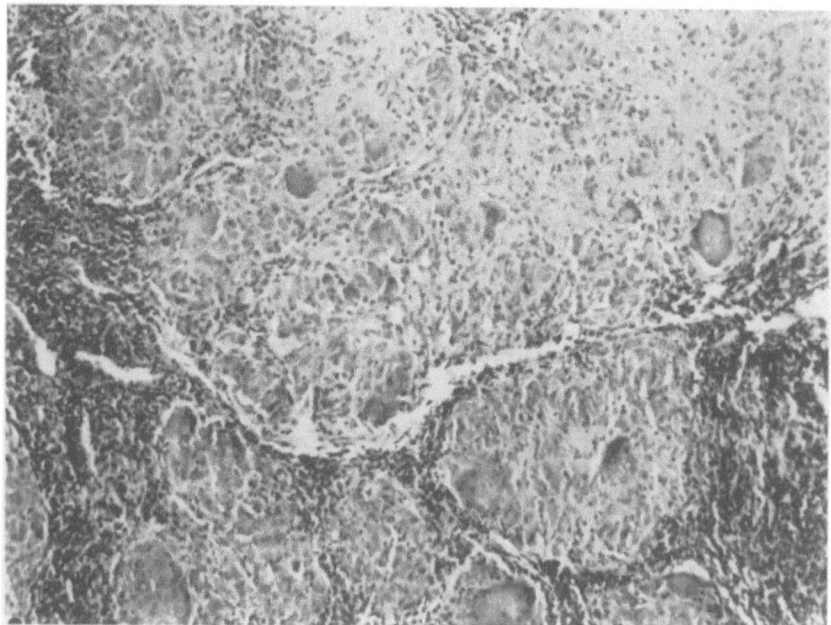

Figure 2.3 Giant cells in lymph-node sarcoidosis. H & E. × 100.

tion, for in the centres of a few tubercles in some typical cases of sarcoidosis eosinophilic granular necrosis, not amounting to actual caseation, may be seen (Fig. 2.2). It is distinguishable from caseation by the persistence of an intact reticulum, demonstrable by silver staining methods; but again this distinction is not absolute. Giant cells are variable in number in tubercles of all sorts, including those of sarcoidosis (Fig. 2.3), and their frequency does not discriminate between the various diseases in which tubercles may be found histologically. In sarcoidosis, certain inclusion bodies may be present in them. Among these, the conchoidal inclusion of Schaumann and crystalline inclusions are more frequent in sarcoidosis than in some other diseases, but they do not constitute a distinguishing characteristic. They are discussed below.

Sarcoid tubercles may resolve completely and leave no detectable residue. They may remain in a pre-fibrotic phase capable of resolution for many years. This is immediately evident in skin sarcoids, many of which eventually disappear completely; even large infiltrations, e.g. of the lupus pernio type, may subside after many years leaving remarkably little scarring (Chapter 7). If they do not resolve, they eventually become converted into a rather characteristic sort of hyaline collagen, which sometimes constitutes extensive featureless masses of avascular acellular fibrous tissue. In tissues in

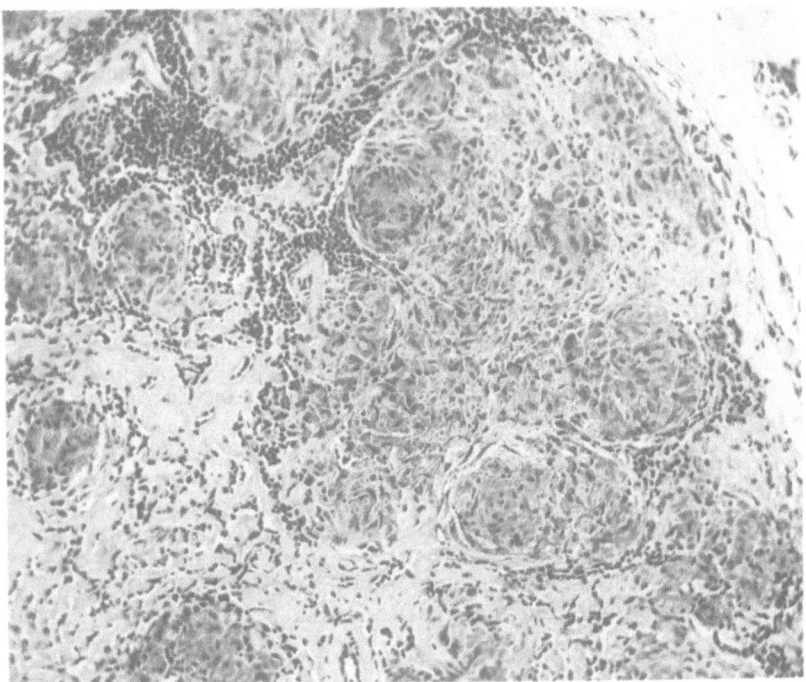

Figure 2.4   Hyaline fibrosis in sarcoidosis of lymph-node. H & E. × 140.

which this process is advancing, there may be some surviving isolated sarcoid tubercles, singly or in small groups, often with the sclerotic process starting at their peripheries, and separated from each other by broad tracts of featureless fibrous tissue (Fig. 2.4). While this sort of dense scarring is a constant finding in sclerosing sarcoidosis, it does not provide an absolute criterion of discrimination from mycobacterial tuberculosis, for it may occur in lesions undoubtedly caused by mycobacterial infection.

There is thus no way in which the histological study of tissue from a single site will permit sarcoidosis to be distinguished with certainty from other diseases in which tubercles can develop; even though a biopsy (e.g. of an extensively involved lymph-node) showing all the essential features and some or all of those which are frequently present strongly supports a diagnosis which seems likely on other grounds. The additional feature which distinguishes sarcoidosis from all the other diseases is the presence of the characteristic 'sarcoid' pattern in all affected organs. Early studies of the histology of sarcoidosis by light microscopy agreed about the widespread uniformity of the changes (Pinner, 1938; Pautrier, 1940; Ricker and Clark, 1949; Longcope and Freiman, 1952; Thomson, 1958). Thus, Longcope and Freiman (1952) reporting on their experiences at the Johns Hopkins and Massachusetts General Hospitals stated:

> The microscopical appearance of the lesions of sarcoidosis reproduces itself over and over with a regularity which has been aptly termed 'monotonous'. Although the skin and lymph-nodes have been the tissues most exhaustively studied, there is abundant evidence to indicate that the fundamental character of the lesion is the same wherever it occurs. In its most characteristic form, it consists of a collection of large palely staining cells with fairly well-defined boundaries which vary from polyhedral to fusiform configuration. The cytoplasm is abundant, slightly granular or homogeneous and sometimes vacuolated. The nuclei are prominent, delicately reticulated and oval, elongated or convoluted. Since there is usually little or no peripheral cuff of non-specific inflammatory cells such as is commonly noted about tuberculous granulomata, these cell clusters tend to stand out in bold relief against such tissue backgrounds as the deeply-staining pulp of lymph-nodes, or appear as inlays between the collagen fibres of the skin. The epithelioid cells in the smaller lesions have no particular pattern, but in larger foci there is often some tendency to whorl formation or concentric arrangement. Some of the cells in such lesions are larger than others and contain several nuclei. Occasionally the central portions of the lesions undergo a form of granular necrosis staining pink with eosin and dark blue with Malloy's phosphotungstic acid-haematoxylin. A few nuclear fragments can occasionally be seen in such areas. This form of necrosis is spotty, rarely involving more than a few scattered lesions and strictly limited to the central portions of the granulomatous foci. It is usually readily distinguishable from true caseation.

And Thomson (1958), studying patients seen in London, summarized the findings as follows:

The histological appearances of sarcoidosis remain characteristically similar in all the body tissues, so that a description of one such area of involvement is exactly mirrored in any other tissue. The essential histological features are the focal collections of epithelioid cells, usually arranged in spherical fashion and surrounded by a variable, but frequently scanty, rim of lymphocytes. These epithelioid cells have pale staining, vesicular nuclei, with pink staining cytoplasm and clearly demarcated cell boundaries. Additional histological features may be present; there are frequently giant cells of either the foreign body or Langhans' type; a variety of inclusions may be visible within these giant cells but they are in no way pathognomonic of sarcoidosis; foci of necrosis may also be present in the epithelioid cell aggregations. This necrosis is never a conspicuous feature; and when present it is confined to the centres of the epithelioid foci and is of the fibrinoid type.

The fibrinoid necrosis that may be seen in sarcoid granulomas was described in detail by Ricker and Clark (1949). It occurs in the centres of individual granulomas, especially where several have coalesced. Affected areas are strongly eosinophilic, fibrillar and acellular apart from a few lymphocytes. Silver staining shows a persistent reticulin pattern though its integrity may be doubtful in border-line cases. Zettergren (1954) found such changes to be more frequent in sarcoidosis known to be of recent onset. Evidence of this sort of necrosis was found in 35% of 300 cases of sarcoidosis from which material was available in the US Army Institute of Pathology (Ricker and Clark, 1949); in 6% of mediastinal lymph-nodes removed for biopsy from patients with sarcoidosis by Carlens *et al.* (1974), who noted that all those with necrosis had presented with a febrile illness; and in open lung biopsies from sarcoidosis patients in 39% of 43 cases by Carrington *et al.* (1976) and in 7.7% of 127 by Rosen *et al.* (1979).

It is now evident that the early descriptions of the histology of sarcoidosis over-emphasized the uniformity of the appearances, probably because they were based mainly upon post-mortem examinations. Biopsy studies, especially of mediastinal lymph-nodes and lungs, frequently show differing patterns of diffuse cellular changes formed granulomas, and fibrosis co-existing (Fig. 2.5). Whether these mixed patterns are due to successive episodes of inception, maturation and resolution or hyalinization of tubercles, or to varying rates of evolution towards these end-points in different parts of a process beginning synchronously may be difficult to determine.

Although the mature sarcoid tubercle characteristically shows limited lymphocytic infiltration only at its periphery, there are two groups of cases in which diffuse inflammatory changes are prominent.

The first consists of cases in which there is conspicuous diffuse cellular infiltration in the vicinity of granulomas in affected organs. Such changes have been observed especially in the lungs and in the meninges; these are considered in Chapters 6 and 14. Rosen *et al.* (1978) found that in open lung biopsies from patients with sarcoidosis, non-granulomatous inflamma-

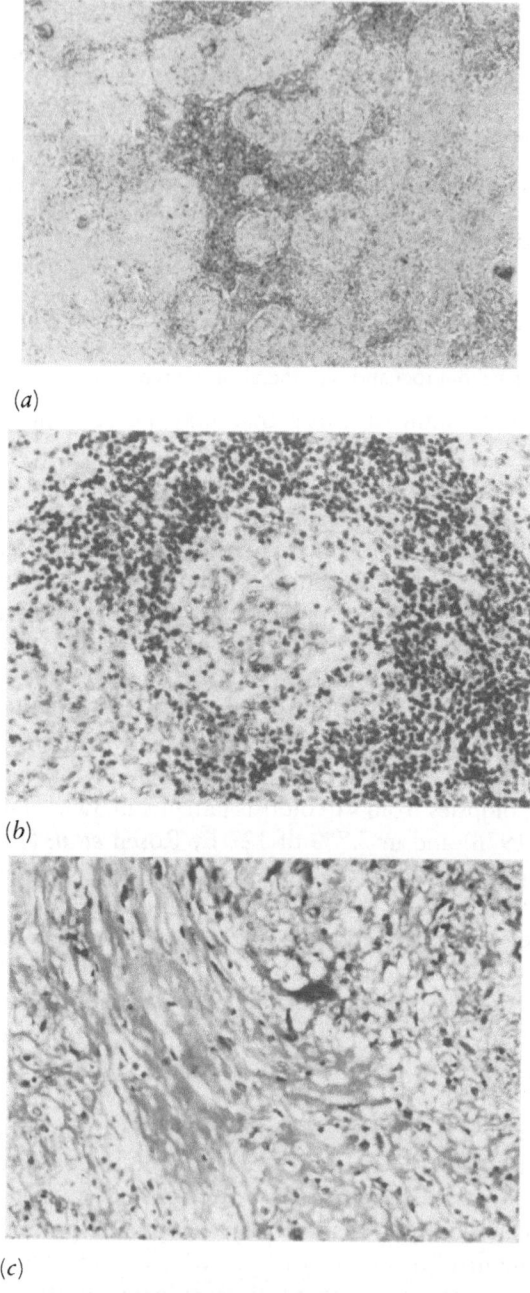

(a)

(b)

(c)

Figure 2.5 Supraclavicular lymph-node from a woman who had had sarcoidosis for six years. H & E. (*a*) × 16, showing both cellular and halinizing granulomas. (*b*) × 72, showing cellular granulomas.(*c*) × 72, showing hyaline fibrosis and remnants of granulomas.

tion tended to be prominent in those at an early stage of the disease, suggesting that changes of this sort antedate the development of granulomas. This is concordant with what is known from experimental studies of the development of granulomas (p. 28), and with studies of pulmonary sarcoidosis by the technique of broncho-alveolar lavage (Chapter 20, p. 435). But the great variability from case to case in the amount of diffuse cellular infiltration accompanying granulomas suggests that factors at present unelucidated determine in individual patients the rate of maturation of granulomas and the duration of persistent pre-granulomatous cellular infiltration.

The second group consists of those cases which have erythema nodosum and/or febrile arthropathy as an early manifestation. Neither of these manifestations shows, or evolves into, sarcoid-type tubercles. The erythema nodosum has the usual histology of this eruption, and resolves spontaneously (Chapter 5); and the febrile arthropathy is also transient, with the clinical features, and in the few cases in which it has been reported the histological pattern, of a non-granulomatous inflammatory arthropathy (Chapter 9). It is probable that the transient anterior uveitis that may occur at a similar early stage of sarcoidosis is, in at least some cases, simply inflammatory (Chapter 8). These well-defined manifestations affect only a minority of patients with sarcoidosis, in whom presumably some special factors not operative in the majority determine their occurrence.

Hyaline sclerosis is more likely to be seen and its extent is likely to be greater in old-standing sarcoidosis, but it is not related constantly to the age of sarcoid tubercles. Granulomas known to be of long duration may remain cellular with little or no hyaline change, and evidently recent granulomas may show it. Hyaline sclerosis usually starts at the periphery of the tubercle, gradually replacing the epithelioid cells. Eventually large tracts of featureless hyaline sclerosis may be all that is left. This process is well seen in lymph-nodes, which may come to consist of a large central zone of hyaline sclerosis with a narrow rim of still recognizable sarcoid tubercles surrounding it (Fig. 2.6). Just as the pattern of the active sarcoid tubercles throughout all organs is characteristically uniform, so is this type of sclerosis the characteristic and universal pattern of scarring in sarcoidosis. Mylius and Schürmann, who published as early as 1929 a detailed account of the pathology in two fatal cases, emphasized the importance of this form of sclerosis in naming the histological pattern 'universelle sklerosierende tuberkulöse grosszellige Hyperplasie'. Teilum (1948) suggested that the hyaline change in the late lesions of sarcoidosis was due to the deposit of a substance related to the globulins of the blood. He named this paramyloid, although it does not take stains for amyloid. Obel and Löfgren (1964) found that in sarcoid lymph-nodes hyaline was formed intracellularly in proliferating reticulo-endothelial cells around granulomas and in islands in the

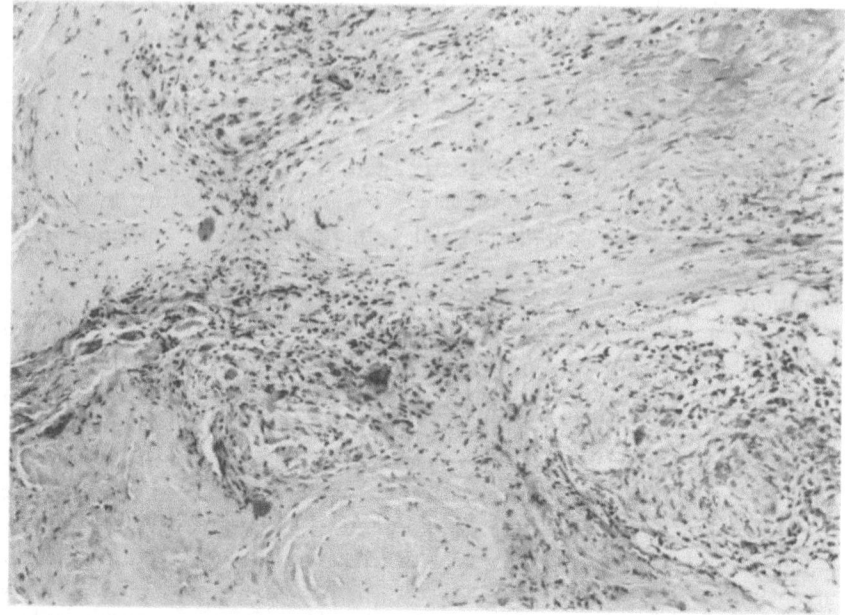

Figure 2.6   Extensive hyaline fibrosis in a sarcoid lymph-node. H & E. × 140.

lymphatic tissue; PAS-positive granules appeared in the cytoplasm and coalesced into large homogeneous masses. The hyaline material resembled amyloid structurally, but was not metachromatic; it gave histochemical reactions for muco- or glyco-protein.

Inclusion-bodies

Several sorts of inclusion have been described in the granulomas of sarcoidosis. Two, crystalline inclusion-bodies and the conchoidal body of Schaumann, occur more frequently in giant cells in sarcoidosis than in other granulomatous diseases. Asteroids and cholesterol clefts may be seen in sarcoid giant cells but are not especially frequent.

The crystalline inclusion consists of colourless doubly refractile crystalline material, varies in size from 1–20 μ, and does not take up stains, except that at the periphery it may take up stains for calcium and iron (Fig. 2.7).

Schaumann described the morphology and development of the conchoidal or concentric inclusion-bodies which generally bear his name in 1941. The smallest are the size of a leucocyte, round or oval. At this stage they are near one pole of a giant cell, single or in pairs, surrounded by a strongly staining membrane, the rest of the inclusion being more or less distinctly refringent. As they increase in size, they move to the centre of the

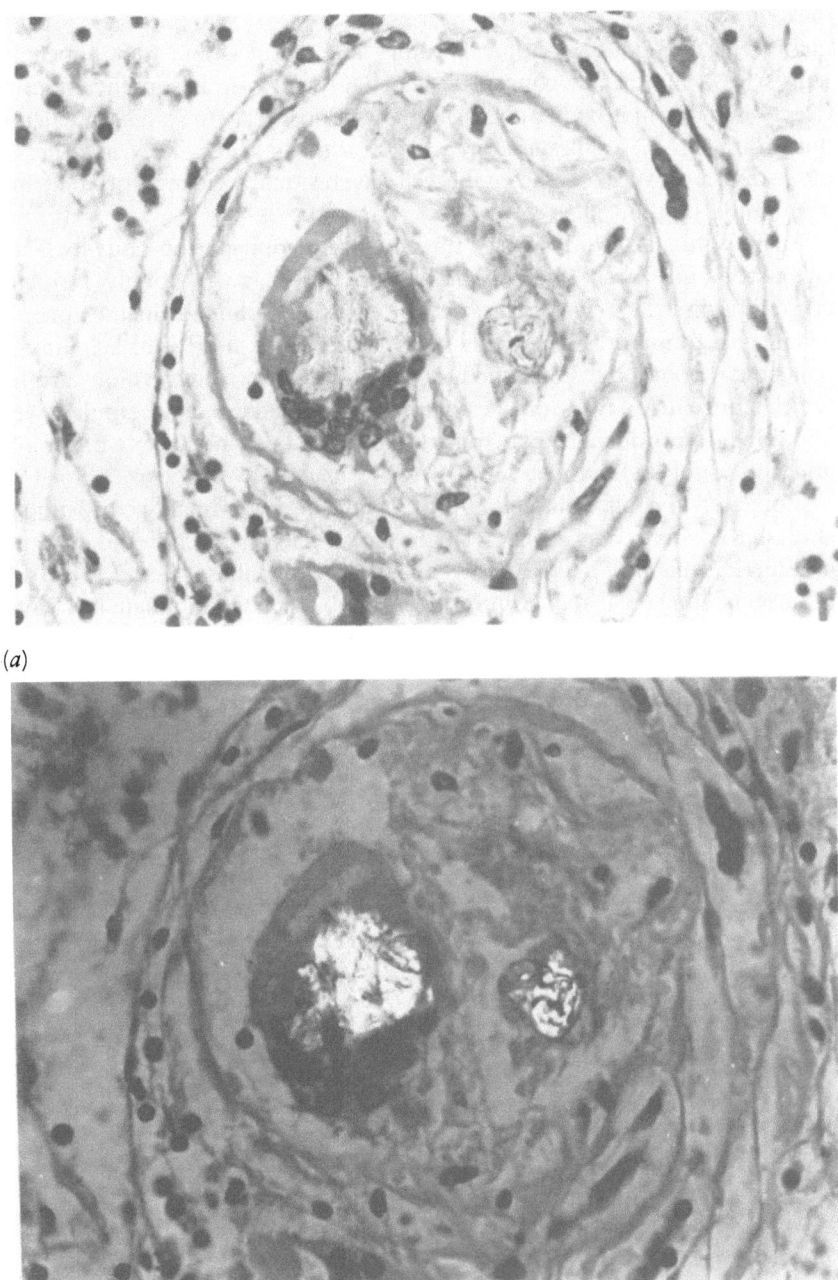

(a)

(b)

Figure 2.7 Crystalline inclusion-bodies. H & E. × 600. (a) normal light. (b) by polarized light, showing birefringence.

giant cells, the double outline becomes less distinct, and they appear to consist of a number of concentric lamellae which are basophilic, staining deeply with haematoxylin, and usually react positively to stains for calcium and iron (Fig. 2.8). They may reach 100 μ in diameter. They may persist after disappearance of the giant cell, as residual evidence of a former granuloma (Fig. 6.41).

Jones-Williams (1960) studied these two types of inclusion-body by histochemistry and X-ray diffraction. He showed that the doubly refractile crystalline inclusion was composed of calcium carbonate in the form of calcite. He found crystals of this sort incorporated in 70% of Schaumann conchoidal bodies. He concluded that the crystals formed the nidus around which concentric layers of a calcium-impregnated protein complex were laid down to produce the conchoidal body. The latter are deeply basophilic and not doubly refractile.

Elongated crystals, soluble in lipid solvents and presumably consisting of cholesterol esters, may be seen in the giant cells of sarcoid and of other granulomas, including those of mycobacterial tuberculosis (Zaki, 1964) and of farmers' lung (Seal *et al.* 1968). Rosen *et al.* (1979) found them in 17% of 127 open lung biopsy samples from sarcoidosis patients. In paraffin-embedded sections for light microscopy they appear as vacuoles. Zaki (1964) found evidence that they, as well as calcite crystalline inclusions, might be the nidus around which Schaumann conchoidal bodies could develop.

Conchoidal bodies were described by Metchnikoff (1893) in gerbils infected with tubercle bacilli, by Wells and Robb-Smith (1946) in natural

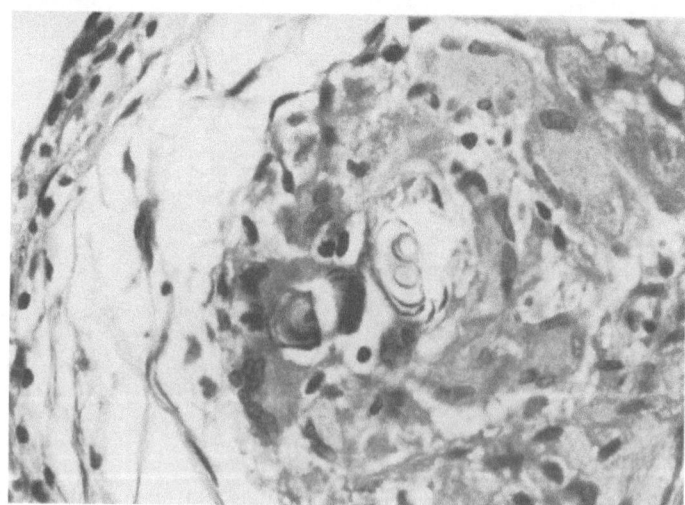

Figure 2.8   Schaumann conchoidal body, H & E. × 320.

and experimental infections with the vole tubercle bacillus, and by Zaki (1964) in cattle after subcutaneous injection of a tuberculosis vaccine. They have been reported in man in lupus vulgaris (Gilchrist and Stokes, 1903), in tuberculosis (Jones-Williams, 1960), in BCG vaccination scars (Zaki, 1964), in beryllium granulomas (Grier *et al.* 1948; Williams, 1960), in giant-cell granuloma of the pituitary (Doniach and Wright, 1951); and in lympho-granuloma inguinale (Rich, 1951). Jones-Williams (1960) found that their composition was the same whether they occurred in sarcoidosis, in chronic beryllium disease or in tuberculosis. The concentric bodies observed by Metchnikoff in tuberculous gerbils and by Wells and Robb-Smith in voles could be shown to contain acid-fast bacilli at their centres, but no compara-ble observation has been recorded in sarcoidosis.

It is evident that the frequency with which inclusion-bodies are found is dependent upon the amount of tissue available and the thoroughness of search. Nevertheless, there is evidence that crystalline and conchoidal inclu-sions are more frequent in sarcoidosis and in chronic beryllium disease, with a granulomatous histology closely resembling that of sarcoidosis, than in other diseases. Jones-Williams (1960b) found crystals and/or conchoidal bodies in 15 (88%) of 17 cases of sarcoidosis, and in 62% of 52 cases of chronic beryllium disease, but in only 6% of 100 cases of tuberculosis. Among the 15 cases of sarcoidosis with these inclusions, six had both types, seven crystals only, and two conchoidal bodies only.

Although the asteroid inclusion-body is usually associated with the name of Wolbach, who described it in 'disseminated granulomatous lesions' in 1911, it was described in 1905 by Lombardo, and later in the same year by Winkler, in Boeck's sarcoid. Wolbach's report concerned 'a new type of cell inclusion' in giant-cell granulomas found at necropsy in lymph-nodes, spleen, liver and lung as incidental findings, death having been due to unrelated causes. The inclusions consisted of a central mass, 2.3–3 μ in diameter with radiating straight or centred spinous projections, the whole being 5–25 μ in diameter. They were insoluble in acids or alkalis, and did not stain with silver nitrate, with stains for fat or iron, by Weigert's method for elastic tissue or with iron-haematoxylin. With Mallory's phos-photungstic acid-haematoxylin they stained deep purple, as does fibrin. The giant-cell granulomas in which the asteroids were found were described too briefly to permit any conclusion about their nature. Hirsch (1935) studied 'radial inclusions of giant cells' found in ten necropsies and 26 surgical specimens: the giant cells were in most instances part of a local granuloma which was an incidental finding, in liver, lungs, spleen or lymph-nodes, in the wall of dermoid cysts, in various scars, in chronic tuberculosis of the lungs, and in goitres. Kay (1950) found typical asteroids in two out of four cases of sarcoidosis of the spleen and Longcope and Freiman (1952) noted that in sarcoidosis, asteroids occur with special frequency in extensively

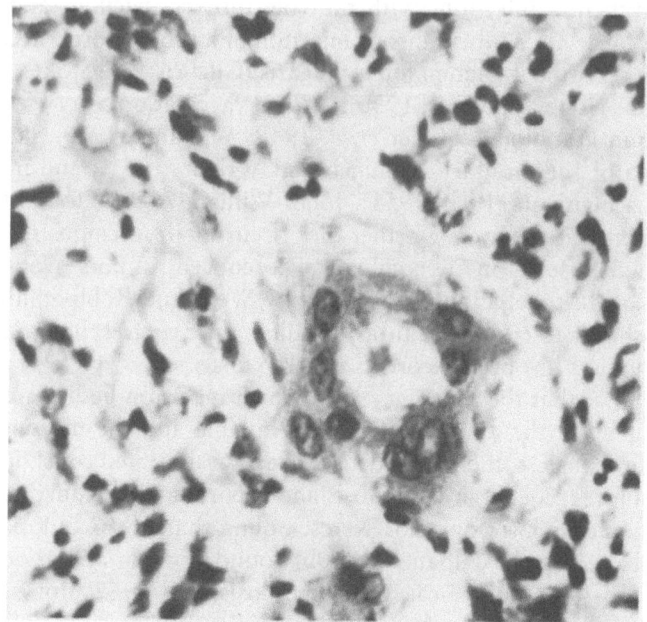

Figure 2.9   Asteroid inclusion body, H & E. × 480.

involved spleens. But they are not a special feature of sarcoidosis in general: Ricker and Clark (1949) noted them in 2% of their 300 cases, and Rosen *et al.* (1978) in 9% of open lung biopsy specimens showing sarcoidosis. A small asteroid appears as a spherical structure with minute spicules inside a vacuole in a giant cell, and stains pink with eosin; larger ones become star-shaped (Fig. 2.9). Friedman (1944) was unable by histochemical methods to determine the composition of asteroids in the spleen in sarcoidosis. Jones-Williams and Williams (1967) suggested from ultrastructural studies that asteroids might be composed in part of collagen fibrils but Cain and Kraus (1977, 1980) have found evidence that they consist of non-collagenous filamentous and microtubular material derived from the cytosphere.

Recently, a number of investigators have drawn attention to the occurrence in the lymph-nodes of patients with sarcoidosis, and other diseases of minute yellow-brown bodies variously called spindle (Hamazaki, 1938), spiral (Wesenberg, 1966), Hamazaki-Wesenberg (Baro and Butt, 1969), curious (Carter *et al.*, 1969) and yellow (Boyd and Valentine, 1970) bodies. These range from 0.5–8 μ in diameter, are yellow-brown in colour, pleomorphic but tending to be oval or spindle-shaped, and histochemically react like lipofuscin. They occur in lymph-nodes both outside and within cells, usually outside granulomas and in the peripheral sinus area. Boyd and Valentine (1970) found them in 15% of lymph-nodes removed for biopsy from various mainly peripheral sites. They noted that in sarcoid nodes, the yellow bodies were found in parts unaffected by the granuloma. Doyle *et al.* (1973) identified these bodies in lymph-nodes from seven of 47 cases of sarcoidosis, and in six out of ten porta hepatis nodes removed at necropsy from patients dying of causes other than sarcoidosis. Rosen *et al.* (1979) found them in 15 of 36 lymph-nodes, mostly mediastinal, and two of 12 open lung biopsy specimens showing sarcoidosis, and in three of 26 non-granulomatous mediastinal nodes. The nature of these structures remains obscure. It has been suggested that they might be budding yeasts or L forms of mycobacteria (Baro and Butt, 1969; Moscovic, 1978), but most observers have concluded that they are giant lysosomes that have become residual bodies (Sieracki and Fisher, 1973; Doyle *et al.*, 1973; Vuletin and Rosen, 1977) and are not specific for any disease.

Calcification

The hypercalcaemia that complicates a small proportion of cases of sarcoidosis may lead to metastatic calcification in previously normal tissues, such as kidneys, the pulps of digits, the conjunctiva and the cornea, and ear-drums (Chapter 19). It was long thought that dystrophic calcification of the chronic lesions of sarcoidosis was very rare. Until 1961, the only references to such calcification were two isolated cases showing radiological evidence of calcification in hilar lymph-nodes (Kerley and Twining, 1951; Scadding, 1960b) and necropsy evidence of calcification in a localized sarcoid deposit in the brain and in hilar lymph-nodes (Ross, 1955). In 1961, Scadding reported that among 136 patients with intrathoracic sarcoidosis followed for at least five years, calcification developed in seven; in both hilar nodes and lung in three, in nodes only in two, and in lung only in two. In none of the patients with this dystrophic calcification had there been evidence of hypercalcaemia, and several in the same series who had hypercalcaemia with metastatic calcification showed no evidence of dystrophic calcification. Israel *et al.* (1961) observed the appearance of new calcification in two of 256 patients; and Sommer (1967) referred to bilateral calcification as a recognized occasional finding in the hilar lymph-nodes of patients with long-standing sarcoidosis. In a case reported by Scadding (1968) it was shown by serial biopsy that calcification had developed in the hyaline connective tissue into which a sarcoid lymph-node had been transformed; a persistent reticulin pattern in the calcified area indicated the absence of caseous necrosis. After prolonged observation of 300 patients, Scadding estimated that about 5% of patients with sarcoidosis involving both lungs and hilar lymph-nodes would develop calcification. Calcification in pulmonary and hilar lymph-node sarcoidosis is considered further in Chapter 6.

Pathogenesis of epithelioid and giant-cell granulomas

Tuberculoid granulomas are the characteristic contribution of cells of the mononuclear phagocyte series to chronic inflammatory reactions. These cells originate in the bone-marrow, circulate in the blood and enter the tissues by amoeboid movement through capillary walls; in the tissues they become macrophages (Van Furth, 1970). Cohn and Benson (1965) found that in culture mouse peritoneal monocytes enlarged without cell-division, developed large numbers of mitochondria and of granules staining with neutral red and giving reactions for acid phosphatase, and showed increased activity not only of this enzyme but also of β-glucoronidase and cathepsin; they thus acquired the characteristics of mature macrophages. Sutton and Weiss (1966) showed that chicken monocytes in culture acquired the ultra-structural characteristics of macrophages in three days, and of epithelioid cells in seven days, and that by 15 days multinucleate giant cells were developing. Papadimitriou and Spector (1971) studied the experimental development of epithelioid cells in mice. They found that macrophages evolved into epithelioid cells if they were incubated without having under-taken phagocytosis, if they had successfully completed phagocytosis, or if they extruded ingested material by reverse pinocytosis. If they had ingested but failed to digest BCG they did not become epithelioid. Epithelioid cells did not phagocytose bacteria and contained no phagolysosomes, but took up colloidal gold or polystyrene by pinocytosis. They showed acid phospha-tase activity in endoplasmic reticulum and in lysosomes, synthesis of RNA in nucleus and cytoplasm, and digestion of ingested protein. Their life-span was normally 1 – 4 weeks, ending in death or in mitotic division into small round cells maturing to macrophages.

It thus seems that when macrophages develop into epithelioid cells, they show further increase in capacity for synthesis of enzymes which marked their evolution from monocytes, while their phagocytic capacity diminishes or is lost. In addition to acid phosphatase, cathepsin and β-glucuronidase, noted above, stimulated macrophages have been shown to produce collage-nase and elastase (Werb and Gordon, 1975 a and b), cytolytic factors (Gallily and Ben-Ishay, 1975; Melsom *et al.*, 1975) and, of special interest in relation to sarcoidosis, lysozyme (Leake and Myrvik, 1971; Sorber *et al.*, 1974; McClelland and Van Furth, 1975; Carr *et al.*, 1978) and angiotensin-converting enzyme (Hinman *et al.* 1979). The experimental induction of granulomas leads to increase in lysozyme levels locally and in the blood, with evidence of secretory activity by cells in the granuloma. In rabbits, Leake and Myrvik (1971) showed that intravenous injection of killed BCG in oil led to change in morphology of lung macrophages to the epithelioid pattern, with increased numbers of dense cytoplasmic granules and corres-ponding increases in lysozyme content of cell extracts and of blood serum;

and Carr *et al.* (1978) studying granulomas induced in rats by BCG followed by Freund's complete adjuvant showed that levels of lysozyme increased in blood and in lymph draining from the granulomatous lesion, and that lysozyme was demonstrable by an immunocytochemical method in macrophages in the established granuloma.

Multinucleate giant cells (MGC) develop by fusion of epithelioid cells. Their numbers are variable, in both experimentally-induced and clinically observed granulomas, and the factors concerned in their formation are unclear. Mariano and Spector (1974) found that MGC appeared on coverslips inserted subcutaneously in mice after three days and rapidly increased in number. Ultrastructural and kinetic studies showed that they developed by progressive fusion of mononuclear cells rather than by mitosis without cell division. Newly arrived macrophages appeared to fuse with older macrophages which might show chromosome abnormalities; possibly the older cells were recognized as effete by the newcomers. The life-span of MGC was estimated at about six days. Most of the early MGC were of the 'foreign body' type with eccentrically grouped nuclei, the Langhans type with peripherally distributed nuclei appearing later. On the other hand, Van der Rhee *et al.* (1978) in similar studies in rats observed that the Langhans type appeared first and seemed to develop into the foreign body type; the distribution of nuclei varied with their number, tending to be peripheral in cells with up to five, and aggregated eccentrically in those with 30 or more. Papadimitriou (1976) in experiments on athymic mice concluded that MGC are not thymus-dependent or thymus-derived. Warfel (1978) showed that in rabbits sensitized with BCG lymphocytes incubated with BCG produced a factor which stimulated alveolar or peritoneal macrophages from normal rabbits to form large MGC *in vitro*.

Inflammatory granulomas experimentally induced by different agents vary in rates of cell turnover by replacement from the circulation and by mitotic division (Spector, 1969). Papadimitriou and Spector (1972) studied three granulomas of differing cell kinetics. Reactions to carrageenan were composed of stable long-lived macrophages with many vacuoles containing material which appeared to be carrageenan. Reactions to *Bacillus pertussis* vaccine showed a labile population of short-lived macrophages maintained by recruitment of new cells from the circulation. Reactions to living mycobacteria (BCG) included after the first week three types of mononuclear cells: young macrophages containing many phagolysosomes, residual bodies and elongated electron-dense inclusions but few recognizable mycobacteria; and epithelioid cells, with prominent endoplasmic reticulum, enlarged Golgi apparatus, many transport vesicles, and elaborate plasmalemma but no phagolysosomes. The life-span of cells in the mouse BCG granuloma was estimated at 1—3 weeks. These observations indicate that in the mouse, long-lived macrophages containing phagocytosed material are the hallmark of low-turnover granulomas, while epithelioid cells with prominent biosynthetic function are characteristic of high-turnover granulomas.

The ultrastructure of sarcoid granulomas

On electron microscopy (EM), the epithelioid cells of sarcoid granulomas show an elaborate convoluted plasmalemma interdigitating with that of adjacent cells, and abundant cytoplasm with variable amounts of endoplasmic reticulum (ER) and Golgi complexes, many mitochondria and lysosomes but few, if any, phagocytic or pinocytotic vesicles. These appearances. suggest a biosynthetic rather than a phagocytic function, and differ only in detail from those of epithelioid cells in other granulomas, including those of mycobacterial tuberculosis, chronic beryllium disease, Crohn's disease and farmer's lung (Hirsch *et al.*, 1967; Jones-Williams and Williams, 1967; Wanstrup and Christiansen, 1967; Greenberg *et al.*, 1970; Jones-Williams *et al.*, 1970, 1972, 1974; Bernaudin *et al.*, 1975; Carr and Norris, 1977).

Jones-Williams *et al.* (1970, 1971) compared the EM appearances of granulomas in a sarcoid spleen with those in non-caseating parts of two tuberculous lymph-nodes. In both, they described two main types of cells, which they designated A and B. Darker-staining A cells contained much lamellar rough ER with cisternae filled with granular material, and moderately abundant Golgi complexes, and irregular nuclei with nucleoli and peripherally located chromatin. Lighter B cells had less organized ER, more abundant Golgi complexes, many vesicles of variable size and shape, some containing lightly-staining granular material, and nuclei of more regular outline, having no nucleoli and diffusely-distributed chromatin. Some cells with intermediate appearances, and a few very light stained cells, possibly degenerate cells of type B, were seen. It was thought that A might be an early, and B a later stage in the evolution of the epithelioid cell. A cells were more numerous in the mycobacterial and B in the sarcoid granuloma. There was little evidence of phagocytosis in either type of cell from either sort of granuloma.

Carr and Norris (1977) found many electron-dense inclusions, presumably lysosomes, in large epithelioid macrophages in sarcoid granulomas in skin and in lymph-node. These had circular or elongated profiles, ranging from 50–250 nm in minimum diameter and contained granules. In places these were arranged in lines with a periodicity of about 8 nm, suggesting a paracrystalline structure. In human macrophages from other sites similar inclusions were seen, but usually lacked the paracrystalline internal arrangement. Some sarcoid epithelioid cells contained vacuoles about 700 nm in diameter resembling the pinocytic vesicles seen by Cohn and Benson (1965) in mouse macrophages incubated in media containing foreign protein. Carr and Norris concluded that of all cells of the macrophage series, the epithelioid cells of sarcoidosis have an ultrastructure most suggestive of a secretory function.

Veien and Kobayasa (1980) studied the ultrastructure of five cutaneous sarcoids in an active stage. Most of the infiltrating cells were of the epithelioid type; about a quarter were classified as macrophages, and a variable small proportion were lymphocytes. Among the epithelioid cells, three types were distinguished. The most frequent type was characterized by well developed granular ER with many ribosomes. The next most frequent type had many lightly stained vesicles thought to be secondary lysosomes. The least frequent was characterized by dense primary lysosomes. The few MGC, amounting to only 1–2% of the cells, had the features of epithelioid cells with many secondary lysosomes. Macrophages were often seen in close contact with epithelioid cells. Most of the blood vessels within the granulomas showed normal endothelial cells, though in a few the luminal surface looked convoluted, with gaps between adjacent cells.

Spector (1975) concluded that the epithelioid and MGC lesions of sarcoidosis are a high-turnover granuloma of macrophages and their derivatives, analogous to that produced experimentally by BCG in mice.

Klockars and Selroos (1977) demonstrated lysozyme immunohistochemically in some but not all epithelioid cell granulomas, free macrophages and MGC in lymph-nodes and Kveim reaction papules of sarcoidosis patients; the amount of specific staining was greater in active lesions, and blood lysozyme levels seemed to vary with the probable amount of active sarcoid tissue. Lobo *et al.* (1978) showed by an immunoperoxidase method and EM that MGC and a few mononuclear cells in a sarcoid granuloma contained lysozyme within cytoplasmic granules. Carr (1980) by similar methods found that sarcoid MGC are rich in lysozyme, which is situated at the centre of the syncytium in dense granules about 200 nm in diameter; the ultrastructure suggested production as well as storage of lysozyme by the MGC. As noted above, lysozyme has been found in cells of macrophage origin in a wide variety of circumstances, and this finding is thus not specially related to sarcoidosis; and proof that lysozyme is being secreted awaits demonstration of the uptake of labelled precursor amino-acids (McLelland and Van Furth, 1975), or of immunoreactive lysozyme in endoplasmic reticulum.

There is evidence that angiotensin converting enzyme (ACE) is present in the cells of the sarcoid granuloma in notably greater amount than in those of other granulomas. Silverstein *et al.* (1979) studied biopsies from lymph-nodes, lungs, liver and skin of patients with sarcoidosis, and compared them with tissue from patients with bacteriologically proved mycobacterial tuberculosis and ileal Crohn's disease. In sarcoid granulomas, ACE was found by an immunofluorescence method in epithelioid cells and MGC, mainly in the peripheral cells of a follicle, central cells often being unstained. This suggested the possibility that the production of ACE might be induced in peripheral cells by interaction with lymphocytes. By contrast ACE was not found in the granulomas of the tuberculosis and Crohn's disease patients.

The immunopathology of the sarcoid granuloma is considered in Chapter 20.

Organ involvement

The frequency of involvement of various organs is discussed individually in the following chapters. In general, it can be expected to vary with the stage of the disease, since there is good evidence that in the early active stage widespread dissemination of granulomas in many organs commonly occurs, causing few or no symptoms and resolving spontaneously in many cases. The experience of morbid anatomists is unlikely to parallel that of clinicians, because some localizations, e.g. in the skin or eyes, are likely to cause symptoms and are not in themselves liable to lead to death, while others, e.g. in the lungs, heart and central nervous system may be fatal. Branson and Park (1954) reviewed 117 cases with necropsy reports: the organs most frequently found to be involved were lymph-nodes (78%), lungs (77%), liver (67%), spleen (50%), heart (20%), skin (16%), central nervous system (8%), kidney (7%), eyes and parotid glands (6%), thyroid gland (4%), intestine (3%), stomach (3%), and pituitary gland (3%). Necropsy findings are of course dependent upon the completeness of the examination and in sarcoidosis especially upon whether macroscopically normal tissues are examined histologically. For instance, Schaumann used the tonsils as a source of tissue for biopsy and found them to be frequently involved, but the tonsils are seldom used for this purpose clinically, or routinely examined at necropsy.

Epithelial and endothelial surfaces are only rarely involved. In the skin, sarcoid infiltration may impinge on the epidermis, but does not invade it; and similarly in the respiratory mucosa, the epithelium usually remains intact over an infiltrated submucosa, though it may show metaplastic changes. For this reason, skin infiltrations rarely ulcerate, except from trauma, and even large long-standing eruptions may resolve leaving little or no scarring. Similarly, because the endothelial surfaces of serous membranes are usually intact, serous effusions occur only rarely.

The distribution of sarcoid tubercles within organs varies from case to case, for reasons that are unclear. Selective distribution may be an important factor in determining the occurrence and nature of functional disturbance; this will be discussed in relation to individual organs. An important example is the occasional prominent involvement of blood-vessels, especially in lungs (Chapter 6), central nervous system (Chapter 14) and kidneys (Chapter 19).

Local 'sarcoid' reactions

Localized groups of epithelioid-cell tubercles of sarcoid type may be observed in a variety of tissues as a response both to foreign bodies of various sorts, and to such infiltrating processes as malignant disease and Hodgkin's disease.

Gardner (1937) showed that silica can stimulate the formation of tubercles closely resembling those of sarcoidosis. There are many reports of granulomas of this sort arising as a result of contamination of wounds of the skin by siliceous material (German, 1940; Ayres *et al.* 1951), or by talc in surgical procedures (Lichtman *et al.* 1946; Eiserman *et al.* 1947; Gruenfeld, 1950). In the active stage of sarcoidosis, old scars may become infiltrated with sarcoid tubercles. Löfgren *et al.* (1955) showed that such infiltrated scars contain siliceous material, presumably introduced at the original injury (Chapter 7, p. 197); and these infiltrations commonly wax and wane with changing activity of the sarcoidosis. But Refvem (1954) found that patients with sarcoidosis did not differ from other subjects in immediate response to intradermal injection of siliceous material. Both normal subjects and patients with sarcoidosis seem to vary widely in their liability to produce such reactions, and the explanation for this inter-subject variation in both groups remains obscure.

Sarcoid-type tubercles may be found in lymph-nodes draining an area containing a malignant tumour (Nickerson, 1937; Nadel and Ackermann, 1950; Gherardi, 1950; Symmers, 1951; Gorton and Linell, 1957) or a bronchial adenoma (Anderson, 1942; Symmers, 1951) and have been found within an ovarian tumour (Schattenburg and Harris, 1946). Nadel and Ackermann (1950) suggested that localized granulomas of this sort may be a stromal reaction to a lipoid produced by the tumour and may depend upon the response-pattern of the subject.

Similar granulomas have been found in association with Hodgkin's disease and other lymphomas (Nickerson, 1937; Kadin *et al.* 1970; Brincker, 1972), both in lymph-nodes and other tissues affected by the lymphoma, and in tissues not so affected. Kadin *et al.* performed multiple biopsies at staging laparotomy in 185 patients with Hodgkin's disease, and found granulomatous reactions in 31 of them; of these, eight were in tissues overtly affected by Hodgkin's disease and 23 in tissues not so affected. Among these 23, granulomas were found in liver in 17, in spleen in 17, and in lymph-nodes in five. In no case was there clinical evidence of sarcoidosis, but long-term follow-up was not reported. Brincker (1972) surveyed 1500 cases of malignant lymphoma and found epithelioid cell granulomas in 19. Of these, five showed evidence of generalized sarcoidosis; the association of sarcoidosis with other diseases, including lymphoma, is discussed in Chapter 24. In the remaining 14, there was no clinical evidence of sarcoidosis during observation for periods up to seven years; granulomas were found in tissues affected by lymphoma in 11, and in unaffected tissues in seven, both showing granulomas in four. In ten of the 14, the lymphoma was classified as Hodgkin's disesase.

The histology of local sarcoid reactions may be indistinguishable from that of generalized sarcoidosis, and may be so extensive within an affected lymph-node as to be misleading (Fig 2.10). Diagnosis depends upon search for evidence of granulomas at other sites, and for possible causes of a local reaction.

Histological criteria for the diagnosis of sarcoidosis

The essential elements in the histology of sarcoidosis are epithelioid-cell tubercles, well circumscribed within the surrounding tissue, with a variable amount of lymphocytic infiltration peripherally. The tubercles show no caseation, though there may be some central eosinophilic necrosis without disruption of reticulin pattern. There is evidence that the number of lymphocytes is higher in the early stage of granuloma formation. In formed tubercles, giant cells are found in variable numbers, but are not essential;

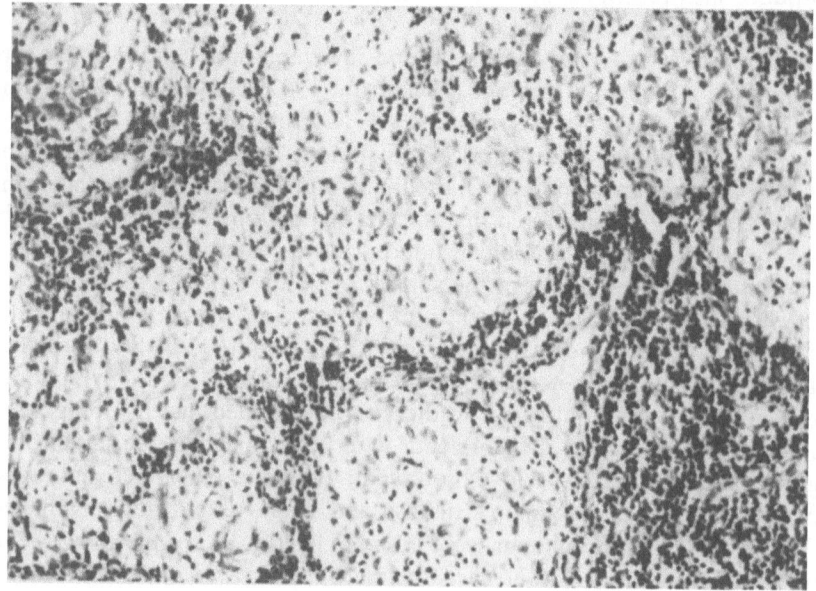

Figure 2.10   Lymph-node obtained by mediastinoscopy from a woman aged 56, showing well-defined sarcoid-type granulomas. She died three months later of anaplastic carcinoma of the bronchus; no granulomas were found at necropsy in other lymph-nodes, lung, liver, spleen or mycocardium. H & E. × 98.

they may be of Langhans or foreign-body type, more commonly the former. They may contain various sorts of inclusion-body; crystalline calcite inclusions and Schaumann conchoidal bodies are more frequent in sarcoidosis and in chronic beryllium disease than in other granulomatous diseases, but may be difficult to find and of no specific significance. Clinical evidence indicates that sarcoid tubercles may remain cellular and capable of resolution for considerable periods. If they do not resolve, they tend to become converted into avascular almost acellular hyaline connective tissue, prominence of which is characteristic of the late stages of sarcoidosis.

At necropsy, the findings of non-caseating epithelioid and giant-cell granulomas and/or their hyalinized remnants as the principal morbid change in scattered locations establishes the diagnosis of sarcoidosis beyond reasonable doubt. Because sarcoid-type granulomas may be an element in the histology of mycobacterial and some other infections and of some other systemic diseases of known and unknown cause, and may occur as a local reaction to foreign bodies or to tumours, the findings of such granulomas at a single site is not in itself diagnostic, and the histology of biopsy material should be reported in descriptive terms; in the presence of clinical, radiological, immunological and other findings compatible with sarcoidosis, together with failure to demonstrate agents known to cause granulomatous diseases, it may be sufficient confirmation of a diagnosis of sarcoidosis. Clinical diagnosis is considered in Chapter 26.

Chapter 3
Definition

Names of diseases appear, at first sight, to refer to agents causing illness; but analysis of the ways in which they are used in medical discourse shows that they have several different sorts of factual implication. Thus the medical concept 'a disease' is logically heterogeneous, though this is not generally recognized (Scadding, 1959, 1963, 1972, 1981b; Campbell *et al.*, 1979). Historically, this heterogeneity has arisen because the characteristics by which individual diseases have been defined have in many instances been changed, explicitly or implicitly, with advances in knowledge. At first, diseases could be characterized only by a distinctive combination of symptoms and signs, and thus were definable only in clinical-descriptive or syndromal terms. If a disease so defined were found to be associated with a specifiable disorder of structure or function, it tended to be redefined in terms of this new knowledge, sometimes with a new name. And when a cause of disease has been identified, causation generally displaces all other criteria as the basis of definition. Consequently, current nosology includes diseases defined in several different ways: by clinical description, by specified disorders of structure or of function, and by cause. This analysis leads to the general statement that in medical discourse the name of a disease refers to the sum of the abnormal phenomena displayed by a group of living organisms in association with a specified common characteristic by which they differ from the norm for their species in such a way as to place them at a biological disadvantage.

Definition, description and diagnostic criteria

When clinicians recognize a group of patients with symptoms and signs which do not conform to the picture of any hitherto described disease, definition initially can only be on the basis of clinical description. To be accepted as being a case of the new disease, a patient must show a stated combination of clinical symptoms and signs. As soon as knowledge has advanced sufficiently to permit a workable definition to be based upon criteria derived from a more objective field of study – anatomical or physiological and eventually aetiological – such a definition may be adopted. A definition based upon morbid anatomy or physiology will usually displace a descriptive one, and one based upon aetiology is generally the most useful when it becomes possible. The evolution of the definition of a disease as knowledge advances is well exemplified by the history of our concept of tuberculosis. At first, the various manifestations of the disease we now call tuberculosis were described under various clinical-descriptive or eponymous names – e.g. phthisis, tabes mesenterica, scrofula, Pott's disease of the spine, etc. – and between them there was at that time no obvious connection. The researches of early morbid anatomists demonstrated the tubercle as the common pathological basis of these, and led to the use of the word tuberculosis, which at this stage had a morbid anatomical connotation. Then the cause of tuberculosis was demonstrated by Koch, and the name tuberculosis, by origin morbid anatomical, was transferred to a disease now defined aetiologically.

At each stage in the development of knowledge, the most appropriate and useful defining characteristics must be chosen. The demonstration of these will indicate beyond doubt that a given example falls into the defined group. But they may not be easily observed directly in the living patient; in such instances, findings that can conveniently be sought clinically and that have been shown to be correlated with the defining characteristic may be adopted as diagnostic criteria, and accepted as indirect evidence of its presence. This is often so even for diseases defined aetiologically; for example, although the most satisfactory definition of influenza is 'the disease caused by the influenza virus', we may quite legitimately make this diagnosis without actually isolating the virus, relying upon indirect evidence from serological tests, or even, during an epidemic, upon clinical evidence only.

When the defining characteristics have been decided, cases in which it has been established, by various means, that they are present should be studied to establish the total description of the disease. This, of course, will include everything that can be discovered about the defined group by all methods of study. While reference to features of inconstant occurrence has no place in a definition – where it serves no useful function, and indeed tends to blur what should be precise – it is essential to a complete description, which should include where possible an estimate of the frequency of all the more important features.

There are thus clear distinctions between defining characteristics, which are those by which, given opportunities of the appropriate type of study, it can be decided beyond doubt whether a case belongs to the defined group; description, which is a summary of established knowledge about the defined group; and diagnostic criteria, which are the considerations upon which a probable diagnosis may be based in practice, and may include characteristics ascertained by any method of study. They will consist of features derived from the total description of the disease which have been found to discriminate between it and other diseases. Only for a disease which is defined on a clinical or syndromal basis will the defining characteristics be an obligatory part of the clinical diagnostic criteria, though even here they will not always be the whole of the possible diagnostic criteria. Whether or not the demonstration of the causative agent is included in the clinical diagnostic criteria of a disease defined aetiologically will depend usually upon the ease with which it can be demonstrated. For diseases defined on other bases – especially morbid anatomical – clinical diagnostic criteria will often be derived in large part from data obtained from methods of study other than that upon which the definition is based. These may give results only partially discriminatory from other diseases, so that their diagnostic significance can be expressed only in terms of probability.

For a disease with a clinical or syndromal definition, we must be prepared to find inconstant morbid anatomy and physiology, and possibly various aetiological factors; and the observed facts about these will be included in the total description of the disease. For a disease with an anatomical definition we shall have, *a priori*, a uniform morbid anatomy, but must be prepared for variability in clinical, functional, and aetiological findings. Sometimes a group defined in one of these fields of study will be found to have specifically distinctive features in another field. We shall no doubt be pleased by this, for it will simplify the problem, especially if a disease defined on some other basis is found to have a specific aetiology, so that it can be redefined aetiologically; but we have no right to expect such convenient findings.

Application of the principles of definition of diseases to sarcoidosis

The foregoing discussion will have made it clear that a definition of sarcoidosis must be a statement of the observations which would lead unequivocally to the diagnosis of sarcoidosis. It is not necessary that these observations should be of a sort that can in practice be made in every case; the definition states the method by which in principle certainty might be reached.

The accounts of the history and pathology of sarcoidosis in Chapters 1 and 2 show that at first the disease now called by this name consisted of a number of independently described manifestations in various tissues and organs; and that the observations which led to these being grouped together as one disease were that two or more of them were frequently observed together in various combinations in the same patient, and that they had a common histological pattern which was present in all affected organs. We have therefore in the histological pattern the unifying feature of the concept sarcoidosis. Although this pattern observed in a single site is not pathognomonic, its presence in all of a variety of affected tissues forms a workable basis for a definition. It will be recalled that all those who have studied the pathology of sarcoidosis have commented on the presence of a relatively narrow range of histological changes throughout affected tissues; and therefore this constitutes the most specific criterion available at present as a defining characteristic of this disease. No difficulty arises over local tissue reactions having a similar histology if it is specified that for the ultimate establishment of the diagnosis of sarcoidosis it is necessary that the defined changes must be present in all affected organs. Since there is no agreement concerning the aetiology of sarcoidosis, nor indeed whether sarcoidosis is an aetiologically homogeneous group, no reference to aetiology can be made in the definition. Even the statement that aetiology is unknown should not be included in the definition, for such a statement not only would result in the abolition of the disease as defined if the aetiology becomes completely known, but also makes it difficult to examine in an unbiassed way at least two tenable hypotheses. One of these is that sarcoidosis represents a possible reaction to more than one external inciting agent. For if this hypothesis were true, and one of the external agents were discovered, the cases shown to be caused by this agent would be excluded by definition from the category sarcoidosis; if a second and a third were discovered, the cases associated with these also would be excluded, until all that was left of sarcoidosis would be those cases which were caused by some other as yet undetected agent, together, probably, with some cases which were really due to one of the identified agents but in which it happened not to have been demonstrated. The other important hypothesis which the inclusion of this statement in the definition excludes from consideration is that sarcoidosis may represent an unusual reaction to an agent or agents already known and normally causing a well-recognized disease, but difficult to demonstrate in the unusual manifestation sarcoidosis. For if this hypothesis were true, it would be expected that the agent would be isolated from only a minority of cases; either this finding would be rejected as an error in the laboratory or elsewhere or explained as due to the supervention of a new disease, or the case would be excluded by definition from the category sarcoidosis. It is of course permissible to state, after the definition has been formulated, that there is at present no general agreement about the aetiology of the disease so defined; but to include this as part of the definition is to fall into a grave error of logic, by introducing as an axiom a proposition which, in addition to excluding *a priori* some hypotheses which should be the subject of empirical inquiry, may confidently be expected to be controverted in course of time.

Some suggested definitions

The definition suggested by the United States National Research Council (quoted by Ricker and Clark, 1949) was:

> Sarcoidosis is a disease of unknown aetiology. Pathologically it is character-
> ized by the presence in any organ or tissue of epithelioid-cell tubercles with
> inconspicuous or no necrosis and by the frequent presence of refractile or
> apparently calcified bodies in the giant cells of the tubercles. The characteristic
> lesions may be replaced by fibrosis, hyalinization, or both. Clinically, the
> lesions may be widely disseminated. The tissues most frequently involved are
> lymph-nodes, lungs, skin, eyes, and bones, particularly of the extremities. The
> clinical course usually is chronic with minimal or no constitutional symptoms;
> however, there may be acute phases, characterized by a general reaction with
> malaise and fever. There may be signs and symptoms referable to the tissues
> and organs involved. The intracutaneous tuberculin test is frequently negative;
> the plasma globulins are often increased. The outcome may be clinical recov-
> ery with radiographic evidence of residue, or impairment of function of organs
> involved, or a continued chronic course of the disease.

The only definite and clear part of this definition is that dealing with the morbid histology, and here the essential requirement that the changes must be present in all of several affected organs or tissues is omitted. The latter part of the 'definition' is entirely permissive, and thus blurs rather than sharpens; it is really part of a description of the disease rather than a definition. In fact, Ricker and Clark in their study adopted histological criteria of diagnosis:

> As this study progressed, there emerged a histologic pattern which was
> adopted as the criterion for pathological diagnosis. Most of this material has
> been selected on the basis of these histologic features. Discrete epithelioid
> granulomas make up the lesions . . . (They) tend to occur in clusters or 'crops'
> of tubercles of the same type of development, resulting in a pattern best
> described as monotonous.

At the second International Conference on Sarcoidosis in 1960, an attempt was made to improve on this; but the difficulty of definition was such that it was concluded that 'a short descriptive paragraph would be more meaningful than a definition'. At the seventh conference in 1975, the matter was reconsidered, and a slightly amended 'description' of sarcoidosis in lieu of a formal definition was accepted (James et al. 1976b):

> Sarcoidosis is a multisystem granulomatous disorder of unknown etiology,
> most commonly affecting young adults and presenting most frequently with
> bilateral hilar lymphadenopathy, pulmonary infiltration, skin or eye lesions.
> The diagnosis is established most securely when clinicoradiographic findings
> are supported by histological evidence of widespread non-caseating epithe-
> lioid-cell granulomas in more than one organ or a positive Kveim-Siltzbath
> skin-test. Immunological features are depression of delayed-type hypersensi-
> tivity suggesting impaired cell-mediated immunity and raised or abnormal

immunoglobulins. There may also be hypercalciuria, with or without hyper-calcaemia. The course and prognosis may correlate with the mode of onset. An acute onset with erythema nodosum heralds a self-limiting course and spontaneous resolution, whereas an insidious onset may be followed by relentless, progressive fibrosis. Corticosteroids relieve symptoms and suppress inflammation and granuloma formation.

Although this statement seeks to disarm criticism by not claiming to be a definition, it is intended to stand in place of one, and must be judged by its aptness for this purpose. One of the few unequivocal statements in it is that sarcoidosis is of unknown cause, which entails the logical difficulties in the study of causation noted above. It lists clinical and other features that may occur. It includes one statement, concerning cell-mediated immunity (as opposed to hypersensitivity), that is probably incorrect. It provides no indication of the way in which, in the final analysis, agreement might be reached in a case over which informed observers disagree. It fails to recog-nize that the difficulties of a histological definition can be avoided by the addition of a proviso that changes of the specified type must be widely disseminated.

What observations would in fact be accepted by all or nearly all informed observers as conclusive of a diagnosis of sarcoidosis in a doubtful case? The answer to this question seems to us to be the demonstration, either by multiple biopsies or at necropsy, in all of several affected organs, of non-caseating epithelioid and giant-cell granulomas, the changes leading to their formation, or their hyalinized remnants. This histological pattern, then, although we may be able to demonstrate it unequivocally only in some cases, must be our defining characteristic; a clinical diagnosis of sarcoidosis is a statement of belief that, if we had the opportunity of looking, we should find widespread changes of this type.

Recommended definition

The following definition is therefore recommended:

> Sarcoidosis is a disease characterized by the formation in all of several affected organs or tissues of epithelioid-cell tubercles, without caseation though fibri-noid necrosis may be present at the centres of a few, proceeding either to resolution or to conversion into hyaline fibrous tissue.

Explanatory notes may be added to this definition, but not as part of it, that the organs most frequently involved are the lymph-nodes, lungs, liver, spleen, skin, eyes, small bones of the hands and feet and salivary glands, though every organ and tissue, with the possible exception of the adrenal gland, has been reported to be involved; that cell-mediated hypersensitivity reactions may be depressed, though in some other respects T-cells are hyperactive; and that no single specific causal agent has yet been identified.

This definition offers the possibility of attaining certainty in the diagnosis of sarcoidosis, even though such certainty can be attained only by a complete necropsy or by an impracticably large number of biopsies. In practice, sufficient knowledge has accumulated about clinical, radiological, immunological and biochemical aspects of cases in which acceptable evidence has been available that they conform to this definition to permit the formulation of diagnostic criteria applicable to the more frequent modes of clinical presentation. These will be discussed when the various clinical manifestations have been described. Some combinations of clinical, radiological and other features, especially if several organs or systems are involved, are so characteristic that they justify a clinical diagnosis of sarcoidosis with little risk of error; and in such instances even this small risk may be eliminated by the observation of a typical histological pattern in tissue removed for biopsy from a single site. In other cases, with less characteristic features, biopsy from a single site, even though it shows a typical pattern, may be insufficient to establish the diagnosis beyond doubt. In general the amount of histological evidence required to support a clinical diagnosis varies inversely with the confidence with which the clinical picture in the individual case is recognized.

Chapter 4

Prevalence, Incidence and Modes of Presentation

There are several reasons why it is difficult to ascertain the number of cases of sarcoidosis in a community. One of these is that since many cases are discovered at screening examinations and follow an asymptomatic course to resolution, it is certain that in the general community many individuals must pass through the whole course of the disease without consulting a doctor. Another is that clinical diagnosis is in some cases a matter of judgement, and it cannot be assumed that standards of diagnosis are uniform. Even death notifications are difficult to interpret, since most of the deaths which result, wholly or in part, from sarcoidosis occur many years after the active stage of the disease, at which time there may be little that is specific in the clinical picture; and thus it is probable that at least some deaths from the late results of sarcoidosis are notified under some other diagnostic label. And finally, the clinical manifestations of sarcoidosis are so various that a patient may come under medical care in various ways. He may come under the care of a respiratory physician because of the discovery of abnormalities in the chest radiograph at a routine examination, or in the investigation of respiratory symptoms; of a general physician because of erythema nodosum or febrile arthropathy, or with symptoms associated with hypercalcaemia; or of a dermatologist, an ophthalmologist, or more rarely a neurologist, a cardiologist, an endocrinologist, or a gastro-enterologist because of symptoms referable to the appropriate system. Information available about prevalence and incidence can be interpreted only after consideration of the ways in which patients with sarcoidosis come under medical care, and of the proportions showing symptoms referable to various localizations of the disease.

Table 4.1 Percentage of patients presenting in various ways in some reported surveys of sarcoidosis.

	Scadding (1967) London		BTTA (1969) Four areas in Great Britain		International study (Siltzbach et al., 1974)				
	Male	Female	Male	Female	London	Paris	New York	Los Angeles	Tokyo
Total number of cases	119	156	224	343	537	329	311	150	282
Percentages presenting with:									
abnormal chest radiograph	38.7	30.8	35.7	28.0	22.2	47.4	39.9	20.0	44.7
respiratory symptoms	29.4	26.3	25.9	18.1	9.1	16.2	19.0	48.7	
erythema nodosum	4.2	16.0	23.2	34.7	27.9	6.7	10.6	9.3	
febrile arthropathy	4.2	1.3	3.6	0.6					
constitutional symptoms	6.7	1.9							
ocular symptoms	6.7	12.2	2.7	5.5	6.9	8.8	7.1	10.0	
skin sarcoids	3.4	7.1	4.0	8.5	9.9	4.3	6.2	12.0	
superficial lymphadenopathy	3.4	3.8	3.1	2.3					
parotid gland enlargement			0.9	0.9					
splenomegaly		0.6	0.4						
dactylitis			0.4						
nervous system changes			0.4						
myositis			0.2						
cardiac symptoms	0.8								
Mode of onset not stated					24.0	16.7	17.4		55.3

FIRST REASONS FOR SEEKING MEDICAL ADVICE

Table 4.1 lists some of the more frequent ways in which sarcoidosis becomes apparent, and indicates the proportions of patients in some published series who presented in these ways. Many reports of large series list manifestations observed at any time during the course, but relatively few refer separately to presenting features. The distribution of these is likely to be affected by the way a series is collected. Of those upon which Table 4.1 is based, Scadding's consisted of 275 consecutive patients under the care of one of us over a 20 year period; the BTTA (1969) study aimed to collect information about all patients diagnosed over a period of five years in four defined areas; and the international study of Siltzbach *et al.* (1974) assembled information supplied retrospectively from five cities. In view of these differing origins, the general similarity in proportions presenting with ocular changes and with skin sarcoids is notable, and contrasts with the wide differences for erythema nodosum. The BTTA study, to which all specialists who might be concerned with patients with sarcoidosis contributed, listed the less common as well as the more usual modes of onset.

Pulmonary and/or hilar lymph-node changes

These changes are the most frequent first overt evidences of sarcoidosis. They may be discovered either by radiography of apparently healthy individuals, or in patients presenting with respiratory symptoms. The relative frequency of these will evidently be affected by the frequency of screening procedures in the relevant populations, as well as by any differences that there may be between populations in liability to symptomatic as opposed to asymptomatic pulmonary sarcoidosis. In common with other manifestations of sarcoidosis, lung changes tend to be more florid in black patients; the high proportion of patients in the Los Angeles series presenting with respiratory symptoms is probably attributable largely to this factor. Israel and Sones (1958), reviewing 160 patients in Philadelphia, of whom 86% were black, found that only 11% were symptom-free, while 72% had symptoms referable to the respiratory system, such as cough, dyspnoea, chest pain or haemoptysis. By contrast, there were much higher proportions of symptomless cases in the BTTA (1969) study, in which all were white, and in Scadding's series in which nearly all were white.

Erythema nodosum

In most European series, the next most frequent presentation was with erythema nodosum or febrile arthropathy, or both of these, with bilaterally enlarged hilar lymph-nodes. This syndrome, which Löfgren (1953) demon-

Table 4.2 Percentages of patients reported to show manifestations referable to various organs in some published series. (Percentages in brackets are based upon less than the total number of patients.)

	Israel and Sones (1958) Philadelphia	Mayock et al. (1963) Personal cases	Mayock et al. (1963) Review of literature	Scadding (1967) London	International study (Siltzbach et al., 1974) London	Paris	New York	Los Angeles	Tokyo
Total number of cases	160	145	1254	275	537	379	311	150	282
Percentages reported to show localization in:									
lungs and/or hilar nodes	95	94	94	98	84	92	90	93	87
peripheral lymph-nodes	69	88	73	31	29	23	37	31	23
erythema nodosum	2	3	(8)	14	31	6.5	11	9	4
skin sarcoids	30	34	(27)	25	25	12	19	27	17
eyes	14	26	(21)	27	27	11	20	11	14
lacrimal glands	3	1.4	(3)						
salivary glands	6	9	(6)	2	6	6	3	6	5
splenomegaly	15	30	(18)	12	12	6	18	15	1
hepatomegaly	19	43	(21)	1.5					
nervous system	3	16	(5)	2	7	6	4	6	5
heart	2	9	(5)	1					
skeletal muscle		2.3	(1.4)						
bone	0.6	3.5	(14)	4	(4)	(3.5)	(9)	(4)	2
upper respiratory tract	1		(5)	1					
pituitary gland			(1.3)						
alimentary tract			(0.7)						

strated to be a frequent early manifestation of sarcoidosis, is discussed in Chapter 5. Reports of its frequency vary greatly, especially among early studies. It was reported in 25% of patients in Stockholm by Löfgren and Stavenow (1961); in 11 and 14% respectively of two series in London by Smellie and Hoyle (1960) and by Scadding and in only 2% of the predominantly black Philadelphia series of Israel and Sones (1958). A similar relative incidence of erythema nodosum was observed in association with primary tuberculosis in Scandinavia, England and Philadelphia when this infection was common (Chapter 5, p. 74), and it may be that populations vary in liability to erythema nodosum, irrespective of precipitating agents. Erythema nodosum occurs in a higher proportion of women than of men with sarcoidosis, though the relative excess among women varies. Where febrile arthropathy without erythema nodosum is recorded separately, there is a considerable excess among men. In Scadding's series, 4.2% of men presented with febrile arthropathy (without erythema nodosum) and 6.7% with constitutional symptoms (malaise, fever, loss of weight), as compared with 1.3 and 1.9% of women; and among men with erythema nodosum, the eruption was in some cases inconspicuous and atypical. It seems likely that though an acute onset with fever and constitutional symptoms occurs in a similar proportion of cases in both sexes, erythema nodosum accompanies these symptoms in a higher proportion of women.

The proportions of patients presenting with various manifestations are likely to be affected by the way a series is collected; there will certainly be fewer with eye or skin changes in a series derived from mass radiographic surveys than in one with a considerable input from an ophthalmological or dermatological department. Similar considerations apply even more strongly to the rarer clinical presentations. Of the studies upon which Tables 4.1 and 4.2 are based, the BTTA (1969) survey of four areas, to which all specialists to whom patients with sarcoidosis might be referred contributed, probably gives the most reliable estimate of the relative frequency of the various ways in which patients with sarcoidosis first came to medical notice.

Among the individuals presenting with symptomless hilar lymph-node and/or pulmonary sarcoidosis, discovered radiographically, an important proportion remain symptom-free and show spontaneous resolution. It is evident, therefore, that many people must go through the entire course of this sort of sarcoidosis undetected. Hagestrand and Linell (1964) reviewed 6706 necropsies in Malmö, Sweden, over a five year period, 1957–62, and found non-caseating granulomas in several locations in lymph-nodes, lungs, liver or spleen, sufficient to justify a diagnosis of sarcoidosis, in 43 cases. In only three was sarcoidosis the cause of death; in the remaining 40, the causes of death were those commonly found, predominantly malignant tumours and cardiovascular disease, the presumed sarcoidosis being an incidental finding. Local sarcoid reactions to malignant disease were found in 14 cases, and distinguished from generalized sarcoidosis. The prevalence of histological evidence of sarcoidosis at necropsy was 0.64%, ten times the prevalence of evidence of sarcoidosis in mass radiographic surveys in the same area.

During the variable course of sarcoidosis, clinical evidence of involvement of many organs may appear, and some organs are more often evidently affected in the later than in the earlier stages. The proportions of cases in a number of published series reported to show various manifestations at any time are summarized in Table 4.2. The figures are certainly dependent upon the duration of observation, the assiduity of investigation, and for some features – e.g. enlargement of the liver – the subjective judgement of the observer.

PREVALENCE AND INCIDENCE

The main sources of information about numbers of cases of sarcoidosis in a community are screening examinations and diagnostic records of hospitals and clinics. Mass radiographic surveys, useful in tuberculosis control pro-grammes in some epidemiological situations, have been the source of some estimates of the prevalence of sarcoidosis. Hospital and clinic records pro-vide information about numbers of diagnoses of sarcoidosis; the frequency of this event in a community can be deduced only if all such records for a defined population can be surveyed. Information from mass radiography and from diagnostic records may be affected by varying diagnostic stan-dards in routine services. A few studies of the incidence of sarcoidosis have sought to apply uniform standards by central review of records.

Mass radiography

Since a high proportion of cases of sarcoidosis show intrathoracic changes, and these generally present characteristic appearances, mass radiographic surveys give some indication of the relative frequency of sarcoidosis in different populations. Most of the information available from this source dates from the time when mass radiography was widely used as a tuberculo-sis case-finding procedure. Policy in the use of this procedure varied. In some areas – e.g. in Scandinavia – the objective was to examine entire populations within certain age-limits; in others, mass radiography was used selectively in groups thought to be themselves at special risk, or to constitute a special risk to others, in surveys at places of work, or in *ad hoc* campaigns in areas of high prevalence. Evidently, surveys designed to cover whole populations are likely to give the most reliable indication of the prevalence of sarcoidosis. Variations in the figures obtained from different sorts of

Table 4.3 Prevalence of changes interpreted as due to sarcoidosis in some mass radiographic surveys (Bauer and Löfgren, 1964). (Figures in brackets refer to reported variations within countries.)

Country	Years	Number of examinations $\times 10^6$	Changes attributed to sarcoidosis per 100 000	Reporter
England and Wales	1958	3.32	20 (10–30)	James and Brett
Scotland	1958–61	1.71	8.2 (6.8–18.0)	Douglas
Northern Ireland	1945–62	1.45	10.3 (4–41)	Milliken
Sweden	1945–53	1.87	55 (4–137)	Bauer and Wijkstrom
	1953–60	1.35	64 (16–72)	
Finland	1960–61	1.43	8.1	Pätiälä et al.
Norway	1954–58	1.45	26.7	Riddervold
Czechoslovakia	?	3.44	3.4 (0–20.7)	Levinsky and Altmann
Germany: West Berlin	1949–62	2.2	14.5	Fried
Leipzig	1960–62	3.02	13.3	Lindig
Netherlands	1952–62	4.59	21.6	Orie and ter Brugge
Switzerland	?	3.16	16.3	Sommer
France	?	0.61	9.5	Turiaf et al.
Australia: Victoria	1959–62	1.57	9.2	Marshman
New Zealand	1952–62	1.08	16 (6.1–24.3)	Reid

survey are illustrated by the findings in England and Wales, where the number of persons per 100 000 examined by mass radiography units in 1959 and found to have abnormalities interpreted as sarcoidosis was 13.8 in men and 19.8 in women, with the highest prevalence in both sexes in the age-group 25–34 years (Ministry of Health Report, 1960) . Among those who attended in response to general publicity, the rates among men and women were 14.4 and 19.6 respectively; among those referred by family doctors, they were 74.0 and 96.8; and among those examined in surveys in factories and offices, they were 9.7 and 11.8. Probably the latter were the nearest approach to a representative sample of a population group, not including a disproportionate number of individuals with symptoms. Rather similar figures for the proportions of mass radiographic examinations showing evidence of sarcoidosis were reported in the years 1962–65 (Hall *et al.*, 1969). In Great Britain, the nearest approach to surveys of entire populations within defined areas has been provided by mass radiographic campaigns. In Liverpool, changes attributed to sarcoidosis were found in nine per 100 000 examinations in such a campaign in 1959 (Semple, 1959). In surveys in Scotland in which nearly 70% of the selected populations were examined, such changes were found in six per 100 000 in 1957, and five per 100 000 in 1958 (McGregor, 1961).

Widely differing figures for the prevalence of sarcoidosis based upon mass radiographic data have been reported from other countries (Bauer and Löfgren, 1964; Levinsky *et al.*, 1976). Some of the findings reported at an international conference in 1963 are summarized in Table 4.3. As noted above, some of the differences are attributable to differing policies in the use of mass radiography, and different diagnostic standards probably are another factor. Perhaps the most interesting differences are those between and within the Scandinavian countries, where both policy and diagnostic standards were similar. In Sweden, surveys in 1945–53 covering between 70 and 98% of the population in selected areas showed 55 cases of intrathoracic sarcoidosis per 100 000 persons over the age of ten years, with a wide variation, six to 137, between areas; and in 1953–60, in another selection of areas, including some of those previously surveyed, 64 per 100 000, varying between 16 and 72 (Bauer and Wijkstrom, 1964). Considerably lower figures have been reported from neighbouring countries. Ridderwold (1964) stated that in Norway in 1954—58, new cases of sarcoidosis were found in 13.1 and 14.4 per 100 000 examinations in men and women respectively, and Selroos (1969) that in Finland the rates for the two sexes combined ranged from 2.3–16.7 per 100 000 in different areas. In Czechoslovakia, Levinsky *et al.* (1976) reported that the number of cases of sarcoidosis found in mass radiographic surveys ranged from less than ten to more than 40 per 100 000 in different areas, and commented that the wide differences between the figures reported from some neighbouring areas raised doubt whether these corresponded to real differences. In Italy, Blasi *et al.* (1974) found that mass radiography revealed 14.9 cases of sarcoidosis per 100 000 examinations in five northern cities, and only 1.3 in four more southerly cities. There is some evidence that in general the prevalence is lower in southern than in northern Europe; Zapatero (1970) stated that in Spain mass radiography revealed only 0.04 cases of sarcoidosis per 100 000. The contributions of differences in diagnostic criteria and in survey procedures to these widely varying reports of radiographic prevalence are unknown.

In the Wellington area of New Zealand, MacKay *et al.* (1964) found evidence of sarcoidosis in 19.4 per 100 000 mass radiographic examinations in the years 1952–57, and in 28.4 per 100 000 in 1958–62; the prevalence was slightly higher in women than in men.

Routine radiography of occupational groups provides further information. Schönholzer (1947) reported that in the Swiss Army, 13 per 100 000 examinations showed changes interpreted as due to sarcoidosis; and Buss and Dörken (1975) that in the West German Army, 28 cases of presumed sarcoidosis were found per 100 000 in routine examinations at induction and at yearly intervals during the years 1965–69.

Data derived from diagnostic records

The other principal sources of data concerning the prevalence and incidence of sarcoidosis are defined populations for which records of disability and death are available in sufficient detail, and with sufficient completeness, and in which it can be assumed that reasonably uniform diagnostic standards have been applied.

In the United States Army, Cooch (1961) reviewed the incidence of sarcoidosis for the years 1953–56 on the basis of records of disability and death. The mean number of cases arising per 100 000 mean strength per year was 11. The highest rate was in the age group 25–29 years. Officers had a slightly lower rate than other ranks, but this may have been due to selection of officers by rigorous medical standards. The rates for blacks were much higher than those for others, averaging 16 times those for all others, the large majority of European origin. Those born in the south-eastern states had about five times the rate of those born in other parts of the United States; the interpretation of this is discussed below. Figures for the United States Navy showing a rather lower rate but similar trends in other respects were reported by Gundelfinger and Britten (1961). The higher mean rate reported in these surveys in the United States than in that of Horwitz in Denmark, noted below, could well be due to two factors; the age distribution of army and navy personnel, which includes the group most liable to sarcoidosis, and the high incidence in blacks in the United States.

In the British Army, Coni (1968) reviewed sarcoidosis over the ten year period 1954–63. The annual incidence of diagnosed sarcoidosis in this predominantly male population was 2.3 per 100 000, with a peak of 5.6 in the age-group 25–29.

In Denmark, Horwitz (1961) estimated the annual incidence of sarcoidosis from the data for the years 1954–7 reported to the Danish Tuberculosis Index by chest clinics throughout the country. The mean annual rate was 5.5 per 100 000; the incidence was uniform except for a great part of Jutland, where it was about three times as high as elsewhere. From 1962 until 1971, a central register of sarcoidosis was maintained (Horwitz *et al.*, 1967; Horwitz, 1971; Fog and Wilbek (1974); Rømer (1977).) During this time, 2563 cases were reported, 1295 in men and 1268 in women, with an average annual incidence of five per 100 000, ranging between four and eight in different years. There was a wide variation between counties, from 1–16 per 100 000. Part of this was due to higher rates in counties that were subjected to mass radiographic screening, in which the rate averaged 14. The peak incidence was in the ages grouped around 25 years, with a second smaller 'hump' of increased incidence, more evident in women in late middle age. Rømer (1967) found that nearly one-third of patients discovered in an intensive study of one area were not recorded on the central register, and noted that many of the unnotified patients were treated in general medical departments for the more severe manifestations of the disease. In this intensively studied area, the annual incidence averaged 10.8 per 100 000.

In Finland, Selroos (1969, 1974) reported that in 12 areas in which all sarcoidosis cases were registered, irrespective of the mode of detection, the annual incidence of new cases between 1961 and 1967 ranged from 3–12 per 100 000, with a mean value of 5.3; no case was detected below the age of 15, and if the number of cases was related to the population over the age 15, the incidence was 6.8 per 100 000. For the period 1968–70, the mean annual incidence was 7.5 per 100 000, or 10.2 per 100 000 over the age of 15. There was a higher incidence among women, who constituted 62.4% of new cases, and the excess was principally due to large numbers of cases in older women, the highest incidence being between 50 and 59 years, with considerable numbers in those over 60 years. Thirty per cent of patients were found in mass radiographic surveys, and the remainder because of symptoms.

In Great Britain, an intensive comparative study of four contrasted areas was undertaken by the British Thoracic and Tuberculosis Association (1969) during the five-year period 1961–66. Since it is well established that an unknown but probably considerable number of individuals go through the entire course of sarcoidosis to resolution without symptoms or overt signs, it is impossible to determine the 'true' incidence of sarcoidosis: indeed this concept is virtually undefinable. The events recorded in this survey were therefore diagnoses of sarcoidosis. All clinicians in the selected areas were asked to submit to a central panel reports of all cases in which sarcoidosis was diagnosed or suspected. The diagnostic opinion of this panel, reached in some cases after a period of observation, was accepted for the purpose of the survey, in order to ensure that comparisons between areas would be valid. The findings are summarized in Figs 4.1 and 4.2. The annual incidence increased from north to south, the range being wider in men, from 2.1 per 100 000 in the most northerly area to 4.1 in the most southerly, than in women, among whom it was 3.5–4.5. Accordingly the female/male ratio of annual incidence was 1.1 in the south and increased to 1.72 in the north. The peak incidence in all areas and both sexes was in the age group 25–34 years. One of the four areas, around Sheffield, is heavily industrialized; the age and sex distribution in this area differed from that in all others in several respects. In other areas, the higher incidence among women was largely attributable to a small rise in incidence in women past the age of 45. In Sheffield, there were very few cases in women or men over the age of 45, and there was an exceptionally high incidence among younger women in the 15–24 year age group. The four areas had few recent immigrants, and all the cases of sarcoidosis occurred in persons of Caucasian stock. Variations in incidence showed no correlations with occupational factors, afforestation, or tuberculosis rates. An account of the ways in which patients in this survey came to light is included in Table 4.1. The only notable difference between areas was in the incidence of erythema nodosum; whereas in North East Scotland and in Cornwall, this occurred as in most other studies, about twice as frequently in women as in men, in Sheffield and East Anglia it occurred with almost equal frequency in the two sexes. This study, in which exceptional efforts were made to ascertain all cases and to apply uniform diagnostic standards within defined areas of a small country, showed important differences in age-and sex-distribution between these areas. The differing incidence in older women is especially noteworthy, in view of the findings in Finland, noted above, of an exceptional incidence in older women in that country. The occurrence of these differences within one country, in areas with few recent immigrants, suggests that they are likely to be due to environmental rather than to genetic factors.

In the Irish Republic, Cummiskey and Dean (1979) estimated from records of mass radiography and hospital admissions for the year 1973 that the annual incidence of new cases was 8.9 per 100 000. Mass radiography discovered 27% of known patients. The sex distribution was unusual, in that there was a slight male excess; in both sexes the highest incidence was in the decennium 20–29 years. Cummiskey and Dean suggested that the higher incidence in Ireland than in Great Britain might account for the disproportionate numbers of cases of sarcoidosis reported among Irish

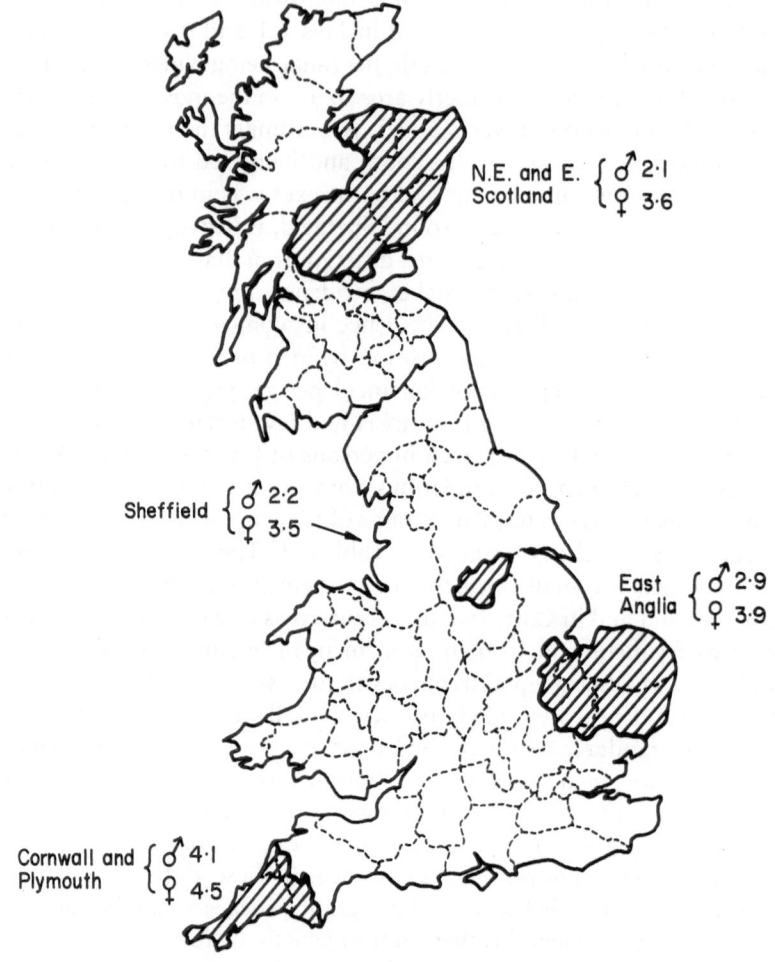

Figure 4.1 Annual incidences of new diagnoses of sarcoidosis in four areas of Great Britain, 1961–1966 (British Thoracic and Tuberculosis Association, 1969). The figures are the annual rates per 100 000 for men and women.

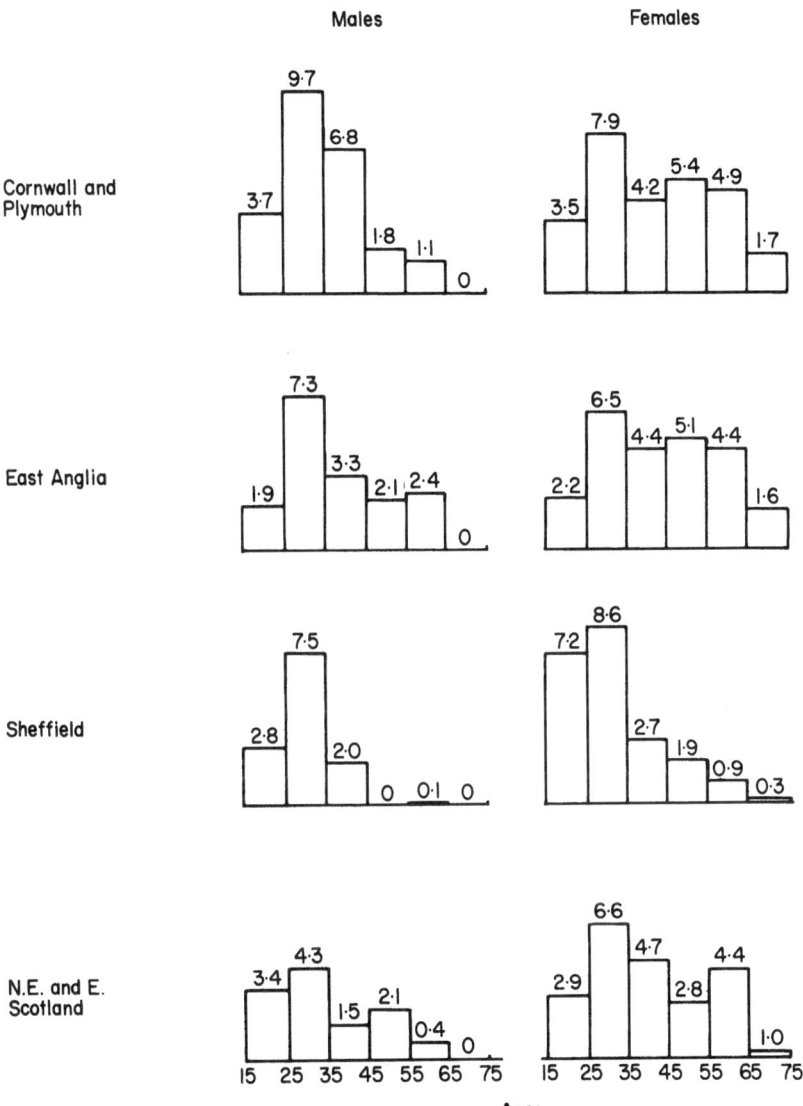

Figure 4.2 Annual incidence of newly-diagnosed sarcoidosis per 100 000 by age in ten-year groups in men and women in four areas of Great Britain, 1961–1966 (British Thoracic and Tuberculosis Association, 1969).

immigrants in mass radiographic surveys in London (Anderson *et al.*, 1963a; James and Brett, 1964; Hall *et al.*, 1969), especially since many immigrants are in the more susceptible age-group.

In Yugoslavia, Goldman *et al.* (1974) estimated the annual incidence of sarcoidosis in two intensively studied areas in 1970 and 1971, using information from all sources; in the area around Ljubljana in the west it was five, and around Novi Sad in the east it was three per 100 000.

In Spain, Morera Prat *et al.* (1983) ascertained all confirmed diagnoses of sarcoidosis during the year 1979 in the Barcelona area; this led to an estimate of 1.2 new cases per 100 000 annually, contrasting with the estimate of 0.04 derived from mass radiography in Spain by Zapatero (1970).

In a survey of histologically confirmed cases in Italy, Mariani (1977) confirmed the impression given by Blasi's (1974) report based on mass radiography that sarcoidosis is more prevalent in the northern than in the southern parts of that country.

In the Cottbus district, with a population of 860 000, north of Dresden in East Germany, Scharkoff (1977) reported that 1647 new cases of sarcoidosis were registered during the years 1961–1975, giving an annual incidence of 13 per 100 000.

Megalif and Brencsone (1977) estimated that the annual incidence per 100 000 of diagnosed sarcoidosis in Latvia between 1958 and 1975 was three in women and two in men. He noted that the female excess was in the older age-groups, the small number of cases in the 10–19 year group showing a 4–1 excess of males.

In Japan, the National Railways provide hospitals and out-patient clinics for employees, and conduct annual radiographic surveys. Since 1961, a register of sarcoidosis has been maintained, and the findings have been reported by Hosoda *et al.* (1974) and Hiraga *et al.* (1974). Among 460 000 workers, of whom 97% are male, 66 cases were notified over ten years, giving an annual incidence of 1.5 per 100 000. Most of the cases were found by routine radiography, only 11 coming to light in other ways. The highest incidence, 6.2, was in the 20–24 year age-group, and the lowest, 0.1, in the 35–39 group. Hosoda *et al.* (1974) combined these findings with those of surveys of hospital records throughout Japan and of records of mass radiography of school children and students to review 2148 diagnosed cases in Japan. Mass radiography is carried out yearly for nearly all school children and students and 40% of the adult population; it was the means of discovery of half the hospital cases. The highest incidence was in the 20–29 years age-group. For those with intrathoracic changes, the incidence in the two sexes was similar, but among those with extrathoracic changes only, women outnumbered men by 3:1. For patients from all three sources, the incidence was highest in the more northern parts of Japan. From hospital records, the incidence in Hokkaido, the northernmost island, was six times that in Kyushu, the southernmost; in mass radiographic surveys, the detection-rates were 4.8 per 100 000 in the city of Sapporo, Hokkaido, and 0.5 in two cities in Kyushu. Hiraga *et al.* (1977) described an exceptionally high incidence in a central mountainous district of Hokkaido, with a female predominance and affecting a generally older age-group than is usual, but were unable to find any possible environmental or genetic explanation for it.

It is a common experience that for a long time after the detection in any area of a relatively uncommon disease which, until recognized in its own right, can be included in a widely-used nosological category, the number of cases recorded increases steadily. It is not surprising, therefore, that in areas with a persistently high incidence of tuberculosis and with limited medical resources, information about the prevalence of sarcoidosis is limited, in some, to individual case reports. Even after allowance has been made for this, there is a strong impression that sarcoidosis is uncommon among the Chinese, and in inhabitants of South East Asia, in black Africans in tropical zones, and in North American Indians. Chapman (1961) stated that in California, with a large Chinese population, no case had been observed in a Chinese at the University Hospital; and that the disease is rare among North American Indians, but noted that the reserves where most of these live are mainly located in dry desert areas in which sarcoidosis seems to be uncommon generally. Hsing *et al.* (1964) reported that in Taiwan, no case of sarcoidosis had been detected in 3 600 000 mass radiographic examinations, and described the first case which had been diagnosed there. This was in a woman aged 33 who had been born in mainland China and moved to Taiwan; she had been trained as a nurse in the United States, and returned to Taiwan; the manifestations of sarcoidosis were a skin infiltration, with biopsy confirmation, pulmonary infiltration and hypercalcaemia. Present and Siltzbach (1967) reported another case in a Chinese woman, born in Hong Kong, who had emigrated to the United States, together with a follow-up report on the patient reported by Hsing *et al.* They stated that only one case of sarcoidosis had been recorded in the Chinese medical literature; and this was an unusual one in an infant with hepatosplenomegaly and pancytopenia leading to removal of the spleen, which showed multiple non-caseating granulomas. Yang and Wu (1974) later reported from Taiwan that only six cases of sarcoidosis had been diagnosed in 15 years in a population of 15 million. Da Costa (1973) reported two cases from Singapore, one of Chinese and one of Indian ancestry, both born in Singapore; no case of sarcoidosis was detected in 500 000 mass radiographic examinations. In Malaysia, Ampikaipakan *et al.* (1983) found 13 cases of sarcoidosis; of these seven were Chinese, five Malay and one Indian.

Lee and Lee (1974) in a search for sarcoidosis in Korea reviewed nearly 50 000 mass radiography films, and found 64 with evidence of bilateral hilar lymph-node enlargement; only 18 could be investigated by Kveim tests, all of which proved negative. Bovornkitti (1974) stated that only seven cases had been reported since 1952 in Thailand, and that no case of sarcoidosis had been detected in over two million mass radiographic and chest clinic examinations. Gupta *et al.*(1982) were able to find reports of 75 cases in India; 34 from Calcutta, 24 from Delhi, and 17 from other places. They gave no information about the prevalence of changes attributed to sarcoidosis in mass radiographic surveys.

Over large parts of Africa, the only information available is from reports of single or a few cases. From West Africa, Ogunlesi and Rankin (1961) reported a single case, and Cook and Carter (1966) three cases. Fletcher (1966) found 17 cases with radiographic evidence of sarcoidosis in pre-employment and subsequent annual examinations of miners in Zambia between 1954 and 1962; the diagnosis was confirmed by biopsy in only two, but the clinical course was compatible in the others. One other case was an incidental finding at necropsy in a man killed in mine accident. During the same period, 780 cases of pulmonary tuberculosis were detected. From Algeria, Larbaqui and Lazib (1977) reported 28 personally observed cases, and stated that about 50 in all had been recorded. From Ethiopia, Tsega *et al.* (1978) reported six clinically diagnosed cases, of which all showed lymph-node enlargement and hepatosplenomegaly and five skin infiltrations; they searched the records of the pathology laboratories in Addis Ababa and found that histological reports of sarcoidosis had been made in 23 cases in two years. In contrast to the findings elsewhere in Africa, Benatar (1977, 1980) in Cape Town found a high incidence among the black population; 110 cases of sarcoidosis were seen in Cape Town from 1969–75; 25 were black, 71 of mixed race and 14 white. The estimated minimal prevalence per 100 000 was 23.2 in blacks, 11.6 in those of mixed race, and 3.7 in whites. As in the United States, sarcoidosis tended to appear in its most florid form in the blacks and those of mixed race, with a high incidence of skin infiltrations and deforming changes in the bones of the hands and feet in the blacks, though hypercalcaemia was more common in whites. It seems likely that there is a real differece in the impact of sarcoidosis on blacks in South Africa and in the rest of Africa, since it is unlikely that the striking manifestations described in them in Cape Town would fail to attract attention elsewhere.

Only limited information is available from South America. In 1961, Purriel and Navarrete found that with 2% of the population of the continent, Uruguay had 34% of the reported cases; differences in medical awareness must be largely responsible for this. In Argentina, Rey *et al.* (1967) reported that from 1963–65, three cases of sarcoidosis had been diagnosed by dermatologists, and none by ophthalmologists; in the years 1961–65, radiographic surveys in the university health service had found seven cases of sarcoidosis and 169 of tuberculosis; and reported 14 confirmed cases, seven found by mass radiography. Castells *et al.* (1970) found that 75 cases had been recorded in general and tuberculosis hospitals in Argentina from 1960–66. Bethlem *et al.* (1983) identified 264 cases of sarcoidosis in Brazil, suggesting a prevalence of known cases of 0.2 per 100 000. Lowe (1980) was able to find 100 cases in Jamaica, with a predominantly black or mixed race population of 2 100 000; both the sex-distribution, with 62% of males, and the age-distribution, widely spread through all adult age-groups, were unusual.

Age- and sex-incidence

The commonest pattern of age- and sex-incidence reported in the studies summarized above is a slightly to moderately higher overall incidence in women than in men, the highest in both sexes being in a young adult age-group, at some point between 20 and 40 years, with a smaller broad 'hump' in the age-incidence in or past middle age in women accounting for most of the excess in the female sex. But there are variations within this pattern, and some exceptions to it. When areas with different patterns have been studied by similar methods and with similar diagnostic standards, reported differences can be accepted as probably corresponding to real differences between the populations studied. Thus, the increasing female–male radio from south to north in Great Britain, and the peculiar age-distribution, especially in women, in the Sheffield area reported in the BTTA (1969) study (Fig. 4.2), and the high incidence in older women in Finland as compared with neighbouring countries (Selroos, 1969) are unlikely to be artefacts. Surveys based entirely on mass radiography or on hospital records are liable to be biased by selective use of medical facilities by different age-groups and by the two sexes. Differences between the sexes in the frequency of some manifestations, notably erythema nodosum, have been discussed above (p. 47).

Children

In most reported surveys, there have been few cases below the age of 15. Nevertheless, sarcoidosis may occur at any age, including the very young. Of the recorded cases below the age of 15, most have been in older children.

McGovern and Merritt (1953) reviewed 104 previously reported cases, and added nine of their own; of these 113 cases, only 28 were below the age of nine years. Among 1050 patients with sarcoidosis, Siltzbach and Greenberg (1968) reported 18 below the age of 15; of these only five were below the age of nine years. Most of the younger children presented with severe symptoms, as did those reported by Jasper and Denny (1968), Kendig (1974), Kendig and Brummer (1976) and Hetherington (1982). The incidence of sarcoidosis in children is difficult to assess for two reasons. First, clinical diagnosis may be difficult. A higher proportion of young children than of adults present with such unusual features as chronic polyarthritis, basal granulomatous meningitis, hepatomegaly and jaundice, purpura, myositis and fever; these are discussed in later chapters. And one of the easily recognized presentations, erythema nodosum with hilar lymphadenopathy, is infrequent in children. Secondly, in most countries, mass radiographic surveys have not included children. But in Hungary and Japan, where schoolchildren have been examined routinely in this way, symptomless bilateral hilar lymphadenopathy (BHL) has been found by this means. Mandi (1964) reported that of 96 cases of sarcoidosis 14 were in children below the age of 15 years, and ten of these had symptomless BHL. Similarly, Niitu *et al.* (1965) found 14 children with changes attributable to sarcoidosis in 225 000 mass radiographic examinations between the ages of eight and 15 years. Later, Hosoda *et al.* (1974) reported that throughout Japan up to the end of 1971, mass radiography had revealed 19 cases of sarcoidosis in 3 185 000 examinations of children between the ages of six and 11 years; 43 in 1 563 000 between the ages of 12 and 14 years; and 39 in 1 202 800 between the ages of 15 and 17 years. Niitu *et al.* (1974b) observed 55 children aged eight to 15 years who had been found to have BHL, six also having evidence of lung involvement. Of 48 followed for one year, 44 showed return to normal radiographic appearances; extrathoracic changes were not described, apart from reference to one child who became blind, presumably from ocular sarcoidosis. Tachibana *et al.* (1974) described the clinical findings in 20 children, 19 of whom were between the ages of ten and 15, and most discovered in radiographic surveys. Three had ocular changes, three enlargement of superficial lymph-nodes, and one was suspected of central nervous system and pituitary involvement. Six were shown to have histological changes in the liver. Most were observed to show improvement in the chest radiographic changes, though three, including two with ocular changes, showed continued activity or relapse of the disease. By contrast, the prognosis reported in most series of children with sarcoidosis, with a high proportion coming under observation with symptoms, is less favourable. For instance, Kendig and Brummer (1976) observed 28 children with sarcoidosis diagnosed in Richmond, Virginia. Only four were initially symptom-free and discovered by radiography; none of these developed serious disease. Of the remaining 24 who presented with various constitutional, respiratory and ocular symptoms, five had serious disabilities at the end of the observation period, although there had been no deaths; of these five, two had visual impairment severe enough to be categorized as 'legally blind', and three had severe respiratory insufficiency. Of the 28 children in this series, 20 were black.

It is evident that in an area where adults are frequently, and children rarely, submitted to chest radiography, the relative frequency of sarcoidosis in children will be underestimated; and at the same time, since the majority of the detected cases in children will be symptomatic, prognosis in children cannot be related to that in adults by direct comparison of statistics of recorded cases. The available evidence suggests that in very young children, sarcoidosis is rare, and when it occurs tends to present in bizarre forms; in later childhood, its frequency increases and it assumes both clinical features and prognosis approximating to that observed in adults.

Racial and geographical differences

As noted above, Cooch (1961) estimated that in the United States Army, the incidence of sarcoidosis in blacks was 16 times that in whites, and in those born in the south-eastern states five times that in those born elsewhere in the United States. Evidence from the records of the Armed Forces Institute of Pathology (Ricker and Clark, 1949) and impressions derived from all large clinical series also indicate a considerably higher incidence among blacks. Several studies also suggested a greater prevalence in the south-eastern states, not explainable by the larger black population in those areas (Michael *et al.*, 1950, Gentry *et al.*, 1955; Cummings *et al.*, 1956). Keller and Dunner (1967) reported data on the birthplace of male patients with sarcoidosis in Veterans Administration (VA) Hospitals in the years 1958–64; they confirmed high prevalence areas in the south-eastern states, and also found evidence of high prevalence in Colorado. Interpretation of these findings is complicated, not only by ignorance of any possible factor responsible for geographical variations in incidence and of its temporal relation to the onset of overt disease, but also by large-scale migration of blacks from the south-eastern to other parts of the United States. Israel (1970) related the numbers of patients with sarcoidosis in VA Hospitals between 1958 and 1964 born in four regions of the United States to the 1935, rather than the contemporary, populations of these regions. In all regions, the ratio for blacks was 12–14 times that for whites, but there were relatively small differences for either groups between regions. Israel concluded that place of birth and residence during infancy did not affect the incidence of sarcoidosis, but the role of factors associated with place of residence later remained undetermined. In a study in the US Navy, Sartwell and Edwards (1974) found that the incidence of sarcoidosis was highest in those with life-long residence in the south-eastern states; the incidence in blacks was 11 times that in whites. Keller (1971, 1973) studied the geographical origins of 420 male patients with a diagnosis of sarcoidosis in VA hospitals between 1960 and 1964, comparing them with controls based on race, age and hospital attributes. The black/white ratio of incidence was 5.3:1. No clear geographical pattern of incidence was found within the continental United States, for either birth-place or place of residence, high incidence in some areas being explicable by a large black population; the only area with a significantly high incidence was Puerto Rico. Thus available evidence suggests a higher incidence of sarcoidosis in blacks in the United States, estimates varying from five to 16 times that in whites; but the evidence suggesting a higher incidence irrespective of race in south-eastern states is less consistent. The clinical experience which underlies the general impression that sarcoidosis is more extensive and follows a less favourable course in blacks in the United States is outlined in disucssion of organ involvement in following chapters; it has been confirmed in comparative studies (Van Ditmars, 1967; Israel and Washburne, 1980).

Cummings *et al.* (1956) noted that the geographical distribution of sarcoidosis which the then available evidence indicated resembled that of pine-forests, and sought a possible explanation for this apparent association. The demonstration that pine-pollen contained an acid-fast lipid and induced epithelioid cell granulomas in tuberculin-sensitive guinea pigs (Cummings and Hudgins, 1958) suggested that exposure to pine pollen might be a causal factor. Much study of the granuloma-producing and immunological activity of pine-pollens followed, with inconclusive results. Studies of the geographical distribution of sarcoidosis in other countries — Denmark (Horwitz, 1961), Scotland (Douglas, 1961), Switzerland (Uehlinger, 1961), Japan (Nobechi, 1961), and Great Britain (BTTA, 1969) — do not indicate any relation between the incidence of sarcoidosis and the distribution of pine-trees. Cummings (1964), after a careful review of the laboratory, epidemiological and clinical evidence concluded that it did not support his hypothesis that there might be a relationship between pine-pollen and sarcoidosis.

In Great Britain, the most obvious differences between racial groups is in the incidence of erythema nodosum and of symptomless changes, principally BHL, found on routine radiography. Anderson *et al.* (1963a) found among persons examined by mass radiography in London that in women of child-bearing age, those of Irish origin showed a prevalence of changes interpreted as sarcoidosis of 200 per 100 000, compared with a general prevalence of 39. Brett (1965) later reported that in London the prevalence of such findings in men born in Ireland was three and a half times, in women born in Ireland nine times, in men born in the West Indies seven times and in women born in the West Indies six times that in persons born in the United Kingdom, for whom the rates in the two sexes were similar. Hall *et al.* (1969) found that the proportions of patients of Irish and West Indian origin among those attending a large sarcoidosis clinic in North London were 2.5 and 2.3 times the proportions of these groups in the general population; erythema nodosum was observed in 34% of the British, 55% of the Irish, and none of 23 West Indian patients, while skin infiltrations and peripheral lymphadenopathy were more frequent in the West Indians. Honeybourne (1980) compared the clinical findings in 36 patients of West Indian and 47 of Caucasian origin with a confirmed diagnosis of sarcoidosis, seen in South London; erythema nodosum was seen among the West Indians only in one woman, and among the Caucasians in three men and 16 women, while skin infiltrations occurred in ten West Indians and only five Caucasians. The disease was generally more widespread, and respiratory symptoms, eye changes and peripheral lymphadenopathy were more frequent in the West Indians. In France, sarcoidosis in immigrants from the Caribbean area has been reported to show similar characteristics (Turiaf *et al.*, 1970; Turiaf and Battesti, 1971). In New York, both black and Puerto Rican patients had a high incidence of skin and eye sarcoidosis; but one-third of Puerto Rican women presented with erythema nodosum and BHL, a rare presentation among blacks (Teirstein *et al.*, 1976b).

Whether the small number of cases of sarcoidosis reported among blacks in tropical Africa is truly indicative of a low incidence among them, or is due to the difficulty of ascertainment in areas with scattered populations, exiguous medical services, and a high incidence of tuberculosis and other infectious diseases is unknown. If there is, in fact, a low incidence among them, the high incidence and the often florid character of sarcoidosis among blacks in the United States and in South Africa would suggest that in these areas they come into contact with a factor or factors to which they are susceptible, and which is uncommon in tropical Africa.

Many studies have suggested that those residing in rural areas are slightly more liable to sarcoidosis than urban-dwellers. Michael *et al.* (1950), Gentry *et al.* (1955) and Cummings *et al.* (1956) in the United States found that sarcoidosis was more frequent in those who had resided in the country, whereas tuberculosis was more frequent in townsmen. Buck and Sartwell (1961) compared 62 sarcoidosis patients with matched controls, and found that a highly significant excess of the sarcoidosis patients had lived for at least six months in the country, and a less significant excess had been born in rural areas. Terris and Chaves (1966) in New York found that a significantly higher proportion of patients with sarcoidosis, but not of those with tuberculosis, than of controls gave a history of having lived on a farm. In the BTTA (1969) survey in Great Britain, the one highly industrialized area (Sheffield) had a much lower incidence of sarcoidosis in the older age-groups than the other three, all with large rural parts. In Denmark, Fog and Wilbek (1974) reported that the annual incidence in the capital city was two, while that in provincial towns and rural districts it was five per 100 000, but found no significant excess among agricultural workers. In West Germany, Buss and Dörken (1975) found that communities of more than 50 000 inhabitants showed about half the incidence found in smaller communities, and that there were comparatively low rates in industrialized regions and big cities. Among regions, Saarland showed the lowest, and Bavaria the highest incidence. In an area north of Dresden in East Germany, Scharkoff (1977) in a study of a population of 860 000 over 15 years found a specially high incidence of sarcoidosis in rural areas. However, Hall *et al.* (1969) found that the proportions of 327 patients with sarcoidosis in London who had been born or had lived for more than ten years in the country were similar to those of 127 control patients with other diseases.

Occupation

Apart from the suggestion from some studies, noted above, of an association of rural residence and agricultural occupations with a high incidence of sarcoidosis, there is no evidence that occupational factors are important. In the BTTA (1969) study, the occupations of sarcoidosis patients seemed to reflect the general patterns in the areas studied; there was no indication of an association of sarcoidosis with occupational exposure to mineral dusts.

Comparisons between incidences of sarcoidosis and of tuberculosis

Historically, the nosological category sarcoidosis has come into general use at a time when in the more affluent areas of the world there has been a striking decline in morbidity and mortality from tuberculosis. It is impossible to judge how far this is due to increasing medical knowledge of a disease cases of which had previously been included in other categories, possibly as unusual variants of tuberculosis, and how far to a real increase in the prevalence of sarcoidosis, irrespective of changes in tuberculosis incidence. Studies in which the contemporary prevalences of sarcoidosis and of tuberculosis in different parts of the same country have been compared have shown no correlations, positive or negative (Horwitz, 1967; BTTA, 1969; Fog and Wilbek, 1974; Goldman *et al.*, 1974; Selroos, 1974). On the other hand, in the United States, blacks are more liable both to tuberculosis and to sarcoidosis than the rest of the population. Terris and Chaves (1966) in

New York found that while tuberculosis patients showed a generally lower level of educational status than controls, sarcoidosis patients resembled controls in this respect; this suggested that socio-economic factors, probably important in increasing the liability of blacks to tuberculosis, were less so in relation to sarcoidosis.

In London, Brett (1965) found in repeated mass radiographic surveys that the prevalence of changes interpreted as due to tuberculosis and to sarcoidosis changed similarly within each of three ethnic groups, but differently between them. Among those born in the United Kingdom, the prevalence of both remained unchanged; among Irish immigrants, both diminished; and among West Indian immigrants, both increased.

Studies of the proportions of patients with sarcoidosis having a history of contact with tuberculosis have given divergent results. Parsons (1960) in London found that 19% of patients with tuberculosis, 12% of those with sarcoidosis and 2% of controls had a history of recent contact with a known case of tuberculosis. Ten Have and Orie (1961) in Holland found that 34% of 150 patients with sarcoidosis and a similar proportion, 30%, of those with pulmonary tuberculosis had a history of contact with open tuberculosis. Bunn and Johnston (1972) in Dundee found a family history of close contact with tuberculosis in 6% of 71 patients with sarcoidosis, 13% of 100 adults with pulmonary tuberculosis, and none of 100 with asthma and bronchitis, the proportions with remote family contact being 21%, 40%, and 11% respectively. On the other hand, Zaki *et al.* (1971) in New York matched 29 patients with sarcoidosis and 29 with asthma for age, sex and race and examined their household contacts, numbering 95 and 82 respectively, and found similar proportions of reactors to five IU of tuberculin, 16.8% and 15.8%, and of radiographic findings interpreted as due to tuberculosis, 10% in both groups; and Hall *et al.* (1969) in London reported that the same proportion, 27%, of 327 patients with sarcoidosis and of 127 patients attending the same hospital and shown not to have sarcoidosis reacted to tuberculin.

Blood groups

Lewis and Woods (1961) found a small excess of blood group A and deficit of group O in 164 sarcoidosis patients at Brompton Hospital, as compared with 894 tuberculosis patients; comparisons of the proportions of groups O and A in various disease groups with the proportions reported for a large sample from London showed that the only possibly significant difference was that for sarcoidosis, which was only borderline at 5%. Addition of patients with sarcoidosis studied at other hospitals in London (Lewis, 1964a) slightly diminished the proportion of group A and increased that of group O, so that the differences from the control series were no longer significant.

Lewis and Woods (1961) and Smellie (1956) found that the proportion of sarcoidosis patients who were rhesus negative did not differ from that of the general population, although Cudkowicz (1956) in a small series had found an unusually high proportion.

Jörgensen and Wurm (1964) studied ABO groups in 518 sarcoidosis patients in Germany. The percentage of group A was 4.8% higher than that of an unspecified German control group, at the expense principally of group B and partly of group O. There was a slight excess of group A in patients with tuberculosis as well as in sarcoidosis. The distribution of rhesus groups was similar in sarcoidosis and controls.

In the BTTA (1969) study of the incidence of sarcoidosis in four areas of Great Britain, ABO groups were compared with those obtained in each of the areas from blood transfusion records. No consistent or significant differences were observed in any area.

Haemoglobinopathies

Greenberg *et al.* (1965) in Philadelphia and Hirschman and Johns (1965) in Baltimore found slightly higher prevalence of haemoglobinopathies in black patients with sarcoidosis that in black control groups in the same cities. Hirschman and Johns speculated that this might be due to a smaller admixture of 'white' ancestry in the sarcoidosis patients.

Familial incidence

Although there are a considerable number of reports of families in which two or more cases of sarcoidosis have occurred, this is a relatively rare event. Among 275 consecutive patients with sarcoidosis seen by one of us (JGS) only two had close relatives known to have sarcoidosis; in both instances two sisters were affected, and the mother of one of these pairs of sisters had suffered from pulmonary tuberculosis. A few studies of familial aggregations have been made.

Jörgensen (1964b) in a survey of 2471 patients with sarcoidosis found that 40 had blood-relatives with the same disease; 21 of these were brothers or sisters and 18 parents, and in one family four of seven sibs, both parents, the father's sister and her daughter were affected. Of the patients surveyed, 15 were twins with a living partner; the partner was affected in two of four monozygotic, and in only one of 11 dizygotic pairs. The British Thoracic and Tuberculosis Association (1973) collected reports of 59 families with more than one case of sarcoidosis in Great Britain. Of these, three contained more than two cases, namely a mother and two daughters; a woman, her sister and her daughter; and a husband and wife and their daughter. In all, there were five twin pairs, four monozygotic and one dizygotic; 28 other sibling pairs; 22 parent–child, and seven husband–wife associations. The total number of affected individuals in these families was 121, with a female/male ratio of 1.6:1.0, at the upper end of the range of sex-ratios found in the study of incidence in Great Britain (BTTA, 1969). There was a significant preponderance of like-sex over unlike-sex pairs among both siblings and parent–child associations. There was also an excess of mother–child over father–child associations, which could be explained only in part by the age-and sex-distribution of sarcoidosis. No explanation could be found for the preponderance of like-sex pairs. Review of 174 published reports of familial sarcoidosis, including that of Jörgensen (1964) showed a similar large excess of monozygotic twins among pairs concordant for sarcoidosis, but only a slight excess of like-sex sibship pairs, and of mother–child over father–child associations. Ito *et al.* (1974) reviewed 16 instances of familial sarcoidosis in Japan, among an estimated total of 2700 diagnosed cases of sarcoidosis; 13 of these were in sibship pairs, one in mother and daughter, one in mother, son and daughter, and one in husband and wife.

A remarkable example of familial aggregation of sarcoidosis has been recorded by Wiman and Beskow (1970) and by Wiman (1972, 1974). This occurred in North Sweden, where the prevalence of sarcoidosis is high, mass radiography showing 100–150 cases per 100 000 examinations, and the sex-ratio is unusual, men outnumbering women by 4:3. In four families, of which three were interrelated, living in a remote area, 21 cases of sarcoidosis were identified in three generations.

James *et al.* (1974) sought for familial associations in 537 cases of sarcoidosis in London, and Sharma *et al.* (1976) added to these a further 150 from Los Angeles. In the combined series of 687 patients, 14 had near blood-relations with sarcoidosis, and there was one husband–wife association. The affected genetically-related pairs were brother–sister in six instances, sister–sister in five, mother–son in two and mother–daughter in one.

Ito *et al.* (1974) reported from Japan one instance of the occurrence of sarcoidosis in husband and wife, and 16 in two or more family-members: five in sisters, two in brothers, seven in brother and sister, one in mother and daughter, and one in mother, son and daughter.

Headings *et al.* (1976) assembled 11 families with more than one case of sarcoidosis from clinical records in Washington, DC All were black. There was an excess of females, with five sets of two sisters and one of three sisters, one brother and sister, one half-brother and half-sister, the offspring of the same unaffected mother, and one pair of twin brothers of unstated zygosity. The daughter of one of an affected pair of sisters and the daughter of an unaffected sister of another affected pair also had sarcoidosis. In the remaining family, the affected members were a woman and two nieces, the daughters of unaffected sisters.

In Hungary, Vezendi and Mandi (1977) among 629 patients with sarcoidosis observed seven families with more than one case; the affected individuals were brothers in two instances, sisters in three, brother and sister in one, and mother and son in one. The sisters included one pair of monozygotic twins.

Other cases of familial occurrence recorded since the review of 174 publications in the BTTA (1973) report include a black mother aged 27 and her son aged six in the United States by Keating *et al.* (1973); a mother and son, and a brother and sister in Italy by Bisetti and Livi (1977); and monozygotic twin sisters in Finland by Selroos *et al.* (1973). Not surprisingly, in monozygotic twins, the disease has generally been noted to become evident at about the same age and to assume similar features. In those reported by Selroos *et al.* (1973), the presentation and course were similar, and the clinical onsets were within four months of each other; the fact that for eight years the sisters had lived in different areas emphasised the probable importance of genetic factors. In many of the other recorded familiar cases, especially those in sibships, the similarity of the clinical manifestations and course has been noted. A striking instance is provided by two sisters reported by Snell and Karlish (1975); the older of these, aged 41, developed a complete Heerfordt's syndrome, starting with uveitis, followed by salivary gland enlargement and then by facial palsy; seven months later, the younger, aged 35, developed erythema nodosum followed by salivary gland enlargement, uveitis, and later facial palsy. But in other instances, the patterns of sarcoidosis observed in family members have shown no such striking resemblance. In a brother–sister pair reported by Salm (1969), the brother's illness started with erythema nodosum and BHL, followed by generalized lymphadenopathy and upper respiratory tract involvement, and terminated in fatal basal meningeal and cerebral sarcoidosis, while the sister had hilar lymph-node and pulmonary sarcoidosis which slowly resolved without residual disability. Taafe and Feinman (1977) reported a family in which the mother had mainly pulmonary and renal changes, a daughter BHL, erythema nodosum and uveo-parotitis, and a son sarcoidosis of the skin. And Mikhail *et al* (1970) described monozygotic twins, one with a pleural effusion, probably tuberculous, and other with sarcoidosis characterized by BHL and a granulomatous response to a Kveim test.

Fewer concurrences of sarcoidosis in husband and wife than in near blood-relations have been reported. Of the 54 families with two or more cases of sarcoidosis in Great Britain reported to the BTTA (1973), there were seven, and among the 174 recorded in the literature reviewed at that time, only three in which husband and wife were affected. The latter figure may be affected by selective reporting of blood-relatives. More recently, cases of conjugal sarcoidosis have been reported by Renner *et al.* (1977), Harrison and Ive (1978) and Gange (1979). In the instance reported by Renner *et al.*, the affected idividuals had similar illnesses, with BHL and pulmonary infiltration subsiding spontaneously, the husband's appearing five months after the wife's. Nevertheless, the small number of reported husband–wife associations suggests that if a transmissible agent is concerned in the causation of sarcoidosis, other factors usually determine the onset of the disease.

The evidence available from collected cases of familial sarcoidosis suggests that the sarcoidosis occurs in blood-relations more often than would be expected by chance. This conclusion is supported by a study in which Buck and McKusick (1961) compared the families of 62 patients with sarcoidosis with those of 62 matched control subjects. There were a total of 14 cases of sarcoidosis in five families of sarcoidosis patients, and none among the families of the control subjects; all the families with multiple cases were black. Familial associations may be due to exposure to common environmental, including infective, factors or to genetic predisposition. The excess of monozygotic over dizygotic twin pairs concordant for sarcoidosis is the strongest evidence suggesting a genetic factor, and the greater frequency of familial aggregations affecting the blood-relations than of husband–wife associations is concordant with this view. Suggestions about the mechanism of inheritance of a presumed genetic factor are speculative. James *et al.* (1974) suggested a recessively inherited susceptibility to sarcoidosis, while Jorgensen (1964) and Headings *et al.* (1976) thought that monogenic modes of inheritance were improbable, multigenic being more likely. The preponderance of like-sex pairs observed in some studies (BTTA, 1973; Headings *et al.*, 1976) is difficult to explain. A similar preponderance was observed by Grufferman *et al.* (1977) among sibling pairs both affected by Hodgkin's disease; of 46 such pairs, 30 were sex-concordant. Grufferman *et al.* also observed relatively few instances of husband and wife both affected by Hodgkin's disease; and their findings in familial aggregations in Hodgkin's disease were in general not unlike those reported in sarcoidosis.

HLA antigens

In view of the suggestive evidence that genetic factors may affect susceptibility to sarcoidosis, and of the importance of immunological reactivity in this disease, several studies of HLA antigens have been undertaken. Such studies are complicated by racial and local variations in distribution of HLA types and by the need to allow for the numbers of antigens tested in assessment of significance of differences from control groups. A high frequency of HLA-B7 was found by Hedfors and Möller (1972) in patients with pulmonary sarcoidosis in Sweden and by McIntyre *et al.* (1977) in black patients with sarcoidosis in South Carolina; but Kueppers *et al.* (1979) in Germany, Neville (1977) and Neville *et al.* (1980) in England, and Eisenberg *et al.* (1978), Al Arif *et al.* (1980) and Newill *et al.* (1983) in blacks in the United States found no association of this antigen with sarcoidosis. In a few studies, excess of some other HLA types has been found among sarcoidosis patients, e.g. B5 and A9 by Akokan *et al.* (1977) in Turkey, and BW15 by Al Arif *et al.* (1980) and AW30 by Newill *et al.* (1983) in blacks in the United States; but the numbers studied were small. Several studies of families with more than one case of sarcoidosis have been reported. Möller *et al.* (1974) studied the large family aggregation in north Sweden reported by Wiman and Beskow (1970) and mentioned above, Turton *et al.* (1980) 59 members of 14 families with more than one case of sarcoidosis, and Al Arif *et al.* (1980) a family in which four siblings were affected; in none of these studies was there evidence of association between HLA and the development of sarcoidosis.

These studies provide no evidence that HLA type affects susceptibility to sarcoidosis; but there is some that it is related to clinical manifestations and prognosis in those who develop the disease. Persson *et al.* (1975) found in Denmark that although HLA-B7 did not affect overall liability to sarcoidosis, among sufferers from the disease it was associated with non-reactivity to tuberculin and with liability to symptoms. Brewerton *et al.* (1977) in London studied 65 patients with sarcoidosis who had uveitis, erythema nodosum (EN), or acute arthropathy, and found a high incidence of B8 in those with arthropathy or EN. Of 45 with uveitis only two (4%) had B27, little different from the 8% in controls, but contrasting with the high proportions found by Brewerton (1975) in patients with acute anterior uveitis and no evidence of other disease (43%), or associated with ankylosing spondylitis or Reiter's disease (86%). Neville (1977) and Neville *et al.* (1980) confirmed the association of B8 with arthropathy and EN; of 107 white patients with various manifestations of sarcoidosis, 40% had this antigen, the proportions among those with arthropathy and with EN being 62% and 89% respectively. A high proportion also had HLA-A1, but this was attributed to linkage disequilibrium between A1 and B8. Neville *et al.* drew attention to a correlation between the frequency of HLA-B8 and the proportion of patients with sarcoidosis having EN in different populations; for instance the frequency of B8 is reported to be 29% in London, 16% in New York and 2% in Tokyo, and the proportions of patients with sarcoidosis having EN in these cities to be 31%, 11% and 4%. Hedfors and Lindström (1983) performed HLA typing in 19 patients with acute-onset sarcoidosis, all having BHL and arthropathy and seven EN, and all following a favourable course. HLA-B8 was present in 67% and DR3 in 90%, compared with frequencies of 24% and 26% in the Swedish population. It was noted that

A1, B8 and DR3 occur in linkage disequilibrium, and that this haplotype has been associated with abornal immune responsiveness.

Smith *et al.* (1981) compared HLA frequencies in 50 patients with fibrotic pulmonary sarcoidosis, in 37 with sarcoidosis that resolved, and in 164 healthy control subjects. B8 occurred in a significantly higher proportion of the group that resolved than of either the fibrotic group or the controls. Of 12 with EN nine, and of two with both EN and arthropathy both had B8. These findings accord with the accepted view that an onset with EN and arthropathy indicates a good prognosis (Chapter 5, p. 93), and suggest that inherited factors, perhaps related to immune response, influence the clinical manifestations of sarcoidosis.

Chapter 5

Erythema Nodosum, Febrile Arthropathy and Bilateral Hilar Lymphadenopathy

Bilateral hilar lymph-node enlargement (BHL) is an important early manifestation of sarcoidosis. It is accompanied in a varying proportion of cases by erythema nodosum (EN). In populations in which chest radiography is a commonly-used screening procedure, the finding of symptomless BHL is one of the more frequent ways in which sarcoidosis is discovered; and except in endemic areas of infections, such as coccidioidomycosis, of which EN is a common feature, a high proportion of cases of EN, certainly of those accompanied by BHL, is attributable to sarcoidosis.

ERYTHEMA NODOSUM

Erythema nodosum, first described in 1808 by Willan, was for a long time regarded as a specific disease, a view that was encouraged by its very distinctive clinical features. There is usually some prodromal malaise, sometimes with pains in various joints, for several days before the rash appears. This takes the form of rounded or oval, slightly raised, tender nodules in the skin and subcutaneous fatty tissue, 1–6 cm in diameter, usually discrete, but sometimes coalescing. They are at first bright red or pink in colour, with shining tense surface. They are characteristically situated on the shins, and are most profuse in this site. If the rash is extensive, it may involve also the ankles, the dorsal surfaces of the feet, and the calves, and may spread over the knees and even to the lower parts of the thighs. Occasionally the forearms, more rarely the upper arms, may be involved. The eruption tends to be symmetrical in distribution. The individual nodules progress, as they subside, from bright red through a dusky pink to a brownish-yellow discoloration resembling that left by a bruise; fresh nodules continue to appear for several days, and occasionally for a longer period, so that nodules at various stages of their evolution are generally seen. They vary greatly in number and size, and in some cases are accompanied by non-nodular elements of a pattern similar to that of erythema multiforme. During the first few days, some fever is usual, but its duration and severity are very variable. The total duration of the eruption varies from one to six weeks, in most cases less than four weeks. Involvement of the joints is also very variable. In some cases, there are no joint symptons; in most, there are flitting pains in joints, especially knees and ankles, without objective signs, and in the most severely affected some periarticular swelling, tenderness or even small effusions into affected joints. Joint symptoms may precede the eruption for several weeks, and may persist after its resolution, and their severity is not related to the extent of the eruption. It has been suggested that a variant of EN can be recognized, in which the nodules are asymmetrically distributed or even unilateral, less tender and cooler and persist longer than usual, some resolving while new ones appear, and are accompanied by little fever, malaise or joint involvement; this has been called 'erythema nodosum migrans' (Bäfverstedt, 1968).

The association with arthropathy led at one time to the view that EN was to be considered as a manifestation of acute rheumatism (Mackenzie, 1886). When the relationship between acute rheumatism and haemolytic streptococcal infection was established, it became apparent that the concurrence of EN and acute rheumatism could be explained by their common association with haemolytic streptococcal infection. That some cases of erythema nodosum were related to haemolytic streptococcal infection was confirmed by immunological and bacteriological studies (Collis, 1932; Coburn and Moore, 1936; Spink, 1937). On clinical grounds, several authors in the nineteenth century suggested that erythema nodosum might be related to tuberculosis; and studies of tuberculin sensitivity and of the frequency of isolation of tubercle bacilli eventually proved this relationship, particularly to primary tuberculosis, and especially in children (Wallgren, 1930; Collis, 1932). It was thus apparent that both haemolytic streptococcal and tubercle bacillus infections could cause erythema nodosum and this gave rise to the concept that erythema nodosum, while a well-defined and uniform clinical syndrome, might be induced, probably through a similar host reaction, by more than one agent (Perry, 1944). Other specific infections provoking EN include leprosy (Wemambu *et al.*, 1969), coccidioidomycosis (Dickson, 1938; Smith, 1940), histoplasmosis (Saslaw and Beman, 1959; Little and Steigman, 1960; Medeiros *et al.*, 1966); blastomycosis (Smith *et al.*, 1955), lymphogranuloma inguinale (Hellerstrom, 1941, Simpson, 1950); psittacosis (Sarner and Wilson, 1965); cat-scratch disease (Daniels and MacMurray, 1954); *Yersinia enterocolitica* infection (Winblad, 1969; Hannuksela and Ahvonen, 1969). As well as sarcoidosis, other diseases of unknown cause which may be associated with EN are ulcerative colitis (Rice-Oxley and Truelove, 1950), Crohn's disease (Crohn and Yarnis, 1958) and polyarteritis nodosa (Churg and Strauss, 1951). Various drugs, including sulphonamides (Löfgren, 1945), penicillin (Hannuksela, 1971), phenacetin (Hannuksela, 1971) and oral contraceptives (Holcomb, 1965; Baden and Holcomb, 1968) may be precipitating factors, though in only some instances has the association been shown to be caused by the recurrence of the eruption on further administration of the drug. More than one of these factors, established or suspected, can be found in some cases of EN, but in others none can; of the 343 reported by Hannuksela (1971) 65 and 75 respectively fell into these two groups, a single factor being identified in 203.

Host factors are evidently important in the pathogenesis of EN. Women are more frequently affected than men, though this difference is not evident before puberty (Löfgren, 1950). Among those exposed to infectious agents known to be potential causes, only an small proportion develop EN, which tends to appear at the time of important changes in immunity; e.g. in tuberculosis and in coccidioidomycosis, soon after primary infection, when hypersensitivity of the kind detected by delayed skin-test reactions has developed. In subjects with EN this hypersensitivity may be very high. The importance of the host reaction is further illustrated by the fact that the frequency of EN in association with primary tuberculosis varies from community to community; for instance, among student nurses, the proportion of those who developed EN soon after becoming tuberculin-positive was reported to be as high as 42% in one study in Scandinavia (Heimbeck, 1950), 2% in Great Britain (Daniels *et al.*, 1948) and less than 1% in Philadelphia (Israel *et al.*, 1941).

ERYTHEMA NODOSUM AND SARCOIDOSIS

In discussion of the relationship between erythema nodosum and sarcoidosis, it is important to use forms of words which keep clear the logical difference between the allocation of a case of erythema nodosum to a group attributed to infection with and named after an identified agent, and its allocation to a group associated with sarcoidosis. It is legitimate to speak of erythema nodosum due to infection with *M. tuberculosis*, with *Coccidiodes immitis* or with haemolytic streptococci. Allocation of a case to one of these categories implies that infection with the named agent was a factor in the causation of EN. But association with a disease whose cause is unknown cannot have this direct causal implication. For sarcoidosis, it implies only that the histological changes of this disease would be found, if sought, in various organs and tissues.

A few reports of EN with radiological evidence of BHL and negative

Table 5.1   Some published reports of the proportions of cases of erythema
nodosum associated with sarcoidosis.

Author	Year of publication	Country	Number of cases of EN	Percentage associated with sarcoidosis
Vesey and Wilkinson	1961	England	70	36
Gordon	1961	England	115	15
James	1961	England	170	74
Wynn-Williams	1961	England	139	41
Macpherson	1961	Scotland	45	11
Macpherson	1967	Scotland	42	17
Macpherson	1970	Scotland	53	13
Löfgren	1946	Sweden	178	8
Löfgren and Lundbäck	1952	Sweden	58	40
Hannuksela	1971	Finland	343	47*

* In 13% of Hannuksela's cases, both sarcoidosis and another known factor were detected.

tuberculin tests appeared from 1935 onwards (Engel, 1935; Vogt, 1939). In
1943, Putkonen reported such a case with histological confirmation of the
diagnosis of sarcoidosis, and about the same time Kerley (1942, 1943)
suggested on radiological grounds that such cases might be frequent. Löfgren (1946, 1953) was the first to make a systematic study of this syndrome,
which is sometimes referred to by his name. Between 1942 and 1944 he
investigated 178 cases of EN in Stockholm, and found evidence of tuberculosis in 104, of streptococcal infection in 30, of sarcoidosis with BHL in 15
(8%), and no infective cause or systemic disease in 29. Later, in 1948–9,
among 58 cases of EN he found evidence of sarcoidosis in a much higher
proportion, 40%, and suggested that BHL, with or without EN, could be
regarded as the primary stage of sarcoidosis. Since then, many reports of the
interrelations of EN and sarcoidosis have been published.

The proportion of cases of EN reported to be associated with sarcoidosis
(Table 5.1) can be expected to be dependent upon the incidences not only of
sarcoidosis but also of mycobacterial, haemolytic streptococcal and fungal
infections in the relevant populations, and upon clinical awareness and the
diagnostic criteria adopted. Selection by reference to a particular hospital or
physician is also likely to introduce a bias; e.g., the very high proportion
(74%) reported by James (1961) reflects his interest in this disease. The
great increase in the proportion of cases of EN associated with sarcoidosis
between the 1946 and 1952 reports from Sweden was almost certainly
attributable not only to diminution of the number due to primary tuberculous infection, but also to new awareness of the EN–BHL syndrome of
sarcoidosis.

Table 5.2   Some published reports of the proportions of cases of sarcoidosis in which erythema nodosum has occurred.

Authors	Year of publication	Country	Number of cases of sarcoidosis	Percentage with EN
James, Thompson and Willcox	1956	England	150	15
Smellie and Hoyle	1960	England	125	12
Scadding (personal series, 1946–66)		England	275	11
BTTA	1969	England:		
		Cornwall	105	24
		England: East Anglia	207	34
		England: Sheffield	156	32
		Scotland: NE and E	99	26
Mikhail, Mitchell, Sutherland and McNicol	1980	England	401	29
Löfgren and Stavenow	1961	Sweden	132	25
Hannuksela and Salo	1969	Finland	283	30
Selroos	1969	Finland	140	30
Lebacq	1964	Belgium	100	25
Würm, Reindell and Heilmeyer	1958	Germany	2177	10
Hurley and Bartholomeusz	1971	Australia	1316	11
Sones and Israel	1960	USA	211	3
Mayock, Bertrand, Morrison and Scott	1963	USA	145	3
James et al.,	1976	Tokyo	282	4

The numbers of cases of sarcoidosis reported to have, or to have had, EN (Table 5.2) must also depend to some extent upon diagnostic awareness and methods, but the very wide difference between parts of the world almost certainly indicate real differences in the incidence of EN as a manifestation of sarcoidosis. Some of the percentages quoted are derived from series of patients observed over periods of years, and thus likely to include an excess of those with chronic disease: since those presenting with EN tend to follow a short course to complete resolution, they are likely to be under-represented in such series. The British Thoracic and Tuberculosis Association (BTTA, 1969) study ascertained the yearly incidences of newly-diagnosed sarcoidosis in four areas over a period of five years. The proportions of patients presenting with EN ranged from 24–34%; this probably represents the most reliable available estimate of the true incidence of EN in diagnosed sarcoidosis, but of course it is valid only for the populations, almost entirely Caucasian, and areas studied. Available evidence suggests that in the United States and in Japan, EN is a much less frequent manifestation of sarcoidosis (James *et al.*, 1976). In the United States, blacks have been found to be less liable to develop EN as a manifestation of sarcoidosis than whites. Sones and Israel (1960) reported that among 211 patients in Philadelphia, 3% of 127 black women, 15% of 13 white women and none of 57 black or 15 white men had EN. On the other hand, EN is frequent among Puerto Ricans with sarcoidosis in New York (Siltzbach, 1958).

Erythema nodosum of all pathogenetic groups occurs more often in women than in men. In Hannuksela's (1971) series of 343 cases in Finland, 89% were female, as were 91% of 2064 cases in seven series which he reviewed. In most studies of sarcoidosis, more cases of EN have been found among women, but the magnitude of the difference between sexes varies greatly. In Sweden, Löfgren and Stavenow (1961) observed EN in 34% of 88 women and 7% of 44 men. In England, one of us (JGS) found a rather lower total incidence of EN and a slightly smaller difference between the sexes; 16% of 156 women and 5% of 119 men. In the BTTA (1969) study, there was a considerable difference between areas in the proportions of men who had EN. These ranged from 11% in Cornwall to 29% in East Anglia, while the proportions among women varied less, ranging only between 30% and 38%. Consequently, the female: male ratio ranged from 1.3:1 in East Anglia and Sheffield to 3.0:1 in Cornwall.

Most patients with EN associated with sarcoidosis have some joint-pains, and in about half of them this is a prominent symptom. The larger joints, especially the ankles and the knees, are most often affected. There may be some swelling in periarticular tissues, apparently inflammatory, but also partly oedema, especially in the ankles in patients who remain ambulant. In some cases, more especially in men, the painful ankle swelling is more prominent than the EN. The clinical picture presented by these cases merges into that presented by a few with this sort of arthropathy, usually febrile, without EN. This is more frequent in men; and has the same place in the natural history of sarcoidosis as does EN. In 275 cases observed by one of us (JGS) 5% of men presented with febrile arthropathy and BHL without EN, as many as presented with EN; among women, arthropathy without EN was much less frequent, occurring in only 1%. In the BTTA (1966) study, arthropathy without EN was similarly more frequent in men, occurring in 4%, as compared with 1% of women.

It seems likely that hormonal factors underlie the differences between the sexes both in incidence of the EN-arthropathy syndrome and in the relative prominence of EN and arthropathy, but this speculation is at present unsubstantiated. The differences in incidence of EN between populations may be due, at least in part, to genetically determined differences in reactivity. As noted in Chapter 4, p. 70). Studies of histocompatibility antigens (HLA) in unselected groups of sarcoidosis patients have shown no consistent differences from control populations; but among sarcoidosis patients those with initial arthropathy or EN have shown a higher frequency of B8, and in one study of DR3, than other sarcoidosis patients or control groups, and there is evidence suggesting that the frequency of this onset of sarcoidosis correlates generally with the frequency of HLA–B8 in a population.

The age-distribution of EN and arthropathy is similar to that of the estimated time of onset of sarcoidosis in general, in most cases occurring between the ages of 20 and 35 years, but with a few outside this, and in some areas an increase among women around the age of 50.

There is no characteristic either of the constitutional illness or of the local eruption which serves to distinguish among cases of EN those associated with sarcoidosis. However, certain associated clinical features and radiographic and laboratory findings usually permit them to be recognized with confidence. The principal points are:

(1) EN in sarcoidosis nearly always occurs at a stage when bilateral hilar lymph-node enlargement is present. Occasionally EN appears in a patient in whom BHL has already been detected radiographically, and a few cases have been reported in which the chest radiograph was normal when EN appeared, and radiographic or other evidence of sarcoidosis was found later (Macpherson, 1970). In a few cases, BHL is accompanied, and in rather more followed, by widespread mottling in the lung fields: e.g. of 30 followed by one of us (JGS), four showed such changes initially and nine more developed them within the following year, usually when the BHL was starting to subside. The radiographic appearances of BHL attributable to sarcoidosis are similar, whether or not associated with erythema nodosum, and are considered below.

(2) The erythema nodosum of primary tuberculosis may be accompanied by evidence of primary tuberculous infection in the chest radiograph; this is discussed below (p. 86). In the erythema nodosum due to tuberculosis, skin sensitivity to tuberculin is always present, and is usually intense. Similarly sensitivity to the appropriate antigen is to be expected in cases due to coccidoidomycosis or histoplasmosis.

Tuberculin sensitivity among patients with the EN–BHL syndrome has generally been found to be lower than that of the populations from which these were drawn, but higher than that of patients with chronic sarcoidosis (Chapter 20). Thus, at a time when 80% of Londoners of comparable age reacted to 100 IU, one of us (JGS) found that 18 (50%) of 36 patients with EN–BHL and 37% of those with more chronic sarcoidosis reacted. Among those with EN–BHL, two reacted to 1 IU and nine to 10 IU. Thus, although persistently low tuberculin sensitivity is significant in excluding an association with primary tuberculosis, and is suggestive of sarcoidosis, it is also compatible with other causes of erythema nodosum, and moderate sensitivity to tuberculin may be found in some, and high sensitivity in a few cases associated with sarcoidosis, certainly in areas with a high level of tuberculin sensitivity.

(3) In cases due to haemolytic streptococcal infection, there may be a history of streptococcal sore throat, from which haemolytic streptococci may have been isolated, or these organisms may be persistent in the throat. Serological evidence of haemolytic streptococcal infection – e.g. a significantly raised or rising antistreptolysin titre – will be found.

(4) The histology of the erythema nodosum itself is in general similar no matter what the cause of the erythema. Löfgren and Wahlgren (1949) studied the histology of 64 cases, divided into groups associated with tuberculosis, with streptococcal infection, with proved or suspected sarcoidosis, and of uncertain association. They found similar changes in all groups, affecting the deep dermis and subcutaneous tissue, the epidermis showing no changes. Early, a few days from the onset, there was hyperaemia, oedema and cellular infiltration, especially of the connective tissue septa of the adipose tissue, chiefly with polymorphs and histiocytes and a few eosinophils. In many cases, there were minute focal collections of histiocytes and lymphocytes, best seen at 5–6 days: later some central necrosis might be seen in these foci. At 8–10 days, there was some fibrinoid degeneration of collagen. Giant cells of foreign body type were found in small numbers in the earlier stages, and became more numerous later. Some veins showed oedema and sparse cellular infiltration of their walls, with intimal swelling.

(5) In some cases, the diagnosis of sarcoidosis is suggested by the finding of extrathoracic manifestations of this disease, concurrently with or appearing soon after EN. These include skin changes (Chapter 7), especially infiltration of scars (Figs 7.24 and 7.27), small nodular sarcoids, and subcutaneous nodules (Figs 5.15 and 5.16); anterior uveitis (Chapter 8); and superficial lymphadenopathy (Chapter 10).

(6) A general approach to the problem of diagnosis in patients with BHL, and the contribution to it of the Kveim test, is discussed below. When BHL is accompanied by EN the likelihood of a granulomatous response to this test is high; e.g. in 94% of the cases reported by James (1961). A negative response does not refute the diagnosis of sarcoidosis, support for which, if required, can be obtained by biopsy from any accessible involved site, including those listed above, or a mediastinal lymphnode. The doubt occasioned by cases of EN without BHL or other possible manifestations of sarcoidosis, but giving granulomatous responses to Kveim tests is more difficult to resolve. Bradstreet *et al.* (1980) tested 278 such patients in London; of these 56 (21%) gave

granulomatous and a further 13 (5%) partly granulomatous responses. Some patients of this sort have been found under further observation to develop other manifestations of sarcoidosis; and it seems probable that of those who do not, most with granulomatous responses (and possibly some with 'negative' responses) have the generalized granulomatosis that characterizes sarcoidosis. But certainty of categorization in the individual case can be obtained only by invasive biopsy procedures: and the course of patients with 'lone' EN is likely to be towards uneventful resolution. In practice therefore, it seems proper to be content with a working diagnosis of 'erythema nodosum, probable (or possible) sarcoidosis' for which appropriate management is symptomatic in the acute stage, followed by periodic review which need be no longer than six months if symptomatic recovery has been complete and no further manifestation has appeared.

BILATERAL HILAR LYMPH-NODE ENLARGEMENT

Although general enlargement of hilar and mediastinal lymph-nodes may result from a variety of infections and neoplasms, such as tuberculosis, coccidioidomycosis, histoplasmosis, lymphomas and metastatic carcinoma, the involvement of the hilar nodes is rarely bilaterally symmetrical in such cases, and evidence of the nature of the disease is usually not difficult to obtain. The characteristics of the BHL which is a manifestation of sarcoidosis are well defined, as a result both of specific studies (Löfgren and Lundbäck, 1952; Löfgren, 1953; Smellie and Hoyle, 1960), and of experience stemming from routine radiography of symptomless individuals.

The separate consideration of those cases of sarcoidosis among a large series which presented initially with radiographic evidence of BHL, is, of course, arbitrary. The following discussion concerns cases in which BHL is not accompanied when first observed either by radiographically evident lung changes or by extrathoracic manifestations of sarcoidosis, e.g. in the eyes. The artificiality of this procedure is obvious, since among patients who in the course of their disease have both BHL and, say, iridocyclitis, those in whom the iridocyclitis gave rise to the presenting symptoms are excluded, while those in whom it developed later are included. Moreover, the presence or absence of an abnormal mottled pattern in the lung fields is an imprecise criterion, since the borderline between normal and slightly abnormal is dependent upon subjective interpretation, and, as will be discussed in Chapter 6 (p. 101), sarcoid BHL is probably always accompanied by some dissemination of granulomas in the lungs, even though the lungs appear normal radiographically. Nevertheless, the separate consideration of cases in which BHL is the only immediately evident finding is justified by the frequency of this finding in routine radiography of apparently healthy individuals or of those with banal respiratory or constitutional symptoms. Of 275 consecutive patients with sarcoidosis under the care of one of us (JGS), 113 had BHL without radiologically evident lung changes when first seen. Of these 17 presented with extrathoracic manifestations of sarcoidosis: uveitis in 14, infiltration of an old appendicectomy scar in one, and enlarged superficial lymph–nodes in three. Of the remaining 96, 42 were symptomless and detected by routine radiography, 19 had various respiratory and constitutional symptoms, and one penicillin dermatitis.

Radiographic appearances

Since it is the detection of BHL by radiography which is the unifying feature of this group of cases, the radiographic appearances will first be described. Typically, the enlargement of hilar nodes is roughly symmetrical (Fig. 5.1), although the mass on the right side often appears larger (Fig. 5.2). This may be at least in part due to the inner part of the left hilar shadow being obscured by the left border of the heart shadow, but there is in many cases probably a real difference in the size of the node mass. This may be

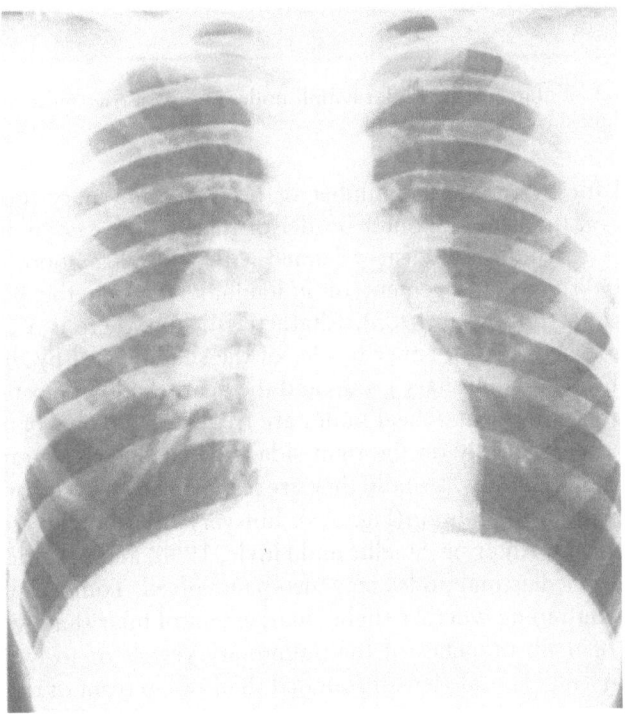

Figure 5.1 Symmetrical discrete enlargement of hilar lymph-nodes in sarcoidosis.

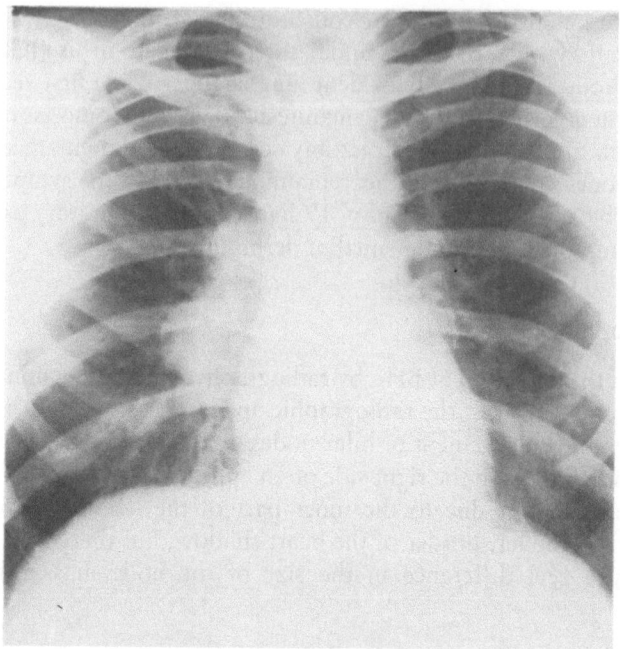

Figure 5.2   Enlargement of hilar lymph-nodes in sarcoidosis, more prominent on the right side.

accounted for by the larger number of bronchopulmonary nodes on the right than on the left. The outer border of the shadow cast by hilar nodes enlarged by sarcoidosis is clearly defined with multiple smoooth contours, suggesting discrete enlargement of individual nodes in the bronchopulmonary group (Rakower, 1963). Characteristically, there is a clear transradiant band between the inner border of the shadow cast by the nodes in the lower bronchopulmonary group and the heart shadow, most evident on the right side. The paratracheal nodes are frequently involved and enlargement of them, especially on the right side is detectable radiographically in more than half the cases. Usually they are less evident than the bronchopulmonary group at the hilum, (Fig. 5.3), but very occasionally they may be more prominent. Anterior (Smellie and Hoyle, 1960) and posterior (Schabel *et al.*, 1978) mediastinal nodes may also be involved. Tomography may be useful in determining whether slight enlargement of hilar shadows is due to dilatation of main branches of the pulmonary vessels or to lymph-nodes. Demonstration in lateral view of rounded shadows in front of the left lower lobe bronchus or in the angle between the right lower lobe bronchus and the middle lobe bronchus strongly suggests lymph-node enlargement, since there are no vessels in these sites. In relation to grossly enlarged nodes, there

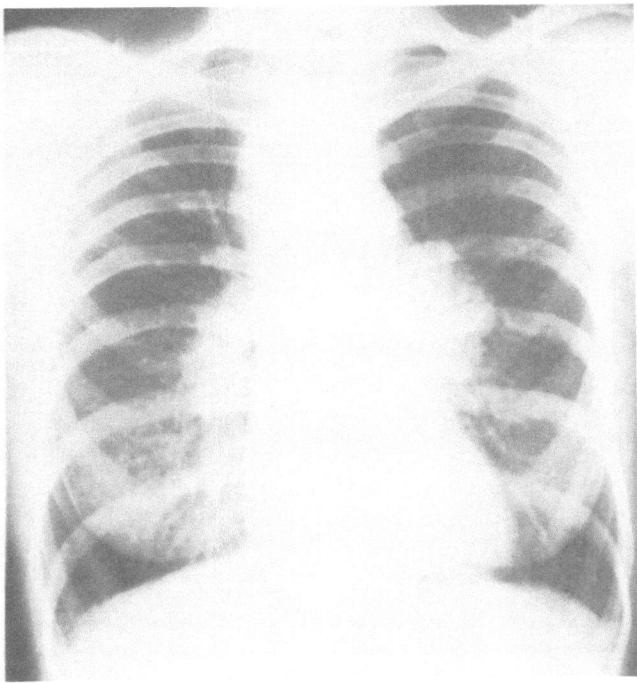

Figure 5.3 Enlargement of right paratracheal and right and left hilar lymph nodes in sarcoidosis.

may be tomographically evident narrowing of large bronchi and widening of the carinal angle, which in a few cases leads to airflow limitation (see below). Occasionally, enlargement of hilar and broncho-pulmonary nodes is massive (Fig. 5.4); substantial or even complete subsidence of these very large nodes is possible (Fig. 5.5).

Although the hilar node enlargement of sarcoidosis is usually bilateral, it is in rare cases apparently unilateral, usually right-sided (Kent, 1965; Mikhail *et al.*, 1980). In two cases mentioned by Löfgren (1953) it was initially unilateral and subsequently became obviously bilateral.

In a few cases of sarcoid BHL, foci of calcification have been observed in the enlarged nodes, presumably having been present before the sarcoid enlargement. Of 39 patients with BHL and EN or arthropathy observed by one of us (JGS), five showed foci of calcification, evident in the postero-anterior radiograph. In four, these were seen in the enlarged hilar nodes. In two of these, there was also a calcified nodule in the related part of the lung, constituting with the hilar calcification a typical calcified primary complex of tuberculosis; one of these patients had a confirmed history of tuberculous peritonitis in childhood. The fifth patient had calcified nodules in the

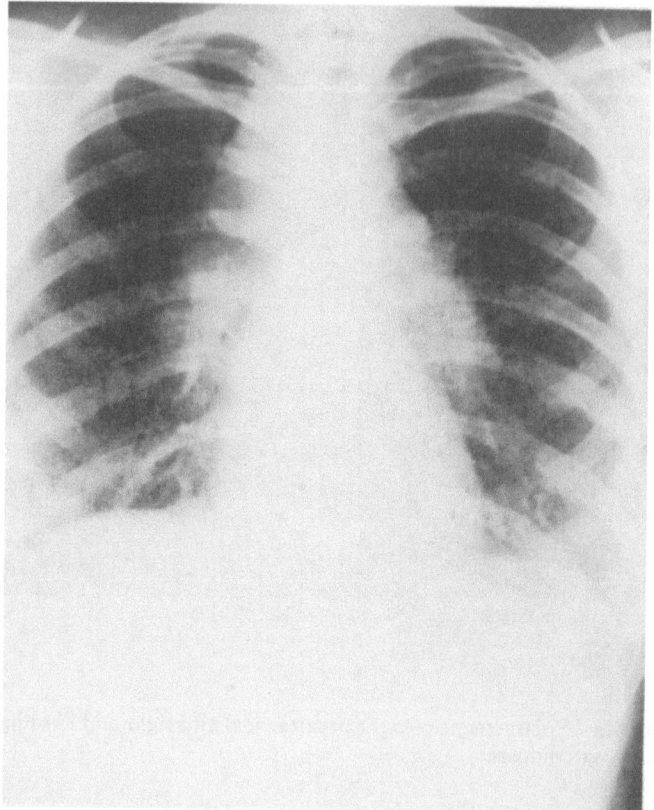

Figure 5.4   Massive enlargement of hilar and paratracheal lymph-node due to sarcoidosis in a woman aged 21.

lung only, at the site of localized pulmonary tuberculosis which had been treated two years previously. Among the 64 other patients who had BHL only when first seen, only two showed calcification; one in the enlarged nodes, and one in small flecks in the upper part of the right lung. There is no reason to doubt that in patients living in England at a time when primary tuberculous infection was frequent, these calcifications represented residues of old healed caseous tuberculosis. The development of calcification under prolonged observation in hilar nodes and lungs affected by sarcoidosis is considered in Chapter 6. It may be noted here that although calcification in hilar nodes develops late in the course of the disease in some patients with both BHL and lung changes, no patient with 'isolated' BHL subsiding without the appearance of lung changes developed calcification in the nodes (Scadding, 1961a).

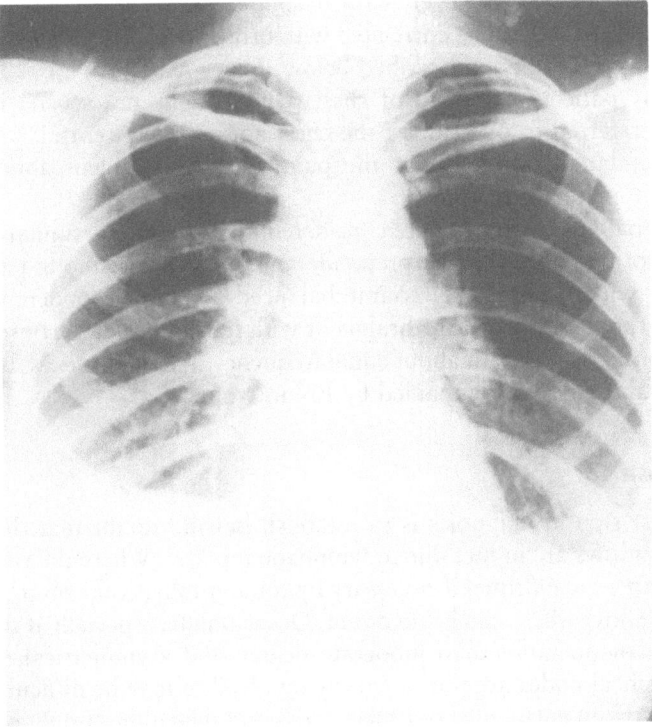

Figure 5.5   The same, two years later, showing spontaneous regression.

Symptoms

Of the patients who present with BHL without EN or arthropathy, a large number have no symptoms, the BHL being discovered at routine radiography. The rest complain of a variety of constitutional and respiratory symptoms.

A few have general malaise and fever, without pronounced joint symptoms or rash. The acuteness and duration of these symptoms vary from a picture resembling that of an acute onset with erythema nodosum or arthralgia except for the absence of these localizing symptoms, to prolonged vague ill-health with occasional evening rises of temperature to just above normal levels, lasting for as long as a year.

Others have symptoms referable to the respiratory tract, such as cough, usually unproductive, dyspnoea, and pain in the chest. Respiratory function in sarcoidosis is discussed in Chapter 7. Here, it may be noted that in most patients with BHL, little functional impairment is found (DeRemee and

Andersen, 1974). However, with dyspnoea at this stage, there is airflow limitation, which can be correlated with bronchoscopic evidence of mucosal infiltration of the type described below (Dines *et al.*, 1978).

A few patients complain of chest pain. Usually not severe, it is nearly always referred to one side of the chest and is rarely central. Its genesis is obscure; lateral reference of the pain when the evident abnormality is central remains unexplained.

If all patients with BHL are considered, the sex-ratio is similar to that for sarcoidosis in general. The preponderance of women among patients presenting with EN is partly counterbalanced by the preponderence of men among those with febrile arthralgia or with fever alone at the onset. Thus an acute onset occurs with about equal frequency in the two sexes, but is much more liable to be accompanied by EN in women.

Diagnosis

The first step in diagnosis is to establish beyond doubt that the enlarged hilar shadows are in fact due to lymphadenopathy. Where the radiographic appearances, confirmed if necessary by tomography, conform to the typical picture above, there can be no doubt. Occasionally, especially if the enlargement is of no more than moderate degree and asymmetrical, and if the paratracheal nodes are not obviously involved, it may be difficult to distinguish between enlargement of hilar nodes and dilatation of pulmonary arteries. In such cases, computerized axial tomography is likely to be helpful; if doubt remains, it can be dispelled, if necessary, by pulmonary angiography.

When it has been decided that the shadows are due to enlarged lymph-nodes, the nature of the lymphadenopathy must be determined. If the patient is free from symptoms, and the lymph-node enlargement is symmetrical and discrete, the probability of sarcoidosis is high. Other common causes of hilar node enlargement which have to be considered are caseating tuberculosis, reticuloses such as Hodgkin's disease and other lymphomas, and metastatic malignant disease. The enlargement of hilar and mediastinal nodes that each of these may cause is rarely bilaterally symmetrical and usually differs in other important respects from the BHL of sarcoidosis.

Most cases of tuberculosis of hilar and mediastinal lymph-nodes arise soon after primary infection as part of the so-called primary complex: a local lesion in the lung at the site of entry of the infecting bacilli with involvement of related lymph-nodes. In those of Caucasian stock, and in others having similar resistance to mycobacterial infection, the lymph-node component tends to be prominent in childhood, but less so when primary infection occurs later in life, and to remain predominantly unilateral. The pulmonary component is usually evident radiologically, and in adults is often the more obvious abnormality. The skin reacts to tuberculin, often strongly; and tubercle bacilli may be found in sputum or in bronchial secretions obtained at bronchoscopy, though culture is usually required. But the development of extensive tuberculosis of mediastinal and hilar lymph-nodes is possible at any time after primary infection, more especially in some racial groups. Such cases must be distinguished from the BHL of sarcoidosis. They occur more frequently among immigrants from Asia, Africa or the West Indies in Great Britain (Ross *et al.*, 1970; Mikhail and Mitchell, 1971) and among blacks in the United States, than among whites. With such extensive lymph-node tuberculosis, the patient is likely to be obviously ill; the various groups of enlarged lymph-nodes are unlikely to be discrete as in sarcoidosis, but are liable to coalesce to form a smooth but ill-defined paramediastinal shadow; there may be evidence of localized lung involvement or of pleural effusion; cervical lymph-nodes are liable to become involved; tubercle bacilli are usually demonstrable without great difficulty; and diagnosis presents no difficulty. But in a few cases there are discordant or equivocal features. The patient may be afebrile and not progressively ill, and may be tuberculin-negative or give only a small reaction to 10 IU or 100 IU. It may be impossible to demonstrate tubercle bacilli, or acid-fast bacilli may be found microscopically with negative

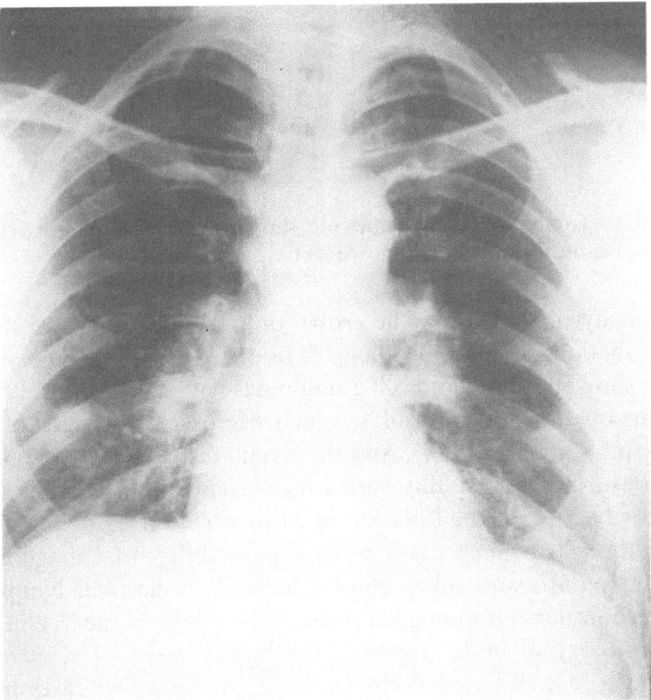

Figure 5.6   BHL with rounded shadow in the right lung in a man aged 28.

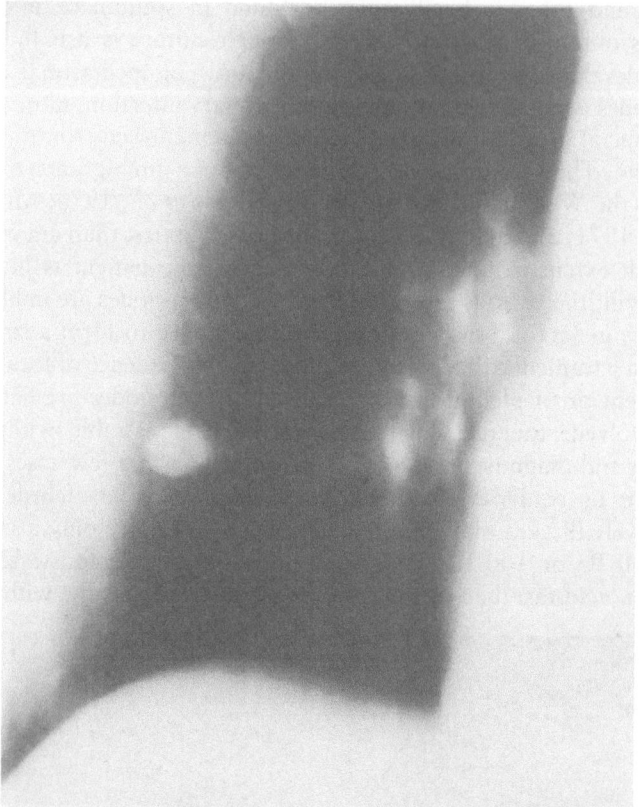

Figure 5.7   Tomograph in the same case, showing calcification both in hilar nodes and in the rounded shadow. See text.

cultures, or mycobacteria may be grown only in small numbers after prolonged incubation. Even the histology of nodes removed for biopsy may be equivocal, showing epithelioid cell granulomas with a little central necrosis, which some observers would call 'granular necrosis' and others 'caseation' (Mitchell and Scadding, 1974). And the Kveim test may give a granulomatous response in cases of this sort which eventually are categorized as tuberculosis because of the isolation of *M tuberculosis*.

Thus, although in most cases in which the differential diagnosis rests between sarcoidosis and tuberculous hilar and mediastinal lymphadenopathy, the clinical and radiological picture, the results of tuberculin testing, and the histology of nodes removed for biopsy and of Kveim test sites should lead to a well-based decision, there remain a few cases in which categorization must be provisional or judgement suspended, as in the following case:

A 28 year old white man was found at a routine examination to have gross BHL, together with a round shadow in the lower zone of the right lung (Fig. 5.6). Tomography showed flecks of calcification in this shadow and in the right hilar nodes (Fig. 5.7). Scalene node biopsy showed close-packed non-caseating tubercles of sarcoid type. A Mantoux test with 3 IU gave a reaction 25 mm in diameter. *M tuberculosis* was cultured from gastric contents. Because of these findings, treatment with streptomycin and isoniazid was started. Within three months, the hilar shadows returned to normal size.

The differential diagnosis from Hodgkin's disease and other lymphomas should rarely cause difficulty. Radiologically, the intrathoracic lymphadenopathy of Hodgkin's disease nearly always differs from that of sarcoidosis in that the well-defined margin with multiple contours of individual nodes or groups of nodes typical of sarcoidosis is not seen, the outline tending to have a single contour; the lower part of the hilar shadow is continuous with the heart shadow, instead of showing a clear band between its inner border and the heart shadow, as in sarcoidosis; and the enlargement is usually

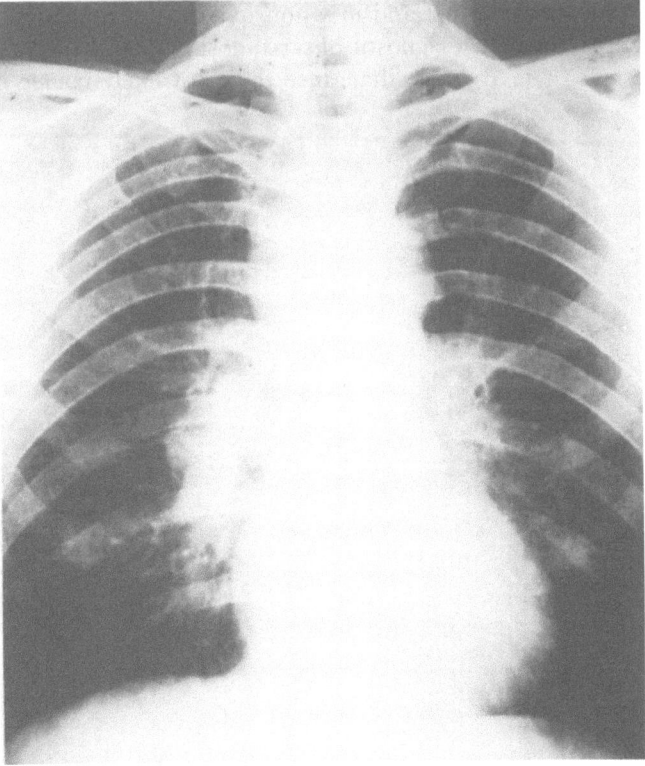

Figure 5.8 Predominantly right-sided hilar and paratracheal lymph-node enlargement, compatible with sarcoidosis, in a man aged 50. Although he had symptoms, investigation was delayed.

asymmetrical. Very rarely, the appearances may for a time mimic those of sarcoid BHL (Figs. 5.8, 5.9). Widespread mottling shadowing in the lung fields is very rare in Hodgkin's disease; the presence of such shadowing in company with symmetrical hilar node enlargement is characteristic, and its appearance under observation, as the hilar shadows diminish, diagnostic of sarcoidosis.

Similarly, metastatic carcinoma in hilar nodes very rarely mimics the symmetrical BHL of sarcoidosis.

The diagnostic procedures that are helpful in doubtful cases include biopsy of lymph-nodes, either accessible enlarged superficial nodes or obtained by mediastinoscopy; biopsy of other possibly involved tissues; and the Kveim test. These are discussed in Chapter 26. The following discussion concerns the special problems of patients with radiological evidence suggestive of sarcoid BHL, with or without symptoms.

Radiologically unequivocal BHL accompanying EN or febrile arthropathy or found by routine radiography in a person who on careful enquiry is found to be symptom-free and in whom physical examination shows no abnormality is virtually diagnostic of sarcoidosis (Winterbauer *et al.*, 1973). In such cases, it is arguable that since the most likely course is towards

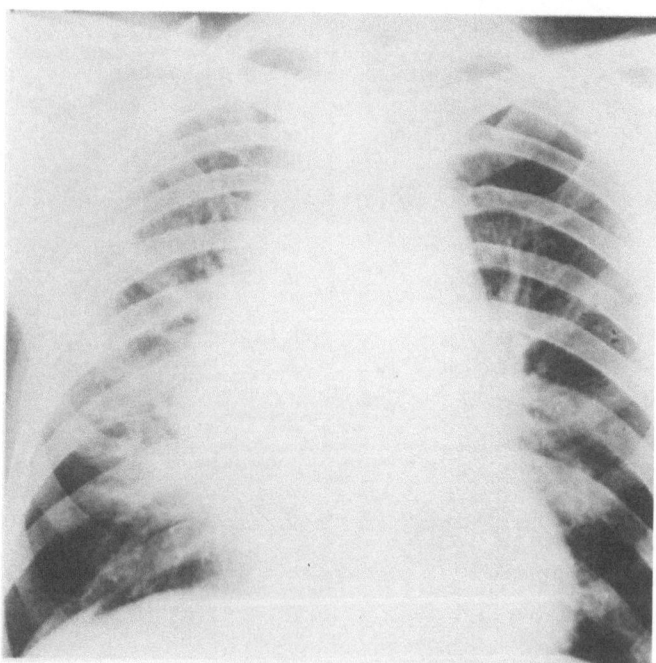

Figure 5.9   The same, 15 months later. The enlarged nodes have coalesced into a single mass. Lymph-node biopsy showed Hodgkin's disease.

resolution and no treatment is required, the interests of the patient are best served by the adoption of a working diagnosis of sarcoidosis in the expectation that continued observation will confirm it. A Kveim test with a satisfactory suspension can be expected to give a granulomatous response in 85–90% of patients with sarcoidosis at this stage, and has been advocated as the least disturbing of the procedures by which histological evidence may be obtained in such cases. A granulomatous response is reassuring, as being in accord with expectation; it will dispel any possible suspicion of Hodgkin's disease, since it is generally agreed that patients with Hodgkin's disease are non-reactive to Kveim test suspension. But it should not be taken to exclude mycobacterial lymphadenitis and some other sorts of lymphadenopathy (Israel and Goldstein, 1971; Mikhail and Mitchell, 1971). And faced with a negative response to a Kveim test, the physician is left with the problem of whether to investigate further the 10–15% of patients in whom the Kveim test is negative, but sarcoidosis remains the most likely diagnosis.

In cases of doubt, including of course all those with radiographic appearances not entirely characteristic of the discrete BHL of sarcoidosis, with constitutional or local symptoms other than those of EN, arthropathy or uveitis, or with significant reactions to skin tests with tuberculin or locally relevant fungal antigens, investigation should be directed towards histology, preferably of an involved lymph-node, and search for evidence of a possibly causal infection.

Careful search for palpable superficial lymph-nodes, and for inconspicuous changes in the skin, subcutaneous tissues, and old scars, which might be sarcoid infiltrations may provide an accessible source of tissue for biopsy. Ophthalmological examination may show evidence of uveitis, or symptomless sarcoid infiltration of the conjunctiva (Chapter 8). But in most cases these approaches are non-contributory. Mediastinoscopy is the least extensive procedure giving access to lymph-nodes in the mediastinum (Carlens, 1964; Ross *et al.*, 1970; Widstrom and Schnurer, 1978) and in experienced hands is safe; it has displaced scalene node biopsy, since it produces useful information in a higher proportion of cases. The finding of unequivocally non-caseating epithelioid and giant-cell granulomas in a lymph-node is strong confirmatory evidence of sarcoidosis, but does not exclude infective granulomatosis (tuberculosis, histoplasmosis, coccidioidomycosis) in cases in which the relevant skin-test is positive. The possibility of local sarcoid reactions to malignancy, either metastatic carcinoma (Symmers, 1951) or lymphoma (Brincker, 1972), in lymph-nodes must be remembered, as must the occurrence of granulomas in lymph-nodes in immune-deficiency syndromes (Sharma and James, 1971). In many cases, including some in which the diagnosis of sarcoidosis is acceptable on assessment of all the evidence and after observation of the further course, there is a variable amount of central necrosis, of a degree which may be

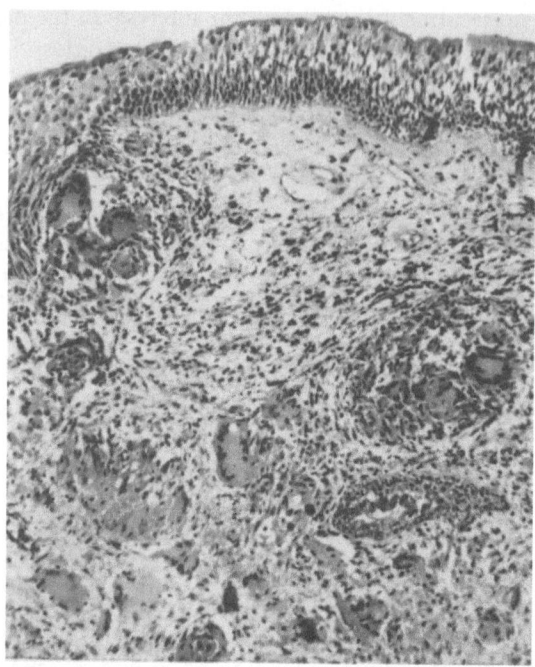

Figure 5.10   Biopsy of bronchial mucosa, which looked normal bronchoscopically, in a man with bilateral hilar lymph-node enlargement. H & E. ×
90.

called by different observers 'granular necrosis' or 'minimal caseation'
(Carlens *et al.*, 1974). In all cases, search for acid-fast bacilli and for
possibly relevant fungi by appropriate staining and microscopy and by
culture is essential.

Bronchoscopic findings in radiographically apparent pulmonary sarcoidosis are considered in Chapter 6, p. 140. In patients with sarcoid BHL
and no radiographically evident lung changes, bronchoscopic appearances
are often normal; but there may be distortion of major bronchi if the nodes
are very large, and the bronchial mucosa may appear thickened and there
may be dilatation of superficial blood-vessels. Biopsy, even of a normal-
looking mucosa, may show infiltration with non-caseating tubercles below a
normal epithelium (Fig. 5.10) Changes of this sort in normal-looking or
only slightly thickened mucosa in patients with BHL only have been reported in proportions ranging from none of nine (Carlens, 1964) to 34% of
63 cases (Liot *et al.*, 1963). The proportion of cases with granulomas in the
mucosa is higher when there is a pulmonary infiltration. In a very few
patients with BHL, but without radiologically evident lung infiltration,
changes in the bronchial mucosa and compression by the enlarged nodes

have been found to be severe enough to cause airflow limitation (Dines *et al.*, 1978). Such changes may be the early stage of the bronchostenoses that are observed in a few cases later in the course of sarcoidosis (Chapter 6, p. 143). There is good evidence that granulomas are present in the lungs of all, or nearly all, patients with sarcoid BHL, even though the lungs are radiologically clear; and transbronchial biopsy during fibre-optic bronchoscopy has been reported to produce tissue containing granulomas in up to 60% of such patients (Koerner *et al.*, 1975; Stableforth *et al.*, 1978). Thus fibre-optic bronchoscopy, with forceps biopsy of both bronchial mucosa and lung, is a useful procedure by which to obtain histological evidence; but the finding of granulomas leaves open the question whether the case should be categorized as sarcoidosis or tuberculosis. The amount of tissue obtained in a single sample is sufficient only for histology, and multiple samples are required to permit culture for mycobacteria and other infective agents. For this reason, and because the finding of a few granulomas cannot exclude malignant disease or lymphoma, a direct approach to involved lymph-nodes by mediastinoscopy may be preferred when the diagnosis is seriously in doubt in a patient with hilar and mediastinal lymphadenopathy.

Course and prognosis

Since BHL, with or without EN, is one of the more frequent modes of presentation of sarcoidosis, the prognosis for patients presenting in this way is worth considering separately, though some patients will develop radiological evidence of pulmonary sarcoidosis, whose prognosis is considered in Chapter 6. One of us (JGS) followed 96 patients presenting with BHL. In 55 of them the lungs remained clear of abnormal shadowing during the period of observation. In 45 of these the nodes returned to normal size, most frequently within one year and nearly always within two years, although in one the enlargement persisted for three years before subsiding, and in three it persisted after more than two years' observation with clear lung fields. In the remaining 41, radiologically evident changes developed in the lungs, within 1–10 months of the detection of BHL, and usually after BHL had started to subside. Of 84 who were observed for more than two years, 66 became free from all radiographic evidence of intrathoracic sarcoidosis; 12 were left without symptoms, but with persistent radiographic abnormality, persistently enlarged nodes in two, enlarged nodes together with minor non-progressive lung changes after 8 years' observation in one, dense non-fibrotic mottling after five years in one, and non-progressive minor fibrotic changes in eight; three had extensive mottled shadowing probably developing some fibrosis and accompanied by dyspnoea; and three had established and disabling fibrosis. Those patients whose illness started with erythema nodosum or febrile arthropathy had a better prognosis than the rest. The proportions attaining a normal chest radiograph were 88% for those presenting with erythema nodosum or febrile arthropathy, 62% for those discovered by routine radiography, and 48% for those who initially had respiratory or constitutional symptoms.

These prognostic trends are similar to those reported from Stockholm by Löfgren (1953), in other series from London by Smellie and Hoyle (1960) and by Walker and James (1972), and by Würm (1974) in Germany. But from Philadelphia, were 87% of their 211 patients were blacks, Sones and Israel (1960) found that only 30% of 71 with BHL only in the initial radiograph attained complete resolution; and similar findings have been reported among West Indians in London (Mikhail *et al.*, 1980).

In a few cases of sarcoid BHL, the nodes remain persistently enlarged, usually after some initial reduction in size, without symptoms and without the appearance of any further manifestation of sarcoidosis. It is probable that in such cases, the major part of the persistently enlarged nodes is occupied by the featureless hyaline connective tissue into which the sarcoid granuloma evolves if it does not resolve. A case in which enlarged hilar and

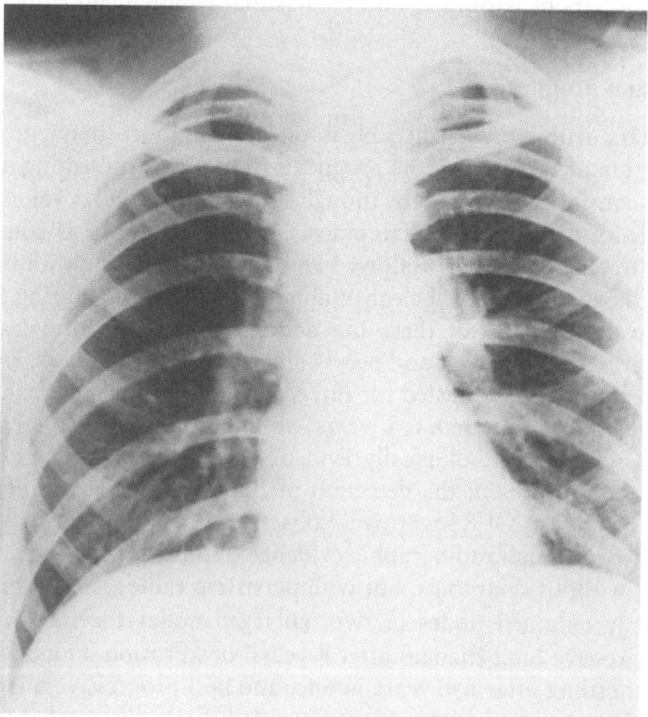

Figure 5.11   Slight enlargement of left hilar and right paratracheal lymph-nodes, known to have been present for four years, in a man aged 22.

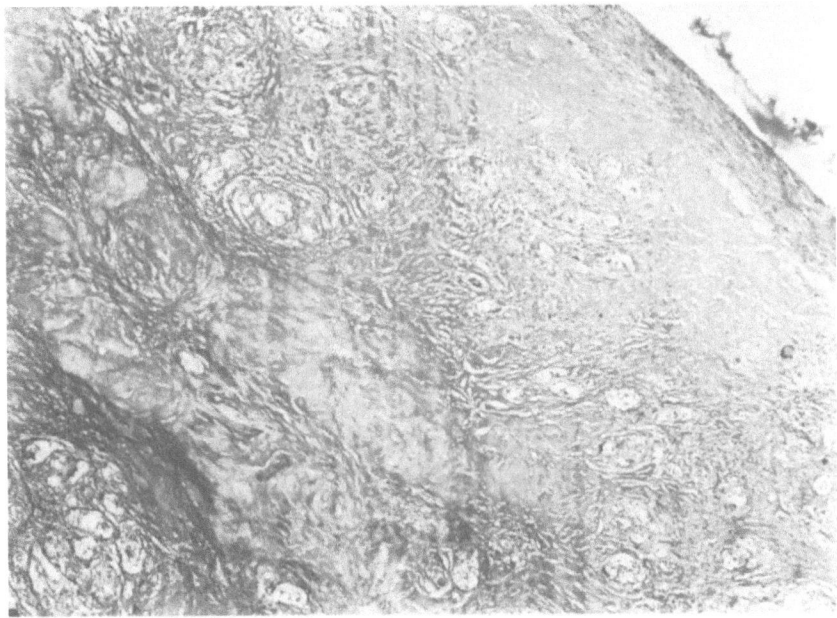

Figure 5.12 Biopsy of left hilar node from the same. The bulk of the node consisted of this featureless hyaline connective tissue. H & E. × 38.

mediastinal nodes had been known to be present without change in radiographic appearance for four years is illustrated in Fig. 5.11. Because of diagnostic doubt, they were removed for biopsy by left thoracotomy, at which 15–20 firm and discrete nodes up to 4 cm in diameter were found at the hilum, freely mobile beneath the mediastinal pleura, and in the fissure overlying the pulmonary artery; histologically, the greater part of them consisted of hyalinizing sarcoid tubercles, with some still cellular tubercles but large tracts of almost acellular hyaline connective tissue (Figs 5.12 and 5.13). In necropsy material from patients dying with extensive chronic sarcoidosis, even more extensively hyalinized lymph-nodes may be found (Fig. 5.14).

Different degrees of cellularity and fibrosis are not infrequently observed in the granulomas of a lymph-node or other tissue obtained by biopsy from patients with clinical evidence of active sarcoidosis, and the amount of hyaline fibrosis present in the lymph-nodes obtained by mediastinoscopy from patients with or without lung mottling correlates poorly with radiographic appearances and with duration of symptoms (Chapter 2). The wide range of histological appearances found in hilar lymph-nodes at Stage I of the usual radiographic classification shows that although this may be a convenient method of referring to radiographic appearances, it must not be

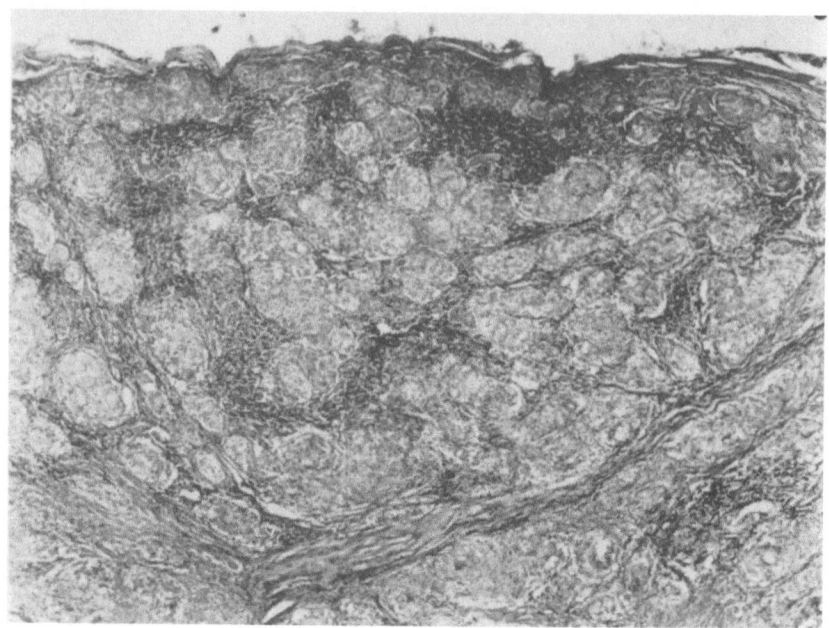

Figure 5.13   The same, showing recognizable hyalinizing sarcoid follicles at the periphery.

assumed to correlate with the duration of disease. Radiographic 'staging' of pulmonary sarcoidosis is discussed in Chapter 6.

When BHL subsides spontaneously and completely without lung infiltration it is extremely rare for further manifestations of sarcoidosis to appear. Lim (1961) reported the case of a woman who had been treated for pulmonary tuberculosis, and subsequently had four episodes of BHL followed by pulmonary infiltration and resolving spontaneously, with iridiocyclitis in the third; in the fourth, scalene node biopsy showed typical sarcoid granulomas. One of us (JGS) has observed one patient, in whom a sarcoid BHL syndrome occurred three times, when he was aged 24, 26 and 32 years, each time with constitutional and abdominal symptoms, and on the third occasion with transitory arthropathy and a limited eruption of erythema nodosum; all the episodes subsided slowly without corticosteroid treatment. MacFarlane (1981) reported the case of a woman who had episodes of EN, BHL and pulmonary infiltration at the ages of 36, 53 and 56, the first two resolving spontaneously and the third after corticosteroid treatment.

The relationship of extrapulmonary manifestations of sarcoidosis to BHL may be illustrated by the experience of one of us (JGS). Adding to the 96 patients, mentioned above, who presented with BHL discovered by routine radiography, or with EN, arthropathy, or constitutional or respiratory symptoms, 14 who presented with uveitis, two with superficial lymphadenitis, and one with infiltration of a scar and were found to have BHL, there were 113 patients for review. At some time during the observed course of these, changes were found in the eyes in 18, in the skin in ten, in the bones of the hands in one, and in the nervous system in one.

The ocular changes tended to occur early in the clinical course; the observation that in 14 cases they were the cause of discovery of BHL suggests this, and is supported by the fact that of the five patients who presented with 'isolated' BHL, two were found to have ocular changes less than one month, one six months, one twelve months, and only one a longer period (six years) after the discovery of BHL.

In the five patients who developed sarcoid lesions of undamaged skin, the time of development tended to be later, between nine months and four years from the discovery of BHL; and in no patient coming under observation for the first time with sarcoids of the skin was BHL without lung changes found.

Subcutaneous nodules and infiltrations of scars, on the other hand, appeared earlier. The three patients with subcutaneous nodules were all

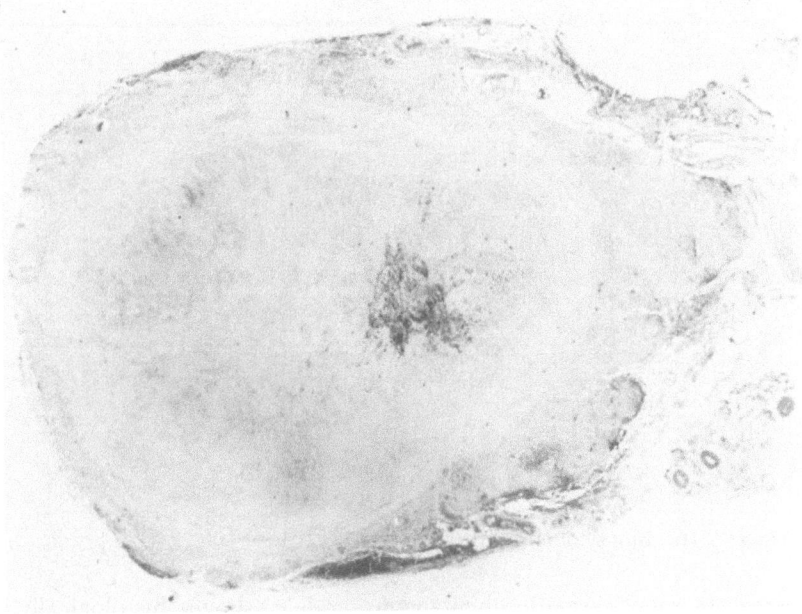

Figure 5.14　A mediastinal lymph-node from a woman aged 48 with sarcoidosis, showing almost complete replacement by hyaline connective tissue, with a small rim which lymphocytes and a few remnants of granulomas were recognizable. H & E. × 11.

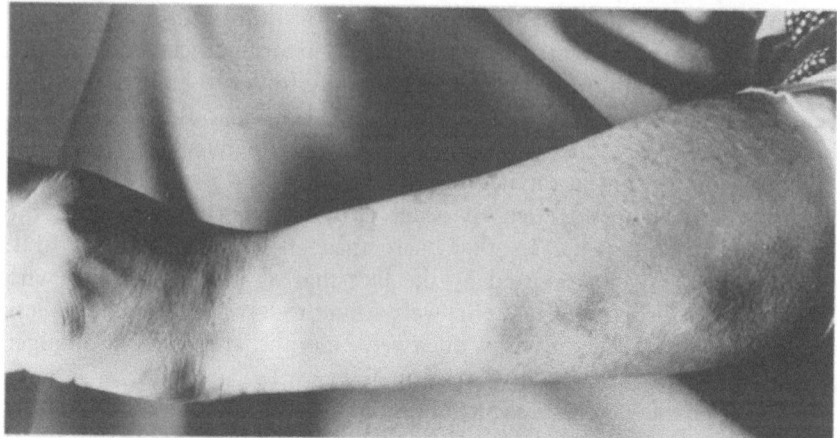

Figure 5.15   Subcutaneous nodules which developed soon after the appearance of erythema nodosum in a woman aged 30.

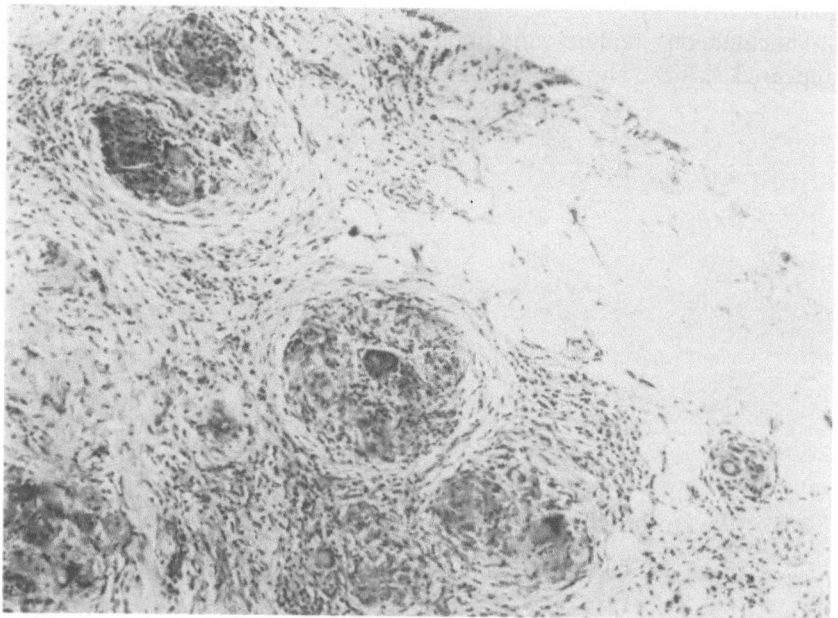

Figure 5.16   Biopsy of one of these nodules, H & E. × 100.

women. In one, a small subcutaneous nodule, shown histologically to consist of sarcoid tubercles, appeared in the cheek three months before EN and BHL. In the other two, the nodules appeared on the forearms, and were first observed shortly after EN, and subsided spontaneously within a year (Figs 5.15, 5.16). Both the patients with infiltrated scars, one on the knee

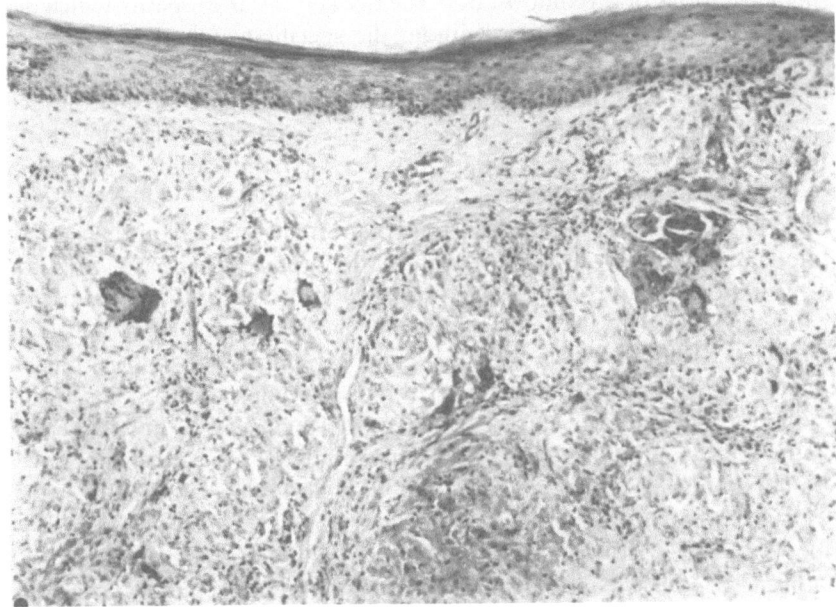

Figure 5.17   Biopsy of a scar on the knee of a man aged 27, which became raised, red and indurated during an attack of erythema nodosum. H & E. × 100.

dating from childhood (Fig. 5.17), and the other an appendicectomy scar, were men; in both, the BHL and scar infiltrations subsided spontaneously.

The place of BHL in the natural history of sarcoidosis

It is clear that BHL is a very frequent manifestation of sarcoidosis. It may be accompanied by no symptoms, by vague disturbances of health, by various unspecific respiratory symptoms, by low fever, by febrile arthropathy, or by erythema nodosum. In cases of sarcoidosis in which BHL is observed, with or without symptoms, it nearly always precedes, even if only by a short time, any other manifestation that may develop. There is some suggestion that there may be a sort of timetable of subsequent developments, changes in the lungs and in the eyes tending to follow closely upon BHL, so that they may be evident when BHL is first discovered, whereas sarcoids of the skin (apart from infiltration of scars) tend to appear later. Löfgren (1953) suggested that BHL might be regarded as 'primary sarcoidosis', and be analogous with the primary stages of such infectious diseases as tuberculosis and syphilis. There are certainly important differences between the phenomena which often accompany BHL as the first clinical evidence, and other manifestations of sarcoidosis. Both the EN and the arthropathy which occur with BHL are inflammatory without the specific histology of sarcoidosis; and uveitis at this early stage similarly appears to have a considerable inflammatory component and tends to resolve completely, in contrast to the chronic granulomatous type that may occur later (Chapter 8). Immunologically, there are differences between the earlier and the later stages, e.g. in the degree of depression of delayed-type skin hypersensitivity reactions. There is thus some justification for the distinction that has been drawn between acute or sub-acute and chronic sarcoidosis, and for a schematic timetable of events in the course of sarcoidosis (James and Thomson, 1959; Siltzbach, 1964c). But two factual questions must be considered: do all cases of sarcoidosis go through the BHL stage? And if not, is there any indication of a possible equivalent in those without a BHL stage?

Both these questions must be answered in the negative. In a few cases of pulmonary sarcoidosis there is evidence that there has been no stage of radiographically detectable BHL, although, naturally, satisfactory evidence on this point is rarely available (Chapter 6, p. 111). The question of a possible alternative syndrome of 'primary sarcoidosis' must therefore be considered. This would presumably consist in enlargement of a group of lymph-nodes corresponding to a route of entry of the hypothetical causative agent other than the lungs. No such syndrome has been described. The factual basis for an analogy with primary tuberculosis or primary syphilis is therefore incomplete.

For these reasons, the term 'primary sarcoidosis' may be misleading, and should be avoided. The phenomena to which it refers can be summarised in the statement that bilateral hilar lymphadenopathy with or without EN and/or arthropathy, usually of a characteristic radiographic appearance, with or without clinical symptoms and signs, is a frequent first manifestation of sarcoidosis.

Chapter 6

Lung Changes

Changes in the lungs, discovered either because they cause symptoms or by radigraphy of apparently healthy individuals, are among the commonest first evidences of sarcoidosis (Chapter 4), and are prominent among the observed features in all reported large series of cases of sarcoidosis.

The proportion of cases found by clinical and radiological methods to have lung changes may be expected to depend upon the source of referral, investigative procedures routinely adopted, and duration of observation. In their survey of 1609 cases of sarcoidosis in five centres round the world, Siltzbach et al. (1974) found that the proportion reported to have lung changes was 46%, ranging from 40–68% in the various centres. But a further 42% had enlarged hilar lymph-nodes, without reported evidence of lung involvement; and it is certain that the large majority, if not all, patients with sarcoid hilar lymphadenopathy have granulomas scattered more or less densely in the lungs. Biopsy of radiographically normal lungs in patients with sarcoid BHL has been found to show granulomas in a proportion of cases increasing with the amount of tissue examined. Eule (1971) performed open biopsies in 38 such patients, and found granulomas in 36, in 25 of whom the lungs appeared grossly normal at thoracotomy. Rosen et al. (1977a) similarly found granulomas in open lung biopsies in 21 consecutive patients with BHL and radiographically clear lungs; the extent of the changes varied greatly, from 'minimal' in seven to affecting more than two-thirds of the tissue examined in one. Transbronchial biopsy has been found to be more productive in such cases the larger the number of samples taken. Roethe et al. (1980), routinely taking ten transbronchial samples, found granulomas in all of ten patients with BHL; in most, only one or two of the samples contained granulomas. It is thus probable that at some time during the course of the disease the great majority of patients with sarcoidosis have granulomas in the lungs, even though in many they are not radio-graphically evident and may resolve without causing symptoms at any time.

In reported necropsy series, the lungs and the lymph-nodes are the most frequently involved organs (Chapter 2). But findings at necropsy cannot be assumed to indicate the proportion of patients showing lung changes during life. Since most deaths from sarcoidosis are directly or indirectly due to chronic changes in the lungs, necropsy figures might over-estimate the proportion of all cases with lung involvement. On the other hand, since it is known that sarcoid granulomas can resolve completely, or undergo hyaline fibrosis with no recognizable residual granulomas, failure to find granulomas in the lungs at necropsy in patients with sarcoidosis dying from an extrapulmonary localization of the disease, from the effects of hypercal-caemia, or from an unrelated disease does not exclude the possibility that the lungs may have been involved at an earlier stage of the disease.

The interrelations of symptoms, pathology, radiographic appearances, and tests of respiratory function in pulmonary sarcoidosis are complex.

SYMPTOMS

Symptoms are widely variable in severity from case to case, and generally non-specific in character, being similar to those produced by a wide range of diseases affecting the pulmonary acini.

As already noted, widespread granulomas in the lungs may be demon-strable only by biopsy, producing neither symptoms nor radiographic changes. Patients with obvious radiographic changes in their lungs may have no, or only trivial, symptoms. Of 275 patients with sarcoidosis observed by one of us (JGS), 34% first came under medical observation because abnormalities had been found when, as apparently healthy indi-viduals, they underwent routine chest radiography. Especially in patients of Caucasian stock, the symptoms of apparently pre-fibrotic sarcoidosis of the lungs tend to be less severe than the extent of radiographic shadows might lead the observer to expect. An example of dense sarcoid infiltration of the lungs in a man who denied symptoms, and in whom standard tests of ventilatory function and carbon monoxide transfer factor were within the predicted range is shown in Fig. 6.1. Symptoms that may occur at an early stage of pulmonary sarcoidosis include dyspnoea on exertion, usually gra-dual in onset, cough, usually unproductive but sometimes with scanty mucoid sputum, ill-defined chest pain, and constitutional symptoms, such as malaise, tiredness, weight loss and fever. Their severity varies greatly, and correlates poorly with radiographic appearances. In a few patients, and especially in those of African and Indian sub-continental ancestry, they develop more rapidly to a disabling level. Among 162 patients observed in Philadelphia, of whom 75 were black and 87 white, Israel and Washburne

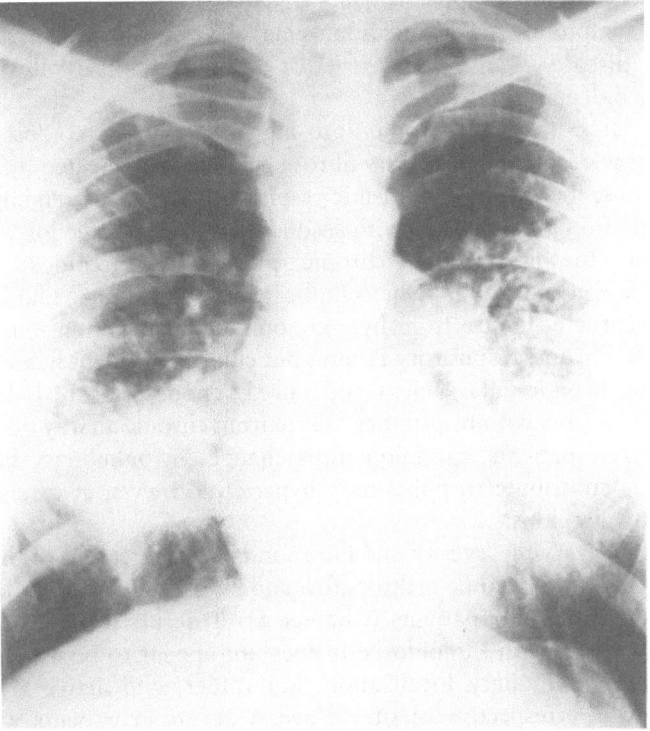

Figure 6.1 Dense sarcoid infiltration of the lungs in a man aged 39 who was symptom-free, with normal carbon monoxide uptake (by steady state method 29 ml min^{-1}mm^{-1} Hg at rest, rising to 48 on exercise).

(1980) found that symptoms were, in general, more severe in black than in white patients. Among the black patients only 4% had no symptoms, while 17% complained of weight loss, 32% of dyspnoea, and 19% were observed to have fever; while the corresponding figures among the white patients were 16% symptom-free, and 1% with weight loss, 15% with dyspnoea, and 10% with fever.

Patients with sarcoidosis who smoke, and who live in areas of general air pollution, must be expected to include the usual proportion susceptible to the induction of bronchial catarrh and persistent airflow limitation by these factors. Cases of pulmonary sarcoidosis may therefore first come to notice during investigation of unrelated respiratory symptoms of these sorts; and since, as noted below (p.140), airways may be involved in pulmonary sarcoidosis, it may be difficult in such cases to assess the relative contributions of sarcoidosis and of air-pollution, private and public, to airflow limitation. Occasionally, a banal acute respiratory infection leads to the discovery of radiographic evidence of sarcoidosis, itself causing no or only trivial symptoms. Atopic individuals may develop sarcoidosis; in such cases, atopic disease – asthma, hay fever or eczema – and sarcoidosis appear to follow independent courses.

The later stages of chronic fibrosing pulmonary sarcoidosis, like other sorts of widespread pulmonary fibrosis, may be complicated by intercurrent infections, the common epidemic respiratory infections tending to lead to exacerbation of symptoms with secondary bacterial infection and purulent sputum. In old-standing chronic pulmonary sarcoidosis, increasing dyspnoea on exertion may be complicated by right ventricular hypertrophy and eventually failure from hypoxic pulmonary hypertension, as in other forms of chronic respiratory failure; but clinically evident heart failure with oedema, hepatic enlargement and raised venous pressure is less frequent than in patients with respiratory failure from chronic airway obstruction. In a very few patients, granulomatous changes in pulmonary blood-vessels (p. 107) contribute to pulmonary hypertension, even at a relatively early stage of sarcoidosis.

Fever of varying severity and duration is a usual feature of the syndrome of erythema nodosum, arthropathy and BHL which marks the onset of sarcoidosis in some patients (Chapter 5). It occurs in only a minority of other patients with sarcoidosis. It does not appear to be associated especially with pulmonary localization, but rather with active and extensive sarcoidosis, irrespective of site. When it occurs in patients with a widespread sarcoid infiltration of the lungs, it may lead to diagnostic difficulty, suggesting such possibilities as tuberculosis, other microbial and fungal diseases, acute extrinsic allergic and cryptogenic fibrosing alveolitis, and collagen-vascular diseases. In a series of 75 patients with a final diagnosis of sarcoidosis, admitted to hospital for investigation, and thus including a high proportion of difficult diagnostic problems, Nolan and Klatskin (1964) found that 60% of blacks and 29% of whites had fever of at least 38.3 °C for at least three days, the difference being significant, $P<0.01$. The duration of fever ranged from a few days to 12 weeks, and was greater than two months in half the febrile patients. Fever might be associated with leucocytosis, counts above 10 000 mm^{-3} being recorded in seven of 31 febrile and only one of 44 afebrile patients. Thus although most cases of sarcoidosis run an afebrile course, fever of limited duration may occur in a few, and especially in blacks.

The symptoms that may arise from pleural involvement, from changes in large bronchi, and from fungus-balls developing in cavities, all of which occur in only a few cases, are considered below.

Diffuse sarcoid infiltration of the lungs characteristically gives rise to no, or inconspicuous, physical signs, especially when it is symptomless. In some cases, more especially those with evident symptoms and a sub-acute onset, fine crackles may be heard over the lungs, but these are generally less than are found in some other diseases affecting the pulmonary acini. In the late fibrotic stages, the physical signs are those to be expected from the structural changes.

Clubbing of the fingers is rarely seen in pulmonary sarcoidosis, and when it occurs is usually associated with long-standing fibrosis, possibly with bronchiectatic changes, cavitation and secondary bacterial infection. In 500 personally observed cases, one of us (JGS) observed drumstick clubbing of the fingers in only one without these complicating factors. This was in a woman, who presented with widespread mottling in the chest radiograph and gradually increasing dyspnoea leading to death five years from the onset. The radiographic shadows persisted diffusely, without the sort of local condensation and development of irregular strand-like shadows and distortion that are more usual; and at necropsy, there was extensive diffuse hyaline fibrosis in the lungs, with only ill-defined remnants of granulomas, and similar changes were found in liver and lymph-nodes. Yancey *et al.* (1972) referred briefly to having seen clubbing of the fingers in four of the 136 patients with sarcoidosis, but gave no detail either of the severity of the clubbing, or of the characteristics of the patients in whom it was observed, beyond that they had evidence of 'bilateral interstitial disease'. Chusid (1980) measured the ratio between the distal phalangeal and the interphalangeal depths of the index finger in 120 patients with sarcoidosis. A value above 1.0, which has been used by Regan *et al.* (1967) and Waring *et al.* (1971) as an index of clubbing, was found in proportions increasing from 7% of 14 with normal chest radiographs to 74% of 23 at conventional radiographic Stage III; but the proportions showing clinically evident clubbing were not stated. West *et al.* (1981) reported briefly the case of a 28 year old black man with widespread sarcoidosis, of three years' duration, affecting superficial and hilar lymph-nodes, lungs, skin and salivary glands, accompanied by migratory polyarthropathy. Eighteen months from the onset, he developed painful clubbing of fingers and toes, without radiographic changes to suggest either sarcoid involvement of bone or hypertrophic osteoarthropathy. The pain responded to colchicine, but there was no long-term follow-up.

PATHOLOGY

Open lung biopsy, which at one time was used almost routinely in some centres for the diagnosis of widespread lung disease whose nature was not otherwise evident, has provided information about some special features of the histopathology of pulmonary sarcoidosis at various stages of its evolution.

Probably the most important of these is the varying prominence of mononuclear infiltration in the vicinity of granulomas, especially in alveolar walls. This has been called 'interstitial pneumonia' by some (Carrington *et al.*, 1976; Rosen *et al.*, 1978, 1979) and 'alveolitis' by others (Roberts, 1981). The principal site of this mononuclear cell infiltration is in alveolar walls, rather than in the very extensive interstitial tissue of the lung generally; and we therefore prefer 'alveolitis'. Used with the conventional limitation of meaning suggested by Scadding (1964), this term denotes an inflammation of pulmonary acini affecting principally alveolar walls, as opposed to 'pneumonia' which refers to inflammatory consolidation by exudation into alveolar spaces. Rosen *et al.* (1978) found non-granulomatous changes predominant in 24% of 128 open lung biopsy specimens from patients with sarcoidosis, prominent in a further 38%, and insignificant in the remaining 38%. These changes consisted of mixed mononuclear cells, mainly macrophages and lymphocytes, infiltrating alveolar walls. Their prominence was inversely related to the profusion of granulomas; it was greater in patients with BHL and radiographically clear lungs than in those with radiographically evident changes; and there was less fibrosis in specimens with predominant alveolitis than in those with predominant granulomas. Similarly in open lung biopsies from 30 patients with

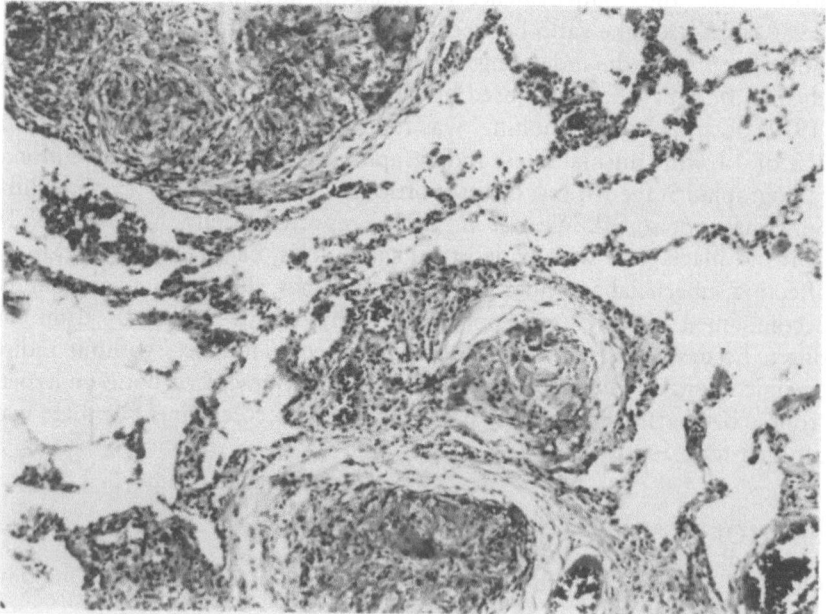

Figure 6.2   Biopsy of lung of a woman aged 30, in whom widespread mottling had been found in the routine radiograph. There are well-formed sarcoid granulomas among the alveoli, intervening alveolar walls being normal. H & E. × 100.

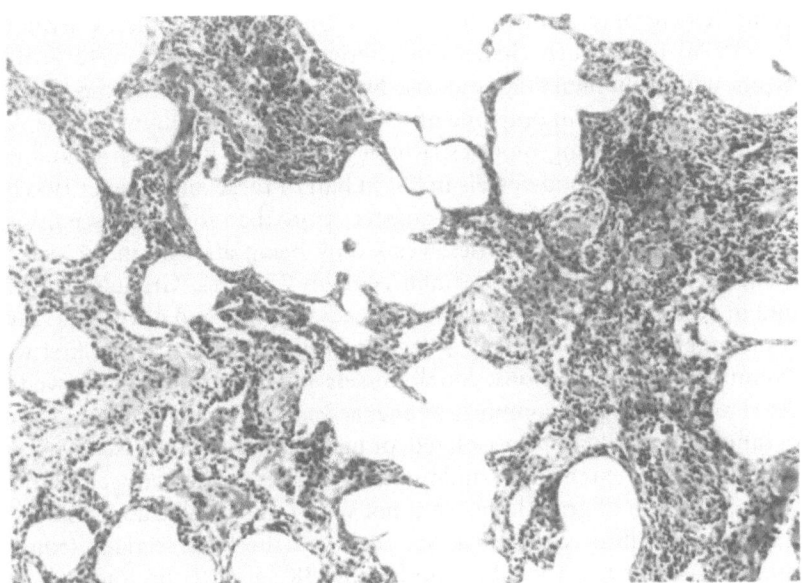

Figure 6.3   Biopsy of lung of a woman aged 21 who presented with arthropathy, increasing dyspnoea and pulmonary infiltration, showing non-granulomatous cellular infiltration of alveolar wall ('alveolitis'). Elsewhere, there were well-formed granulomas. H & E. × 70.

sarcoidosis, Lacronique *et al.* (1983) found both infiltration of alveolar walls by inflammatory cells, mainly lymphocytes, and formed epithelioid and giant-cell granulomas, and studying the relative extent of these changes by a point-counting method, showed that there was an inverse relation between them. These findings suggest that alveolitis is an early stage of the process, antedating and resulting in the formation of granulomas; they are consistent with experimental studies of granuloma formation (Chapter 2, p. 28) and with the immuno-cytological studies made possible by broncho-alveolar lavage (Chapter 20, p. 435). Figure 6.2 shows discrete granulomas of sarcoid type with normal-looking alveoli between them in a woman who admitted to only slight dyspnoea on exertion after widespread mottling had been found in a chest radiograph; by contrast, Figure 6.3 shows extensive cellular infiltration of alveolar walls in a woman with a short history of arthropathy and increasing dyspnoea on exertion, formed granulomas being found elsewhere in the biopsy section.

A few cases in which extensive granulomatous changes were found at necropsy in pulmonary blood-vessels in patients with sarcoidosis have been reported (Bottcher, 1959; Michaels *et al.*, 1960; Thompson, 1966), possibly causing pulmonary hypertension (Levine *et al.*, 1971); but the frequency of granulomatous angiitis throughout the course of pulmonary sarcoidosis has become evident only from studies of open lung biopsy samples. Carrington *et al.* (1976) found such changes in arteries, veins, or both in 42% of 48 patients with pulmonary sarcoidosis; by contrast, granulomatous changes in vessels were found in only one of 15 with chronic beryllium disease. In a study of 128 open lung biopsies, Rosen *et al.* (1977b) found granulomas within the walls of blood-vessels in 88; in half of these, only one or two foci of angiitis were seen, while in one-quarter, more than four were seen. Veins were affected more than arteries, veins only being affected in 54, arteries only in seven, and both arteries and veins in 27 cases. Granulomas were found in vessels of various sizes, and in media, intima and adventitia. Serial sections might show that changes evident in only one coat in the first were transmural in other sections. Small vessels might be much narrowed by these changes, but no thrombosis or aneurysmal dilatation was seen. Vascular granulomas might appear isolated, or be in continuity with extravascular granulomas. The extent of granulomatous angiitis correlated well with the general profusion of granulomas, but not with radiographic appearances or the amount of fibrosis. Rosen *et al.* reviewed the lung sections from 15 necropsy cases of miliary tuberculosis, and 98 surgical specimens of pulmonary tuberculosis of other sorts, and found two cases, one from each of these groups, with granulomatous pulmonary angiitis similar to that seen in their sarcoidosis patients.

Bronchiolar and peribronchial granulomas are frequent, and seem to be so placed in some cases as to be likely to narrow small airways (Carrington *et al.*, 1976). Changes in larger bronchi are considered below (p. 140).

The varying prominence of vascular involvement in the granulomatous process in pulmonary sarcoidosis, and the varying balance between granulomas and non-granulomatous alveolitis, may lead to difficulty in diagnostic interpretation of lung biopsies. Prominence of alveolitis suggests the possibility of chronic beryllium disease (Chapter 22), or of extrinsic allergic alveolitis, in which inflammatory changes with a variable granulomatous element occur in alveoli and small airways as hypersensitivity reactions to organic dusts, such as mouldy hay and other agricultural products, environmental moulds, and bird droppings (Emanuel *et al.*, 1964; Seal *et al.*, 1968); or of a few rarer diagnostic categories currently definable only in terms of pulmonary histopathology, such as lymphomatoid granulomatosis (Liebow *et al.*, 1972). Prominence of granulomatous angiitis may suggest Wegener's (1939) granulomatosis, in either its generalized or apparently localized forms (Carrington and Liebow, 1966), schistosomiasis or reactions to other pulmonary parasites, or certain rare histopathologically defined categories, such as necrotizing sarcoidal angiitis and granulomatosis (Liebow, 1973, Stephen *et al.*, 1976; Churg *et al.*, 1979) and benign lymphocytic pulmonary angiitis and granulomatosis (Saldana *et al.*, 1977). Where lung biopsy appearances are equivocal, the diagnosis of sarcoidosis must depend upon recognition of generally compatible clinical features and/or evidence of sarcoid-type granulomatous changes in other organs or in response to a Kveim test (Chapter 26).

RADIOLOGY

Although tests of lung function, lung biopsy, and more recently broncho-alveolar lavage have added greatly to knowledge of pulmonary sarcoidosis in the past 20 years, changes in the chest radiograph are often the first evidence of sarcoidosis; and because radiology was the chief means by which knowledge of the course in intrathoracic sarcoidosis was obtained, and still provides the most convenient way of following it, it has become customary to group patients suffering from it according to radiographic appearances for purposes of description. Scadding (1961b), in a study of prognosis, divided patients into four descriptive groups, according to the radiographic findings at the beginning of the observation-period, as follows: Group I, BHL with radiographically clear lungs; Group II, apparently non-fibrotic lung changes with concurrent or previously observed BHL; Group III, apparently non-fibrotic lung changes, without BHL, either currently or previously observed; and Group IV, lung changes interpreted as fibrotic. Grouping of this general sort has been rather widely adopted, usually with the groups renamed stages, and with Group II including only cases with concurrent BHL and lung changes, and Group III consisting of those with lung changes and without concurrent BHL, whether or no BHL has been observed previously; and sometimes with the addition of a 'Stage 0' to refer to cases in which the chest radiograph is normal. The use of the term 'stage' to refer to descriptive groups is unfortunate, since it implies, unjustifiably, that the numbering O–IV corresponds to a necessary temporal sequence. Although the sequence BHL, appearance of lung infiltration, subsidence of BHL with persistence of lung changes occurs in many cases, there are important exceptions to it. A lung infiltration without BHL may be the earliest detected change, occasionally in patients who have had a normal chest radiograph so recently that preceding BHL is unlikely; in rare cases, BHL with radiographically clear lungs persists indefinitely (Chapter 5, p. 94), and may be accompanied by progressive granulomatous changes in other organs; as noted above, it has been shown that radiographically clear lungs with BHL usually contain granulomas, and with or without BHL may contain granulomas at various stages of their evolution to fibrosis. Moreover, the correlation of radiology with histopathology made possible by biopsy has shown that fibrotic elements may be present without any of the accepted radiographic evidences of fibrosis, such as distortion of vascular, septal and other shadows, localized emphysema, and displacement of mediastinum, ribs or diaphragm. Thus, although grouping by radiographic appearances is convenient for descriptive purposes, it should not be thought of, or called, staging, and should be based on radiological criteria only. In the definitions of Scadding's (1961b) Groups II and III, 'apparently non-fibrotic' should be interpreted as, or replaced by 'without distortion of vascular shadows of displacement of mediastinal structures or ribs'. Estimates of duration and chronicity can be made only by consideration of all available evidence, and radiological grouping, apart from Group IV, should carry no necessary implications in these respects.

For those reasons, the radiographic appearances will be described without reference to 'stages', except where necessary in discussion of reports in which this terminology has been used.

Pulmonary infiltration

The most frequent radiographic appearances of sarcoidosis of the lungs early in its course is a widespread mottled shadowing, distributed either more or less uniformly, or tending to be rather denser in the middle thirds of the lung fields. In the following discussion, the term 'sarcoid infiltration' will be used to refer to shadows distributed widely in the lung fields and attributed to sarcoidosis.

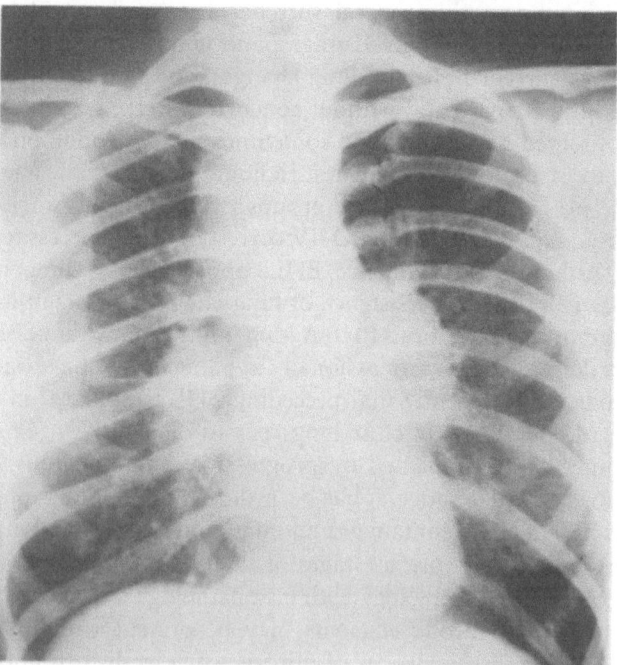

Figure 6.4   Bilateral hilar and right paratracheal lymph-node enlargement in a woman aged 32.

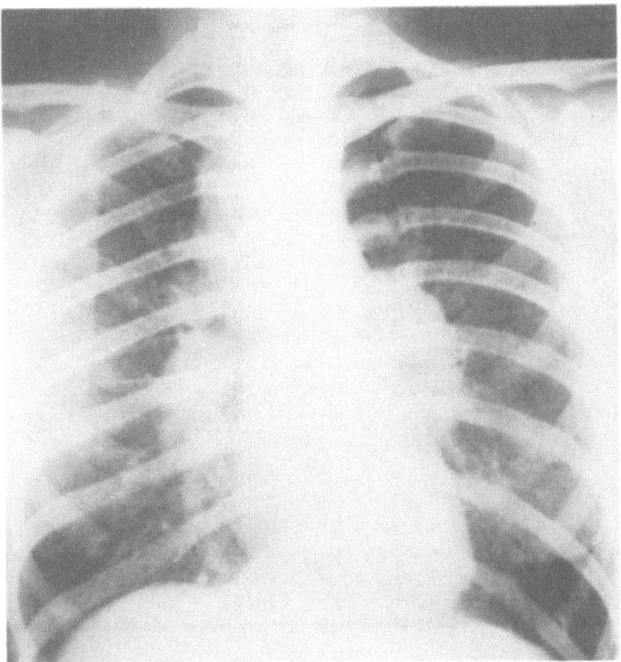

Figure 6.5   The same, 18 months later; lymph-nodes much smaller, widespread mottling in both lungs. One year later, lung fields and hilar shadows were normal.

Relation to BHL

In a high proportion of cases, sarcoid infiltration of the lungs is accompanied at the time of its discovery by enlargement of hilar lymph-nodes on both sides, with or without paratracheal nodes (BHL) of the type described in Chapter 5. When associated with BHL, it frequently appears as the BHL starts to subside, and reaches its full development after the BHL has subsided (Figs 6.4 and 6.5). Occasionally BHL and lung mottling coexist for months or even years (Fig. 6.6), but it is exceptional for the BHL in such instances to remain prominent.

In some cases, the first evidence of pulmonary sarcoidosis is a widespread shadowing in the lung fields, without enlargement of hilar shadows. In these cases, either there has been in fact no stage of BHL, or such a stage has passed without symptoms and therefore without detection. The concept of BHL as a necessary stage in the evolution of pulmonary sarcoidosis (p. 99) would imply the latter. But in all reported series, a proportion of cases of

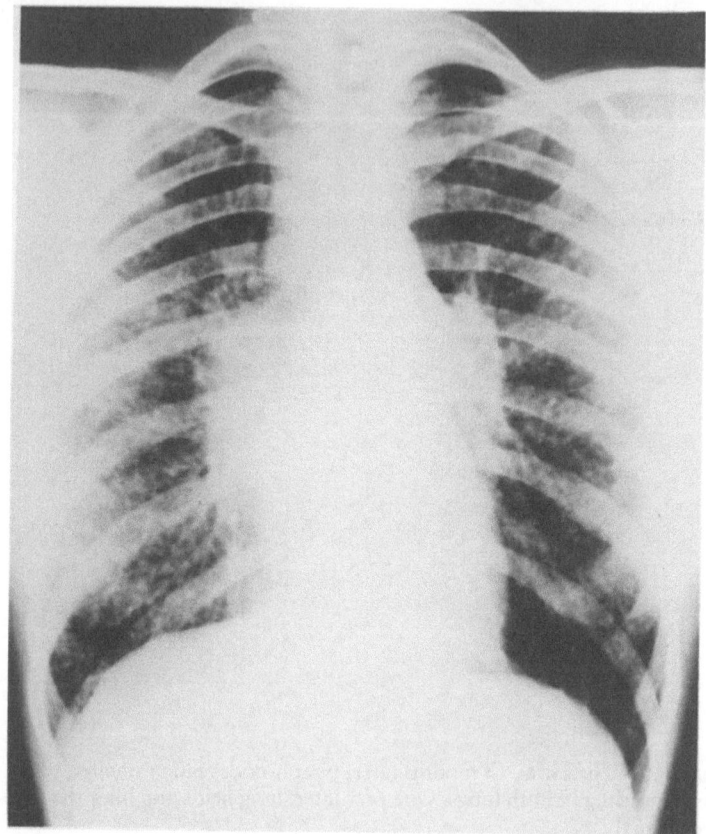

Figure 6.6   This mottling and BHL was known to have been present for more than two years without symptoms.

pulmonary sarcoidosis have had pulmonary infiltration without BHL when first seen; and although this proportion is likely to over-estimate their frequency, cases without BHL at any time certainly occur.

Of 136 patients reviewed after five years' observation by one of us (Scadding, 1961), 77 had apparently non-fibrotic lung changes at the beginning of the observation period. Of these, 40 either had at that time or were known in the past to have had BHL, and 37 had no present or available past evidence of BHL. It was of course not possible to be certain that none of the patients in the latter group had ever had BHL; but three of them had had normal chest radiographs within one year before the first abnormal one, and ten others were symptom-free at the time of the detection of the abnormality. The average estimated duration of the disease in those first seen with lung changes without BHL was about the same as that in those with BHL. The proportions with erythema nodosum at the onset and with ocular involvement were widely different in these two groups. Of those with BHL, seven had erythema nodosum and nine eye changes, as compared with one and three respectively in those without detected BHL. Thus the presence or absence of BHL was accompanied by other differences between these two groups. The numbers of patients without detected BHL in other reported series have varied, probably in part at least because of differing criteria for the diagnosis of hilar node enlargement. In another study in London, Smellie and Hoyle (1960) reported that of 125 patients only nine had infiltration without BHL when first seen; while Sones and Israel (1960) in Philadelphia reported that of 128 patients, 56 had no obvious hilar lymphadenopathy in the earliest radiograph. In a later report from Philadelphia, Freundlich *et al.* (1970) reviewed 300 cases with radiographic evidence of pulmonary sarcoidosis, and found that BHL had been detected at some time in three-quarters, but not in one-quarter of them. Kirks *et al.* (1973) in San Francisco found similar proportions; among 150 patients with sarcoidosis and an abnormal chest radiograph, 65 had BHL alone, 61 BHL and lung infiltration, and 24 lung infiltration alone, the latter figure constituting 28% of those with radiographic evidence of lung infiltration.

Radiographic appearances

Sarcoid infiltration of the lungs usually involves large parts, up to the whole, of the lung-fields more or less symmetrically. Most commonly it has a mottled or stippled quality, consisting of elements from 1–5 mm in diameter. But the possible range of radiographic patterns is wide. In a few cases, there are scattered rounded or irregularly-shaped shadows of larger size, and rarely a few larger shadows of more or less uniform density.

Description of widespread mottled or stippled patterns is difficult. The quality of such patterns in a radiograph can vary with variations in radiographic technique. Most authors have been content to describe them in terms of the coarseness of the pattern in available radiographs, as judged by the size of individual elements in the pattern.

Nitter (1953) divided sarcoid infiltrations of the lungs into nodulation, with densities varying from 3–5 mm in diameter, and miliary lesions, with densities about 1 mm in diameter, and found that resolution was more frequent in those with miliary shadows.

Smellie and Hoyle (1960) described the readiographic appearances in 94 patients with pulmonary sarcoidosis judged to be pre-fibrotic in four categories; 26 had coarse nodular shadows 3–5 mm in diameter, 50 fine nodular shadows 1–3 mm in diameter, eight fine stippling, less than 1 mm in diameter, and ten scattered or localized patches.

One of us (JGS) analysed the radiographic patterns in 71 cases of pulmonary sarcoidosis showing no evidence of fibrosis. Fifty-two showed more or

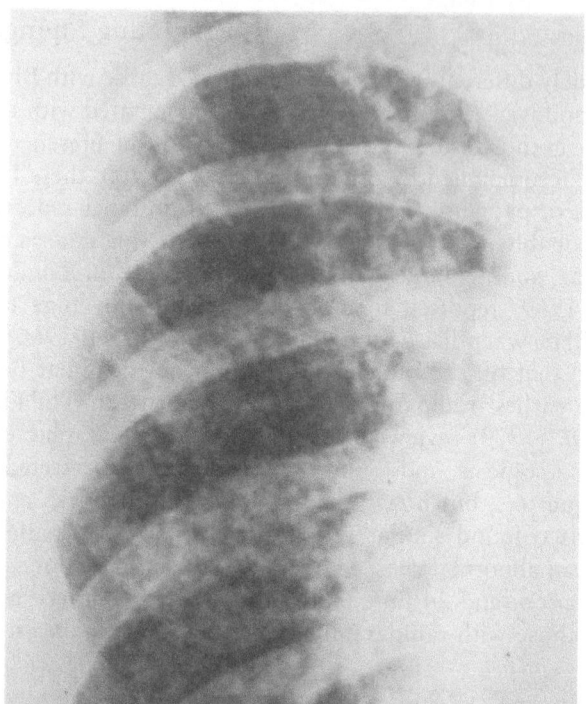

Figure 6.7 'Mottling': most elements exceed 2 mm in diameter.

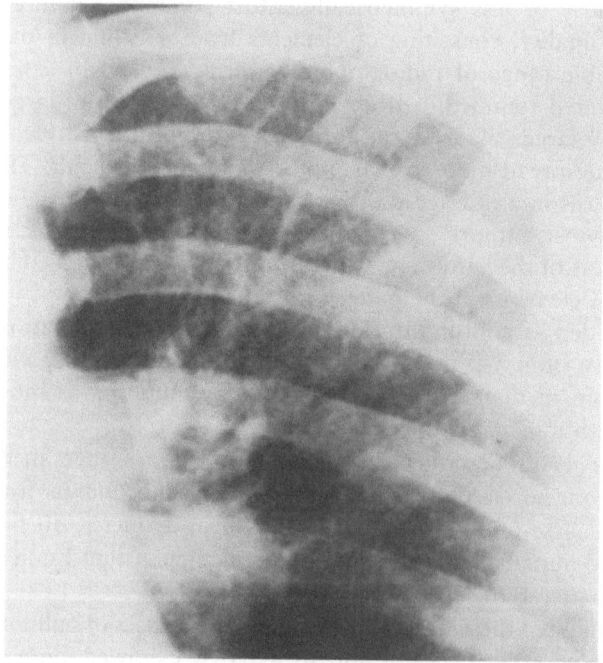

Figure 6.8 'Stippling': most elements less than 2 mm in diameter.

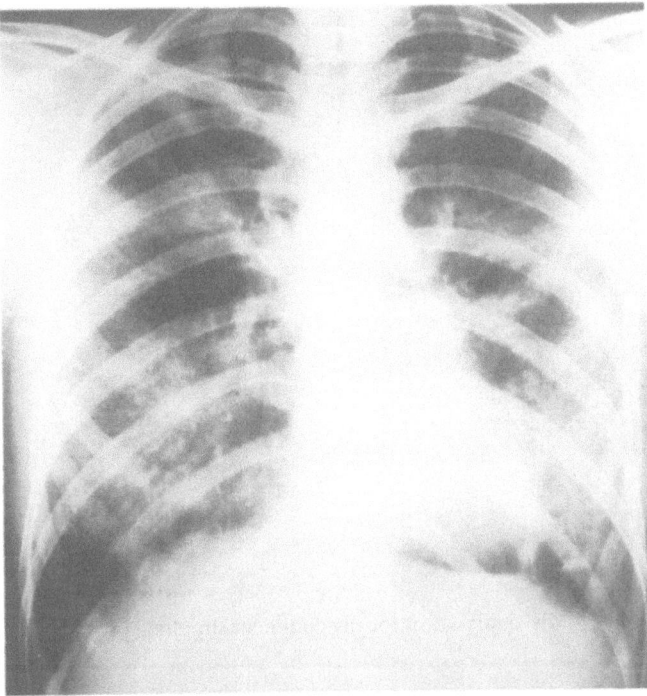

Figure 6.9   'Cloudy shadowing', for description see text.

less uniform scattering over major parts of the lungs of small rounded
opacities, up to 5 mm in diameter with poorly or moderately well-defined
margins. Individual opacities varied in size, but it was usually possible to
distinguish cases in which many of them exceeded 2 mm in diameter, from
those in which most were below this size. The coarser pattern of large
opacities, called 'mottling'. (Fig. 6.7), occurred in 34 cases; the finer pattern,
called 'stippling' (Fig. 6.8) occurred in 18. The appearance for which the
name 'cloudy shadowing' was adopted occurred in 17 cases. It was
composed of shadows, of substantially uniform density, up to 5 cm or more
in diameter, with poorly defined margins and scattered irregularly through
the lungs. Close inspection of these, especially at their edges, showed
stippling, usually very fine, the individual elements being less than 1 mm in
size (Fig. 6.9). The distinction between mottling and stippling, and between
partial confluence of stippling and cloudy shadowing was in the borderline
case arbitrary. It may be that stippling, especially of the very fine sort seen at
the periphery of 'cloudy shadows' is indeed acinar in origin, in the sense in
which this word was used by Ziskind *et al.* (1963), and that these shadows
are caused by confluence of acinar elements. The remaining two cases
showed more clearly defined localized shadows. In one, multiple irregularly

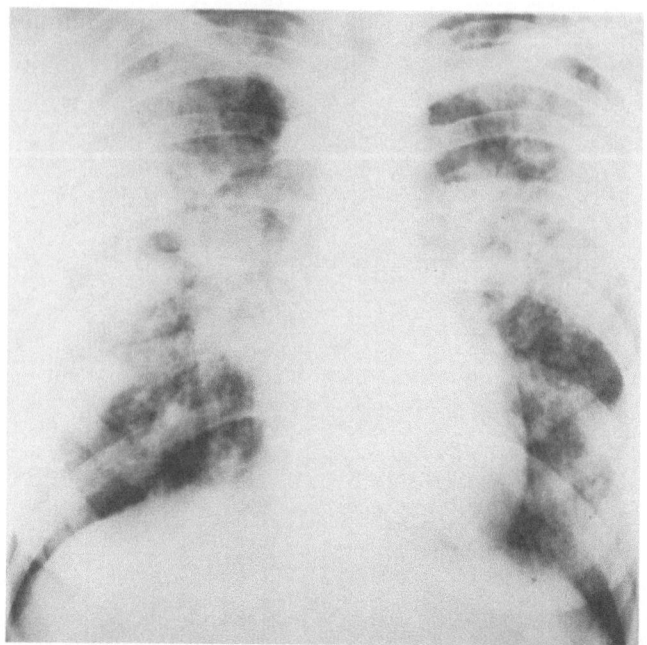

Figure 6.10 Dense cloudy shadows, or locally confluent stippling, in a woman aged 43.

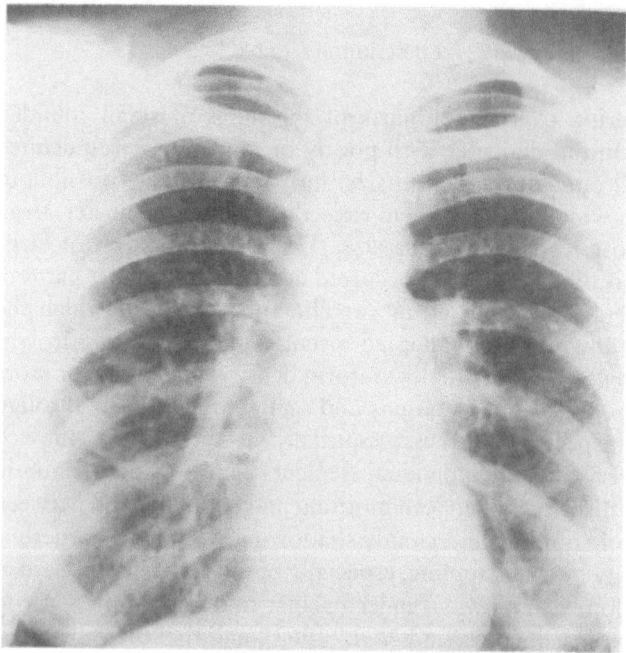

Figure 6.11 The same, 18 months later, showing spontaneous clearing.

shaped opacities, up to 2 cm in greatest diameter, of only moderate density, were scattered through both lungs; they resolved under observation. In the other, there was a localized shadow at the apex of the right lung in a patient with BHL and erythema nodosum, which also resolved spontaneously. There was no indication of any difference in course between those with mottling and those with stippling, half of those with stippling and rather more than half of those with mottling having resolved completely during the observation periods which, though variable from case to case, were similar for the three main groups. Cloudy shadows seemed to have a worse prognosis, only rather less than one-third resolving, and nearly one-half showing evidence of fibrosis within the observation period. Nevertheless, the lesion associated with such shadows sometimes resolved (Figs 6.10 and 6.11).

Rarely, a widespread infiltration may be accompanied by one or more localized uniform opacities. Such a shadow may resolve spontaneously (Figs 6.12–6.15).

A few cases present with multiple well-defined shadows suggesting pulmonary nodules without a background generalized infiltration. Sharma *et al.* (1973) reported six young black patients with pulmonary sarcoidosis presenting in this way; five of them had concurrent BHL. Large nodular

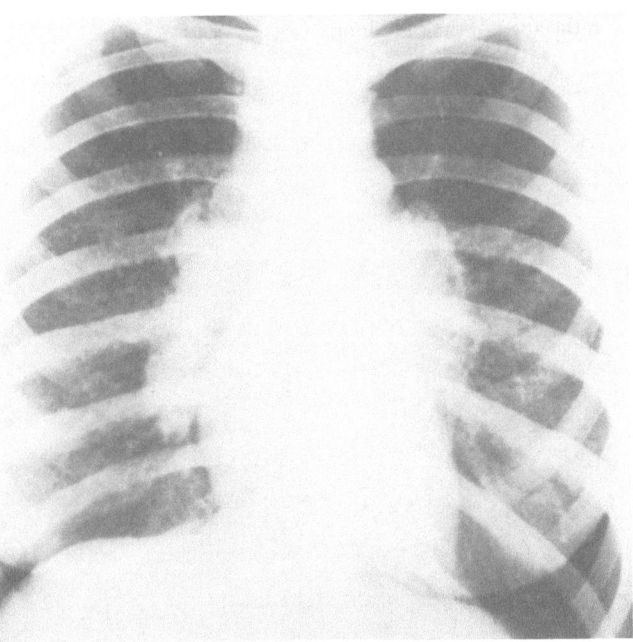

Figure 6.12   BHL and middle zone mottling in a woman aged 24 who presented with anterior uveitis.

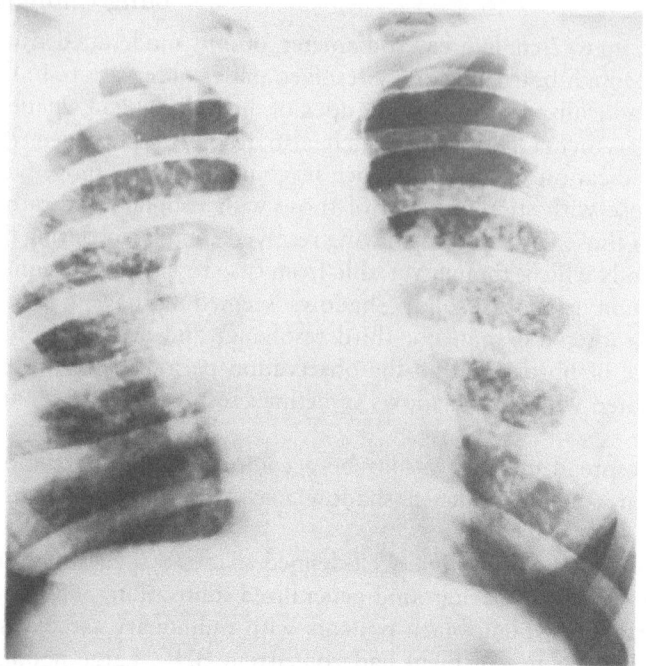

Figure 6.13 The same, one year later, showing much denser mottling and a localized shadow at the apex of the right lung.

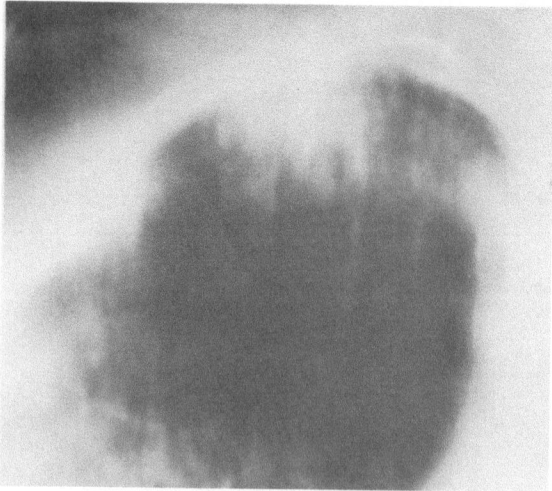

Figure 6.14 Tomograph defining the localized shadow.

shadows were found in three of 103 patients by Kirks *et al.* (1973) and in three of 89 by Littner *et al.* (1977); Kirks *et al.* estimated that pulmonary

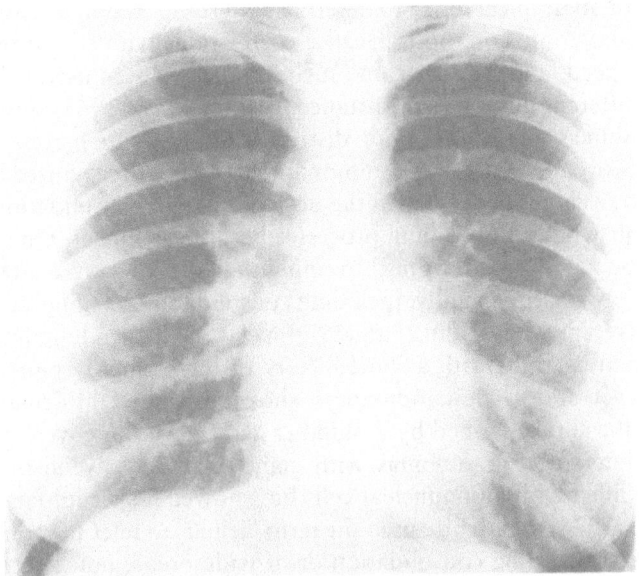

Figure 6.15 The same case, one year later, showing almost complete spontaneous resolution; the uveitis had also resolved.

sarcoidosis presented in this way in 4% of young black patients. Rømer (1977) reported that two of 126 Danish patients with intrathoracic sarcoidosis initially showed multiple large opacities simulating pulmonary metastases; in one, a normal chest radiograph had been obtained six weeks before the first abnormal one, and in both patients radiographic resolution was observed. Other cases with multiple well-defined opacities have been reported by Talbot *et al.* (1959); Dhakhwa *et al.* (1976) and Tellis and Putnam (1977). In some of these reported cases, 'air bronchograms' have been observed within the otherwise uniform shadows, suggesting confluent filling of acinar air-spaces with normal airways. Diagnostic difficulty may arise in patients with scattered 'nodular' opacities, if changes are limited to the lungs, especially in the minority in which hilar nodes are not enlarged, and coalescence of granulomas infiltrating the lung generally, but radio-performed, granulomas have generally been found not only coalescent in the nodule but also scattered elsewhere in the lung. Chrisholm and Lang (1966) resected part of the lower lobe of a black woman aged 58, who presented with BHL and a localised shadow at this site; in addition to a granulomatous mass 5 cm in diameter, the lung contained multiple small nodules. It seems likely that localized well-defined shadows are due to local profusion and coalescence of granulomas infiltrating the lung generally, but radiographically inapparent elsewhere, and thus represent the extreme of the patchy localization which leads to 'cloudy shadowing'.

The use of anatomical terms to describe patterns of radiographic shadowing may cause confusion, both because correlations with structure are not generally agreed, and because some such terms have been used in different senses by different authors. For instance, Ziskind et al. (1963) showed that in at least some cases fine stippling distributed in a rosette pattern was due to opacities occupying discrete pulmonary acini. They recognized that this acinar pattern might be a stage in the development of consolidation, which would result when acinus-filling processes became confluent. On the other hand, Felson (1967) used 'acinar' to imply that shadows were attributable to alveolar processes generally, including consolidation, as opposed to those affecting alveolar walls. Sahn et al. (1974) performed open lung biopsy in a black woman aged 26 with a short history of increasing dyspnoea, cough and low fever and a chest radiograph showing a bilateral acinar rosette pattern of the sort described by Ziskind et al. (1963); there were peribronchial and interstitial granulomas with giant cells, and alveoli in affected areas were filled with mononuclear cells but showed no granulomas. Shigemitsu et al. (1978) apparently used the term 'acinar' to refer to radiographic appearances suggesting consolidation or, if widespread, not describable as 'reticulo-nodular'. They found that 20% of 101 patients showed changes of these sorts, in all accompanied by BHL; in open lung biopsies, the 'acinar' pattern so defined was correlated with granulomas and macrophages in alveolar spaces. Battesti et al. (1982) found that 33 (4.4%) of 746 patients with pulmonary sarcoidosis showed localized opacities more than 15 mm in diameter, and called these opacities 'alveolar'. In 17 cases the appearances suggested large nodules with ill-defined margins, usually multiple and bilateral; and in 16 they were more diffuse, in some with an air bronchogram. In 20 the localized shadows were accompanied by a reticulo-nodular pattern. Lung biopsy in four cases showed confluence of granulomas at sites of localized shadows, but no other unusual features. Clinical findings and pattern of functional disorder did not differ from those found in patients with more usual radiographic patterns.

Widespread apparently non-fibrotic sarcoid infiltration tends to affect the two lungs approximately equally, and the middle or the middle and upper zones more than the lower, though there are exceptions to both these rules. One of us (JGS) analysed the distribution in 70 cases of this sort, and found a pattern similar to that reported by Smellie and Hoyle (1960). The two lungs were involved equally in 60, the right being more densely affected in eight and the left in two. The zonal distribution was more or less uniform in 40; the middle and upper zones were affected in 14, and the middle zones only in 15. The lower zones were least often involved in unevenly distributed infiltrations, being affected with the middle zones in one case, and predominantly in a generalized infiltration in one. Infiltrations limited to the middle zones were nearly all of the quality described as mottling (ten) or stippling (four), only one of those described as 'cloudy shadowing' having this distribution.

A few variant patterns of widespread radiographic shadowing can be accepted as due to predominantly non-fibrotic pulmonary sarcoidosis because they may be observed to resolve. One, which occurs in a few cases at the stage of BHL, usually when the BHL is prominent, consists in a varied mixture of mottling and streaky linear shadows, more or less radiating from the region of the central hilar shadow in each lung (Fig. 6.16). This shadowing is densest centrally, and therefore blurs the outlines of the enlarged hilar and paratracheal lymph-nodes, and obliterates the clear band which is usually seen, especially on the right side, between the inner border of the lower part of the hilar lymph-node shadow and the heart shadow. One of us (JGS) noted three or four examples of appearances of this sort, or intermediate between them and the more frequent well-defined hilar node shadows among 275 patients reviewed. Rabinowitz *et al.* (1974) suggested the apt name 'hilar haze' for it. Another is that described, e.g. by Turiaf and

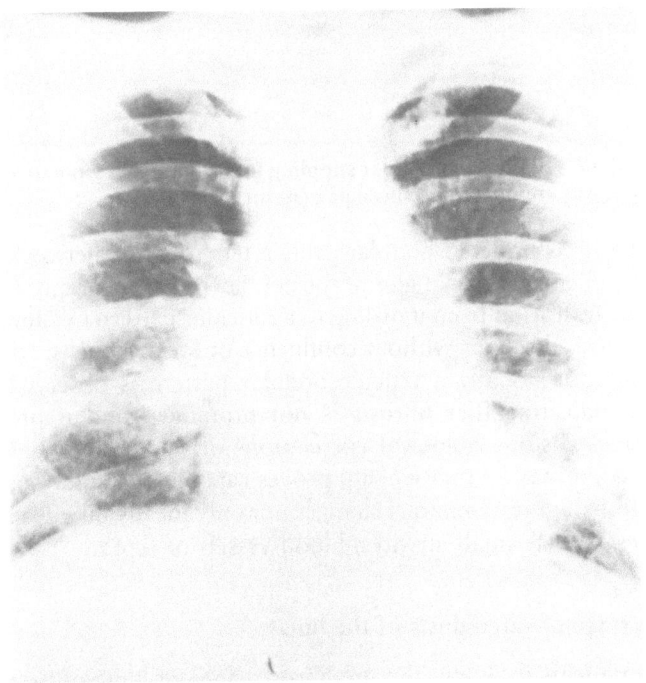

Figure 6.16   BHL with para-hilar mottling, blurring the usually distinct outlines of the enlarged lymph-nodes in a man aged 40, who also had hepatosplenomegaly and enlarged iliac lymph-nodes. Prednisolone treatment was given for relief of symptoms for two and a half years. Five years from the onset, he was well, with an almost clear chest radiograph.

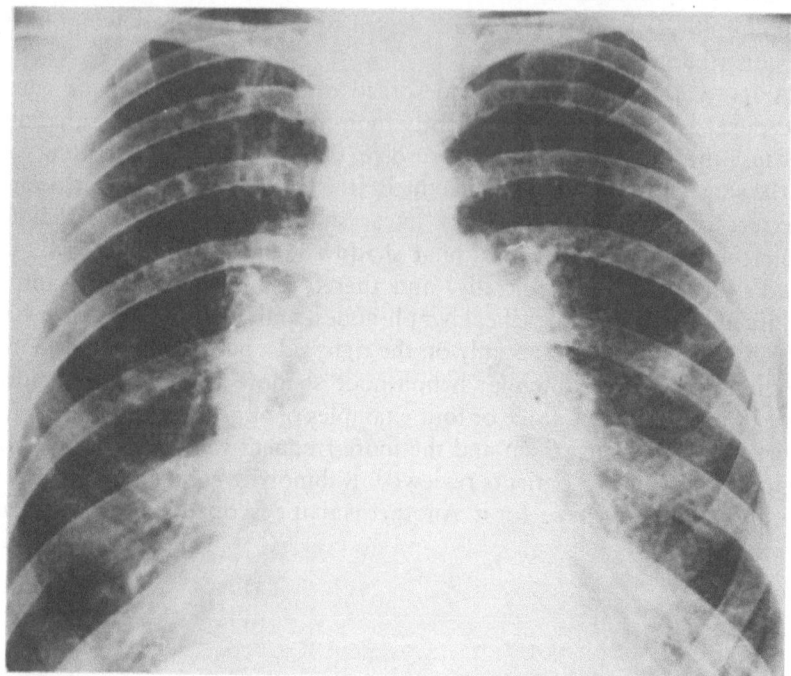

Figure 6.17   BHL with irregular stippling in the lungs in a woman aged 36; the BHL was known to have been present for two years.

Brun (1955), as 'reticulo-nodular'; this refers to a fine network with small punctate opacities at the angles of the net. Such an appearance may develop during the transition from mottling to a reticular pattern in a few patients in whom fibrosis develops without confluence of focal changes, which is more usual. But occasionally a reticulo-nodular pattern is observed early, and resolves, indicating that fibrosis is not prominent and if present is not progressive. Histopathological correlations of this pattern have not been established; it may be that when it proves capable of resolution, it is due to distribution of granulomatous changes not only focally but also along linear structures such as small airways, blood-vessels or septa.

Fibrotic stage of sarcoidosis of the lungs

In those patients in whom the pre-fibrotic stage of lung infiltration fails to resolve, progress towards fibrosis is insidious. It is made manifest clinically by the development of dyspnoea in previously symptom-free patients or increasing dyspnoea in those in whom a pre-fibrotic infiltration has caused this symptom, and by certain changes in the radiographic appearances. These are not always correlated. Development of some local fibrosis while the greater part of the infiltration resolves may cause a recognisable radio-

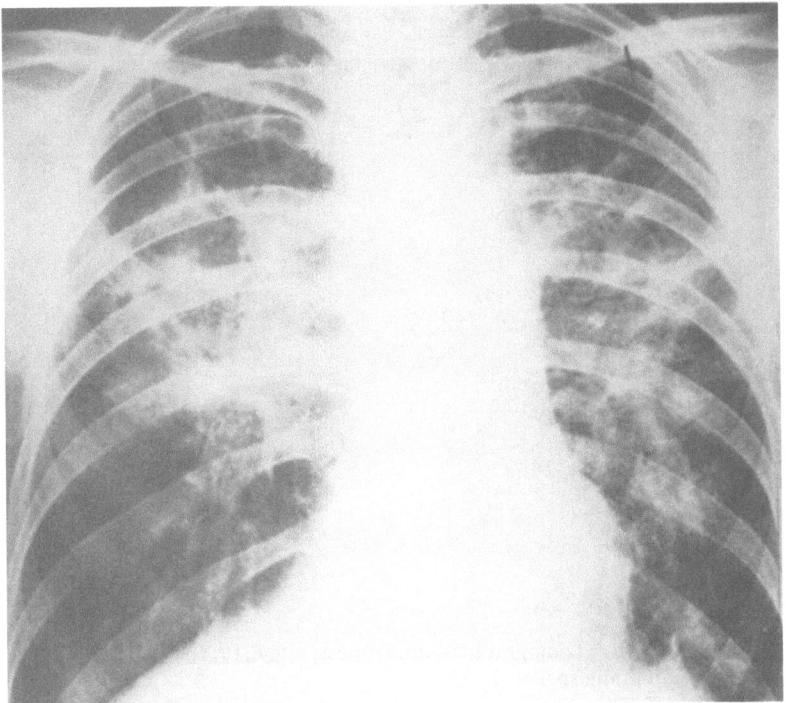

Figure 6.18   The same, three years later; BHL has subsided, and the lung infiltration evolved into the characteristic appearance of fibrosis predominantly in the middle and lower parts of the upper zones of the lungs, with basal and apical emphysema.

graphic shadow but no symptoms, especially in a patient with a sedentary habit of life. On the other hand, as noted below, in rare cases with uniform fine infiltration of the lungs, fibrosis may develop focally without coalescence of the sarcoid tubercles into confluent masses, and in these cases a disabling fibrosis may be accompanied by apparently trivial radiographic changes. Furthermore, dyspnoea due to advancing fibrosis may appear before there is much change in the radiographic appearance of a widespread infiltration, and, as noted above, a dense and widespread infiltration may cause dyspnoea although it eventually resolves with little fibrosis and with diminution of dyspnoea. The longer infiltration persists, the more likely is fibrosis to result; but the clinical and radiographic evidence of fibrosis develops insidiously, at a variable pace, and sometimes with long periods during which the whole process appears static. If resolution is eventually to be complete, the radiographic shadows nearly always start to become less dense and extensive within a year of their appearance, although occasionally a dense infiltration which shows little change for several years may clear remarkably, leaving much less fibrosis than might have been expected.

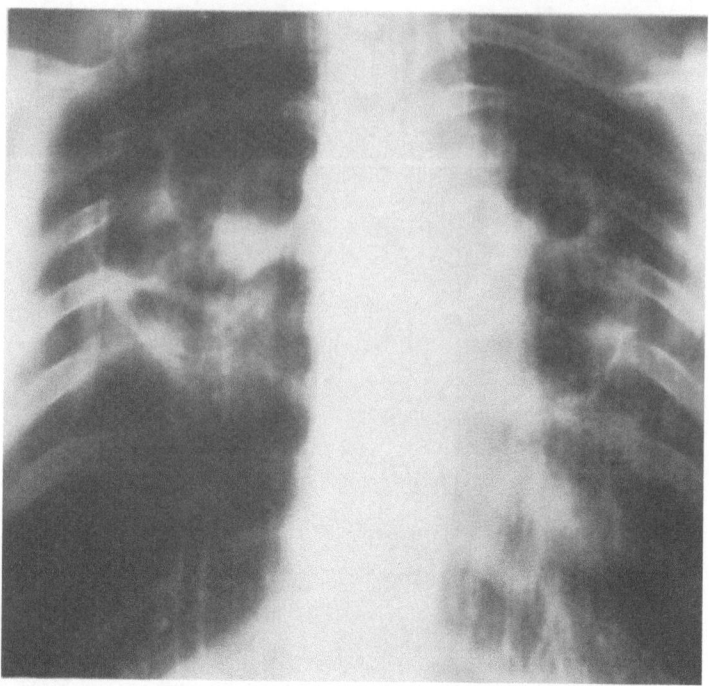

Figure 6.19 Tomograph at same time as Fig. 6.18, showing large irregular air-containing spaces.

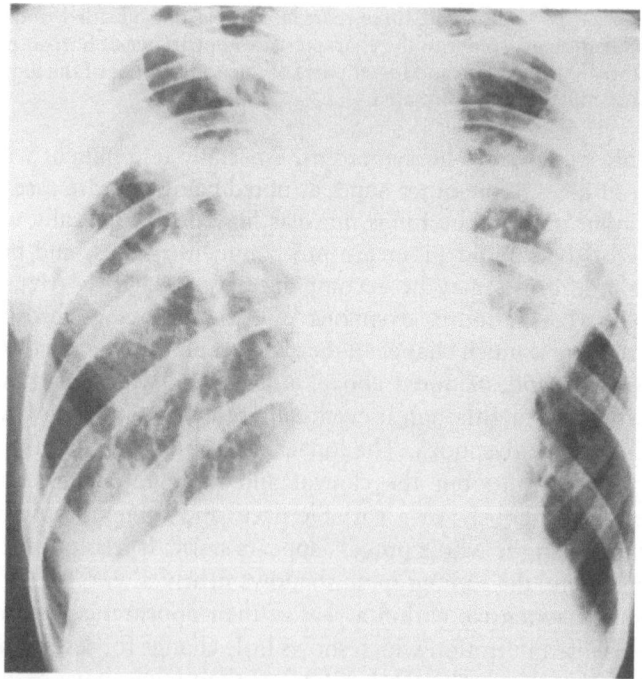

Figure 6.20 The same, three years later, showing further contraction of the fibrotic parts of the lungs.

The most frequent pattern of radiographically evident fibrosis is predominantly localized near the middle of the lung fields, usually around the upper part of the middle third. The mottled shadowing indicative of sarcoid infiltration, as already noted, is often densest in the middle zones. In cases in which this sort of fibrosis is developing, the middle zone mottling becomes denser, while that at the apices and bases may be diminishing, as if the individual elements in the mottling were coalescing into the middle third of the lungs, and in some cases being pulled up towards the apices. Established sarcoid fibrosis of this middle-zone distribution presents an almost pathognomonic radiographic picture. Dense shadows near the hila with strand-like linear opacities spreading out from them into the upper part of the middle zones are accompanied by distortion of vascular patterns, often by elevation of the hila, and by areas of transradiancy in the upper and lower zones indicative of emphysema, which may be evidently bullous. Tomography of the area of denser shadowing in the middle zones often shows evidence of large air-containing smooth-walled spaces between the strands of fibrosis; these presumably may represent either bullous emphysema between tracts

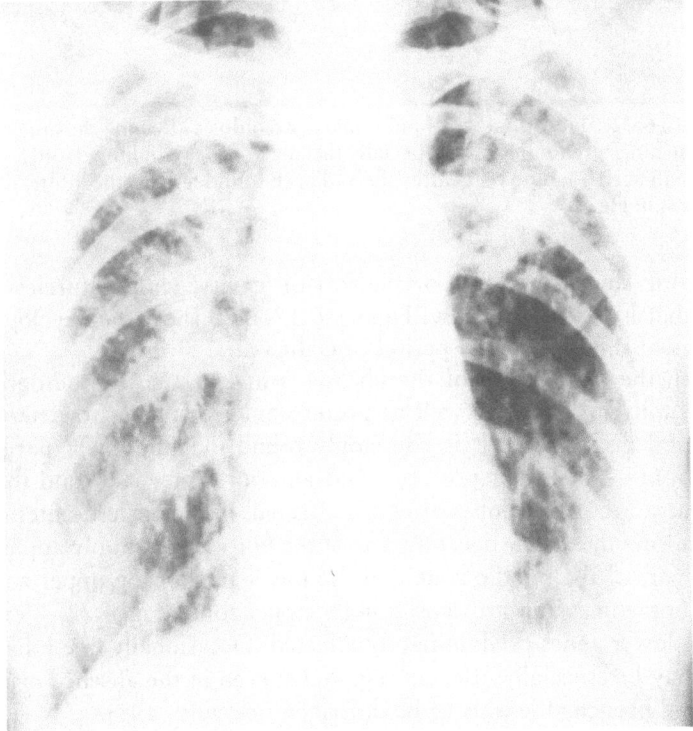

Figure 6.21   Fibrosing stage of pulmonary sarcoidosis in a woman aged 55, showing most prominent changes in the middle zones and the lower parts of the upper zones of the lungs.

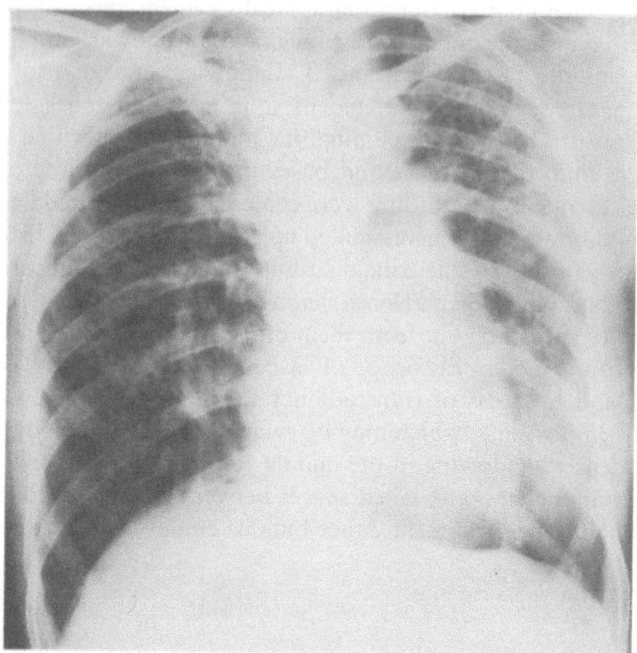

Figure 6.22   Fibrotic stage of pulmonary sarcoidosis affecting the upper parts of the lungs predominantly, especially the apex of the right lung; from a woman aged 44, nine years after she had been found to have the infiltration shown in Fig. 6.9.

of fibrotic contracted lung, or the sort of 'cavity' with featureless fibrous walls that is described below. Figures 6.17–6.20 show the development of changes of this sort over a period of eight years.

When the distribution of the fibrosis is investigated by radiography or tomography in lateral as well as postero-anterior planes to determine its segmental distribution, it is commonly found that the lower parts of the upper lobes – i.e., their posterior and anterior segments – and the apical segments of the lower lobes are most affected. In the postero-anterior view, the shadows due to the densest parts of the fibrosis commonly appear in the upper part of the middle zone and the lower part of the upper zone (Fig. 6.21). Sometimes they are densest in the upper zones (Fig. 6.22). Very rarely are the lower zones predominantly affected. Occasionally one lobe or segment may be especially affected (Fig. 6.23) even in the absence of the rare stenosing bronchial lesions to be described below (p. 143).

Dense local shadows developing during the evolution of pulmonary sarcoidosis to fibrosis, with emphysema elsewhere in the lungs may simulate the progressive massive fibrosis of coal-miners' pneumoconiosis (Fig. 6.24).

In some cases, a widespread infiltration appears to undergo fibrosis

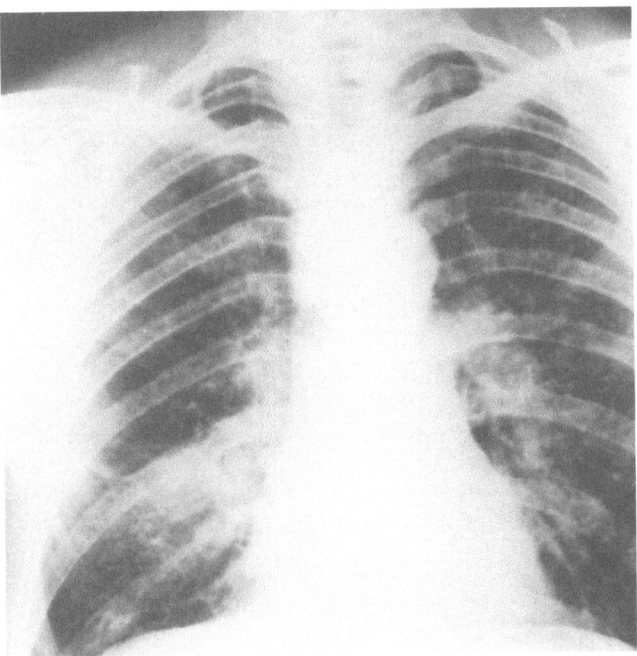

Figure 6.23 Pulmonary sarcoidosis in a man aged 35, with confluent shadowing in the right lower zone, shown in the lateral view to be in the middle lobe.

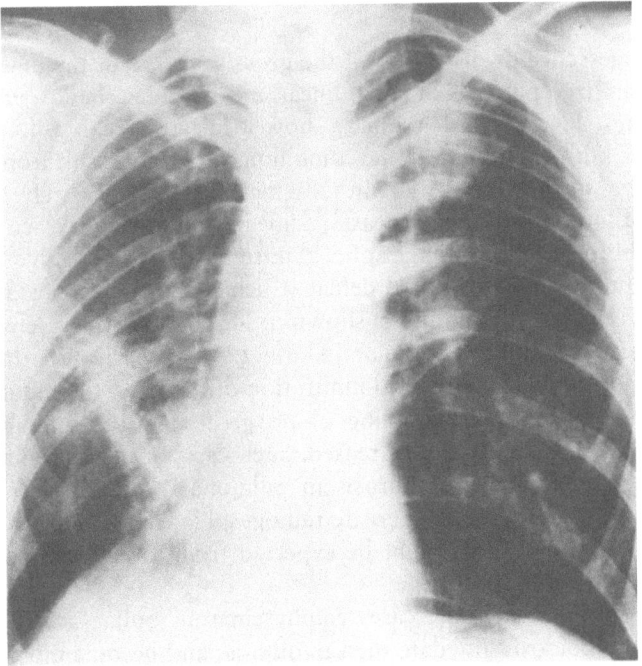

Figure 6.24 The same three years later, showing the development of further localized shadows in the left upper and right middle zones.

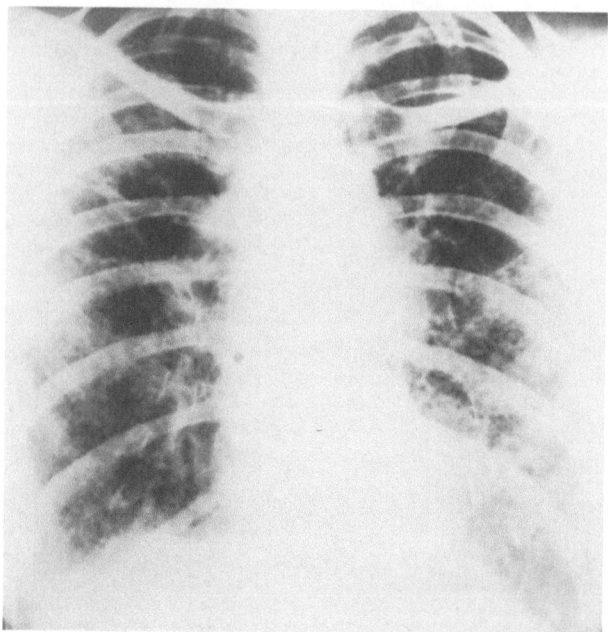

Figure 6.25   Widespread 'reticulo-nodular' fibrosis in a woman aged 51 known to have had pulmonary sarcoidosis for at least eight years, with increasing respiratory disability.

without coalescence or distortion of the gross structure of the lung, giving rise to generalized patterns of small linear and irregular shadows throughout the lungs (Fig. 6.25). These may show local areas with a honeycomb appearance, but generalized 'honeycomb lungs', as may result from fibrosing alveolitis, histiocytosis X or mesodermal dysplasia, is rarely or never the result of sarcoidosis. In a few cases, a fine infiltration gives place to a fine pattern of fibrosis with a radiographic abnormality less impressive than the severe symptoms and functional deficit which it causes. For instance, the patient whose chest radiograph is shown in Fig. 6.26 was severely breathless, with signs of right ventricular failure; 12 years earlier she had been found to have widespread sarcoid infiltration of the lung, the radiographic pattern being a very fine stippling of no great density, with moderate dyspnoea, which had steadily increased. Such cases are exceptional; more usually, the development of fibrosis in pulmonary sarcoidosis produces well-marked and rather characteristic radiographic changes, and disability in many cases is less than might be expected from the obvious extent of these changes.

It is possible that in some cases emphysematous bullae accompanying pulmonary sarcoidosis antedate the sarcoidosis, and become more evident and increase in size as a result of the sarcoid changes in the lung.

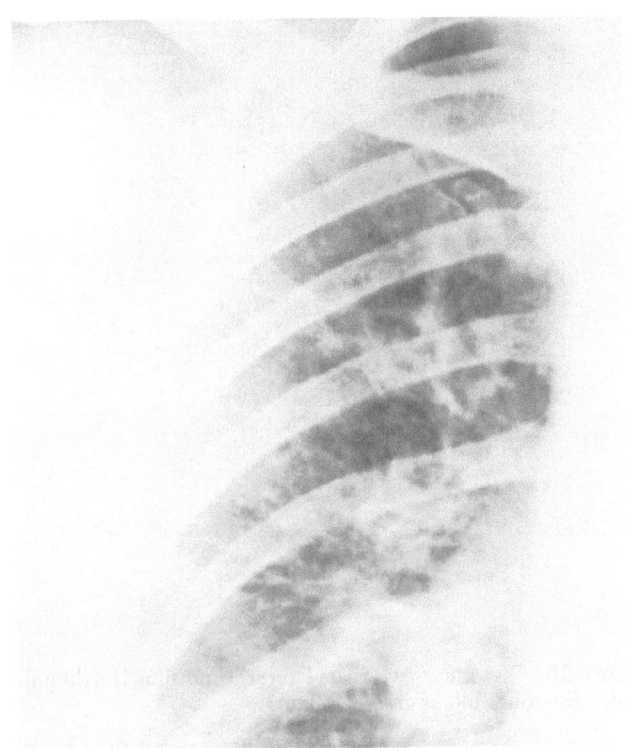

Figure 6.26 Widespread fine fibrosis causing severe disability in a woman aged 52, known to have had pulmonary sarcoidosis with inconspicuous radiographic changes for at least 12 years.

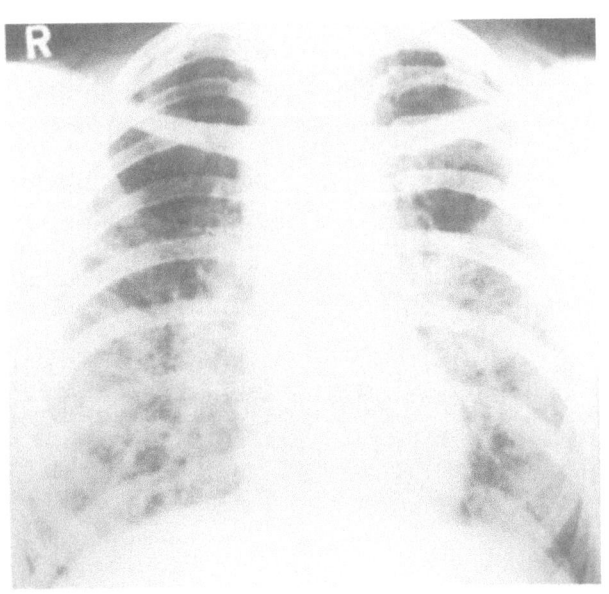

Figure 6.27 BHL and mottling in a woman with lupus pernio; there is a small emphysematous bulla at the apex of the left lung.

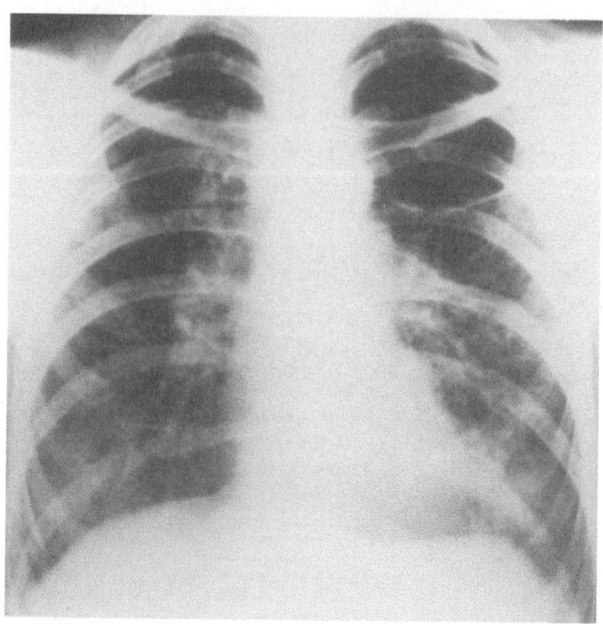

Figure 6.28 The same, two years later; the mottling has diminished and the emphysematous bulla is greatly inflated.

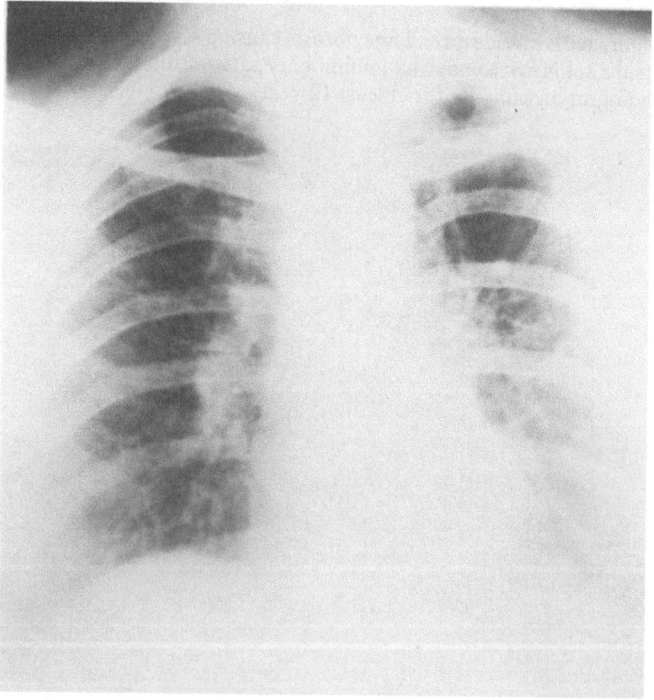

Figure 6.29 The same, two years later still: the bulla has disappeared.

A woman aged 40 developed lupus pernio of the left great toe with radio-graphic changes in the phalanges (Fig. 7.13). BHL with mottling in the lungs was found soon afterwards (Fig. 6.27). At this time a group of small emphyse-matous bullae was evident at the apex of the left lung; these presumably were of old standing and antedated the sarcoidosis. Two years later, the infiltration was giving place to a diffuse fine fibrosis, and the bullae had inflated grossly (Fig. 6.28). She was treated with prednisolone, because of the increasing fibrosis and the painful toe, with good effect. The bulla remained variably inflated for another two years, and then almost disappeared (Fig. 6.29). Presumably in this case changes in the patency of the airways leading to the bullous area caused the changes in its size.

Thick-walled air-containing spaces may appear not only in lungs densely fibrotic from long-standing sarcoidosis, as noted above, but also very rarely in nodules of more recent origin. Cavities of this sort may cause suspicion that overt tuberculosis has supervened; but when there is no change in tuberculin sensitivity and no tubercle bacilli can be found, and especially if there are extrathoracic localizations of sarcoidosis, this is unlikely. The possibilities that then remain are (i) that the 'cavities' are emphysematous bullae whose walls have been thickened by secondary bacterial infection; (ii)

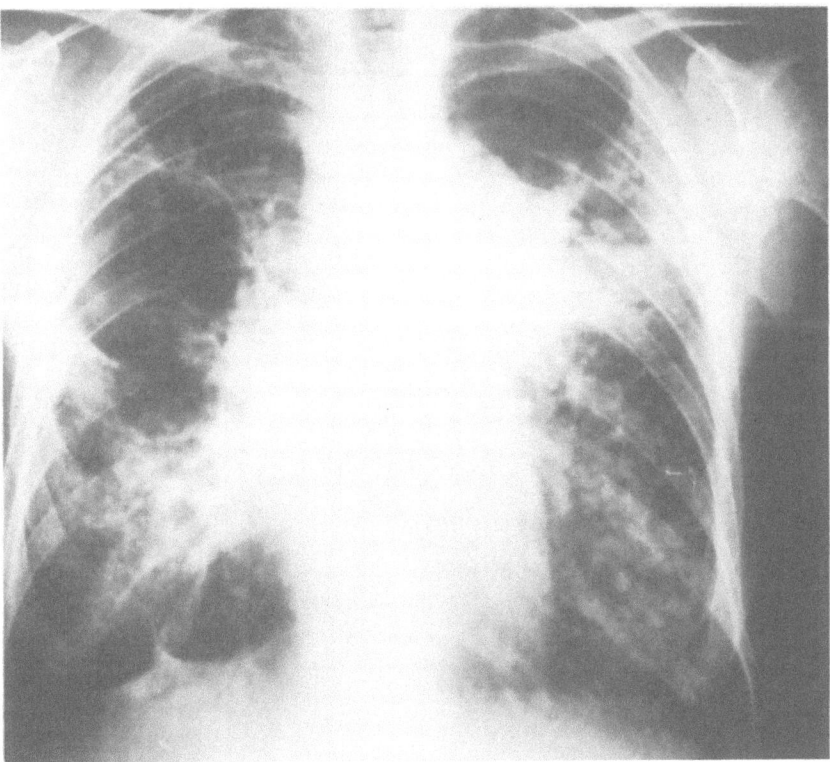

Figure 6.30   Fibrotic pulmonary sarcoidosis in a woman aged 41, showing large irregular air-conditioning spaces.

that they are intercurrent pyogenic lung abscesses; and (iii) that they result from necrosis at the centres of large masses of confluent sarcoid granulomas. The first two possibilities can in many cases be excluded because there has been no evidence of secondary bacterial, infection. It seems likely that the third possibility is the correct explanation of most thick-walled cavities in chronic sarcoidosis, in which the available evidence suggests that necrosis has occurred in areas of dense hyaline fibrosis. Necropsy findings in such cases have been reported by Tice and Sweany (1941), Ustvedt (1948), in a Clinico-Pathological Conference (1950) on a patient under the care of one of us, by Uehlinger (1955), Löfgren and Lindgren (1959) and Adamson *et al.* (1960). In these reported cases, the sarcoidosis was of old standing with much hyaline fibrosis forming large nodules; the lymph-nodes have frequently shown almost complete replacement by such fibrosis; and the cavities have been lined by fibrous tissue, without specific elements, and without epithelium. These features were especially striking in Case 2 of

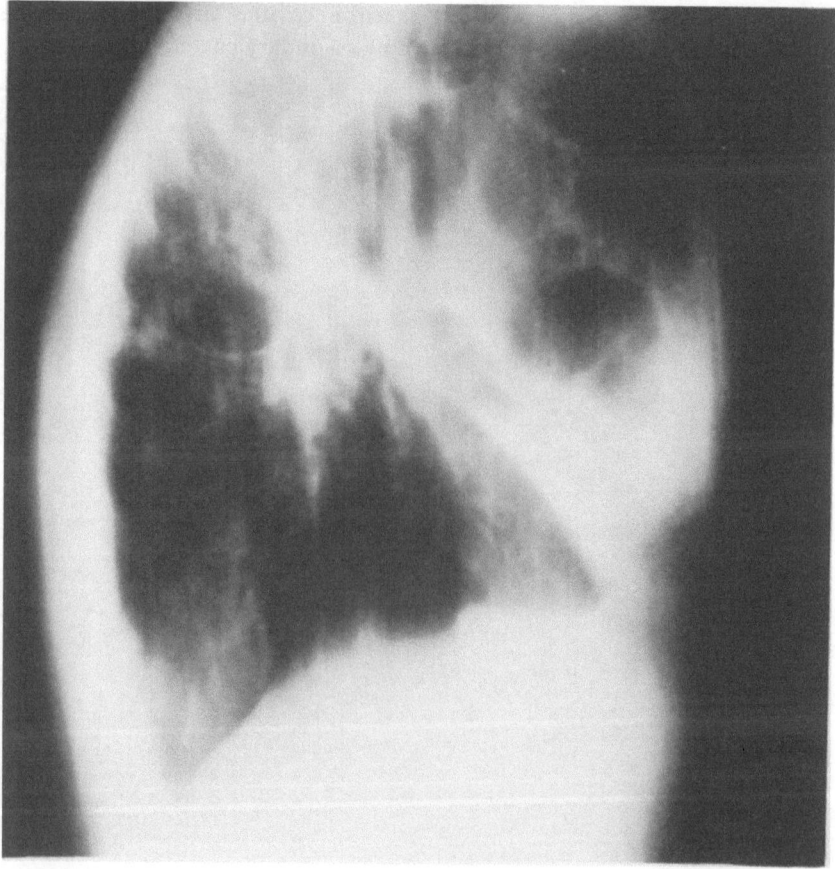

Figure 6.31   Right lateral tomograph of the same.

Ustvedt (1948). A woman aged 39 died with chronic fibrotic changes in the lungs with smooth-walled cavities lined with hyaline fibrous tissue; the large mediastinal lymph-nodes showed massive hyaline fibrosis, but no specific changes. Eleven years before death she had had a typical uveoparotitis with bilateral hilar adenopathy and a negative tuberculin test, leaving no doubt of the diagnosis of sarcoidosis though all specific granulomata had been replaced by hyaline fibrosis at the time of death.

The patient whose case was discussed at the Clinico-Pathological Conference (1950) was aged 41 at the time of death. She had presented clinically with extensive fibrotic changes in both lungs, principally in the middle zones, and large multiocular air-containing spaces with thick smooth walls (Figs 6.30 and 6.31). Her skin was non-reactive to tuberculin. Biopsy of a palpable supracla-

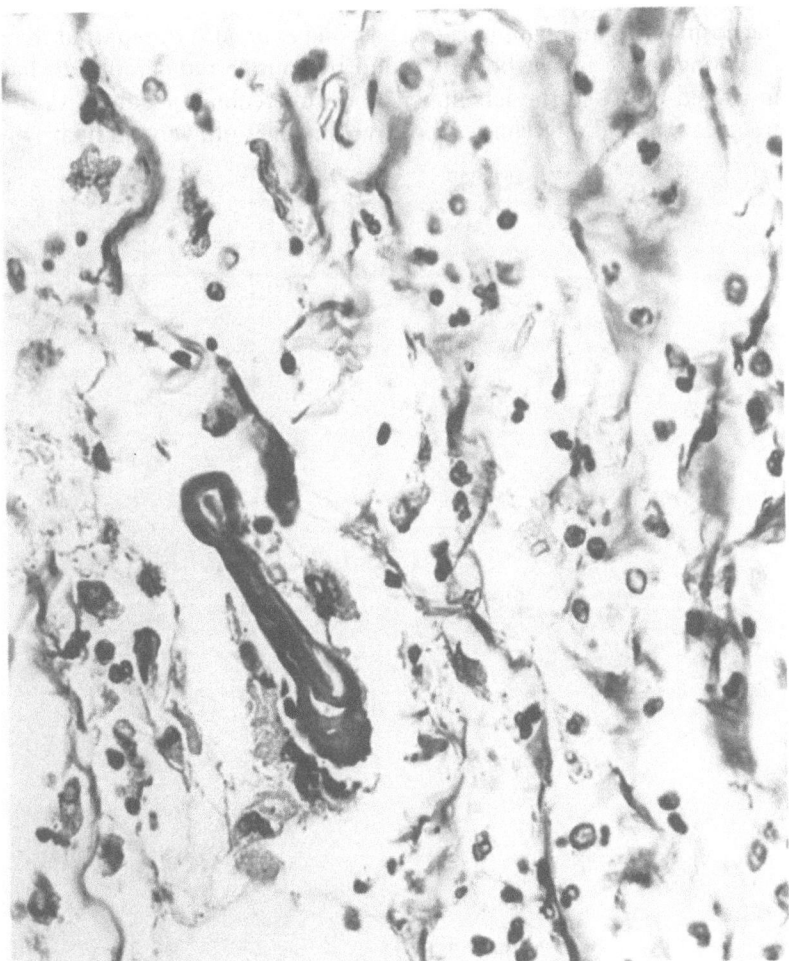

Figure 6.32   Section of the wall of the air-containing spaces, showing irregular fibrous tissue with a dumb-bell shaped body, presumably originally an inclusion-body.

vicular lymph-node showed a central zone of dense hyaline collagen, with a peripheral rim of recognizable sarcoid granulomas. At necropsy, it seemed that at least one of the 'cavities' might have originated as an emphysematous bulla; but others had thick fibrous tissue walls without epithelial lining. This fibrous tissue was unremarkable, except that it contained some dumb-bell shaped bodies, that might originally have been intracellular inclusions (Fig. 6.32). The liver contained large nodules consisting of hyaline connective tissue with a fringe of sarcoid granulomas, and some of these nodules had necrotic centres. It seemed likely that similar changes at the centres of hyalinized nodules in the lungs were the origin of the thick-walled air-containing spaces.

A very few cases have been reported in which nodules at an apparently earlier stage of sarcoidosis have shown radiographic evidence of cavitation. Hamilton *et al.* (1965) reported the histology of the biopsy specimen of the wall of such a cavity; it was composed of epithelioid and giant cells with some eosinophils and lymphocytes. Bistrong *et al.* (1970) reported the case of a young white man who was found by routine radiography to have a thin-walled cavity in the left upper lobe; tuberculin and fungal skin tests were negative, and a Kveim test positive. Biopsies of liver and hilar lymph-

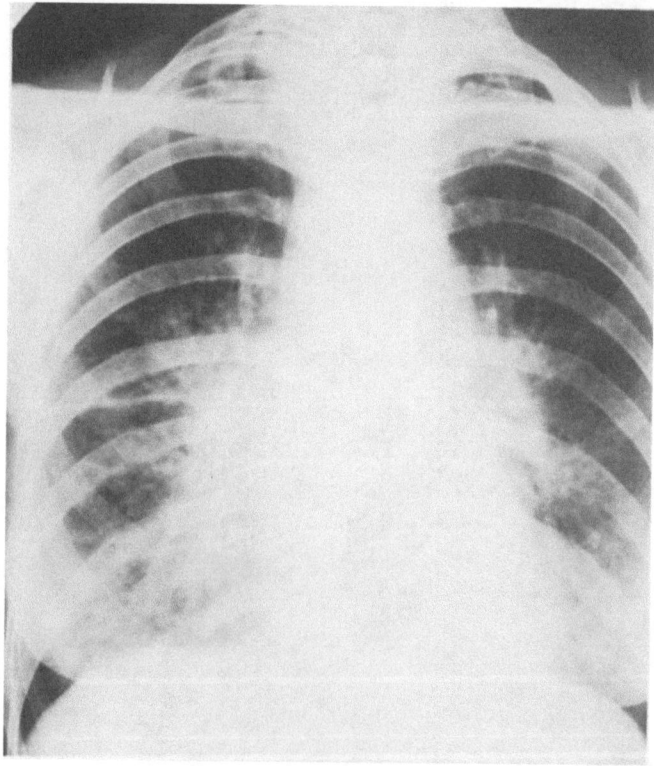

Figure 6.33   Sarcoidosis of hilar lymph-nodes and lungs in a woman aged 38.

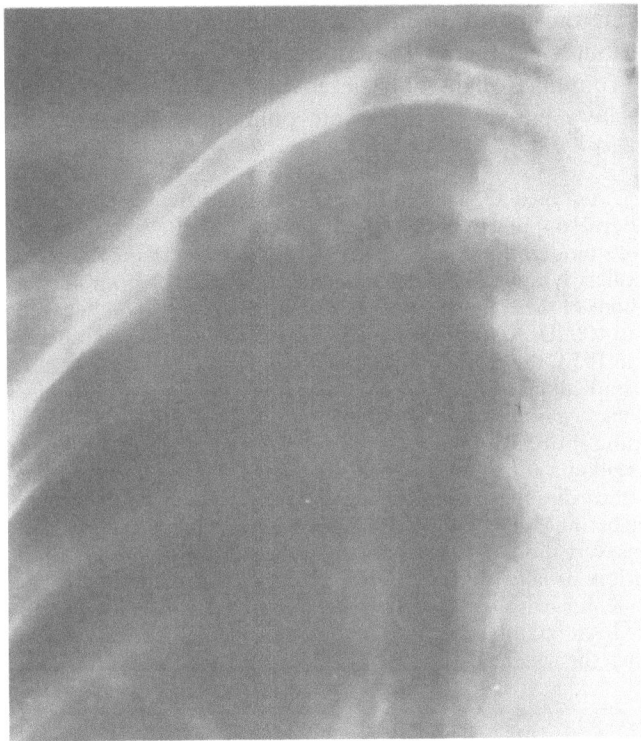

Figure 6.34 Tomograph of the apex of the right lung, showing an air-containing space.

nodes showed non-caseating granulomas, and of the wall of the cavity coalescent granulomas with dense fibrosis. Followed 18 months, he remained symptom-free. Tellis and Putnam (1977) described the case of another asymptomatic young white man who was found to have multiple nodular shadows in a routine chest radiograph, some of which showed appearances of cavitation: biopsy of one of the nodules showed many granulomas, but no cavitation; partial resolution occurred during six months' observation.

Colonization of cavities by Aspergillus ('aspergilloma')

Occasionally cavities in chronic fibrosing sarcoidosis, like other long-standing cavities in the lung, become colonized by *Aspergillus*, usually the species *fumigatus*, giving rise to the formation of a mass of mycelium eventually occupying the greater part of it, the so-called aspergilloma or *Aspergillus* mycetoma (Hinson *et al.*, 1952; Campbell and Clayton, 1964; BTTA, 1968, 1970). In such cases, productive cough and haemoptysis are frequent symptoms, but it is difficult to determine how much the aspergilloma contributes to them. The aspergilloma may produce no evident symptoms, coming to light only because of typical radiographic changes developing in a patient with chronic pulmonary sarcoidosis, as in the following case:

A woman, then aged 38, was found in 1949 to have enlargement of hilar lymph-nodes, stippling in both lungs, especially in the lower two-thirds (Fig. 6.33), and a moderately thick-walled cavity at the apex of the right lung (Fig. 6.34). Axillary lymph-nodes were moderately enlarged on both sides, and biopsy of one of these showed typical sarcoid tubercles. The skin gave a small reaction to 100 IU. No tubercle bacilli were isolated in many cultures of sputum. In 1953, the cavity was seen to be filled with a solid mass, surrounded by a transradiant crescent of air (Fig. 6.35), the typical appearance of an aspergilloma. A. *fumigatus* was found intermittently in the sputum, and later precipitating antibody to this mould was found repeatedly in the blood serum. The aspergilloma at first increased in size (Fig. 6.36), and then waxed and waned, nearly disappearing in 1970. Later the cavity in the upper part of the right lung became bilocular, with small fungus balls in both (Fig. 6.37). Symptoms were those to be expected from the pulmonary fibrosis, with exacerbations usually precipitated by intercurrent infections in the winter. From 1968 onwards these tended to be complicated by haemoptysis, and control of bacterial infection by antibiotics was helpful. She survived until 1981, when she was aged 70.

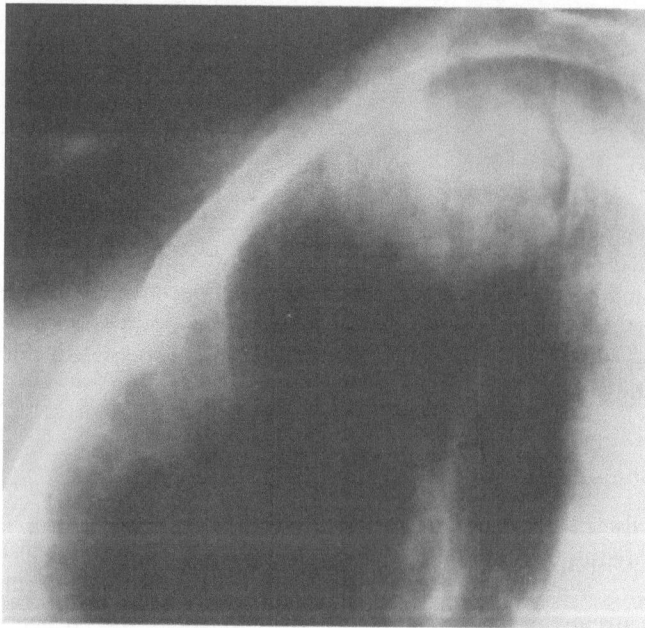

Figure 6.35 Tomograph of the same area four years later, showing the cavity filled with an aspergilloma.

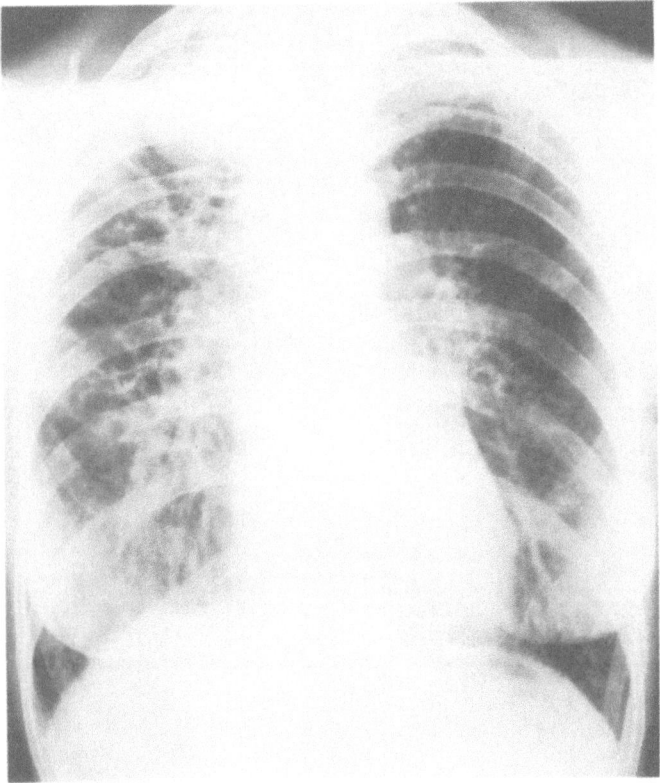

Figure 6.36   The same, 13 years after Fig. 6.35, showing increase in size of the aspergilloma.

The serum of patients with a mycetoma generally contains precipitating antibody to antigens of the causal fungus, giving rise to multiple precipitation lines in Ouchterlony double gel diffusion tests. The fungus is demonstrable in sputum, but may appear only intermittently. While *Aspergillus* species are most commonly found, *Allescheria boydii* has been recorded as the cause of a mycetoma in a patient with sarcoidosis by Belitsos *et al.* (1974).

Israel and Ostrow (1969) reviewed ten patients with chronic pulmonary sarcoidosis who developed mycetomas. 'Cystic' cavities in the upper lobes were the usual sites, unilaterally in five and bilaterally in five. Haemoptysis was noted in nine patients. Three died, two of respiratory failure and one after haemoptysis. *Aspergillus* species were cultured in eight, and identified as *fumigatus* in four and *niger* in two. Later, Israel *et al.* (1982) reported observations on the role of surgery in the treatment of 38 patients with *Aspergillus* fungus balls complicating pulmonary sarcoidosis. In all, respiratory function was moderately or severely impaired. Surgery was undertaken

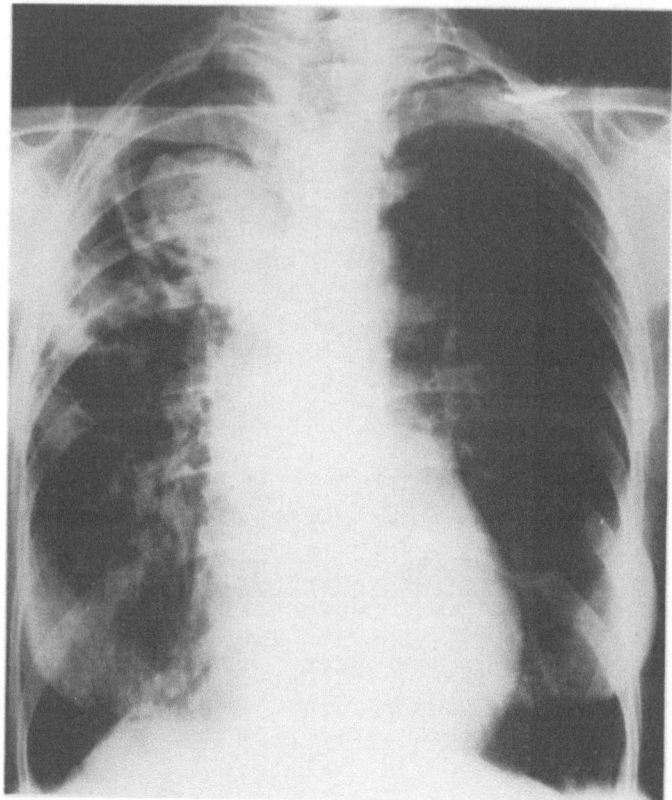

Figure 6.37   The same, three years later, showing a second fungus ball in the lower part of the now bilocular cavity.

for the control of haemoptysis in 14. Results were largely dependent upon the severity of functional impairment. Of seven with only moderate impairment, six had a good result and one died; while of seven with severe impairment, only four survived surgery and three of these died one, 11 and 27 months later of respiratory failure. Kaplan and Johns (1979) detected mycetomas in 12 of more than 600 retrospectively reviewed patients, of whom 80% were black; only one with mycetoma was white. Haemoptysis occurred in 11 and was managed conservatively with success on all but one occasion, when it contributed to death in a black man with severe pulmonary, cardiac and hepatic sarcoidosis. Two other deaths occurred from respiratory insufficiency. The remaining nine patients were surviving three–14 years after the diagnosis of mycetoma. Except in one patient who had a mycetoma in the middle lobe together with mycetomas in both upper lobes, only the upper lobes were involved, bilaterally in six. In no case was there evidence of extracavitary disease caused by the fungus.

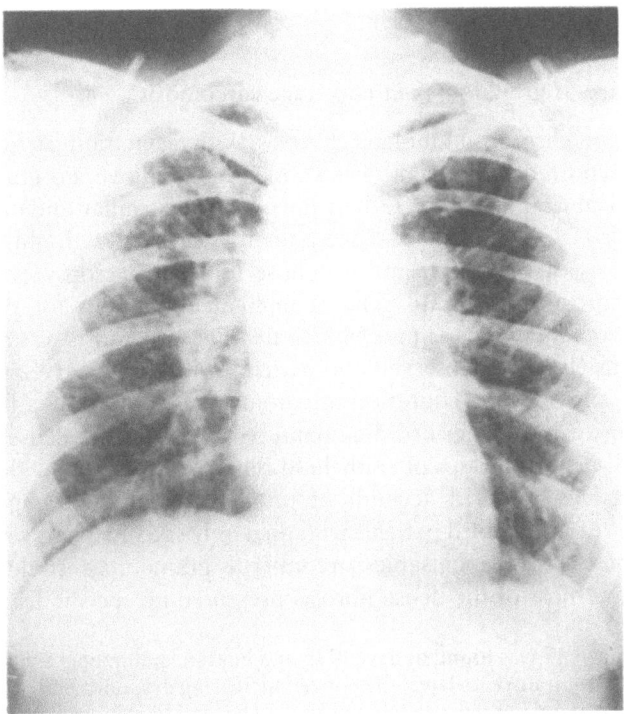

Figure 6.38   Sarcoidosis of hilar lymph-nodes and lungs in a woman aged 37.

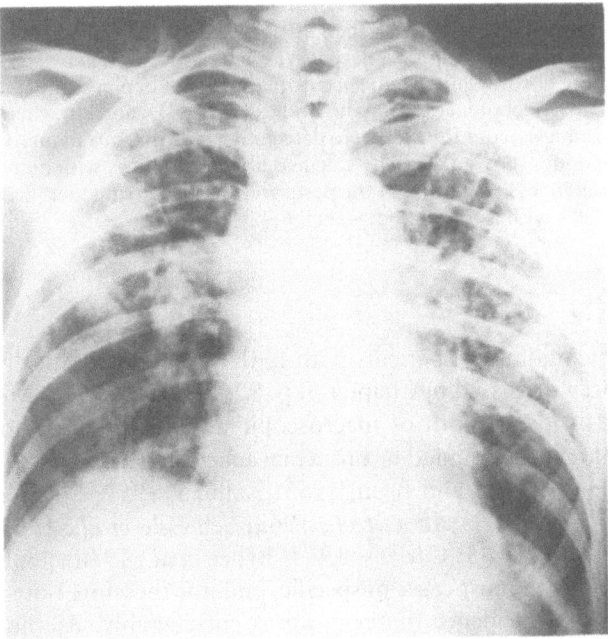

Figure 6.39   The same, six years later, showing fibrotic changes.

Disappearance of granulomas in end-stage sarcoidosis

In the case of chronic pulmonary fibrosis with cavitation attributed to sarcoidosis reported by Ustvedt (1948), mentioned above, no granulomas were recognizable at necropsy. Others have reported similar findings. Smellie and Hoyle (1960) mentioned three patients who died with old-standing sarcoid fibrosis of the lungs, and in whose lungs at necropsy only dense hyalinized fibrosis was found. They commented that but for preceding evidence it would have been impossible to tell that sarcoidosis was responsible. One of us (JGS) has observed two patients with pulmonary sarcoidosis of 30 years' and 15 years' duration in whom at necropsy only a few giant cells, some inclusion bodies of Schaumann type persisting in dense fibrosis, and scanty ill-defined groups of epithelioid cells were left to show the nature of the disease. A detailed account of one of these has been published (Scadding, 1968). In a third patient, who died only six and a half years from the apparent onset, recognisable sarcoid-type granulomas could still be found, though most of the dense fibrosis presented no specific feature:

A woman aged 37 was found to have BHL and bilateral pulmonary infiltration (Fig. 6.38); four years later, she noticed increasing dyspnoea and dry cough; the skin did not react to tuberculin, 100 IU, and liver biopsy showed non-caseating tubercles. Six years from the onset, she was completely disabled by dyspnoea; radiographically, there was an irregular pattern of dense opacities and rounded transradiant areas (Fig. 6.39), which tomography suggested might be emphysematous bullae (Fig. 6.40). She died six and a half years after the first abnormal radiograph. At necropsy, the lungs showed extensive fibrosis; most of the fibrosis showed no specific features, but in places the fibrosis included many conchoidal Schaumann bodies (Fig. 6.41), and elsewhere a few still recognizable sarcoid follicles were detectable in the fibrous tissue. The mediastinal nodes showed partially calcified fibrous scarring, with no remnant of sarcoid tubercles except that at the periphery of the scarring there were some giant cells with asteroid bodies (Fig. 6.42).

BRONCHI

Bronchoscopic findings in patients with BHL and radiographically normal lungs have been discussed in Chapter 5, p. 92. In patients with evident lung changes, the incidence both of macroscopic abnormalities and of microscopic granulomatous change in bronchial mucosa is higher than in those with BHL alone (Turiaf and Brun, 1955; Kalbian, 1957; Friedman *et al.*, 1963; Huzly *et al.*, 1963; Liot *et el.*, 1963; Schiessle *et al.*, 1963; Ståhle, 1963; Turiaf *et al.*, 1963; Carlens, 1964; Bybee *et al.*, 1968). Macroscopic abnormalities are in most cases unspecific, and it is therefore not surprising that the reported incidence of them varies considerably. At the stage of BHL, some thickening of the mucosa especially of the main bronchi is found

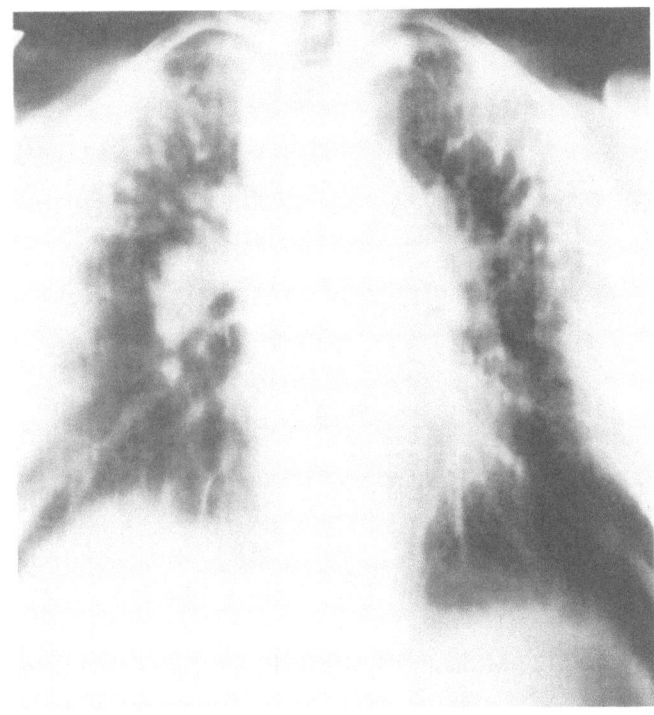

Figure 6.40   Tomography at the same time as Fig. 6.39; persistent hilar node enlargement; irregular air-containing spaces.

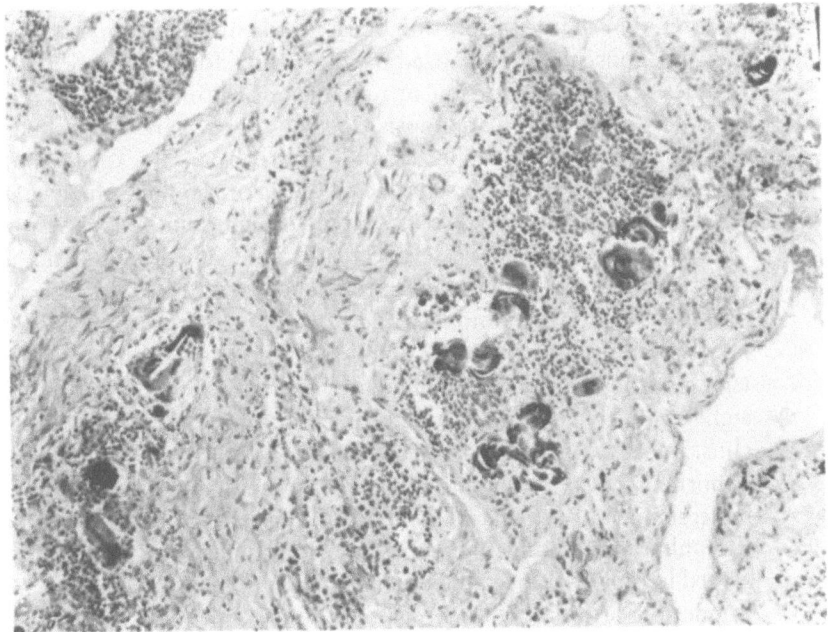

Figure 6.41   Lung at necropsy; dense fibrosis with groups of Schaumann conchoidal bodies as the only remnant of granulomas H & E. × 100.

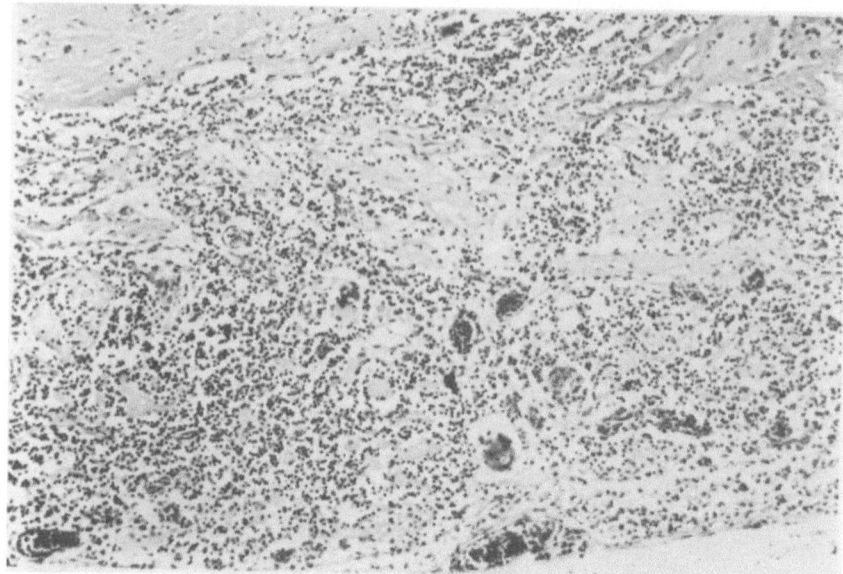

Figure 6.42   Mediastinal lymph-node, with giant cells as the only remnant of granulomas.

in about half the cases, with localized dilatations of venules in a few. In the presence of an active pulmonary infiltration, these changes are more marked and found in a large proportion of cases, and in a few, more specific-looking changes, consisting of localized papilloma-like formations, or flat yellowish plaques are seen; distortion or narrowing of bronchi may be seen. In the later fibrotic stage of sarcoidosis, specific changes are less frequently seen, the mucosa tending to be atrophic rather than thickened, but fibrotic stenoses may rarely be present (see below). For instance, Huzly *et al.* (1963) described in detail the bronchoscopic findings in 294 cases. Localized dilatations of mucosal vessels were frequent at all stages; nodules were reported in the mucosa in one-sixth of those with BHL alone, in two-thirds of those with active pulmonary infiltration, and in more than half those with fibrosis; and plaques in only one with BHL, none with fibrosis, and one-eighth of those with active pulmonary infiltration. Stenoses were observed in eight cases, four of upper lobe bronchi and four of the middle lobe bronchus. Bybee *et al.* (1968) reviewed bronchoscopic studies in 55 patients; no abnormality was observed in 20. The commonest gross abnormality was hyperaemia and oedema of the mucosa, observed to regress on remission of the pulmonary changes in some cases; granularity or nodularity was observed in only two cases, superficial erosion in one and atrophic appearance in one; distortion of bronchi was seen in 19 and some narrowing in eight.

Biopsy studies have shown granulomas in the bronchial mucosa in varying proportions, up to 60%, of patients with BHL and radiographically clear lungs (Chapter 5, p. 92); and in presence of evident lung changes, most observers have reported similar, perhaps rather higher, proportions.

Kalbian (1957) reported biopsies of bronchial mucosa in ten patients with hilar node and pulmonary sarcoidosis; three showed non-caseating tubercles and three a thickened mucosa with giant cells. Friedman *et al.* (1963) found that 15 of 18 biopsies from thickened or otherwise abnormal mucosa, and seven of 17 from normal-looking mucosa showed specific changes. Huzly *et al.* (1963) in 294 cases at all stages of sarcoidosis found bronchial biopsies positive in 36%. Liot *et al.* (1963) found that 70% of 61 cases of pulmonary sarcoidosis showed specific changes in bronchial biopsies, including five of 18 with normal-looking mucosae. Schiessle *et al.* (1963) reported positive findings in 78% of 126 cases with active pulmonary infiltration and in 50% of 60 with fibrotic changes. Ståhle (1963) found lower proportions, 44% of 27 and 17% of 19 respectively. Turiaf *et al.* (1963) found specific changes in bronchial biopsies from 22 of 41 cases with active pulmonary infiltration, although only one had shown a specific-looking abnormality on inspection; they noted that granulomas might persist in bronchial mucosa in spite of apparent clearing of hilar node and lung changes, in one case as long as 13 years after such clearing. Carlens (1964), performing three biopsies in each case, found granulomas in only six of 35 with active pulmonary infiltration and five of 12 with fibrosis. Bybee *et al.* (1968) found granulomas in eight of 34 adequate bronchial mucosal biopsies in patients with pulmonary sarcoidosis, and noted that in three the granuloma-containing mucosa looked normal.

Bronchostenosis

It is thus apparent that infiltration of the bronchial mucosa is frequent, but in most cases symptomless. However it may narrow bronchi sufficiently to limit airflow.

A very few cases have been reported in which functionally important narrowings of large bronchi were found at an early stage, contemporary with BHL (Benedict and Castleman, 1941; Hadfield *et al.*, 1982). In Cases 1 and 4 of Hadfield *et al.*, there was good evidence that multiple narrowings of segmental or sub-segmental bronchi were contemporary with recently-developing BHL, accompanied by EN in Case 1; the narrowings were shown by bronchography to be more widespread than was suggested by bronchoscopy, at which the mucosa presented a cobble-stoned appearance, and on biopsy was found to be infiltrated with sarcoid granulomas.

Most of the reported cases of bronchostenosis have been detected later in the course of sarcoidosis, and have affected principally the proximal parts of segmental or lobar bronchi, and occasionally main bronchi (Fig. 6.43). Histologically, epithelioid cells and giant cells tend to be rather diffusely scattered through a thickened submucosa with a general infiltration with round cells and fibroblasts and more or less mature fibrous tissue (Fig. 6.44); well-defined granulomas may be rare. As would be expected, this condition produces dyspnoea out of proportion to the density of any pulmonary infiltration that may be evident, and often with prolongation of inspiration and a faint inspiratory as well as expiratory stridor; it may also lead to recurrent or persistent inflammatory collapse-consolidations in the segments whose bronchi are narrowed. If this clinical picture is accompanied by the typical bronchographic appearance of proximal segmental stenoses, the diagnosis of chronic stenosing sarcoidosis of the bronchi is very probable, although bronchial biopsy may show only a rather uncharacteristic giant cell granulomatous change. Citron and Scadding (1957)

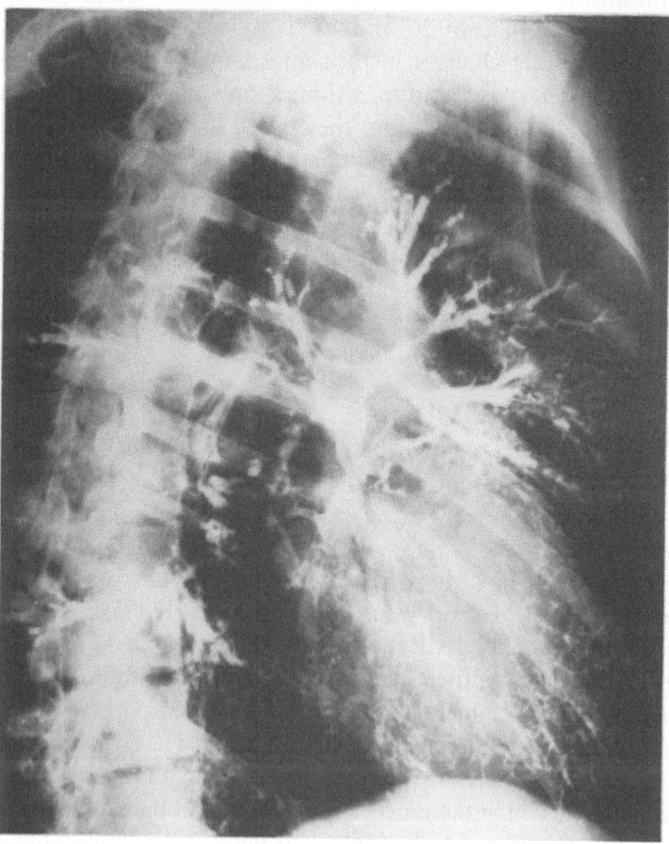

Figure 6.43   Bronchogram showing narrowing of segmental bronchi of left upper lobe near their origins in a man aged 31.

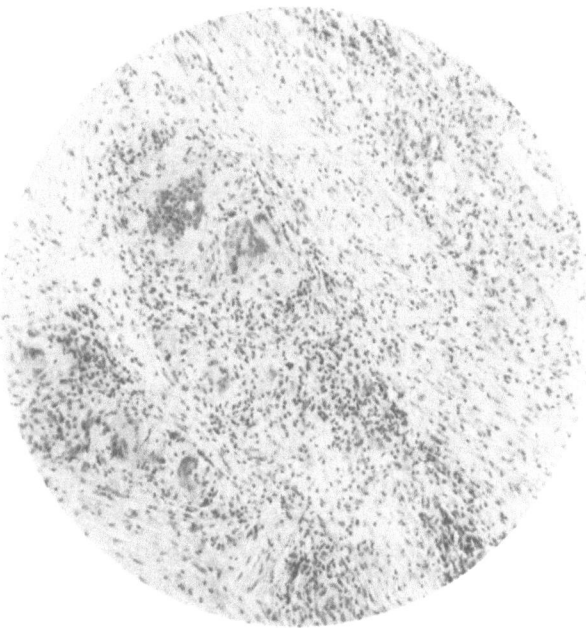

Figure 6.44 Biopsy from mucosa of narrowed bronchus in same case, slowly fibrosing with giant cells, some epithelioid cells and scattered round cells. H & E. × 90.

reported three cases of multiple bronchial stenosis of this sort. One showed also typical sarcoid tubercles in biopsies of liver, of a mild granulomatous conjunctivitis and of a Kveim test nodule; one showed also a positive Kveim test with histological confirmation; and one showed typical non-caseating sarcoid-type tubercles in mediastinal and cervical lymph-nodes and in an infiltrated scar. There could thus be no doubt of the diagnosis of sarcoidosis although the histological changes in the bronchi alone would not have been diagnostic. Similar cases have been reported by Brun and Viallier (1948), Siltzbach and Som (1952), Kalbian (1957), Honey and Jepson (1957) and Smellie and Hoyle (1960). Cases in which an early non-stenosing bronchial mucosal infiltration was observed to progress to stenosis have been reported by Turiaf *et al.* (1952) and Grimminger (1955).

Among 275 patients with sarcoidosis under the care of one of us (JGS), seven showed evidence of bronchostenosis. In four, this was of the sort described above, involving the proximal parts of several segmental bronchi, with some general narrowing of one or both main bronchi. In three there was stenosis of a lobar bronchus, all on the right side, those to the upper, the middle and the lower lobe each being affected in one case. A similar stenosis of the right upper lobe bronchus occurred in Case 3 of Hadfield *et al.* (1982). In all there were relevant symptoms and signs, either of inspiratory and expiratory airflow limitation, or episodes of lobar or segmental collapse-consolidation. Bronchograms in seven patients with extensive pulmonary sarcoidosis without either of these features showed equivocal changes in only one, the others showing bronchi of normal calibre. Narrowing of large bronchi is thus an infrequent feature of chronic pulmonary sarcoidosis. Atelectasis due to bronchostenosis was mentioned by Freundlich *et al.* (1970) in three of 200, and by Kirks *et al.* (1973) in one of 150 patients with pulmonary sarcoidosis. Atelectasis of the right middle lobe with histological confirmation of granulomatous change in the narrowed middle lobe bronchus was observed in two of 300 patients with sarcoidosis by Katsouros (1971), and has been reported in single cases by Di Benedetto and Ribaudo (1966) and Poe (1978). It seems possible that in Case 8 of Talbot *et al.* (1958), in which 'migratory pneumonitis' without eosinophilia was observed in a black man with sarcoidosis, there were multiple proximal bronchostenosis; in their case 2, right middle lobe atelectasis was due to sarcoid bronchostenosis. Olsson *et al.* (1979) reported a high incidence of bronchostenosis found on bronchoscopy in 98 Swedish patients with pulmonary sarcoidosis; eight showed severe narrowings of major bronchi, multiple segmental orifices being involved in three, a single segment in three, the right upper lobe in one and the right middle lobe in one. Granulomas were found in mucosal biopsies in 32 of the whole series and in six of the eight with stenoses. The ages of the patients with stenoses ranged from 37–71 years.

Especially when the middle lobe is involved, differential diagnosis from mycobacterial tuberculosis must be considered. Lobar or segmental collapse-consolidation, especially of the middle lobe, is a well-recognized comlication of primary tuberculosis; the course of the right middle lobe bronchus predisposes it to compression by enlarged broncho-pulmonary lymph-nodes, and to granulomatous inflammation by direct extension from them. In Case 3 of Citron and Scadding (1957), there was evidence of *M tuberculosis* infection concurrently with a clinical, radiological and histological picture typical of sarcoidosis with multiple bronchostenoses (Chapter 23, p. 506).

PLEURA

It is probable that some granulomas are present in or immediately under the visceral pleura in many cases of pulmonary sarcoidosis, but symptoms attributable to pleural involvement are rare. A few necropsy reports have mentioned striking changes in the pleura as an incidental finding. For instance, Nickerson (1937) found flat white nodules 1–4 mm in diameter, coalescing to form irregular plaques up to 1.5 cm in diameter, scattered over the parietal pleura of the right lung, and the parietal pericardium in a black woman aged 58 who died of 'acute sarcoidosis'. Wilen *et al.* (1974) reviewed lung biopsies from 11 patients with pulmonary sarcoidosis who showed no radiographic evidence of pleural changes, and found pleural granulomas in four. In Cases 3 and 4 of Beekman *et al.* (1975) lung biopsies from patients presenting with radiographic abnormalities in the lungs but no clinical or radiographic evidence of pleural involvement showed granulomatous changes in pleura as well as lung.

Pleural sarcoidosis becomes clinically evident most frequently by leading to pleural effusion. Effusions not attributable to some other cause, and presumed or in some cases confirmed by biopsy to be related to sarcoidosis have been reported in no more than 3% of most large series of patients with sarcoidosis; in one of 275 reviewed by one of us (JGS), in two of 160 reported by Longcope and Freiman (1952), in four of 200 by Freundlich *et al.* (1970), in five of 150 by Kirks *et al.* (1973) and in seven of 950 by Chusid *et al.* (1974). The diagnosis was confirmed by biopsy in three of the effusions observed by Kirk *et al.* and in five of the seven by Chusid *et al.* The series of 227 patients surveyed for pleural involvement by Wilen *et al.* (1974) in New York showed an exceptionally high proportion with radiographically evident pleural changes: 15 showed pleural effusions, pleural biopsies in seven of these showing granulomas. These effusions usually resolved within eight weeks, but in two left some pleural thickening. In eight patients with long-standing pulmonary sarcoidosis, pleural thickening was observed, biopsies in five showing fibrosis with interspersed granulomas. Among 150 patients in Los Angeles, of whom 80% were black, reviewed by Sharma and Gordonson (1975), six, all black, had pleural effusions at some time. The effusions were small in all cases, and bilateral in two. Open biopsy showed granulomas in the visceral pleura, as well as the lung, in one case; in the others needle biopsy of the pleura showed only non-specific changes. In all cases, the effusions cleared, spontaneously in three and after corticosteroid treatment in three. Two presented with pleural effusions, the others developing them at intervals of four months to six years from the original diagnosis of sarcoidosis. Sharma (1980) later extended this series to 250, of whom 12 had pleural effusions at some time.

Small pleural effusions accompanying active intrathoracic sarcoidosis, resolving spontaneously or in response to corticosteroid treatment, and showing no evidence of other cause, can be accepted as a manifestation of sarcoidosis, even without biopsy confirmation of the presence of granulomas in the pleura. Needle biopsy cannot be relied upon, since in the presence of an effusion it produces only a small sample of parietal pleura. A number of the reported cases have occurred at an early stage of the disease, with BHL with or without evident lung changes, often without local symptoms, though sometimes with pain of pleuritic type, and of limited duration. We have seen several cases of this sort, and others have been described by Selroos (1966, Cases 1, 2 and 3), Beekman (1975, Cases 1 and 2), Sharma and Gordonson (1975, Cases 2 and 4) and de Vuyst *et al.* (1979). In Case 3 of Sharma and Gordonson, a small right pleural effusion preceded the discovery of BHL by six months, at which time, small effusions were present on both sides. In Case 4 of Selroos (1966) pleural effusion recurred with recurrent activity of pulmonary sarcoidosis: a middle-aged man had bilateral effusions accompanying BHL and lung infiltration, clearing within a year; two years later the lung shadows reappeared, with a left pleural effusion, bronchial biopsy showing granulomas, but needle biopsy of the pleura only non-specific changes.

In a few cases, large pleural effusions have constituted a prominent clinical feature. Berte and Pfotenhauer (1962) reported the case of a black woman aged 28 who developed a large left pleural effusion one year after the diagnosis of sarcoidosis causing BHL and uveitis; the effusion continued to accumulate after repeated aspirations, leading to pleurectomy; the thickened pleura and the lung contained many epithelioid and giant-cell granulomas; four months after operation, the lungs were radiographically clear and the patient was well. Kovnat and Donohue (1965) described two young black patients with established diagnoses of sarcoidosis, who developed large pleural effusions, left-sided on one and bilateral in the other, shown by biopsy to be due to granulomatous infiltration of the pleura. Mikhail *et al.* (1976) reported the case of a 37 year old black man who presented with a large right pleural effusion, and no radiographic evidence of hilar lymphnode enlargement; pleural biopsy showed thickening with non-caseating granulomas; in spite of a negative tuberculin test and failure to demonstrate acid-fast bacilli, anti-mycobacterial treatment was started, together with a short period of corticosteroid treatment. The pleural effusion disappeared, but on cessation of the corticosteroid, it recurred and later a widespread pulmonary infiltration appeared. Mediastinal lymph-node biopsy now showed non-caseating granulomas and a Kveim test gave a granulomatous response; antimycobacterial treatment was stopped and reinstitution of corticosteroid treatment was followed by clearing of the effusion, and diminution of the infiltration.

Persistence of pleural effusions for long periods has been reported in a few patients with chronic pulmonary sarcoidosis. Macquet *et al.* (1965) described the case of a woman found to have pulmonary sarcoidosis at the age of 59, which was still present five years later; needle biopsy showed a thickened pleura with a focus of mononuclear cells and a giant cell, and bronchoscopy showed thickened mucosa containing an epithelioid cell granuloma. Brun *et al.* (1963) reported the case of a woman with established sarcoidosis for several years, who developed a large left pleural effusion, reaccumulating rapidly after paracentesis, and at one time frankly bloodstained. The histology of the pleura was not studied; the patient had had phlebitis of leg veins. It must remain speculative whether this effusion was related to sarcoidosis.

Pleuritic pain was a presenting symptom in cases reported by Gardiner and Uff (1978) and by de Vuyst *et al.* (1979). The first of these was that of a white man aged 47 who had recurrent left pleural pain, accompanied by pleural rub; radiography showed BHL, and fine pulmonary infiltration; open lung biopsy showed many granulomas, especially under the pleura, and in hilar lymph-nodes; there was a prompt response to corticosteroid treatment. The patient whose case was described by de Vuyst *et al.* was a man aged 50 who presented with bilateral pleural pain, and was found to have bilateral pulmonary infiltration with small pleural effusions; mediastinoscopy showed many large lymph-nodes, biopsy of which showed epithelioid and giant-cell granulomas.

Pleural thickening in the later stages of pulmonary sarcoidosis cannot be attributed with certainty to sarcoidosis without histological confirmation; nevertheless, Wilen *et al.* (1974) found pleural thickening for which no other cause was evident in eight of 227 patients with sarcoidosis; all eight had chronic and extensive pulmonary sarcoidosis; and biopsies in five of them showed fibrotic pleura with interspersed granulomas. They noted that in two of their 15 patients with pleural effusions attributed to sarcoidosis, resolution of the effusion left some residual pleural thickening.

In some reported cases, there has been an association between pleural changes and involvement of major bronchi on the same side (Macquet *et al.*, 1965; Selroos, 1966, Case 1; Voog *et al.*, 1969). A woman aged 50 under the care of one of us had clinical and radiological evidence of thickening of the pleura at the base of the right lung. The skin persistently failed to react to tuberculin, 100 IU: biopsies of the mucosa of the right lower lobe bronchus and of an axillary lymph-node both showed non-caseating tubercles.

Most of the published reports giving information about the characteristics of effusions attributed to sarcoidosis have described them as exudates, with specific gravities ranging from 1.018–1.035 and protein contents from 4.0–6.0 g dl^{-1}; cells have been predominantly, up to 100%, lymphocytes. Exceptionally, Wilen *et al.* (1974) in eight patients with active sarcoidosis and transient pleural effusions, in six of whom biopsies showed pleural granulomas, found that the effusions had the characters of transudates, with specific gravities between 1.011 and 1.016, and protein contents between 1.3 and 2.3 g dl^{-1}; no cells were found in five and a few lymphocytes in three.

Two cases reported by Mikhail (1970) illustrate difficulties that may arise in deciding whether a pleural effusion is to be classified as associated with sarcoidosis, or due to mycobacterial tuberculosis. These occurred in Irish twin brothers aged 21 shown by blood-group studies to be probably monozygotic, who came to England at the same time, and lived in the same household. One presented with a pleural effusion, biopsy showing epithelioid and giant-cell granulomas with some caseation in the pleura; and a tuberculin test with 10 IU was positive, though no mycobacteria could be found on culture of the fluid. The effusion cleared under anti-mycobacterial treatment for 18 months, with an initial month of corticosteroid treatment. At the end of treatment, a Kveim test gave an unequivocally granulomatous response. The other twin, examined as a contact of his brother, was found to have symptomless BHL; a lymph-node removed at mediastinoscopy showed confluent granulomas with hyalinization; a Kveim test gave a granulomatous response; and a tuberculin test with 10 IU was positive. On the evidence of the tuberculin tests, both twins had had a mycobacterial infection; and both gave granulomatous responses to Kveim tests. On balance of evidence, most observers would probably categorize the first as having a tuberculous pleural effusion, in spite of the Kveim test; and the second as showing the typical syndrome of sarcoid BHL, in spite of the tuberculin test. But in neither case would it be unreasonable to hold another view.

Pleural changes due to intercurrent infective inflammatory episodes may of course occur in the course of sarcoidosis, especially in the fibrotic stage; associated symptoms and signs of broncho-pulmonary infection usually leave little doubt of their nature.

Spontaneous pneumothorax has been reported in a small proportion of most large series of patients with pulmonary sarcoidosis: e.g. in four of 200 by Freundlich *et al.* (1970), in four of 150 by Kirks *et al.* (1973), in seven of 250 by Sharma (1980), and in 14 of 617 by Johns *et al.* (1980). Most of these – e.g. all reported by Kirks *et al.* and by Johns *et al.* – occurred in patients with old-standing fibrotic and emphysematous changes, evidently the cause of the pneumothorax. Occasionally, spontaneous pneumothorax has occurred at an earlier stage, e.g. in cases reported by Voight-Richter (1965), by Fein *et al.* (1980) and by Ross and Empey (1983). In the latter case, left- and then right-sided pneumothorax appeared and were present simultaneously in a West Indian man who was receiving corticosteroid treatment for active pulmonary and hilar lymph-node sarcoidosis. In view of the rarity of this association, it is arguable that it is coincidental, since spontaneous pneumothorax is not infrequent in otherwise healthy young adults.

Among 275 patients followed by one of us for periods up to 20 years, five were observed to have spontaneous pneumothoraces. One youth, aged 18, developed pain in the chest while he had BHL shortly after erythema nodosum, and was found to have a right spontaneous pneumothorax, which expanded without incident. One man, aged 23, had two episodes of spontaneous pneumothorax during the resolution of mottled infiltration in the lungs after BHL. One man, aged 33, had a single episode while he had an infiltration of cloudy shadowing type which later progressed to fibrosis. All these episodes occurred in young men at the age at which 'idiopathic' spontaneous pneumothorax is frequent, and in all the pneumothorax absorbed uneventfully. In the remaining two, both women in the early forties, the sarcoidosis was in a late fibrotic stage with bullous emphysematous changes, gross in one. Both of these had recurrent attacks, involving both sides on different occasions, with urgent symptoms necessitating the insertion of intercostal tubes and suction drainage; clearly in these cases leakage from emphysematous bullae was the immediate cause of the pneumothorax.

CALCIFICATION IN INTRATHORACIC SARCOIDOSIS

Many reviews of large series of cases of sarcoidosis mention the presence from the beginning of calcification in the hilar nodes or in the lungs. Riley (1950), describing 52 cases observed in New York, stated that nine showed

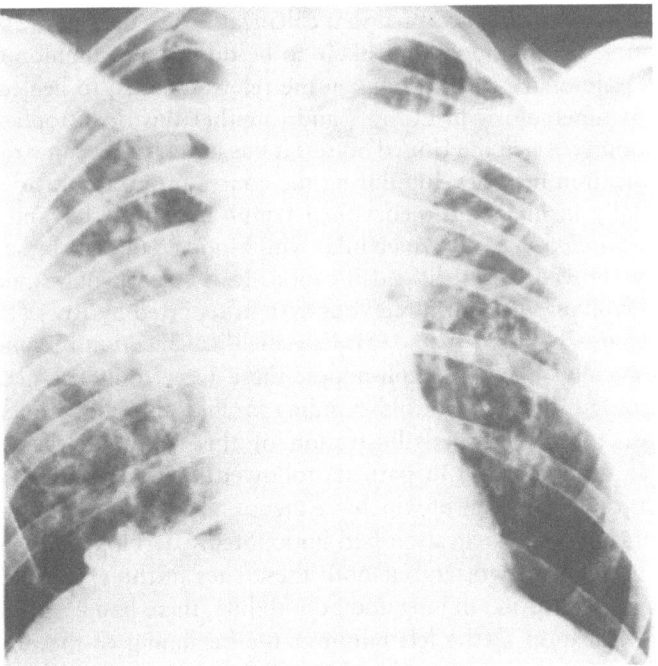

Figure 6.45 Chronic pulmonary sarcoidosis in a man aged 43 with extensive old calcification at the base of the right lung and in right hilar lymph-nodes.

calcified foci either in the hilar nodes or in the lungs. Cowdell (1954) stated that five of 90 patients observed in Oxford had calcified hilar or mesenteric lymph-nodes. Wurm *et al.* (1958) found calcified foci in lung and hilar nodes in 11% in lung only in 6% and in hilar nodes only in 13% of 243 cases in Germany. Ten Have (1958) found 'manifest' calcification in 9% and 'dubious' calcification in 14% of 150 patients in Holland. Israel *et al.* (1961) found calcification of hilar nodes or in the lung of 10.1% of 256 patients with sarcoidosis in Philadelphia. In 136 patients in London whose radiographs were specially surveyed for the presence of calcification, Scadding (1961) found acceptable evidence of calcification at the beginning of observation in 16 (11.8%); at the hilum in nine, in the lung in three, and at both these sites in four. Figure 6.45 shows typical chronic sarcoid infiltration of the lung with large, evidently old-standing, calcifications in the lower zone of the right lung and in right hilar lymph-nodes. The diagnosis of sarcoidosis was confirmed by the presence of a generalized superficial lymphadenopathy, biopsies of cervical and epitrochlear nodes showing typical histology, by total non-reactivity of the skin to tuberculin and by response to corticosteroid treatment. In one sputum specimen, acid-fast bacilli were found, but cultures of this and many others for mycobacteria were negative.

It would be generally accepted that calcifications evident at the beginning of the course of sarcoidosis are likely to be due to the common causes of hilar and pulmonary calcifications in the relevant areas; to healed caseous residues of tuberculosis in Europe, and to either this or histoplasmosis or coccidioidomycosis in the United States. It has gradually become recognized that calcification may develop during the course of intrathoracic sarcoidosis, especially in hilar and mediastinal lymph-nodes. Kerley and Twining (1951) mentioned a case in which hilar lymph-nodes enlarged by sarcoidosis eventually showed 'egg-shell' calcification. In a case of long-standing sarcoidosis involving the central nervous system reported by Ross (1955) and mentioned in Chapter 14 (p. 315), 'egg-shell' calcification became evident radiographically in hilar lymph-nodes; these were found at necropsy to show histologically 'active or old-standing sarcoidosis with calcification but no necrosis'; the published illustration of this shows extensive hyaline fibrosis. In a survey of 136 patients followed for at least five years, the findings at the beginnings of which are mentioned above, Scadding (1961a) found that in seven calcfication had undoubtedly developed, at the hila in two, in the lung in two, and at both these sites in three; in one of those developing calcification in lung and at both hila, there had been some small foci of calcification at the left hilum at the beginning of the observation period. In one of these cases, tubercle bacilli had been isolated from a single sputum specimen late in the course of the disease, with a change from

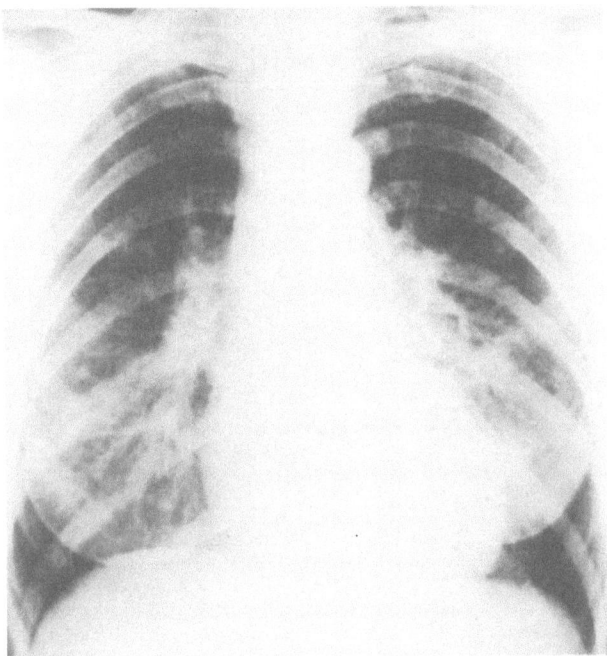

Figure 6.46   Moderate BHL and scattered pulmonary infiltration in a woman aged 47 with lupus pernio.

tuberculin insensitivity to sensitivity to 10 IU; but in the others the course remained entirely characteristic of sarcoidosis. Israel *et al.* (1961) reported shortly afterwards that two of 256 patients with sarcoidosis had been observed to develop intrathoracic calcification under observation; one of these had evidence of infection with chromogenic acid-fast bacilli, and also had multiple calcified nodules in the liver.

The following case illustrates the development of calcification:

A housewife aged 47 presented with lupus pernio affecting the middle fingers of both hands and later the first and second toes of the right foot, with lattice-like rarefactions of the underlying bones. The chest radiograph (Fig. 6.46) showed enlargement of hilar shadows, and irregular scattered opacities in the lungs, with no calcification. The skin gave no reaction to tuberculin, 100 IU. Axillary lymph-node biopsy showed non-caseating tubercles. Corticosteroid treatment was given to relieve symptoms arising from the changes in the fingers and toes, and needed to be continued in moderate dosage for nearly four years, when it was withdrawn without return of symptoms. Calcification gradually developed at the site of sarcoid involvement in the hilar nodes, and in a few small nodules in the middle zones of the lungs (Fig. 6.47). Other manifestations in this patient included a typical sarcoid infiltration of an old scar on the knee and a positive Kveim test.

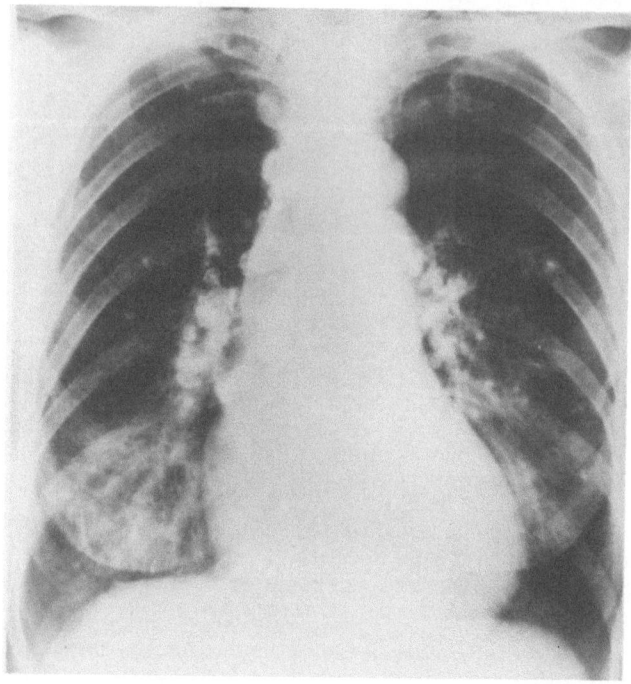

Figure 6.47   The same, seven years later, showing calcification in hilar and paratracheal lymph-nodes.

In a later review, Scadding (1968) reported five more instances of the development of calcification in hilar nodes, in some also in lungs, late in the course of sarcoidosis. He observed it only in patients in whom there was in the active stage radiographic evidence of both lung and hilar node involvement, and noted that calcification in hilar and mediastinal lymph-nodes in a generally symmetrical distribution resembling that of the active stage of sarcoidosis was highly suggestive of late-stage sarcoidosis (Fig 6.48). In most cases, calcification involved the discretely enlarged lymph-nodes throughout, sometimes patchily; a peripheral 'egg-shell' pattern was seen in some of the affected lymph-nodes in some cases. In one, a calcified lymph-node was studied histologically. A woman aged 53, in whom BHL had been discovered six years earlier, presented with gradually increasing dyspnoea on exertion together with mottled shadowing in the lung fields for two years, with persistent BHL (Fig. 6.49). Biopsy of a supraclavicular lymph-node showed non-caseating epithelioid and giant-cell granulomas with small areas of hyalinization (Fig. 6.50). Treatment with prednisolone was started, with improvement; it was found necessary to maintain it for three years, when it was withdrawn without relapse, the lungs being radio-

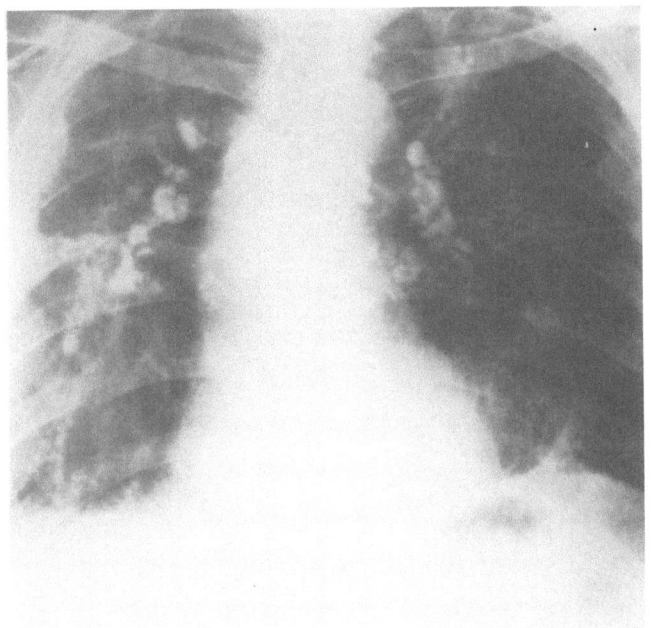

Figure 6.48 Symmetrical calcification in hilar lymph-nodes, with a distribution similar to that of sarcoid BHL, in a man aged 60 who had had lupus pernio of fingers and toes since the age of 25.

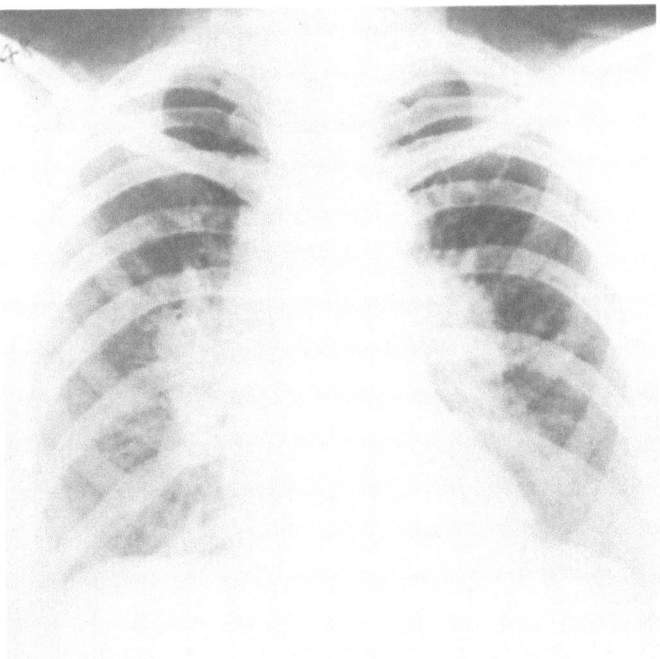

Figure 6.49 BHL, first discovered four years earlier, and pulmonary infiltration in a woman aged 51.

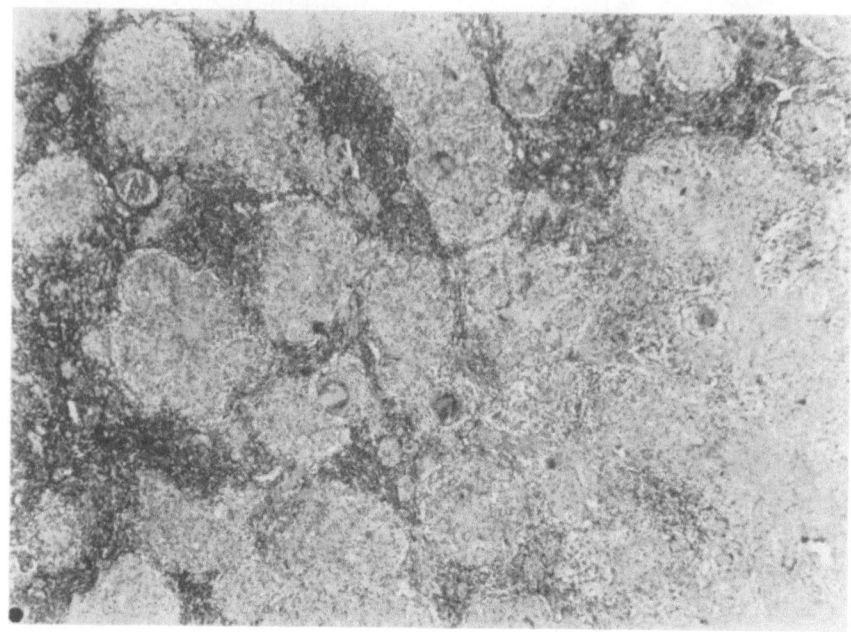

Figure 6.50 Supraclavicular lymph-node biopsy showing sarcoid tubercles, in places coalescent and undergoing hyalinisation H &E. × 38.

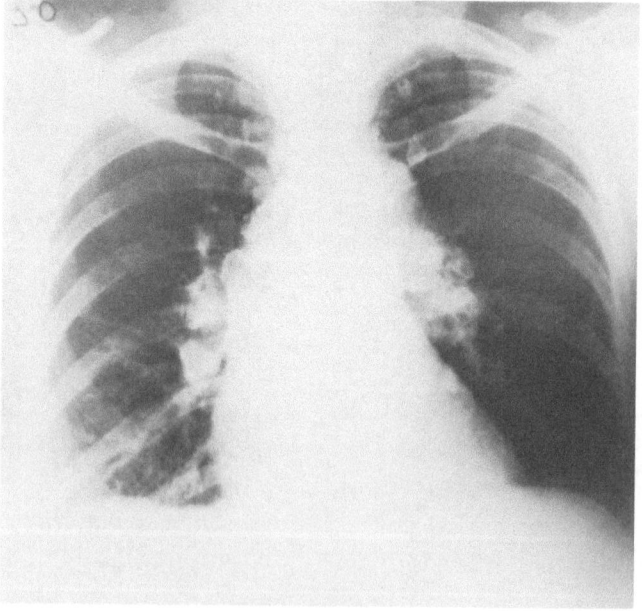

Figure 6.51 Chest radiograph eight years later, showing symmetrical calcification in hilar nodes and also in left supraclavicular nodes.

graphically almost clear, with some persistent enlargement of hilar shadows, in which some calcification had become evident. Over the next few years, this increased at both hila, and also behind the left clavicle, the site of the lymph-node biopsy (Fig. 6.51). Seven years after the first, a second lymph-node was removed from this site for biopsy; it was almost completely replaced by fibrous tissue undergoing calcification, only a small subcapsular zone of lymphocytes and no recognizable granulomas persisting (Fig. 6.52a). A reticulin stain showed that the reticulin pattern persisted in the calcified areas (Fig. 6.52b), suggesting that the avascular connective tissue had become calcified without undergoing necrosis.

Voog *et al.* (1969) reported the histopathological changes in partly calcified mediastinal lymph-nodes removed by mediastinoscopy from a man aged 58 whose chest radiograph showed extensive symmetrical calcification, some of 'egg-shell' distribution, in hilar lymph-nodes. Follicular sarcoid lesions were juxtaposed with well demarcated fibro-hyaline tissue without caseation, in which calcification had occurred.

Kirks *et al.* (1973) observed the development of calcification in hilar lymph-nodes during observation in five of 150 patients with pulmonary sarcoidosis. McLoud *et al.* (1974) described three patients with sarcoidosis who had persistent lung changes and BHL, in which calcification was noticed between five and seven years from the onset, and 2–4 years later had assumed an 'egg-shell' distribution in the hilar lymph-nodes.

In a group of 111 patients followed for at least ten years, Israel *et al.* (1981) observed the development of calcification, principally in hilar and mediastinal lymph-nodes in 23. The group studied included a high proportion with persistent and symptomatic disease, since it was derived from clinical follow-up. Calcification tended to be a late event, developing in the first decade of observation in only three, in the second in 11, and in the third in nine. It appeared in hilar and mediastinal lymph-nodes in 22 and in lungs in three. Calcification appeared in two of 19 patients who had presented with BHL and had never shown radiographic evidence of lung infiltration; in 20 of 69 in whom both hilar nodes and lung had shown radiographic changes; and in only one of 20 who had shown radiographic changes in the lungs only.

Scadding (1968) reported one patient in whom typical symmetrical hilar node calcification appeared and then disappeared during prolonged observation. A woman aged 32 presented with uveitis, BHL and pulmonary infiltration; treatment with corticosteroids was required for the control of symptoms intermittently for several years, but eventually the pulmonary changes became quiescent, leaving only minor residual shadows. Eight years from the onset, calcification with a tendency to 'egg-shell' distribution was obvious in the hilar nodes. During five years' further observation, the lung shadows cleared further, and the hilar calcification diminished, leaving only

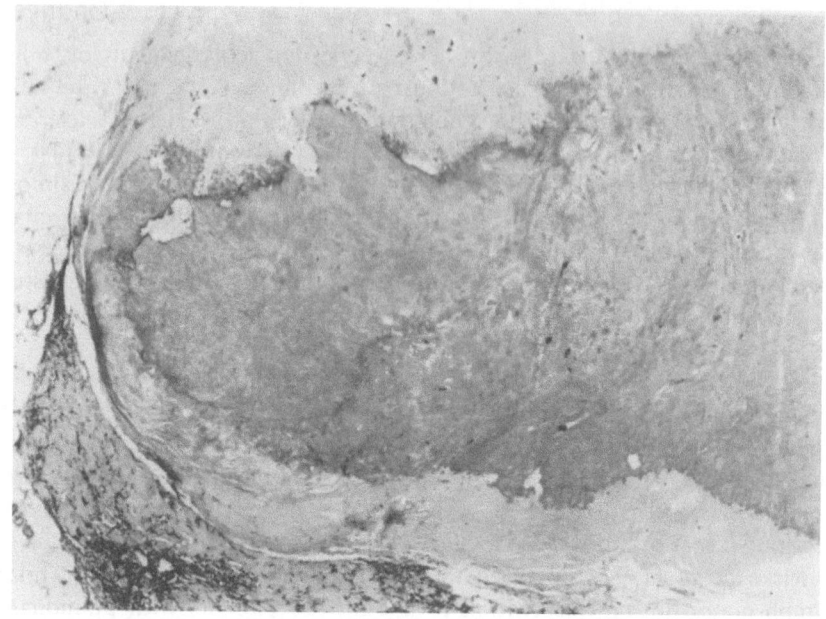

(a)

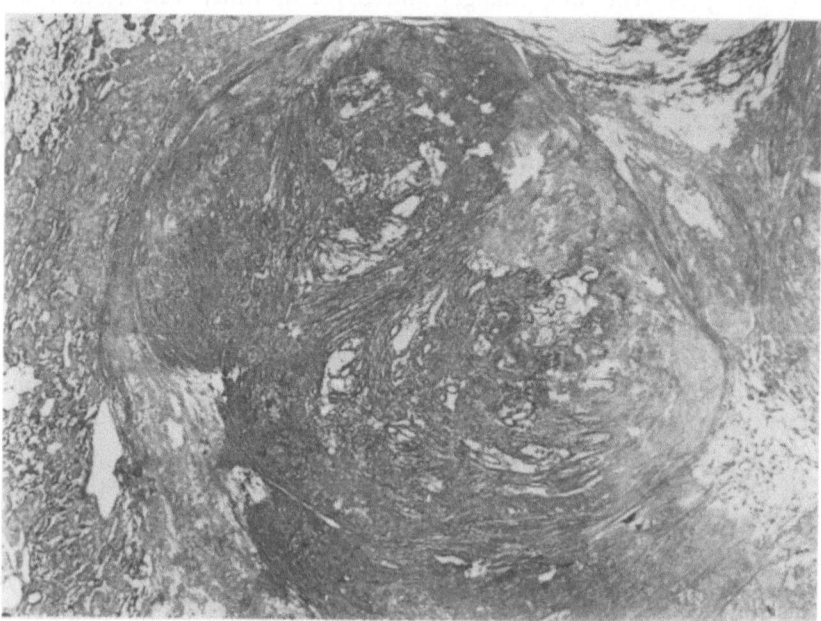

(b)

Figure 6.52 Biopsy of calcified supraclavicular lymph-node; sections cut after decalcification. (a) Most of the node consisted of hyaline connective tissue, in which calcification had occurred (darker-staining part) H & E. × 38. (b) Reticulin stain, × 38, showing persisting reticulin pattern throughout.

a few flecks. Israel *et al.* (1981) observed no instance of diminution in density of calcification among their 23 patients.

It is evident that calcification in affected hilar and mediastinal lymph-nodes is a not infrequent late event in patients with sarcoid BHL which has been slow to subside, and especially in those who have also an indolent pulmonary infiltration. There is evidence that it occurs in the avascular hyaline connective tissue into which large parts of persistently enlarged sarcoid lymph-nodes may become converted. More rarely, minor focal calcification may occur in persistent lung changes, but it is uncertain whether this develops in hyaline tissue or in foci of necrosis. It remains possible that in some instances, calcification develops in caseating foci of pre-existing or concurrent mycobacterial tuberculosis.

Special radiographic techniques

Findings by computed axial tomography (CT) in intrathoracic sarcoidosis have been described by Solomon *et al.* (1979), Putnam *et al.* (1977), and Yotsumoto *et al.* (1980). Although it rarely showed lymphadenopathy in patients in whom it was not evident in radiographs, it might show enlarged nodes in sites difficult to explore by radiography. Solomon *et al.*, among 34 patients found lymphadenopathy by radiography in 15 and by CT in 16; enlarged nodes were found only by CT in the anterior mediastinum in four and behind the right main bronchus in three. Yotsumoto *et al.*, found that CT did not increase the number of patients found to have lymphadeno-pathy, but among 24 with lymphadenopathy showed affected nodes not evident otherwise in the anterior mediastinum in three, along the aorta in 13, and below the carina in nine. In the lungs, CT delineates the cross-sectional distribution of the changes, tending to be peripheral, and may define bullous changes and solitary nodules. Solomon *et al.* found bullae not otherwise evident by CT in four of their 34 patients; in three in which the radiograph showed short irregular lines at the bases, CT showed a coarse network suggesting honeycombing. Minor pleural changes were evident in the radiograph in nine and by CT in three more; in two of these, the CT appearances suggested small effusions. An incidental finding by CT was abnormal density of vertebral bodies in three cases; this remained unex-plained.

McKusick *et al.* (1973) noted that extensive uptake of gallium-67 in the lungs of a patient with recent active sarcoidosis diminished dramatically with clinical and radiographic improvement after treatment with predni-sone. Line *et al.* (1981) correlated gallium-67 scans with clinical radio-logical, functional and broncho-alveolar lavage findings in 41 patients with pulmonary sarcoidosis. Uptake was increased in 65%; it correlated only weakly with clinical radiographic and function test findings, but very strongly with the numbers of lymphocytes and of T-lymphocytes recovered by broncho-alveolar lavage. Gallium-67 uptake thus reflected the activity of T-lymphocytes in the lung process.

CHANGES IN RESPIRATORY FUNCTION

Many studies of respiratory function in pulmonary sarcoidosis (e.g. Riley *et al.*, 1952; Marshall *et al.*, 1958; Svanborg, 1961; Marshall and Karlish, 1971) were concerned with correlations with radiographic appearances, usually including appraisal of the amount of fibrosis. The abnormalities most often found in standard tests are diminution in total lung capacity and its subdivisions, mainly restrictive defect of ventilatory capacity, impaired gas transfer (diffusing capacity), and low compliance. Among patients with BHL alone, many give results within predicted ranges, and mean values are only slightly or moderately outside them, though a few show more severe deficits. Those with recent infiltration, usually with BHL, show only slightly more abnormalities. With increasing duration of apparently non-fibrotic infiltration, abnormalities tend to increase, and evidence of airflow limitation may be found. With the appearance of radiographic changes interpreted as fibrotic, abnormal results in one or more tests are found in nearly all, and mean values are well outside predicted ranges, though a few patients show little disability. But there are important exceptions to any generalizations. Young *et al.* (1966) drew attention to disparities between radiographic and physiological findings, reporting some patients with normal or only slightly abnormal lungs radiographically who showed considerable reduction in carbon monoxide diffusing capacity (DL_{CO}), and others with grossly evident pulmonary infiltration who had DL_{CO} within normal limits. And the wide variation in tests of function within a group defined on clinico-radiological criteria is illustrated by the findings of Sharma *et al.* (1966a) in 18 patients with BHL and radiographically normal lungs, among whom DL_{CO} varied between 42% and 115% of predicted values; one-third showed low lung compliance, and one-third high airways resistance. These discrepancies are not surprising, in view of the inconstant correlations between radiographic appearances and histopathology, noted above, and of the variability of distribution of histopathological change in relation to alveolar walls, airways and blood-vessels.

Studies in which it has been possible to correlate function tests with structural changes as shown by lung biopsy (Young *et al.*, 1967; Young *et al.*, 1968; Carrington *et al.*, 1976; Huang *et al.*, 1979) have shown more congruity. Young *et al.* (1967) performed open lung biopsies in 22 black patients within one week of a standard set of lung function tests. All were found to have a restrictive ventilatory defect, and most uneven matching of ventilation and perfusion; a diffusion defect was demonstrated in one-third.

Involvement of small airways was frequent. Granuloma density correlated with tidal volume, and, less, with minute volume and alveolar ventilation. Four patients with BHL and radiologically normal lungs had discrete granulomas, the profusion of which correlated with the severity of relatively minor functional defects. Young *et al.* (1968) performed percutaneous needle biopsies of the lung in 34 patients, and found granulomas in 95% of 22 with disease of less than one year's duration, and 45% of 12 with a longer duration; alveolar membrane thickening was frequently found. The only measures of function that correlated well with the severity of histological change were the arterial oxygen pressure (PaO_2) on exercise and the DL_{CO}; though there was some correlation of function test findings with radiographic changes, there was a large range of values in all radiographic groups. Carrington *et al.* (1976) in a review of lung biopsy findings in 47 patients with sarcoidosis and 13 with chronic beryllium disease found that the function tests that correlated best with pathology were PaO_2, alveolar-arterial O_2 differences and, less, DL_{CO}; among structural changes, interstitial cell infiltration correlated best with function test abnormalities. Correlations between radiographic appearances and both function and histopathology were poor, except in severe cases. Bronchiolar and peribronchiolar granulomas were common, and, as noted above (p. 108), granulomatous angiitis was seen in 42%; selective localization of granulomas at these sites seemed likely to affect V/Q ratios. In a systematic study, Huang *et al.* (1979) correlated the findings in open lung biopsies with lung function tests and radiographic findings in 81 untreated patients with sarcoidosis. The profusion of granulomas, and the extents of 'interstitial pneumonitis' (cellular infiltration of alveolar walls), of granulomatous angiitis, and of fibrosis were graded. Strong correlations were found between tests of gas transfer (DL_{CO} and PaO_2 on exercise) and granuloma density, interstitial pneumonitis and a composite estimate of overall pathology. There was no correlation between hypoxaemia at rest and any single test, or between lung function tests and grades of granulomatous angiitis. A composite estimate of function correlated very strongly with overall pathology, strongly with extent of granulomas and of interstitial pneumonitis, and less strongly with fibrosis. While there was a general correlation of the conventional radiographic 'stages' I, II and III with extent of granulomas and of interstitial pneumonitis and with pulmonary function tests, especially tests of gas transfer, there were important discrepancies, especially in 'Stage I'. While normal function tests and radiographically clear lungs were associated with minimal histopathological changes and no fibrosis, conventional 'Stage I' might be associated with extensive, possibly fibrotic, changes. Among function tests DL_{CO} correlated best with both pathology and radiology.

The high proportion of patients with apparently non-fibrotic sarcoidosis of the lungs who show low values for DL_{CO} was confirmed by Miller *et al.*

(1976) in a study of 25 patients with conventional Stage I and 19 with Stage II. In Stage I patients, mean values for static dynamic lung volumes and exercise arterial O_2 pressure were normal, but that for DL_{CO} was low. Mean values for all tests in Stage II patients were low. The transfer factor for carbon monoxide can be shown to be dependent both upon the rate of transfer of gas from alveoli into alveolar capillaries (the membrane component, D_M) and upon the rate of uptake by the red cells in the capillaries, the latter being chiefly dependent upon the volume of blood in the alveolar capillaries, Q_c (Roughton and Forster, 1957). Studies of the relative importance of these two components in small numbers of patients by McNeill *et al.* (1958), Bates *et al.* (1960) and Johnson *et al.* (1961) gave discordant results. Saumon *et al.* (1976) studied three groups of patients (i) 19 with BHL only, (ii) 49 with infiltration later shown to clear under corticosteroid treatment, and (iii) nine with infiltration possibly with radiographic evidence of fibrosis that proved unresponsive to treatment. Mean values for DL_{CO} were slightly but significantly reduced in groups (i) and (ii), and more severely in group (iii). In groups (i) and (ii), mean D_M was within the predicted range when related to body surface area, but reduced when related to estimated alveolar area, while in group (iii) both these measures of D_M were reduced. Mean Q_c did not differ from predicted in groups (i) and (ii), though five of the 49 in group (ii) had low values; Q_c was very significantly reduced in group (iii). It thus appeared that in groups (i) and (ii) the reduced DL_{CO} was due to low D_M, to V/Q inhomogeneity or to both of these. In group (iii) low Q_c was an additional factor, and the pattern of functional impairment became similar to that found in a group of patients with diffuse interstitial fibrosis.

Attention has been drawn to the functional effects of airway involvement in sarcoidosis by a number of investigators. Miller *et al.* (1974) studied 16 patients with fibrotic pulmonary sarcoidosis by conventional indices of airflow, flow-volume curves and nitrogen wash-out, and found that nearly all showed impaired distribution of inspired air and 75% airway obstruction. De Remee and Anderson (1974) reviewed 107 patients, 39 with radiographic changes of conventional Stage I, 14 Stage II, and 37 Stage III. Dyspnoea was noted in none at Stage I, three at Stage II and 19 at Stage III. It was associated with slowing of expiratory flow-rate and distorted radiographic patterns. Levinson *et al.* (1977) studied 18 patients, 16 with BHL and infiltration and two with chronic changes with bullae; all had low lung volumes, low DL_{CO}, and high static transpulmonary pressures. All showed abnormal small airway function by at least one test; upstream airway resistance was high in 16, closing volume was increased in 16; frequency dependence of compliance was found in eight. But only six showed a low FEV_1/FVC ratio, the lowest being 60%, and two, both with bullae, low airway conductance. That these changes could not be attributed to smoking was indicated by the observation that the proportions showing abnormalities were similar in the seven who were non-smokers and in the 11 smokers. Rizzato *et al.* (1980) investigated airway function in 25 non-smokers with sarcoidosis, most with conventional Stage III radiographically, and found evidence of increased resistance to flow in small airways in nearly all, and in large airways in some. In a group of 15 patients with chronic pulmonary sarcoidosis selected because they complained of exertional dyspnoea and wheezing, Sahetya *et al.* (1980) likewise found evidence of high resistance to flow in both small and large airways; seven of their patients were non-smokers. Of four patients with localized airway narrowings demonstrable by bronchography reported by Hadfield *et al.* (1982), the one with the longest history had a flow-volume loop suggestive of intrathoracic large airways obstruction, while the other three had loops typical of small airways obstruction.

Clinical evidence of haemodynamic effects of pulmonary sarcoidosis are considered in Chapter 15 (p. 346). Like other forms of pulmonary fibrosis, the fibrotic stages may give rise to pulmonary hypertension (McClement *et al.*, 1953; Svanborg, 1961; Emirgil *et al.*, 1969; Rizzato *et al.*, 1980), in the causation of which granulomatous angiitis is unlikely to be important. At the earlier stages, some elevation of pulmonary artery pressure in a few cases has been reported, but its relation to granulomatous angiitis is uncertain. Svanborg (1961) in his study of 37 patients found slight to moderate elevation of pulmonary artery pressure in eight of 15 with moderate to severe fibrosis, but no sign of right ventricular failure; in 11 with BHL and radiographical normal lungs, cardiovascular function was normal at rest and on exercise; and in 11 with non-fibrotic infiltration, the only abnormality found was slightly elevated pulmonary vascular resistance on exercise in four.

Changes in pulmonary function tests in the course of sarcoidosis, with or without corticosteroid treatment, show only partial correlation with changes in radiographic appearances. Marshall *et al.* (1958) found persistent reduction in DL_{CO} in five of six patients in whom infiltrations had resolved completely. Winterbauer and Hutchinson (1980) have reviewed some subsequent publications (Boushy *et al.*, 1965; Sharma *et al.*, 1966b; Stone and Schwartz, 1966; Emirgil *et al.*, 1969; Johns *et al.*, 1976; Colp, 1977). In general, vital capacity (VC) and DL_{CO} showed parallel changes, being discordant in only 5%. Among untreated patients, VC and DL_{CO} improved or showed no change in those who improved radiographically, while they showed no change or diminished in those with unchanging or worsening appearances, with the exception of a few with improved VC. Of those with radiographic improvement after corticosteroid treatment, 65% showed increase and 4% fall in VC, and 52% improvement and 10% fall in DL_{CO}; while of those with unchanged or worse radiographic appearances,

48% showed increase and 17% fall in VC, and 41% increase and 19% fall in DL_{CO}. Combining treated and untreated patients, 67% of those with radiographic improvement had a coincident increase in VC and 45% in DL_{CO}, and less than 5% a fall in either of these.

DIAGNOSIS OF PULMONARY SARCOIDOSIS

The diagnosis of sarcoidosis and the measures, including biopsy procedures, that may be useful in establishing it are considered in Chapter 26. The following discussion concerns only some points of differential diagnosis in patients presenting with widespread pulmonary infiltrations.

Infiltration with BHL

The differential diagnosis of BHL is considered in Chapter 5, p. 86. When typical BHL is accompanied by pulmonary infiltration, no difficulty arises. Other disesases that may present with enlarged hilar nodes and pulmonary infiltration include tuberculosis, fungal infections causing granulomatous inflammation, lymphomas, and lymphagitis carcinomatosa; but in all of these, clinical and radiological features generally differ from those typical of sarcoidosis.

A few patients with BHL and pulmonary infiltration present confusing combinations of features of sarcoidosis with others suggestive of mycobacterial tuberculosis. Most of those reported from North America are black (Haroutunian *et al.*, 1964), and in Great Britain many are of West Indian, Asian or African origin. These patients are usually symptomatic, with low fever, constitutional symptoms, slight dyspnoea and cough. The hilar lymphadenopathy has ill-defined margins in the chest radiograph, without the well-defined polycyclic outline more often seen in sarcoidosis, and is sometimes asymmetrical; and the infiltration may be patchy. Superficial lymphnodes, especially supraclavicular and axillary, may be enlarged. In lymphnodes removed for biopsy, and sometimes in lung, the granulomatous change is accompanied by some central necrosis, which may be called either granular necrosis or caseation, depending upon the histologist's final opinion. The skin may react to tuberculin. Acid-fast bacilli may be seen on microscopy, and perhaps one of a series of cultures produces a few colonies of mycobacteria. In the presence of findings of these sorts, especially positive cultures, a diagnosis of tuberculosis (defined aetiologically) is likely to be made, and the 'sarcoid-like' features attributed to an unusual reaction to a mycobacterial infection. But the Kveim test frequently gives a granulomatous response in such cases, and in some extrathoracic changes of 'sarcoid' type, such as uveitis and granulomatous infiltrations of the skin are present or appear during the later course. Faced with such apparently discordant features, observers who regard it as unthinkable that mycobacteria may have a role in the causation of sarcoidosis may (i) reject the diagnosis of sarcoidosis, in spite of overtly 'sarcoid' features, in favour of tuberculosis (Kent *et al.*, 1970); (ii) dismiss the isolated bacteriological findings as laboratory or other errors, and accept the diagnosis of sarcoidosis; or (iii) conclude that the patient is suffering from both tuberculosis, caused by *M tuberculosis*, and sarcoidosis, about whose causation they admit ignorance, apart from the certainty that it is not related to mycobacterial infection. Our view is that in cases in which clinical and radiological features of sarcoidosis with compatible histology on biopsy of affected tissue or a granulomatous response to a Kveim test are accompanied by isolation of *M tuberculosis* or other mycobacteria, diagnostic categorization should refer to both these features, leaving open the question of possible relationship between them (Chapter 23).

Hodgkin's disease and other lymphomas can cause hilar node enlargement, but the character of this is different from that of the BHL of sarcoido-

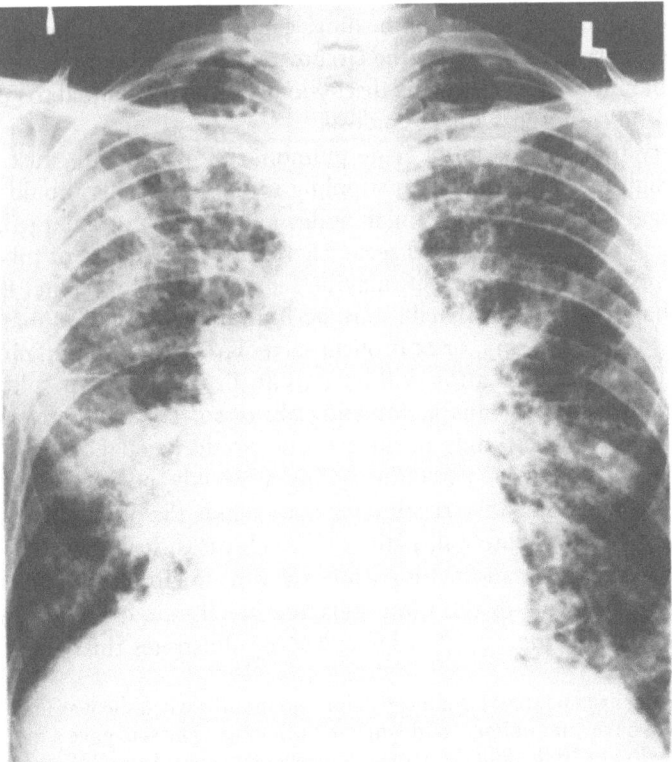

Figure 6.53 Lymphangitis carcinomatosa; note similarity to pattern of chronic pulmonary sarcoidosis shown in Fig. 6.18.

sis (p. 89); and although these diseases occasionally cause infiltrations of the lungs, these rarely have the widespread and generally symmetrical distribution of a sarcoid infiltration, and are likely to be accompanied by constitutional symptoms. Lymph-node biopsy is the definitive diagnostic procedure.

In lymphangitis carcinomatosa, the hilar nodes are generally bilaterally enlarged, and this with the widespread reticular and linear pattern of shadowing in the lungs may simulate the appearance of a diffuse sarcoid infiltration undergoing fibrosis with persistent BHL (Fig. 6.53). However, in lymphagitis carcinomatosa there will be a brief history of rapidly increasing dyspnoea becoming much more severe than would be expected with sarcoidosis causing a similar radiographic picture.

Infiltration alone

The list of conditions which may be considered from a radiological viewpoint in the differential diagnosis of widespread mottled, stippled or reticulo-nodular shadowing in the lungs can be extended with ingenuity to a great number; but in practice the circumstances of the individual case limit the probabilities. The following discussion is therefore limited to conditions likely to be confused with sarcoidosis.

Miliary tuberculosis in its acute pulmonary form should cause no difficulty. High fever with uniform stippling in the lung fields should immediately suggest that diagnosis; hilar nodes are usually not enlarged, though unilateral enlargement may be seen. There may be evidence of tuberculosis elsewhere. Choroidal tubercles may be seen. The cerebro-spinal fluid may show changes. Tubercle bacilli may be found on direct examination of a smear of sputum, if any, or of broncho-alveolar aspirate; but in most cases, bacteriological confirmation will have to await the results of cultures, and will therefore not be available for six weeks or so. Tuberculin tests may not be helpful; a very strongly positive result would be suggestive of miliary tuberculosis as against sarcoidosis, but a weakly positive result is not significant, and a negative result does not exclude the possibility of miliary tuberculosis in an acutely ill patient. In such cases, it is advisable to start antimycobacterial chemotherapy while awaiting the results of bacteriological cultures. But it is in the rarer subacute or chronic cases that difficulty arises. The following case (Scadding, 1960b) illustrates this:

A woman, aged 61, had been feverish for two months when she was first found to have faint miliary shadowing in both lungs. The skin gave a moderate reaction to 10 IU. Full doses of streptomycin, isoniazid and PAS were given, but fever persisted up to 101 °F (38.3 °C), the shadowing in the lungs became steadily denser (Fig. 6.54), and the early cultures failed to grow tubercle bacilli. After three months of apparently ineffective treatment, the

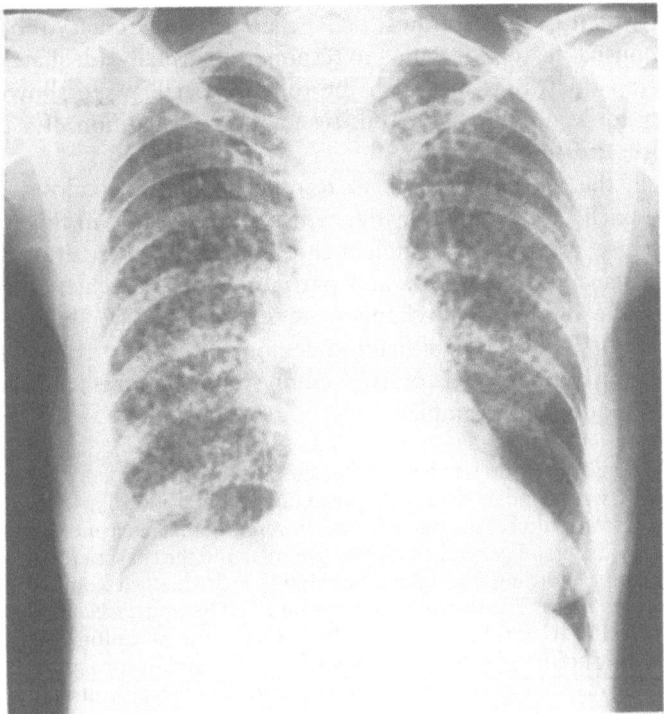

Figure 6.54 Chronic miliary tuberculosis in a woman aged 61, failing to respond to specific chemotherapy until prednisolone was added.

diagnosis was reviewed, and the possibility of sarcoidosis was considered. A liver biopsy showed many epithelioid and giant-cell tubercles without caseation. Prednisolone was added to the chemotherapy, with the thought that whether the disease was finally labelled sarcoidosis or caseating tuberculosis, corticosteroid treatment covered by effective antituberculosis chemotherapy was at that stage indicated. This was followed by immediate defervescence, and progressive clearing of the shadows from the chest radiograph. About this time, reports were received that cultures of two sputa collected six weeks previously had produced tubercle bacilli sensitive to all three drugs; and a choroidal tubercle was seen for the first time in the right fundus oculi. The prednisolone treatment was continued for six months and then gradually withdrawn without reappearance of the miliary shadows, and antituberculosis chemotherapy was given for a total of twenty months. The patient made a good recovery with slight dyspnoea on exertion and some reduction in the diffusing capacity of her lungs as the only residua of this remarkable illness. She remained well when last seen six years from the time of her first admission to hospital.

In this case, if less intense efforts had been made to find tubercle bacilli, or if it had happened that bacilli had not been found in the specimens examined, the diagnosis of sarcoidosis would certainly have been difficult to controvert. As it is, the case must be labelled subacute miliary tuberculosis with the unusual feature of failing to respond to normally adequate doses of chemotherapeutic drugs to which the tubercle bacilli were shown in the laboratory to be fully sensitive, but responding on addition of a corticosteroid to the treatment.

Although the apparent failure to respond to antituberculosis drugs to which the bacilli were fully sensitive which was observed in this patient is extremely rare, cases of very indolent chronic miliary tuberculosis with low tuberculin sensitivity and slow and partial response to chemotherapy as judged by the radiographic changes are rather less rare. In such cases, tubercle bacilli may be very difficult to demonstrate, being isolated in small numbers from perhaps one or two among large numbers of specimens cultured. To quote an example:

> A woman, aged 55, who had been rather short of breath with a dry cough for one month, was found to have widespread radiographic mottling in the lungs. Laryngeal swab cultures for tubercle bacilli were negative. Five months later, she remained in good general condition, afebrile, and the chest radiograph showed coarse mottling throughout both lungs, little changed from the initial findings (Fig. 6.55). The skin did not respond to 10 IU, and gave a moderate response to 100 IU of tuberculin. Liver biopsy was normal. Culture of gastric contents now produced a growth of tubercle bacilli. Antimycobacterial chemotherapy was followed by slow partial resolution of the lung infiltration.

In this case, the diagnosis of chronic miliary tuberculosis would not have been possible without the finding of tubercle bacilli, and these were found only after a large number of negative examinations. In the absence of this finding, the alternative diagnosis of sarcoidosis might well have been accepted, even after the rather slow and partial resolution which followed the antibacterial treatment. Thus the differential diagnosis between sarcoidosis and chronic miliary tuberculosis may involve an arbitrary element. If tubercle bacilli are found, the case would normally be called chronic miliary tuberculosis; if they are not found, there may be no factual basis for a decision whether to give it this label or label it sarcoidosis. The significance of this situation in relation to the problem of the aetiology of sarcoidosis is discussed in Chapter 25.

Pneumoconiosis should rarely be confused with sarcoidosis if a proper industrial history is taken. The special case of chronic beryllium disease which on a histological definition of sarcoidosis might be regarded as a variety of sarcoidosis whose aetiology is known, is considered in Chapter 22. In the common forms of pneumoconiosis, in addition to the history of exposure, the absence of hilar lymph-node enlargement, the uniform distribution of the radiographic shadowing, and in the case of some dusts, features that are associated especially with the relevant form of pneumoconiosis, may be helpful. On the whole, it is unlikely that changes discovered in the lungs of a man known to be exposed to dust will be misinterpreted as sarcoidosis; a more likely error is to misdiagnose changes in fact due to sarcoidosis as pneumoconiosis because the affected individual has been exposed to dust. Even if initial clinical examination does not reveal features discordant with the diagnosis of pneumoconiosis in such a case, the course of the disease, either to resolution of the radiographic changes or to their evolution in a way unexpected in pneumoconoisis, with possibly the appearance of extrathoracic manifestations, should eventually lead to the correct diagnosis.

Chronic phases of extrinsic allergic alveolitis (hypersensitivity pneumonitis), caused by hypersensitivity reactions to organic dusts in the pulmonary acini, may be confused with sarcoidosis. The first of these to be described was farmer's lung, due to exposure to mouldy hay (Fuller, 1953; Studdert, 1953; Dickie and Rankin, 1958; Hapke *et al.*, 1968). Acute and chronic phases can be recognized. Acute exposure leads after about six hours to tightness in the chest with dyspnoea but usually no wheezing, headache and fever with crackles at the lung bases, sometimes with widespread fine mottling of variable density in the chest radiograph. This illness usually clears within 24 hours, or longer in severe episodes, and is unlikely to be

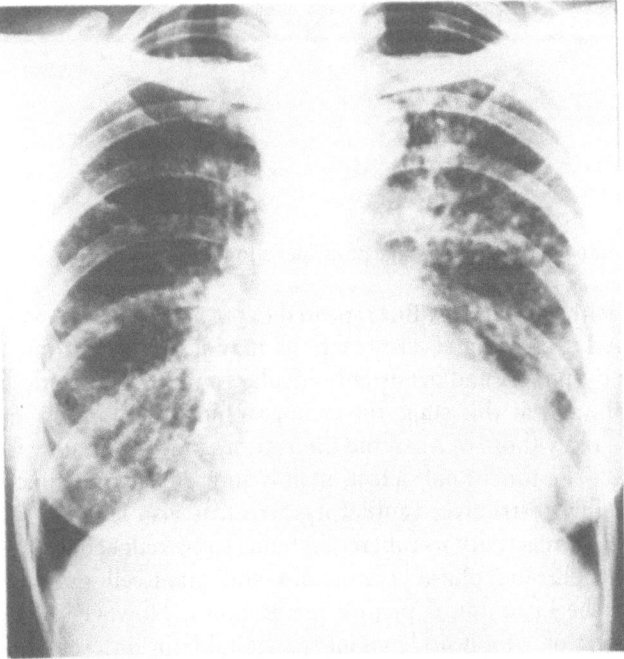

Figure 6.55 Indolent disseminated pulmonary tuberculosis in a woman aged 55, with a tuberculin reaction only to 100 IU.

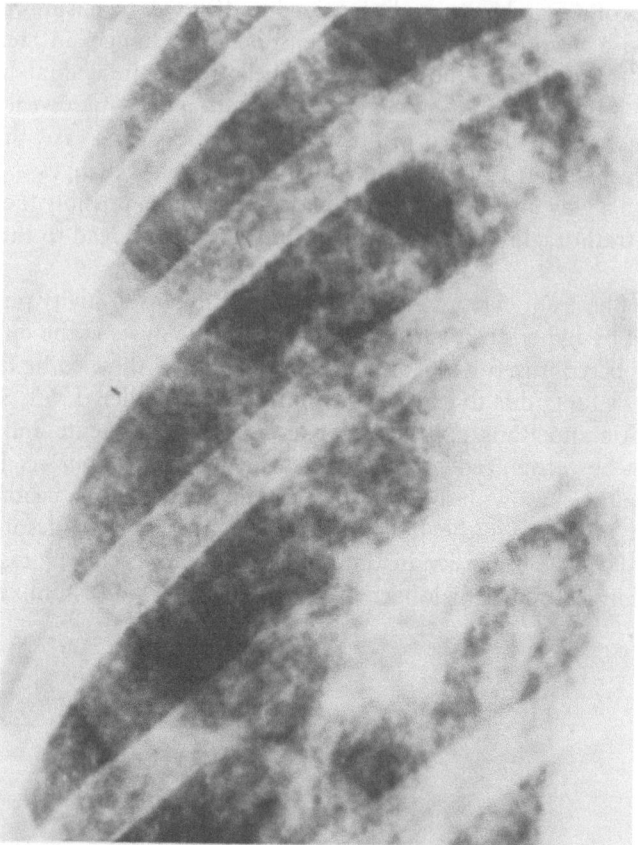

Figure 6.56   The chronic stage of farmer's lung.

confused with sarcoidosis. But repeated exposure, or heavy exposures leading to slowly resolving severe reactions may lead to a chronic stage, with
persistent dyspnoea, and persistent reticular or mottled opacities in the chest
radiograph, and at this stage the radiographic picture and symptoms may
resemble closely those of a sarcoid infiltration undergoing slow focal fibrosis
(Fig. 6.56). The functional defect, mainly in gas exchange function, with a
mixed, mainly restrictive, ventilatory defect, is also similar. Moreover, in
farmer's lung, reactivity to tuberculin tends to be reduced as in sarcoidosis,
and in the chronic phase, epithelioid and giant-cell granulomas are a
feature of the histological picture in the lungs. However, the absence of
extrathoracic or lymph-node changes is notable in differentiation; and an
occupational history is even more helpful in this group than in other
pneumoconioses, since there may have been acute episodes related to work
with mouldy hay. Precipitating antibody to extracts of mouldy hay or to

thermophilic actinomycetes which are the source of the causal antigen is demonstrable in the blood serum (Pepys *et al.*, 1962). Extrinsic allergic alveolitis has been described in response to a large number of other organic dusts (Pepys, 1977). Among these, those encountered as a result of exposure to birds, especially budgerigars which are kept as pets in the house (Hargreave *et al.*, 1966), and to air-conditioning contaminated by growth of moulds (Banaszak *et al.*, 1970; Sweet *et al.*, 1971), are especially liable to give rise to slowly progressive widespread fibrosis, since exposure is to small concentrations over long periods. This leads to changes mimicking those of chronic fibrotic pulmonary sarcoidosis (Fig. 6.57). Diagnosis depends upon the history, and the demonstration of precipitating antibody to the relevant antigen in the serum, though this may be found in some exposed but not affected individuals; and in doubtful cases carefully performed challenge tests (Hargreave and Pepys, 1972). A rare variety of extrinsic allergic alveolitis, that caused by pituitary snuff (Pepys *et al.*, 1966), is important in the differential diagnosis of diffuse lung changes accompanying diabetes insipidus, in which sarcoidosis must also be considered (Chapter 16, p. 350).

Pulmonary involvement in histiocytosis X (Thannhauser, 1950; Lichtenstein, 1953) has been reviewed by Lewis (1964b) and Basset *et al.* (1978). In its earlier stages, its radiographic appearances may mimic a sarcoid infiltration, though in its later stages it is one of the causes of generalized

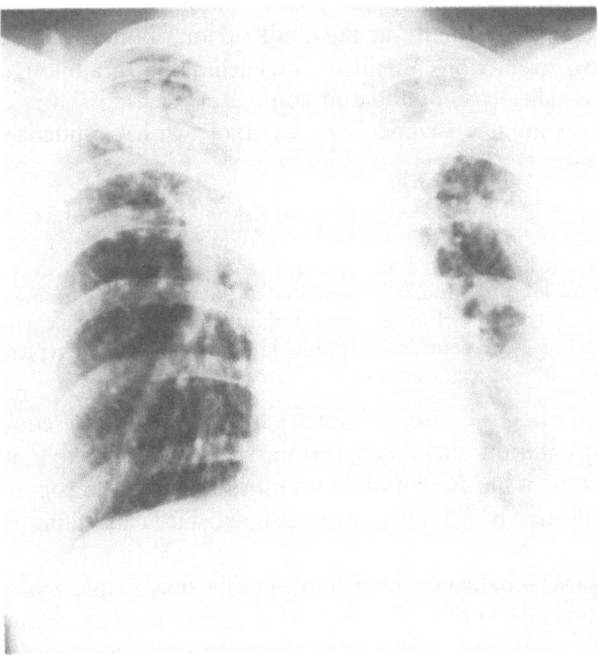

Figure 6.57   Budgerigar fancier's lung.

'honeycomb lungs' (Oswald and Parkinson, 1949; Parkinson, 1949), with distinctive radiographic appearances. It is a systemic disease, with possible involvement of several organs and tissues; from the point of view of the diagnosis of the lung changes, involvement of the bones is the most important association, though it is observed in only a minority of the cases that present with lung changes; even more rarely diabetes insipidus from pituitary involvement may accompany the changes in the lungs (Spillane, 1952; Grant and Ginsburg, 1955; Pongor and Viragh, 1959). In its early stages, pulmonary histiocytosis X shares with non-fibrotic sarcoid infiltration a relative paucity of symptoms, and indolent course; but while there may be long periods during which the condition remains stationary, progression to an irreversible 'honeycomb' stage at which respiratory function is inevitably impaired, is usual. At this stage, liability to recurrent spontaneous pneumothorax is characteristic. Before generalized honeycombing is evident, the points which may suggest the diagnosis of pulmonary histiocytosis X are the limitation of the lesions to the lungs, with the possible exception of certain bone changes or, rarely, diabetes insipidus; reactivity to tuberculin-type antigens is not impaired; and very often, even when the lung changes are first detected, there is at least a tendency to the development of multiple small cyst-like air spaces which eventually leads to the picture of widespread honeycombing. It is only in a minority of cases that bone changes will be present. These consist radiologically of localized well-defined rarefactions usually in the skull or long bones; histologically the areas of these rarefactions are filled with eosinophilic granuloma, composed of reticulum cells, eosinophils and some giant cells. If bone changes are present they enable a diagnosis to be made with confidence, as in the following case:

> A boy aged 18 had noticed excessive tiredness and slight loss of weight for one year. A chest radiograph (Fig. 6.58) showed widespread reticular shadowing. He said that he had had an operation four years previously for a cyst of the bone near the left hip. Inquiry showed that at this operation a granuloma had been curetted from just above the acetabulum, and the resulting cavity filled with bone chips, with satisfactory result. The curetting had the typical structure of an eosinophilic granuloma.

When, as is often the case, pulmonary histiocytosis X presents as the only clinical manifestation, diagnostic certainty may be attainable only by lung biopsy; recently, it has been found that ultrastructurally-recognisable histiocytosis X cells may be present in broncho-alveolar lavage fluid (Basset *et al.*, 1977).

A rarer variety of generalized honeycomb lung is that associated with mesodermal dysplasia of the type of which other manifestations are tuberous sclerosis, adenoma sebaceum, subungual fibromata and multiple tumours of the kidneys (Oswald and Parkinson, 1949; Dawson, 1954). It

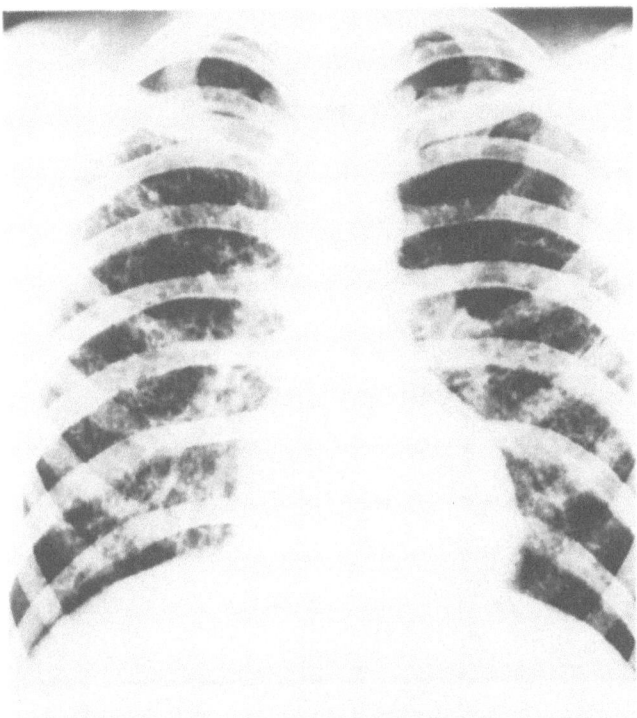

Figure 6.58 Histiocytosis X.

appears that with this condition, as with histiocytosis X, one of the possibly affected systems tends to be predominantly affected. Thus Dawson (1954) reported that of 72 patients in mental hospitals because of the effects of cerebral tuberous sclerosis, only one was found to have the lungs affected; while of 13 recorded cases with pulmonary changes, only three were mentally defective, one of them with fits, and two others had fits but were not mentally defective. In the later stages of the lung changes, with established honeycombing, confusion with sarcoidosis is very unlikely to arise; earlier, before the changes are so extreme, the radiographic appearances may be confused. The chief differential points are the absence of other evidences of sarcoidosis, and the possible presence of the typical rash of adenoma sebaceum on the face, of subungual fibromata, and of renal tumours demonstrable by pyelography.

Diffuse pulmonary alveolar fibrosis of unknown cause (cryptogenic fibrosing alveolitis, interstitial pneumonia) occasionally mimics pulmonary sarcoidosis. Rarely, it presents in an acute form (Hamman and Rich, 1944), which affects especially young adults. More frequently it is sub-acute or chronic (Grant *et al.*, 1956; Scadding, 1960) affecting all age-groups, but

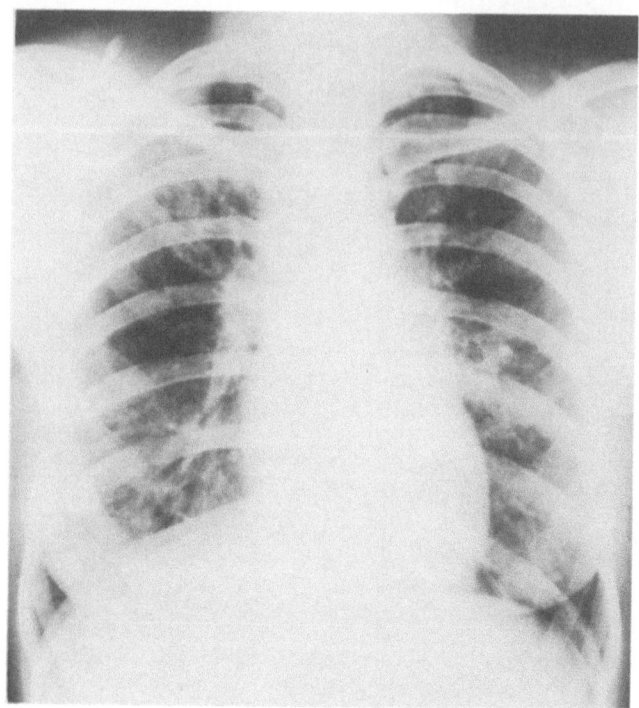

Figure 6.59   Cryptogenic fibrosing alveolitis radiographically simulating chronic pulmonary sarcoidosis.

most frequently middle-aged or older adults, and correlations between histopathological, clinical, radiological, functional, immunological and other features have been extensively studied (Liebow *et al.*, 1965; Scadding and Hinson, 1967; Carrington *et al.*, 1978; Turner-Warwick, 1978). Lung changes of this sort may occur in the course of a number of 'connective tissue' diseases, notably rheumatoid arthritis, systemic sclerosis, and Sjögren's syndrome, or be associated with various diseases of other organs having auto-immune features. It is principally the sub-acute or chronic cases, without evident systemic disease, which may be confused with sarcoidosis. Characteristically, the leading feature in such cases is increasing dyspnoea on exertion, out of proportion to the prominence of the radiographic changes; persistent fine to medium crackles are audible at the bases of the lungs; clubbing of the fingers, often gross, is often present by the time the patient first comes under medical care, and nearly always develops as the condition progresses; the radiographic appearances in the lungs, though variable, tend to be most prominent at the bases, and to have a fine reticular pattern, though there may be mottling or stippling with little suggestion of this pattern; and from the beginning, the functional picture is one of well-maintained ventilatory capacity, with a tendency to hyperventilation at rest and even more on exercise, impaired diffusing capacity, arterial hypoxia possibly at the rest and certainly after exercise with normal or low carbon dioxide tension. In such a typical case fibrosing alveolitis should not be confused with sarcoidosis. However, in a few cases, the earlier stages are less typical; clubbing may not develop until later, the radiographic shadowing may be distributed uniformly or even involve the upper parts of the lungs more than the lower, and the pattern of disordered function, while predominantly a diffusion defect, may be mild and compatible with a sarcoid infiltration.

Figures 6.59 and 6.60 show the changes over three and a half years in the chest radiographic appearances in a woman who initially complained only of a dry cough, and was found to have no abnormal physical sign except crackles audible over both lungs, no clubbing of the fingers, and a slight gas transfer defect with normal ventilatory function. Gradual deterioration with increasing dyspnoea was not arrested, though possibly slowed, by corticosteroid

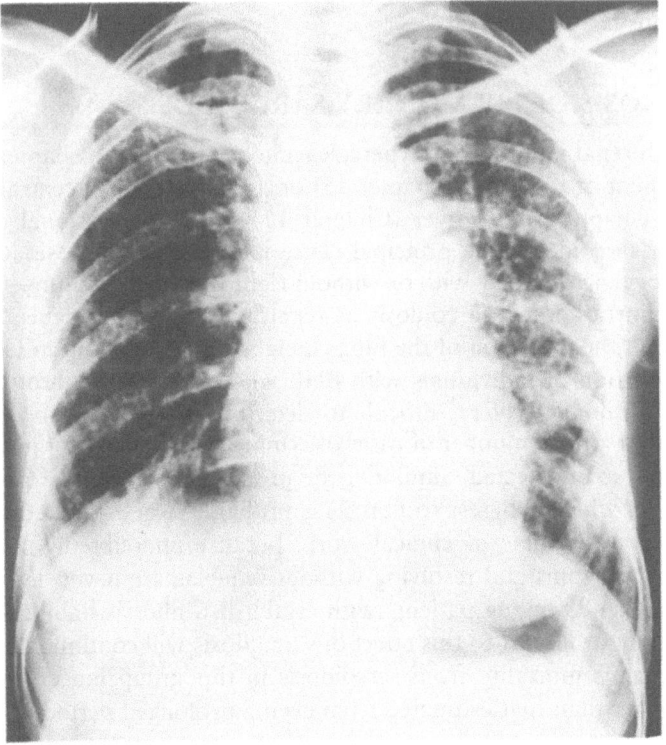

Figure 6.60   The same, three and a half years later, when the lungs showed 'honeycombing', and the clinical picture had become characteristic of cryptogenic fibrosing alveolitis.

treatment. Clubbing became evident five years from the onset; she died six years from the onset, and necropsy confirmed fibrosis alveolitis in an advanced 'honeycombed' stage.

In fibrosing alveolitis, broncho-alveolar lavage typically shows increase in the proportion of polymorphonuclear leucocytes, while in sarcoidosis, lymphocytes are increased (Chapter 20, p. 436). Transbronchial lung biopsy should serve to distinguish between fibrosing alveolitis and sarcoidosis, though open biopsy is more informative in the categorization of fibrosing alveolitis.

Blood-borne metastases of malignant tumours may be widely disseminated in the lungs, but usually cast shadows larger and more distinct than the elements even in the coarser sorts of mottling produced by sarcoid infiltration. Very occasionally, multiple small metastases from a tumour of low malignancy may produce few or no symptoms and grow extremely slowly, thus mimicking a sarcoid infiltration. Adenocarcinomas of low malignancy may present with pulmonary metastases of this sort, the primary tumour producing no symptoms and sometimes being discovered only at necropsy.

PROGNOSIS OF PULMONARY SARCOIDOSIS

Although renal failure from hypercalcaemic nephropathy (Chapter 19) and involvement of the heart (Chapter 15) or, more rarely, the central nervous system (Chapter 14) or liver (Chapter 11) are very occasional causes of death in sarcoidosis, the principal cause is pulmonary fibrosis leading to respiratory insufficiency with or without right ventricular failure. The prognosis of intrathoracic sarcoidosis as regards life therefore depends principally upon the evolution of the lung changes. As pointed out in Chapter 5, the proportion of individuals with BHL who develop pre-fibrotic infiltration of the lungs is very difficult to determine, principally because it is certain that a large number of cases of symptomless BHL must pursue their entire course undetected. Similarly, the proportion of cases of pre-fibrotic infiltration which progress to fibrosis is probably over-estimated by observations in the course of clinical work, because undoubtedly some cases without symptoms and resolving without sequelae are never detected. On the other hand, among patients with established fibrosis liability to death due entirely or in part to this effect of sarcoidosis will continue throughout life, and thus mortality from sarcoidosis in this group must be expected to be higher than that estimated from even a prolonged period of observation.

For these reasons, gross figures for mortality reported in different series have little meaning without knowledge of the way the series was collected, and the sorts of case included in it. Series collected from chest clinics dealing with a large number of out-patients will be likely to include more patients with symptomless pre-fibrotic changes, including BHL, and thus to show a lower mortality, than series composed of patients treated in hospitals. Thus, among 700 cases collected from records of chest clinics in Holland, Ten Have (1958) estimated mortality at only 2%; while Nitter (1953) found that of 90 patients observed in hospitals in Oslo, 13 (14.4%) died of sarcoidosis.

Carr and Gage (1954), using a life-table method, estimated survival rates for 194 patients, of whom only nine were black, studied at the Mayo Clinic. The ten-year survival rate was calculated to be 80%, as compared with 90.6% for an unselected population of the same age distribution. Of 17 known deaths, only three were known to be due to sarcoidosis and one to tuberculosis; eight were known to be due to unrelated causes; and in five the cause of death was not determined. The material upon which they based these observations was clearly not a representative sample, since their patients, with a mean age of just over 41 years, were on the whole older than those in other large published series. Moreover, they had been referred from a distance to the Mayo Clinic, and may therefore have contained a high proportion of the more severely affected. The first of these considerations, and probably also the second, would tend to cause their estimate to exceed the true mortality of sarcoidosis as a whole. Sones and Israel (1960), using a similar method, calculated that the survival rate for their patients ten years after diagnosis was 84.8%, compared with a normal expectancy for a population of the same age distribution of 95.2%, suggesting a mortality of rather over 10% from sarcoidosis within ten years. Their series included 184 blacks, among whom during the observation period 50 deteriorated and 20 died, whereas among 27 patients of European stock only four deteriorated and none died. This is in accord with the general impression that in North America the course is less favourable in blacks than in whites. They found fewer deaths among those with BHL only at the beginning of observation (5.6% of 71) than among those with BHL and infiltration (12.5% of 72) or with infiltration alone (12.5% of 56), but this difference did not attain statistical significance.

Smellie and Hoyle (1960) described the natural history of pulmonary sarcoidosis based upon the study of 125 patients observed in London for varying periods from two to more than 20 years. It may be calculated from their data that the mortality in patients who at first observation had, or subsequently developed, pulmonary infiltration was about 9%. Also in London, Scadding (1961b) assessed prognosis from a study of 136 patients all observed for at least five years. Thirty-two of them had had BHL only when first observed, and of these ten developed infiltration while under observation; 40 had BHL and infiltration, and 37 had infiltration only, making a total of 87 patients who were observed with apparently non-fibrotic lung changes. Of these 87, 25 were judged to have developed fibrosis by the end of five years' observation, and none had died within this time. Of 27 patients who had established fibrosis at the beginning of the observation period, when the estimated mean duration of the disease had already been five and a half years, six died of sarcoidosis during the five years' observation. From these two proportions it was deduced as a tentative estimate that between 6 and 7% of patients who came under medical observation with pre-fibrotic sarcoid infiltration of the lungs were likely to die of the disease within 10–15 years.

Among 617 patients with sarcoidosis, of whom 80% were black, observed by Johns *et al.* (1980) in Baltimore, between 1960 and 1977, there were 46 deaths, 39 of which were attributed to sarcoidosis. The localizations of sarcoidosis held responsible for death were the lungs in 31, the myocardium in five and the liver in four.

Factors affecting prognosis

Since lung changes are frequently the most important manifestation of sarcoidosis, the prognostic significance of involvement of other organs is of some interest. Sones and Israel (1960) in Philadelphia, and Smellie and Hoyle (1960) and Scadding (1961b) in London, correlated proportions showing spontaneous radiographic improvement in lung changes with the presence or absence of some common extrathoracic manifestations. In both the London series, the good prognostic import of an onset with erythema nodosum (Chapter 5, p. 93) was confirmed, as was the trend towards worse prognosis with greater extent of extrathoracic involvement. Smellie and Hoyle (1960), whose patients included an unusually high proportion with chronic ocular sarcoidosis, found that those with eye changes did worse than those without. Scadding's (1961) series, with fewer patients with severe eye changes, did not show this difference; but a significantly higher proportion of those with than of those without sarcoidosis of the skin failed to attain a clear chest radiograph. The conclusion that the presence of skin sarcoids implies a worse prognosis for the lung changes, while the presence of eye changes has little effect upon the prognosis for the lung changes, was in general agreement with the findings of Sones and Israel (1960). They found that the difference in prognosis between patients with and without cutaneous involvement remained significant regardless of race and involvement of other systems. Scadding (1972), reviewing a series of 500 patients of whom 82 had a sarcoid infiltration of the skin at some time during the observed course, found that these infiltrations fell into two groups in relation to their prognostic implications for the lungs. Large persistent infiltrations, including lupus pernio, were associated with chronic irreversible lung changes, only one of 35 patients with such skin changes showing radiographic clearing of lung changes; smaller transient skin sarcoids, subcutaneous nodules and infiltrations of old scars without other skin sarcoids were observed in 47, and did not affect prognosis, since in 21 of them lung changes cleared under observation. The rarity of erythema nodosum in patients with large persistent infiltrations (Chapter 7, p. 203), but not in those with other sorts of sarcoidosis of the skin, correlates with this difference in prognostic significance.

In a review of 2510 patients with chronic sarcoidosis, Wurm and Rosner (1976) found that prognosis for the lungs was worse with increasing age of onset; better in those who were initially tuberculin-positive; and better in those with normal gamma-globulin levels. It seemed to be little affected by sarcoidosis of the skin, but no distinction between various sorts of skin involvement was made.

In Scadding's (1961) study, there was a suggestion that those patients with infiltration and BHL did better than those with infiltration and no detected BHL; 58% of the former and 43% of the latter attained clear chest radiographs. Among those with BHL, the incidence of skin lesions was higher (20%) than in those without detected BHL (11%) a factor which, on the experience of the series as a whole, would have been expected to lead to a trend of prognosis in relation to the lung changes opposite to that which was actually observed. The incidence of eye changes was also lower in those without detected BHL.

Development of caseating tuberculosis

Many investigators in the past have agreed that a greater proportion of cases of sarcoidosis develop overt tuberculosis than would be expected among the population from which they are drawn, though the reported incidence of this event varies greatly. Ustvedt (1948), reviewing 59 reported necropsies in cases of sarcoidosis, found that tuberculosis was the cause of death in 11. Riley (1950) reported that 13 of 52 black patients with sarcoidosis in New York developed overt tuberculosis; and later Reisner (1967), also in New York, following 86 consecutive patients, of whom 80% were black, for a mean period of eight years found that 11 developed bacteriologically confirmed pulmonary tuberculosis and two others extra-pulmonary tuberculosis at intervals ranging from 2–21 years from the diagnosis of sarcoidosis. Sones and Israel (1960) reported that seven of their 211 patients developed tuberculosis, but Smellie and Hoyle (1960) observed this terminally in only one of 125 patients. Of 230 patients reviewed by Scadding (1960b), five produced overt evidence of mycobacterial infection during the course of sarcoidosis. On the other hand, and especially in more recent reports, many authors have reported that in their experience the incidence of mycobacterial tuberculosis in their patients with sarcoidosis was no higher than that of the population from which they were drawn. Figures of this sort are so dependent upon the criteria used for the diagnosis both of sarcoidosis and of tuberculosis that they are difficult to interpret without consideration of the individual case records. Reported associations between sarcoidosis and mycobacterial tuberculosis are reviewed in Chapter 23.

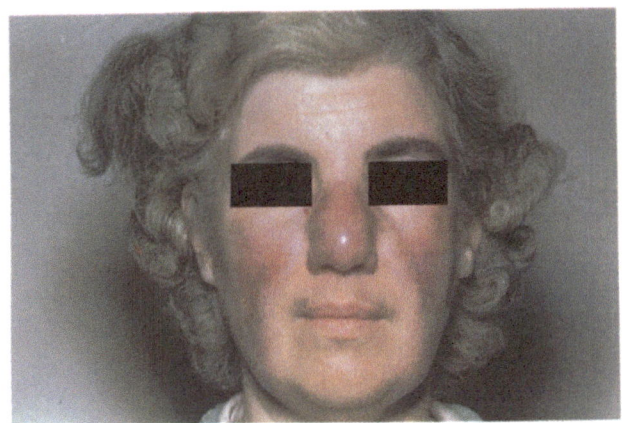

Plate 1

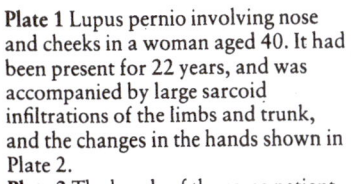

Plate 1 Lupus pernio involving nose and cheeks in a woman aged 40. It had been present for 22 years, and was accompanied by large sarcoid infiltrations of the limbs and trunk, and the changes in the hands shown in Plate 2.

Plate 2 The hands of the same patient, showing swellings of the second, third and fourth fingers on the right and the fifth on the left, with dystrophy of the nails of two of the affected fingers, and erythema and swelling of soft tissues of the dorsum of the right hand. Phalanges of the affected fingers showed lattice-like rarefactions.

Plate 3 Flat plaque of sarcoid infiltration on the shin; same patient as Fig. 7.7.

Plate 4 Indolent plaque of sarcoid infiltration on the ulnar side of the forearm of a woman aged 59.

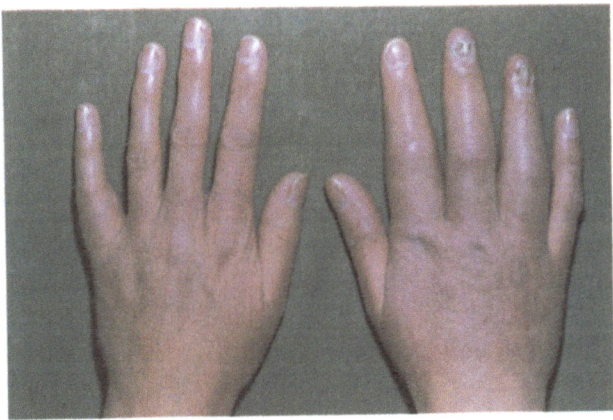

Plate 2

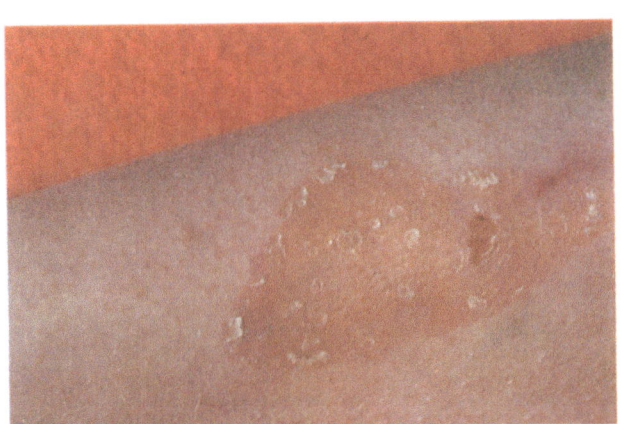

Plate 3

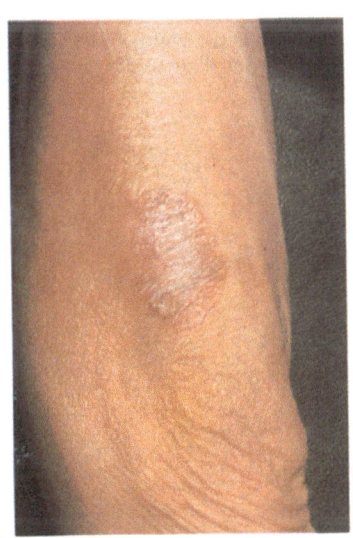

Plate 4

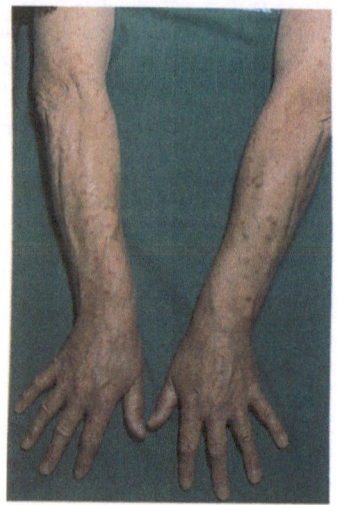

Plate 5

Plate 5 Multiple papulo-nodular
sarcoid infiltrations of the skin of a
woman aged 61.
Plate 6 The same, close-up view.
Plate 7 Papular sarcoid infiltrations in
the skin of the neck of a West Indian
woman, aged 37. These, with similar
papules on the eyelids, and small
infiltrations of the skin of the limbs
and of scars in the elbows and knees,
erupted six months after the
withdrawal of prednisolone which had
been given for one year for pulmonary
sarcoidosis.
Plate 8 Scarring at the site of a large
nodular sarcoid which had persisted
for 30 years before regressing
spontaneously; from the patient with
lupus pernio illustrated in Plates 1
and 2.

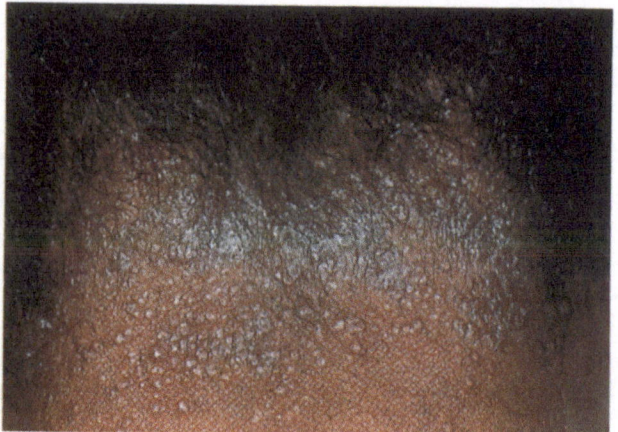

Plate 6

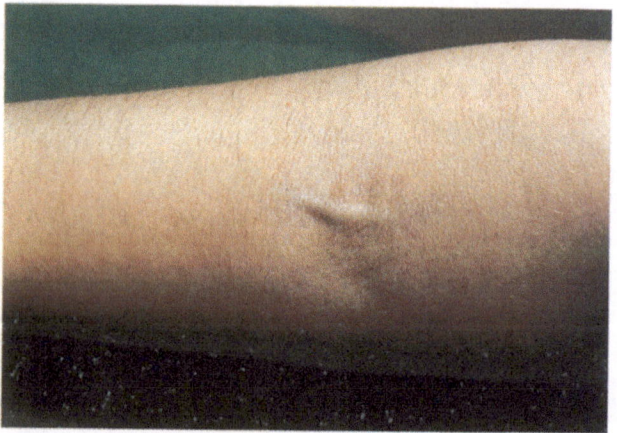

Plate 7

Plate 8

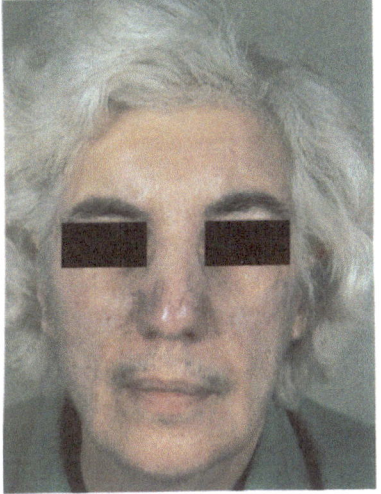

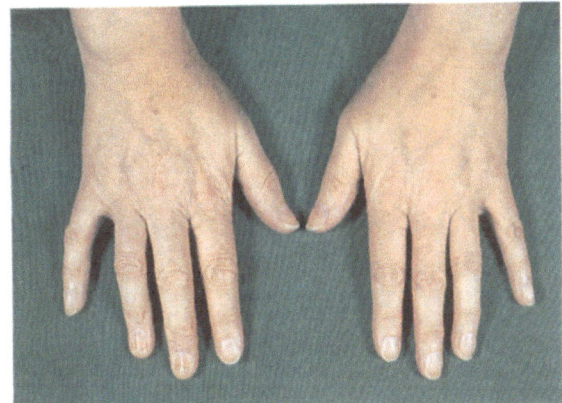

Plate 9

Plate 10

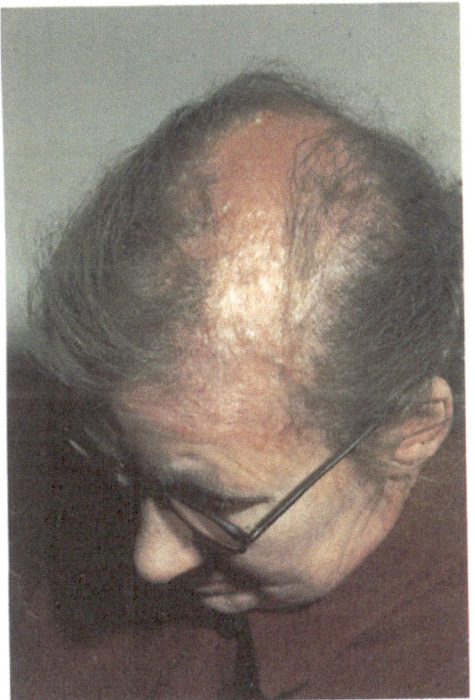

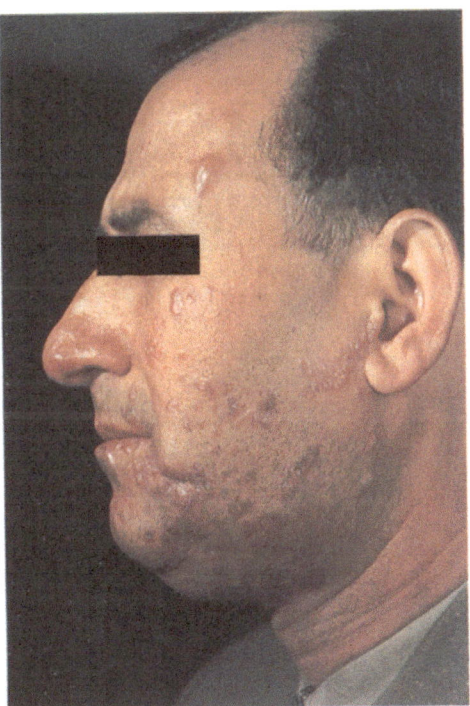

Plate 11

Plate 12

Plate 9 Slight scarring after spontaneous regression of lupus pernio; 16 years after Plate 1, and more than 30 years after its onset.

Plate 10 The hands of the same patient, showing resolution of the changes in fingers, dorsum of hand and fingernails shown in Plate 2.

Plate 11 Scarring of the scalp with alopecia where a sarcoid infiltration presenting no unusual features on the forehead has involved the hairy scalp; the patient also had multiple small sarcoid infiltrations of the skin of the trunk (Fig. 7.8).

Plate 12 Sarcoid infiltration of scars on the face resulting from explosion of a mine in desert warfare.

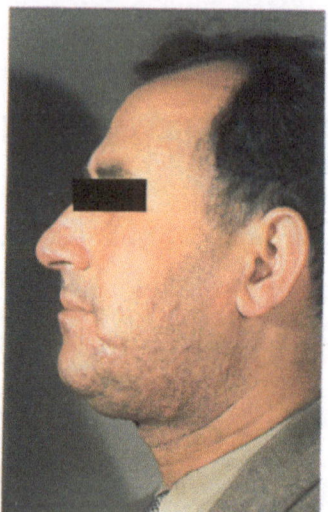

Plate 13

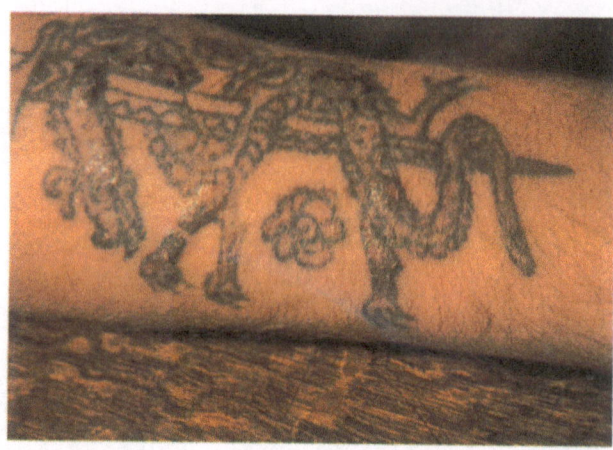

Plate 14

Plate 13 Spontaneous regression of the scar infiltration shown in Plate 12.
Plate 14 Nodules of sarcoid infiltration in a tattoo on the arm of a man aged 30, coincident with erythema nodosum and BHL.
Plate 15 Psoriasis in a woman aged 60; this disease had followed a typical variable course for 18 years.
Plate 16 Small sarcoid infiltrations of the skin which had been present for three months in the same patient; they were accompanied by a lung infiltration and splenomegaly.

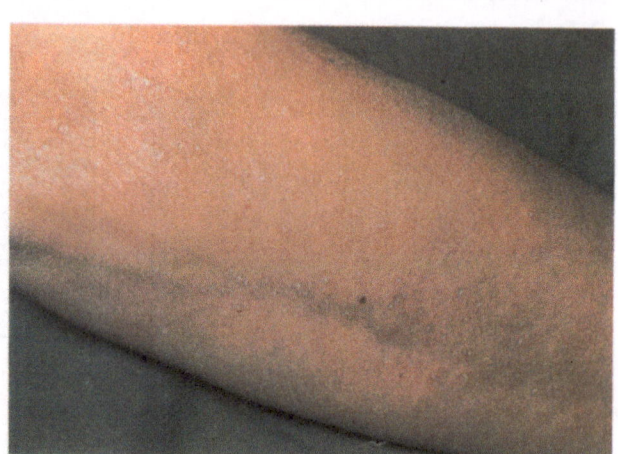

Plate 15

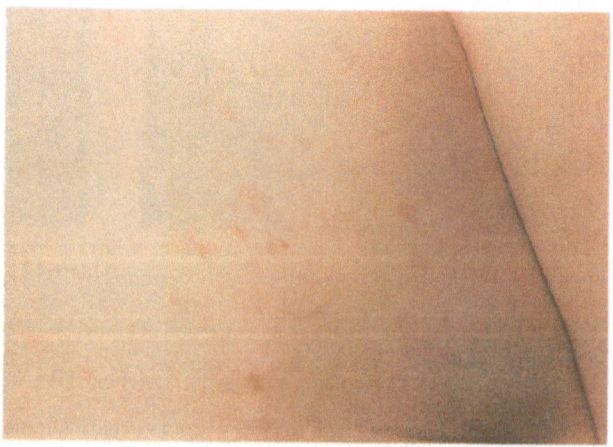

Plate 16

Chapter 7

Sarcoidosis of the skin

The history of our knowledge of sarcoidosis starts with the first descriptions of the skin changes (Chapter 1), and for a long time the disease was regarded as the special concern of dermatologists. Nevertheless, after Schaumann first pointed out in 1914 that lupus pernio and skin sarcoids were part of a generalized disease which might affect other organs without affecting the skin, it gradually became clear that sarcoid infiltrations of the skin occur in only a minority of detected cases of this disease, in some as the presenting or most prominent feature, but in most as part of a complex clinical picture.

A sharp distinction must be drawn between the infiltrations of the skin by sarcoid granulomas discussed in this chapter, and the erythema nodosum that occurs in some cases of sarcoidosis, usually at the onset, and is indistinguishable histologically from erythema nodosum associated with other diseases (Chapter 5). Skin infiltrations and erythema nodosum seem to have different places in the evolution of sarcoidosis; inter-relations between the various sorts of skin infiltration and erythema nodosum are considered below (p. 203).

FREQUENCY OF SKIN INFILTRATION

As with other manifestations, the proportion of cases of sarcoidosis found by an observer to have skin changes varies with the source of his patients. Among the 142 cases reported from two hospitals by Longcope and Freiman (1952), 22.5% of those seen at the John Hopkins Hospital, Baltimore, had skin lesions, while at the Massachusetts General Hospital, where many patients were referred from a skin clinic, the proportion with skin lesions was 63.4%. Among 212 cases of 'primary' pulmonary sarcoidosis – i.e. BHL with or without infiltration of the lungs – reported by Löfgren (1953) in Stockholm, only four were found to have infiltration of undamaged skin, four infiltration of scars, and two subcutaneous nodules; this low incidence is clearly related to the early stage of the disease at which these patients were observed. James (1959b) found that among 200 patients with sarcoidosis in London, 27 (13.5%) had skin lesions and six infiltration of scars. Smellie and Hoyle (1960) reported a similar incidence in London patients, 17 (14%) of 125 patients having shown skin changes. Sones and Israel (1960) in Philadelphia found that 26.5% of their 211 patients had skin involvement. A high proportion of the Philadelphia patients (87%) were blacks, among whom skin involvement was especially frequent, occurring in 28.8% of them, as compared with 11.1% of other patients.

In 500 patients observed for periods of up to 20 years, Scadding (1972), working at both a general and a special chest hospital, observed granulomatous infiltrations of the skin at some time during the course of sarcoidosis in 82 (16.4%). They were present at the time of first diagnosis in 49 (9.8%), but only 26 of these patients (5.2% of the whole series) sought medical advice because of the skin changes; in the remaining 23, the skin changes were incidental findings, sometimes unnoticed by the patient. In 33 (6.6%) skin infiltrations appeared in patients already under observation with sarcoidosis (Table 7.1). Stahl *et al.* (1980) reported a series of 125 patients with biopsy-confirmed sarcoidosis referred to a dermatological clinic in Denmark; every abnormality found on scrutiny of the entire skin surface and suspected to be a sarcoid infiltration was examined by biopsy. The selected character of this series is indicated by the fact that in 30 patients, the skin changes were the only clinically apparent localization; and in view of this, and the intensive investigation, it is not surprising that as many as 80 (64%) were found to have skin infiltrations of various sorts.

Table 7.1   Skin infiltrations observed in 82 of a series of 500 patients with sarcoidosis, listed by principal morphological type and time of appearance during the course of the disease (Scadding, 1972).

	At onset		Appeared during observation	Total
	Presenting	*Incidental*		
Lupus pernio	7	1	3	11
Plaques	3	1	5	9
Large nodular infiltrations	5	2	8	15
Small nodular infiltrations	3	9	12	24
Subcutaneous nodules	5	3	1	9
Scar infiltration	3	7	4	14
Total	26	23	33	82

There is a general tendency for most varieties of sarcoid infiltrations of the skin to occur in rather older patients than other common manifestations of sarcoidosis; and for some of the more chronic varieties to affect women more frequently than men, especially in those of Caucasian stock. Because there is evidence that these tendencies differ for different types of skin infiltration, age- and sex-distribution will be discussed after the commoner morphological patterns of skin infiltration have been described. This description is complicated by the wide variety of these patterns, the varied terminology, and the not infrequent concurrence of more than one of them in the same patient. Occasionally, sarcoidosis of the skin mimics a common skin disease, and a number of cases have been reported under names which refer to this resemblance.

MORPHOLOGICAL PATTERNS OF SKIN SARCOIDOSIS

The commoner patterns of sarcoid infiltration of the skin may be described under the headings lupus pernio, the separate description of which is justi-fied both historically and by its distinctive and easily recognized features; nodular infiltrations, which are of varying size and shape, slightly raised, with a variably defined margin, both visible and palpable, usually dis-coloured, and sometimes with epidermal scaling or desquamation; plaques, which are flat discoid lesions, sometimes with a raised infiltrated margin, when they may be described as annular; papules, which are small well-defined, palpable, slightly elevated thickenings of the epidermis or upper dermis; subcutaneous nodules, which are palpable and may be visible under normal overlying skin; and infiltrations of old scars. A number of rarer patterns, some simulating common skin diseases, have also been described; in such cases diagnosis is dependent entirely upon biopsy.

Most patients with skin sarcoidosis show a fairly uniform morphological pattern, but a minority show lesions of more than one type. Among the 82 reported by Scadding (1972), 17 showed mixed patterns. Lupus pernio and large nodular infiltrations were more frequently associated than other pat-terns of infiltration of unscarred skin, whereas plaques and small nodular infiltrations tended to be the sole pattern. Scar infiltrations were sometimes associated with infiltrations of unscarred skin, and these might be of any pattern.

Lupus pernio

The chilblain-like swellings of lupus pernio may affect the face, the hands or the feet. Fully developed lupus pernio of the face presents a striking appear-ance (Plate 1). It affects the nose, the cheeks, especially over the cheekbones, sometimes the forehead and the ears. The affected parts are greatly swollen, of livid purple-red colour, with a shining surface, often with dilated venules especially over the bulbous tip of the nose. The margins of the affected area are moderately well defined, giving place over a zone of diminishing infiltration only a millimetre or so wide to normal skin. To the touch, their consistence varies; commonly they feel firm, blanching momentarily after pressure, and giving an impression of a thin superficial soft vascular layer overlying deeper induration. Some scaly desquamation may be seen, and there may be a few small superficial erosions. On the hands and feet, similar changes in the skin may occur, especially over the dorsal surfaces; affected digits may be swollen (Plate 2). Phalanges of swollen parts of digits usually show radiographic evidence of sarcoid changes (Chapter 9, p. 231), with multiple lattice-like rarefactions. When the terminal phalanx of a digit is involved, the nail usually becomes thickened, opaque and brittle, ridged and deformed. Lupus pernio of the face is often associated with granulomatous changes in the nasal mucosa and nasal bones (Chapter 13 p. 292).

Lupus pernio is typically a persistent and slowly-evolving eruption, and associated with chronic manifestations of sarcoidosis elsewhere. Not surprisingly, it is the first overt evidence of sarcoidosis in a high proportion of those suffering from it.

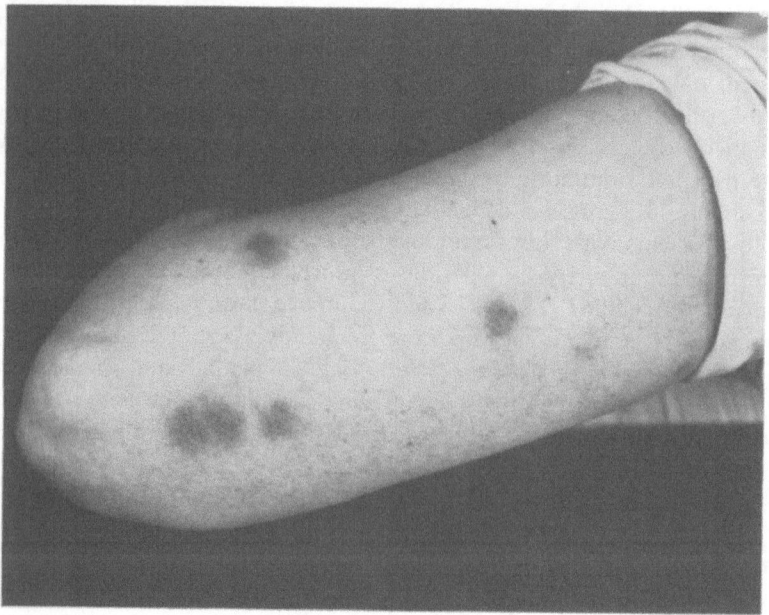

Figure 7.1   Nodular sarcoid infiltrations of the skin of a woman aged 30. Similar lesions were present on all four limbs.

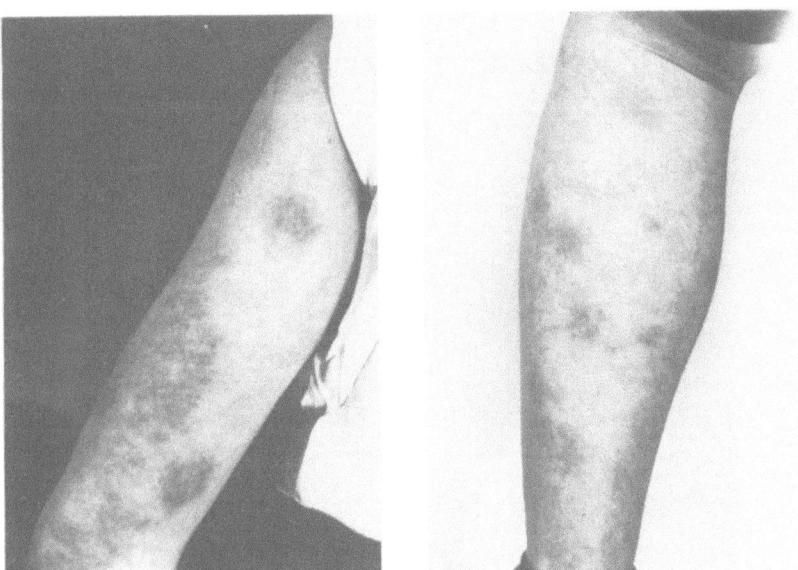

Figure 7.2 Multiple sarcoid infiltrations of the skin at various stages of their evolution in a woman aged 35.

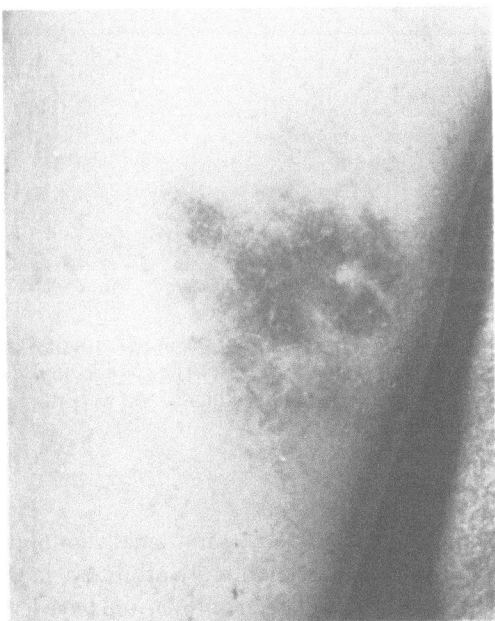

Figure 7.3 Sarcoid infiltration with irregular outline on the upper arm of a woman aged 41.

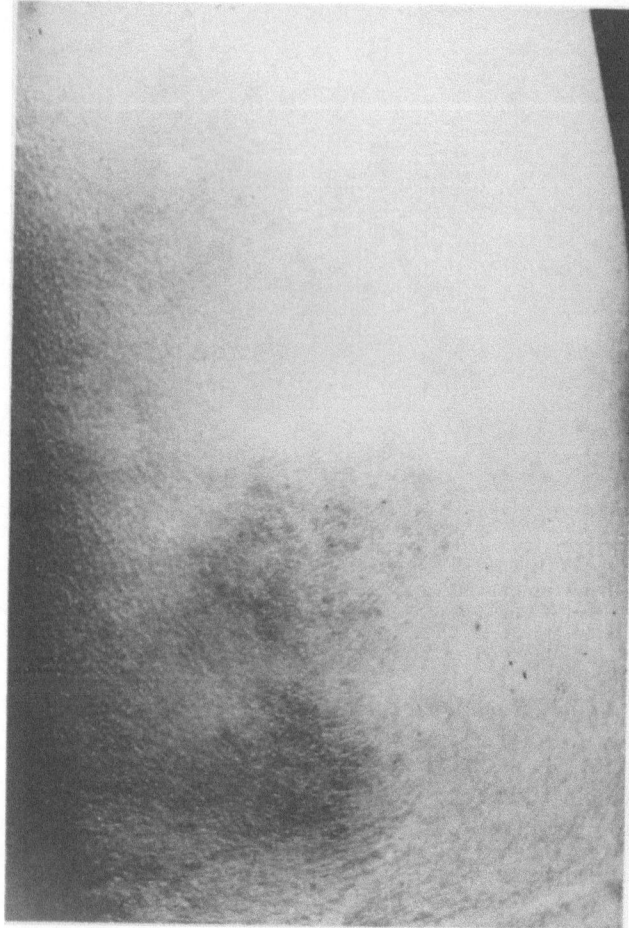

Figure 7.4   Sarcoid infiltration of the skin of the upper arm of a woman aged 44 who also had mild lupus pernio of the nose. The changes in the upper arm were evident only as an irregular area of erythema, and were not palpable.

Large nodular infiltrations

It is useful to distinguish between large and small nodular infiltrations. Although the distinction by size is admittedly arbitrary, large infiltrations tend to be deeper, and may be irregular in outline, and have less well-defined margins than those less than 1 cm in diameter; and there is evidence, outlined below, that the prognostic significance of large and small nodular infiltrations is different.

Large nodular infiltrations are observed most frequently on the proximal parts of the limbs, the buttocks, the trunk, and the face, usually multiple and often scattered over several sites. They are raised above the surrounding normal skin and usually palpable. They may be fairly regular in outline, round or oval and of uniform colour. When such infiltrations first appear their surface is pink or red and smooth; later it becomes brownish- or purplish-red with fine superficial desquamation (Fig. 7.1). On the limbs they may undergo a slow evolution, and some may resolve while others appear, infiltrations at different stages of their evolution being present at the same time (Fig. 7.2). Sometimes, especially when they involve soft skin and subcutaneous tissue, such as that of the upper arms, they are irregular in shape and present a mottled appearance (Fig. 7.3), and may be impalpable (Figs. 7.4 and 7.5). When skin overlying bone, with less subcutaneous fat, is involved, the infiltrated area is flat, as in Fig. 7.6, which shows an infiltration of the forehead of the same patient as Fig. 7.7. Infiltrations of this sort merge imperceptibly into plaques.

Plaques

A plaque is generally rounded or oval in shape, sometimes with a slightly irregular edge. At the periphery is a narrow rather nodular slightly raised rim, of a pinkish-brown colour, generally darker than the normal skin, and sometimes with a little scaling. Within this the skin is soft and smooth and

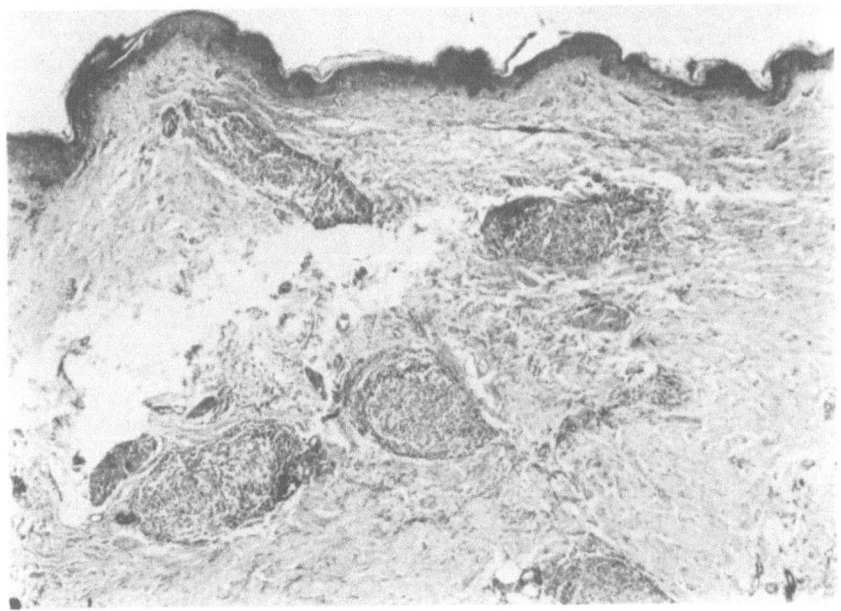

Figure 7.5　Biopsy of the infiltration shown in Fig. 7.4. H & E. × 38.

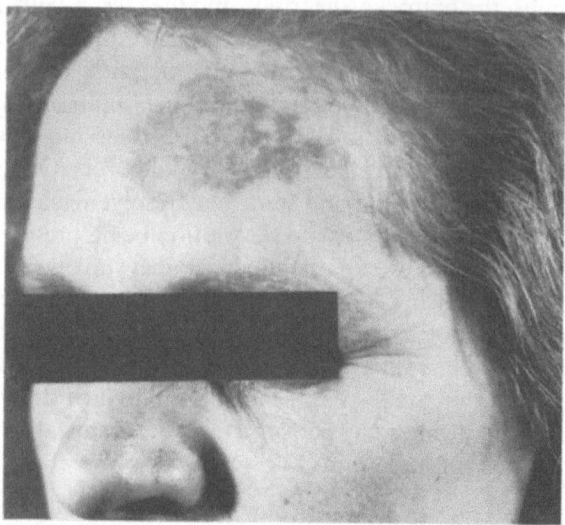

Figure 7.6   Infiltration of the skin of the forehead and of the tip of the nose in the patient whose upper arm is illustrated in Fig. 7.3.

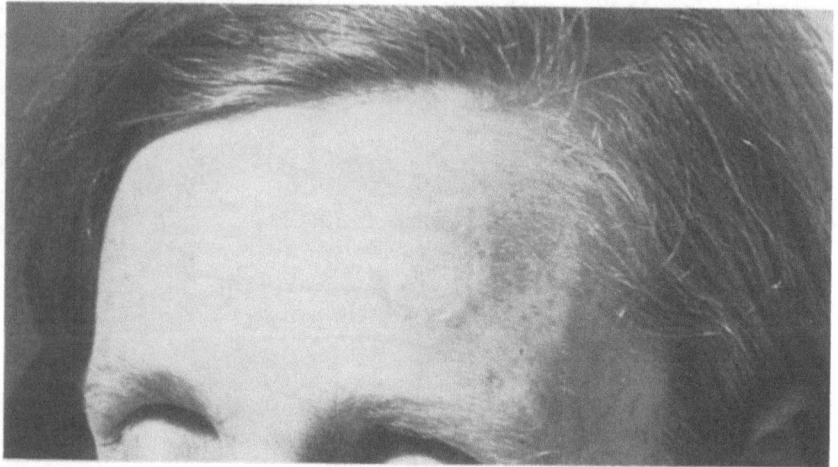

Figure 7.7   Sarcoid infiltration of the skin of the forehead of a woman aged 45, in the form of a slowly spreading plaque with a raised nodular rim.

does not feel infiltrated, but is a little thinner and paler in colour than the normal skin. It looks as though the plaque has started as a small superficial infiltration which has extended centrifugally, clearing centrally with a little atrophic scarring as it spreads peripherally. Pautrier (1940) described and illustrated this sort of lesion, and regarded it as a late stage of

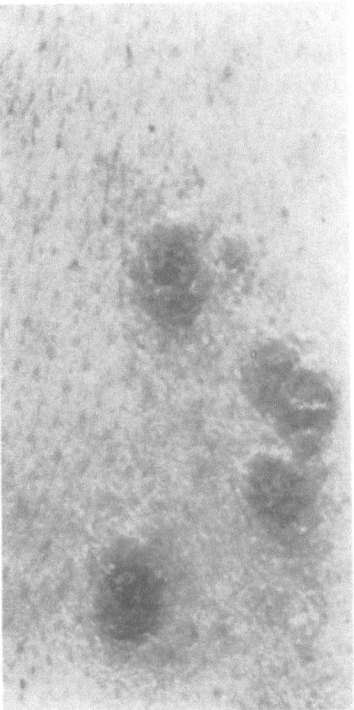

Figure 7.8   Small sarcoid infiltrations of the skin of the back of the trunk of a woman aged 54, who also had a plaque on the forehead extending into the scalp (Plate 11).

a large nodular infiltration; but we have not observed a large nodular infiltration evolve into a plaque. Although this sort of sarcoid infiltration occurs most frequently in skin overlying bone, especially on the forehead (Fig. 7.7), the shins (Plate 3) and the ulnar side of the forearm (Plate 4), they may be seen elsewhere. The resemblance of this sort of infiltration to granuloma annulare, and, more remotely, to necrobiosis lipoidica, may give rise to diagnostic difficulty, discussed below (p. 200).

Small sarcoid infiltrations

Sarcoid infiltrations of below 1 cm in diameter vary widely in number, in conspicuity and in distribution. Characteristically, they start as smooth pinkish slightly raised areas, and later become brownish-pink with some superficial scaling. They may accompany larger infiltrations. Figure 7.8 shows small nodular sarcoids of the skin of the back, which accompanied

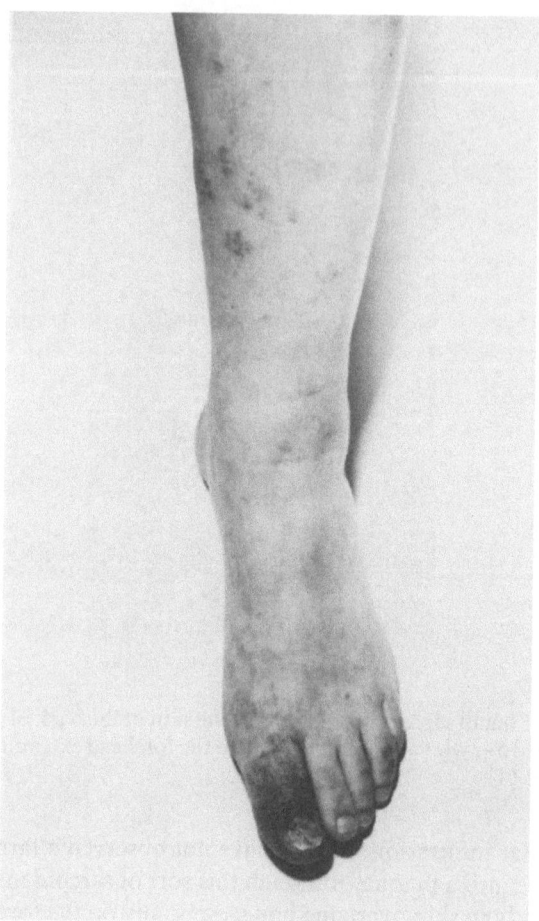

Figure 7.9   The left foot and lower leg of a woman aged 42, showing lupus pernio of the great toe and small sarcoid infiltrations of the skin of the lower leg.

the large plaque on the forehead and scalp of a woman aged 54, illustrated in Plate 11; and Fig. 7.9 small sarcoids of the lower legs and lupus pernio of the great toe in a woman aged 42 who also had lupus pernio of the nose. When small nodular infiltrations are the only form of skin sarcoidosis, they tend to be less persistent than large infiltrations, and may appear in crops.

Infiltrations of this sort may be numerous and widely scattered (Plates 5 and 6). In some cases they appear as closely-packed papules in such areas as the eyelids and adjacent areas and along the hairline (Plate 7). But they may be sparse (Fig. 7.10) and inconspicuous, appearing as a few insignificant-looking papules or even macules, and detectable only by careful inspection and palpation, followed by biopsy of suspected areas (Figs. 7.11 and 7.12.)

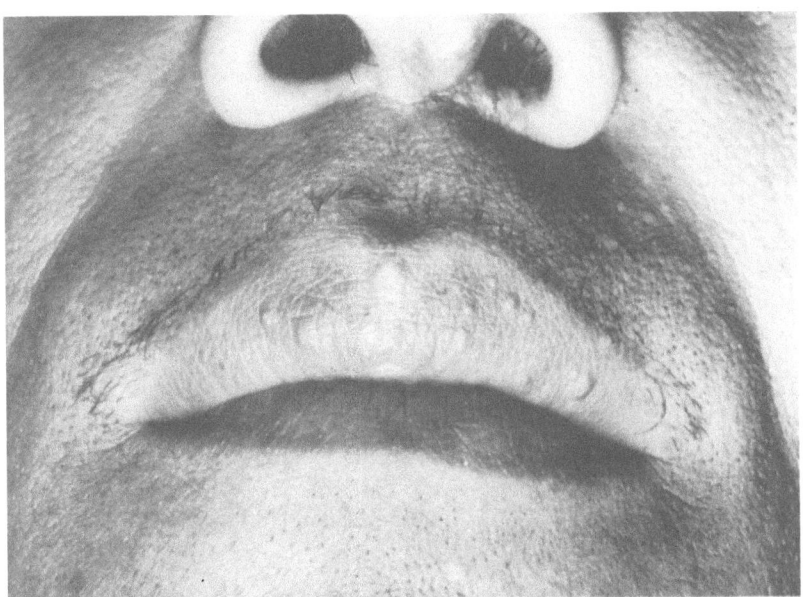

Figure 7.10 Papular sarcoid infiltrations on the upper lip involving also the left nostril in a West Indian aged 40.

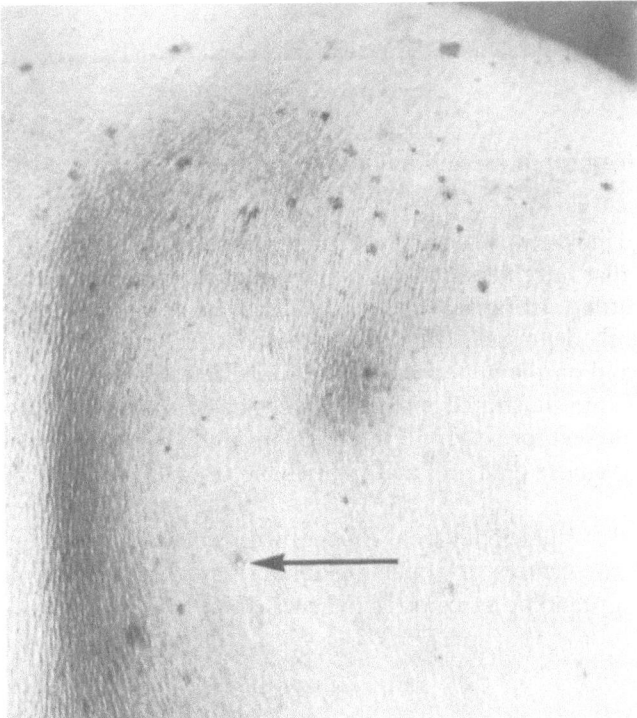

Figure 7.11 Small papular sarcoids on the back of a sandy-haired man aged 33. The most prominent is marked with an arrow. At first sight, they were easily missed among the freckles.

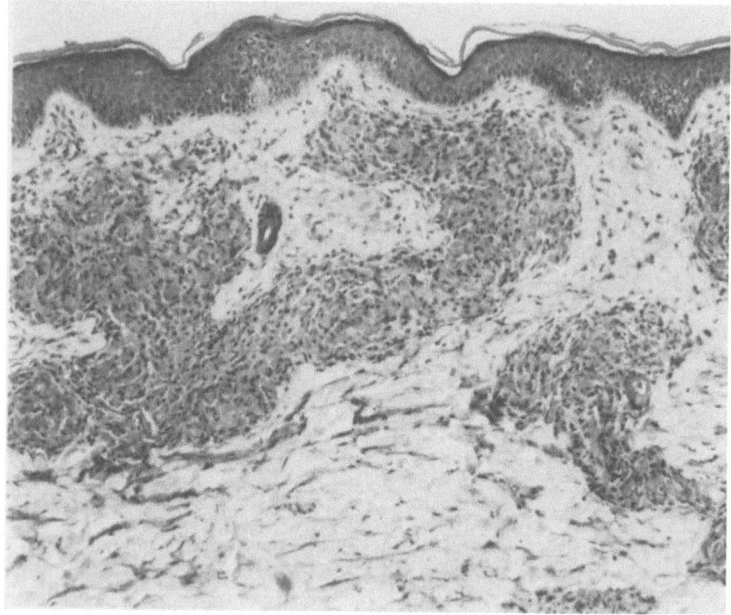

Figure 7.12   Biopsy of one of the papular sarcoids shown in Fig. 7.11. H & E. × 100.

Occasional features of sarcoid infiltrations of the skin

Scarring

Small sarcoid infiltrations generally resolve without scarring, and even large infiltrations that have persisted for long periods may eventually heal with remarkably little scarring, leaving only a slightly atrophic pale area of skin, possibly slightly depressed. Plate 8 shows such a scar at the site of a large nodular sarcoid on the upper arm of the sort illustrated in Plates 1 and 2. The lupus pernio illustrated in these plates subsided spontaneously after having been present for nearly 30 years, leaving only slight atrophic scarring at the tip of the nose (Plate 9), and virtually no residue on the hands (Plate 10).

Widespread atrophic epidermal changes with some telangiectasis, of the type seen at the centres of annular plaques, may occur in patients with extensive long-standing sarcoidosis (Michel *et al.*, 1968; Chevrant-Breton *et al.*, 1977).

Ulceration

Ulceration is exceptional, apart from superficial erosions on extensive infiltrations of the lupus pernio and larger nodular types.

There are a few reports of deeper ulceration of exuberant sarcoid infiltrations of the skin. As noted in Chapter 1 (p. 3). Besnier's original patient with lupus pernio showed extensive ulceration of affected parts of the ears; no histological studies were made. Schaumann (1924) observed ulceration of lupus pernio on the face in two patients from the northern, coldest part of Sweden. Ulceration in extensive sarcoids of the skin of the face and limbs in black patients has been reported by Cottenot *et al.* (1977) and Schiffner and Sharma (1977).

Ulceration in sarcoids of the lower leg has been reported by Simpson (1963), Brodkin (1969, two cases) Bazex *et al.* (1970), Hopf and Krebs (1974), and Meyers and Barsky (1978). In some of these cases, it seems likely that hypostasis was a factor in determining ulceration. One of Brodkin's patients, a black woman aged 52, had had persistent swelling of one leg since pregnancy at the age of 20. Simpson's patient was a man aged 66 with extensive lymph-node sarcoidosis, who had had oedema of the feet for several months before painful ulcers whose base was shown to consist of sarcoid tissue appeared on the lower legs; he also had large sarcoid plaques on the thighs. In the cases reported by Bazex *et al.* and by Hopf and Krebs, ulcerations developed in long-standing sarcoid infiltrations in women aged 62 and 63. On the other hand, in the case reported by Meyers and Barsky, painful ulcerating sarcoids appeared in the pretibial areas in a black woman aged 35 with a three year history of sarcoidosis of the skin of the face and uveitis shortly after cessation of corticosteroid treatment which had controlled the uveitis.

In some of the reported cases with ulceration, there has been an admixture of features of sarcoidosis with those of caseating mycobacterial sarcoidosis.

Multiple papular infiltrations, in places coalescent, with irregular small ulcerations, simulating papulo-necrotic tuberculides were described by Irgang (1955) in a black woman, aged 25, who also had some subcutaneous nodules, splenomegaly, peripheral lymph-node enlargement, and lung changes. The diagnosis of sarcoidosis was suggested by a negative reaction to 1:100 OT, and failure to find tubercle bacilli in sputum or discharge from an ulcer; biopsies of skin showed granulomas and ulceration, and of two subcutaneous nodules epithelioid cell granulomas with much fibrosis in one and some necrosis in the other.

In a case reported by Lewis (1961) multiple sarcoid infiltrations of sarcoid type appeared on the limbs of a woman with pulmonary sarcoidosis, confirmed by scalene node biopsy, three months after cessation of prednisolone treatment which had caused temporary regression of the pulmonary infiltration; her sister also had histologically confirmed pulmonary sarcoidosis. Three months after they had appeared, the infiltrations ulcerated, tubercle bacilli were isolated both from the ulcers and from gastric contents, and the tuberculin test, previously showing a reaction only to 100 IU, became positive to 1 IU.

Verrucous and papillomatous changes

Such changes shown histologically to be associated with granulomatous infiltrations of the skin in young black men with extensive sarcoidosis were reported by Irgang (1952) and Shmunes et al., (1970).

Simulation of other generalized skin diseases

Sarcoidosis of the skin may present appearances simulating those of psoriasis, with scaly follicular lesions (Costello, 1961; Burgoyne and Wood, 1972; Greer et al., 1977, Case 3); ichthyosis (Kauh et al., 1978; Kelly, 1978; Matsuoka et al., 1980, three cases); and lichenoid eruptions (Pautrier, 1940; Wolf, 1946; Waldman and Stiehm, 1977; Gange et al. 1978, two cases). In Boeck's (1899) first case, there was an area on one thigh in which the eruption presented a lichenoid appearance with numerous very small flat papules.

Schaumann (1924) and Pautrier (1940) described erythrodermic changes, without tactile evidence of deep infiltration, on the lower limbs of patients with extensive sarcoids of the lupus pernio or large nodular type elsewhere. Wigley and Musso (1951) reported a case in which extensive erythrodermic areas were a presenting feature of skin sarcoidosis, and reviewed eight previously published cases. Morrison (1976) described the case of a six year old boy with universal erythroderma and exfoliation, together with multiple small papules, biopsies from six areas showing granulomas in the papillary dermis and involving the epidermis; there was generalized lymphadenopathy and splenomegaly and evidence of old uveitis and fibrotic lung changes; and the eruption was suppressed by corticosteroid treatment. In this case, and in that of Wigley and Musso (1951) in an adult, some areas showed follicular spiny keratosis.

Alopecia

A few cases in which plaques of sarcoid infiltration involving the scalp caused cicatricial alopecia have been reported. Such a case is illustrated in Plate 11. In this patient, the transition from the almost unscarred plaque on the hairless part of the forehead to severe scarring of the hairy scalp was striking, so that doubt arose about the nature of the scalp lesion; but a biopsy from the central part of the scarred area confirmed that it was of sarcoid histology. This patient also had multiple nodular infiltrations of the trunk, principally the back (Fig. 7.8). Golitz et al. (1973) reported four patients, all black women, with sarcoidosis causing cicatricial alopecia, and reviewed 13 previously published cases. Other cases have been described by Brodkin (1969, Case 1) and Andersen (1977), who emphasized the difficulty of differential diagnosis from necrobiosis lipoidica affecting the scalp. Alopecia without scarring, associated with granulomas located close to pilo-sebaceous units was described by Greer *et al.* (1977, Case 2) in a white woman aged 34, who had had sarcoidosis, initially involving cervical lymph-nodes, for two years; during six months' observation, hair grew again in the area first affected, while another area became involved.

Pruritus

Skin sarcoids are usually not itchy, but a few exceptional cases have been reported. Fong and Sharma (1975) described the case of a black man aged 41 who had had a widespread pruritic maculo-papular eruption for 20 years before biopsy of the skin showed sarcoid-type granulomas; there was some enlargement of cervical and inguinal lymph-nodes, and biopsy showed sarcoid granulomas; the rash and pruritus responded to prednisone, but large doses were required initially. Powell and Smith (1976) reported the case of a 47 year old woman who was under treatment for long-standing fibrotic pulmonary sarcoidosis, and had been treated by surgery and radiotherapy for four squamous-cell carcinomas at various sites; she developed a widespread severely pruritic rash, at first thought to be a reaction to one of her medications, but persisting after cessation of all of them; biopsy showed granulomatous infiltration of the skin, and there was a prompt response to prednisone treatment.

Pigmentary changes

Cornelius *et al.* (1973) reported four, and Clayton *et al.* (1977) eight black patients with sarcoidosis in whom hypopigmentation was a prominent feature of skin changes. Clayton *et al.* studied biopsies by electron microscopy in two of their patients, and found changes in melanocytes similar to those found in other acquired hypopigmentary conditions.

Palms of the hands and soles of the feet

These areas are very rarely affected. Pautrier (1940) described one case in a patient with iridocyclitis, parotid gland enlargement, facial palsy, large nodular infiltrations of the skin of the arms and thighs, and infiltration of the lungs. The palms showed patchy erythema, and the soles of the feet irregular areas of erythema covered with scaly desquamation, suggestive of psoriasis, and biopsy of the skin of the sole showed infiltration with well-demarcated collections of epithelioid cells. In the child with extensive erythrodermic sarcoidosis, reported by Morrison (1976) and mentioned above, there was pitting on the palms and soles shown by biopsy to be due to parakeratosis with granulomas in the mid-dermis. In Case 3 of Greer *et al.* (1977), a man with extensive plaques of skin sarcoidosis, the palms and soles were involved, biopsy confirming that the palmar changes were sarcoid in nature; whereas the changes elsewhere caused no subjective symptoms, those on the palms and soles were painful. In the patient whose multiple papular skin sarcoids are illustrated in Plate 7, discoloured, poorly defined, slightly indurated areas appeared on the palms and soles simultaneously with the eruption elsewhere, but biopsy was not thought to be justified.

Subcutaneous nodules

The occurrence of subcutaneous nodules in association with erythema nodosum and BHL has been described in Chapter 5, p. 97; such nodules usually resolve spontaneously.

More chronic subcutaneous nodules may occur during the course of sarcoidosis. One of us (JGS) has observed a woman aged 52 who noticed painless nodules in the pulps of both thumbs and several fingers. Biopsy of one of these showed typical collections of non-caseating tubercles. Radiography of the chest showed indefinite soft mottling in the lungs with collapse-consolidation of the middle lobe of the right lung. Bronchoscopy showed thickening of the mucosa of the right bronchus with narrowing of the middle lobe bronchial orifice; biopsy showed fibrosis of the mucosa with atypical tubercles, of the sort commonly seen in chronic stenosing sarcoidosis of the bronchi (p. 143). Under observation, the bronchial infiltration resolved, leaving cicatricial stenosis of the middle lobe bronchus, with clear lungs apart from the atelectatic middle lobe. The subcutaneous nodules in the thumbs and fingers were still evident after six years' observation. Marten and Warner (1967) reported two black patients who presented with multiple subcutaneous nodules, on the arms in one, and on the arms, legs and thighs in the other. Both had BHL and gave granulomatous responses to Kveim tests, and no response to tuberculin, 100 IU: the nodules were shown to consist of epithelioid cell granulomas by biopsy. Clayton and Wood (1974) described the case of a black man aged 41 who presented with painless nodules up to 0.75 cm in diameter under the skin of the limbs, cheeks forehead, abdomen and back, parotid gland enlargement, generalized superficial lymph-node enlargement, BHL and anterior uveitis. Biopsies of lymph-node, liver, subcutaneous nodule and Kveim test site showed granulomas; in the node biopsy there was some caseation, and in the subcutaneous nodule some acid-fast bacilli were seen, but no mycobacteria were found on culture, and tuberculin tests with up to 2000 IU were negative.

Kroll *et al.* (1972) reported a case in which dystrophic calcification developed in persistent subcutaneous nodules. This was observed in a Puerto Rican woman aged 52, in whom the nodules appeared on the left arm, and were followed by fever, polyarthropathy, parotid gland swelling, cough and dyspnoea; four years later, a further crop of painful subcutaneous nodules appeared on both arms. She also had BHL and a pulmonary infiltration appeared as this subsided. A Kveim test was positive. Biopsies of the nodules initially showed discrete and confluent granulomas in the subcutaneous tissue, the dermis being unaffected. Later, some of the granulomas were hyalinized, and foci of calcification were seen in the hylanized tissue. Calcifications became evident radiographically for the first time four years from the onset, and two years later had increased slightly in number and size. Serum and urinary calcium levels were found to be within the normal range.

Scadding (1972) observed the evolution of subcutaneous nodules to involve the skin in four patients. In one, a man aged 58, irregular mottled shadowing was found in a chest radiograph. Nine months later, he noticed small lumps under the skin. Biopsy of one of these showed sarcoid granulomas. Six weeks later, there were pea-sized subcutaneous nodules scattered over the limbs and the back of the trunk, some visible as prominences under the skin. One on the back of the arm and one on the trunk had started to infiltrate the skin and had assumed the usual appearance of a skin sarcoid with a dusky red shiny surface. In the other three, solitary small subcutaneous nodules on the face, appearing in one a few weeks before the eruption of erythema nodosum, extended to cause visible changes in the skin before ultimately resolving completely.

Infiltrations of scars

In the active stages of sarcoidosis, old scars may become raised, red and indurated, and on biopsy be found to be infiltrated with sarcoid-type granulomas; in appearance they resemble keloids, but are generally less indurated on palpation. Scars on any part of the skin surface may be affected, including those that most people carry on their knees from child-hood falls, those resulting from surgery, and tattoos. Infiltrated scars may be the only evident skin involvement, or may accompany infiltrations of the unscarred skin.

In a series of 500 patients reviewed by Scadding (1972) and mentioned above (p. 182), 24 had infiltrations of scars at some time during the observed course. In 14, these were the only form of skin infiltration, and in ten they accompanied sarcoidosis of unscarred skin; lupus pernio in two, large nodular infiltrations or plaques in four, small nodular infiltrations in three, and subcutaneous nodules in one. Unlike sarcoids of unscarred skin, scar infiltrations as the only skin involvement occurred in a higher proportion (3.9%) of men than of women (1.8%). They tended to occur at an early stage of the disease, and the infiltration waned with the cessation of activity, the scar reverting to its former flat pale appearance; for instance, in two young men, old appendicectomy scars became infiltrated simultaneously with the detection of symptomless BHL, both subsequently subsiding spontaneously.

Löfgren *et al.* (1955) studied 23 patients with sarcoidosis who developed granulomas in scars. In all but two there was the possibility of contamination by mineral particles; and in all but one of those where this possibility existed, foreign bodies were found histologically. In some cases these were shown by X-ray diffraction to be talc, in scars of surgical procedures, and quartz, in those due to road accidents. In five patients, the granulomas developed in the scars of scalene node biopsies which had confirmed the diagnosis of sarcoidosis; these appeared three months to three years after the biopsy procedure. In the rest, the granulomas appeared at much longer intervals, varying from 3–27 years, after the wound, which had presumably preceded the development of sarcoidosis. It seems clear, from these experiences, that during the active phase of sarcoidosis, scars may become infiltrated with sarcoid granulomas; that this is more apt to occur in scars that have been contaminated with quartz or talc; that scars without such contamination may become infiltrated, but more rarely; and that infiltration of scars is likely to follow a course parallel to that of sarcoidosis elsewhere in the body. The development of infiltration of scars, without other skin involvement, does not seem to have any prognostic significance.

A striking case in which old scars, almost certainly contaminated by siliceous material, became infiltrated during the active phase of sarcoidosis is illustrated in Plate 12. In 1948, this man received multiple wounds of the left side of the face from the explosion of a mine in desert warfare. These healed, leaving unremarkable scars. In 1956, the scars became swollen, red and firm. At the same time, lymph-nodes below the jaw on both sides, in the rest of the right anterior triangle of the neck and in the right axilia were found to be enlarged, and in the chest radiograph mottling was observed at the bases of both lungs, although he had no respiratory symptoms. Biopsy of the skin showed infiltration with sarcoid tubercles (Fig. 7.13). Treatment with prednisolone was followed by a rapid return of the scars to a normal appearance, but on its cessation they equally rapidly reverted to their infiltrated state. About six months later, spontaneous resolution started, and by 1960, the scars presented an unremarkable appearance (Plate 13) and the shadowing at the bases of the lungs had become much less evident. A similar case has been reported by Artz (1955).

Tattoos

A number of cases have been reported in which red raised indurations of parts of old tattoos have proved to be due to infiltration of the tattooed skin with sarcoid-type granulomas, and has been the first evidence of sarcoidosis

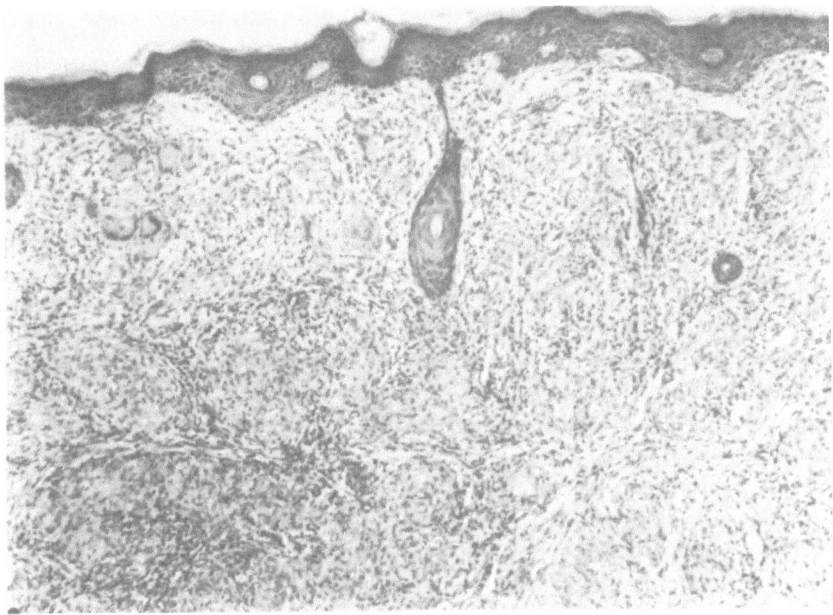

Figure 7.13.   Biopsy of one of the infiltrated scars shown in Plate 12.
H & E. × 100.

(Obermeyer and Hassem, 1955; Dickinson, 1964; Weidman *et al.*, 1966;
Iveson *et al.* 1975; Kennedy, 1976; Farzan, 1977). In these cases, chest
radiographs have shown BHL, with or without pulmonary infiltration, and
in one (Farzan, 1977) the changes in the tattoo accompanied erythema
nodosum. In those cases in which the course was reported, spontaneous
improvement or clearing has been observed. These seems to be no special
predilection for any one pigment, although in some of the reported cases,
areas with one or two of several pigments used were selectively affected.
Plate 14 shows a tattoo on the arm of a man aged 30, in which nodules
appeared; at the same time there were joint-pains and three weeks later
erythema nodosum. Biopsy showed sarcoid infiltration of the affected part
of the tattoo, and a chest radiograph showed BHL. All manifestations
subsided spontaneously.

CONCURRENCE WITH OTHER SKIN DISEASES

As noted above, the very wide range of appearances presented by sarcoid
infiltration of the skin include some which simulate various well-recognized
skin diseases. In such cases, differential diagnosis is complicated by the
possibility of concurrence of sarcoidosis and another skin disease, and of

secondary infiltration by sarcoid granulomas of pre-existing lesions of other diseases.

A few cases have been recorded in which patients with psoriasis have developed sarcoidosis, and the lesions of the two diseases have been co-existent in the skin (Farmer and Winkelmann, 1960). One of us (JGS) has observed a patient with long-standing psoriasis (Plate 15) who developed multiple small papular and nodular sarcoids of skin (Plate16), and pulmonary sarcoidosis; the diagnosis of both sorts of skin change was confirmed histologically. Burgoyne and Wood (1972) reported the case of a 71 year old woman in whom a psoriasiform eruption accompanied BHL and lung infiltration; skin biopsies showed psoriatic changes together with granulomatous infiltration of the dermis; they concluded that sarcoid granulomas had localized in psoriatic lesions.

Interrelations between sarcoidosis and lymphoma in the skin in cases reported by Attwood *et al.* (1966, Case 1) and Kahn *et al.* (1974) are similarly difficult to interpret. In the first of these, it appeared that mycosis fungoides developed independently six years after plaques and papules of cutaneous sarcoidosis; but at necropsy five years after the diagnosis of mycosis fungioides, only lymphomatous changes were found, no sarcoid granulomas remaining. In the patient reported by Kahn *et al.*, multiple skin plaques, initially showing the histology of sarcoidosis, waxed and waned over a three year period, when one of them enlarged rapidly and on biopsy showed a malignant lymphoma without granulomas; radiotherapy and chemotherapy were only locally effective, and the patient died after a few months. There was no necropsy. The authors speculated that the granulomatous changes were a reaction to lymphoma rather than sarcoidosis.

Lockman (1980) reported the case of a black woman, aged 38, in whom porphyria cutanea tarda (PCT) was associated with granulomatous changes in liver and bone marrow, radiographic changes in the lungs, and raised angiotensin converting enzyme level in the blood. There was a prompt response to corticosteroid treatment, and it was thought that sarcoid changes in the liver had precipitated the manifestations of PCT.

Persistent sarcoid plaques may have a partially atrophic centre (Plate 4) and then resemble granuloma annulare or necrobiosis lipoidica, which are localized to the skin, and, except for the possible association of necrobiosis lipoidica with diabetes, are not accompanied by changes in other organs. They tend to resolve after a course of variable duration, and are little affected by treatment (Wells and Smith, 1963). The lesions of granuloma annulare may be solitary or multiple; histologically, the characteristic appearance is of necrobiotic changes in collagen in the dermis surrounded by a granulomatous reaction of lymphocytes, histiocytes and giant cells arranged in palisade fashion. Borrie (1957) described a case in which skin changes having the macroscopic and histological features of necrobiosis lipoidica appeared in a woman aged 49, six years from the onset of extensive sarcoidosis involving lymph-nodes, eyes, and nervous system; he accepted the skin changes as an unusual variant of skin sarcoidosis. Dicken *et al.* (1969), in a review of 26 cases of widespread granuloma annulare, mentioned two in which skin changes interpreted as granuloma annulare were accompanied by evidence of generalized sarcoidosis; and Umbert and Winkelmann (1977) reported five cases in which granuloma annulare and sarcoidosis were thought to co-exist. In such cases, the diagnosis of granuloma annulare depends upon histology; and the hypothesis that the observed histological pattern is a variant of that of sarcoidosis of the skin seems at least as acceptable as the hypothesis that the patient is suffering from two aetiologically distinct diseases.

Biro *et al.* (1968) and Singh *et al.* (1971) have reported cases in which there was suggestive, but not unequivocal, evidence that widespread papular eruptions with granulomatous histological features were due to secondary syphilis modified by sarcoid infiltration; in both cases, penicillin treatment led to resolution.

CORRELATIONS WITH OTHER FEATURES OF SARCOIDOSIS

In correlations of skin infiltrations with other features of sarcoidosis, including their prognostic implications and age- and sex-distribution, it has been found useful to disinguish between large infiltrations of the lupus pernio, large nodular and plaque type, which tend to be persistent, and small nodular and papular infiltrations, scar infiltrations and subcutaneous nodules which are in many cases transient (James, 1959b; Scadding, 1972).

All varieties of sarcoid infiltrations of the unscarred skin are more frequent in women than in men. Among the 500 patients reviewed by Scadding (1972) 19.5% of women and 6.6% of men had skin infiltrations at some

Table 7.2 Sex incidence of skin infiltrations in 500 patients with sarcoidosis (Scadding, 1972).

	Male	*Female*
Total number of patients	228	272
Lupus pernio	2	9
Plaques	1	8
Large nodular infiltrations	5	10
Small nodular infiltrations	5	19
Subcutaneous nodules	2	7
Total number with infiltrations of unscarred skin	15 (6.6%)	53 (19.5%)
Infiltrations of scars only	9 (3.9%)	5 (1.8%)
With other infiltrations	3	7

Table 7.3 Prognosis for skin infiltrations and for lung changes related to principal type of skin infiltration (Scadding, 1972).

Principal type of skin infiltration	Course of skin infiltration			Course of lung changes			
	Persisted > 2 years	Cleared < 2 years	Duration unknown	Persisted > 2 years	Cleared < 2 years	Duration unknown	Never found
Lupus pernio	10		1	10		1	
Plaques	8		1	8		1	
Large nodular	12	2	1	13	1	1	
Small nodular	4	17	3	12	8	1	
Subcutaneous nodules	2	6	1	2	6		
Scar only		12		5	7		2

time during the observed course. On the other hand, infiltrations of scars as the sole sarcoid involvement of skin occurred in 3.9% of men and only 1.8% of women (Table 7.2). Of 27 patients with sarcoid infiltrations of the skin reviewed by James (1959), only four were men. A rather smaller preponderance of women was reported by Gilg (1955) among 191 patients seen in the Finsen Institute in Copenhagen; 69% were women. The mean age at the first evidence of sarcoidosis tends to be rather greater in those presenting with skin changes than in others (James, 1959; Scadding, 1967).

PROGNOSIS

James (1959b) made the important observation that lupus pernio and large infiltration tend to be persistent for long periods, and to be associated with chronic changes in other organs, while smaller infiltrations are frequently transient and associated with resolving changes in other organs. This finding was confirmed in Scadding's (1972) review, in which lupus pernio, plaques and large nodular infiltrations nearly all persisted for more than two years and in many cases very much longer, and were generally associated with persistent lung changes; whereas small nodular infiltrations and subcutaneous nodules in most cases, and scar infiltrations in all, cleared within two years, and were associated with lung changes of which more than half cleared within two years (Table 7.3).

Both Sones and Israel (1960) in Philadelphia and Scadding (1961) in London observed that the presence of skin sarcoids makes it more likely that sarcoidosis of the lungs will proceed to fibrosis. The more detailed analysis of the skin changes into groups shows that it is the 'fixed' lesions, lupus pernio, plaques and large nodular infiltrations which carry this unfavourable prognostic implication; the occurrence of transient small nodular infiltrations probably has no effect on long-term prognosis.

RELATION TO ERYTHEMA NODOSUM

Though small skin infiltrations of the small nodular type, subcutaneous nodules, and infiltrations of scars may appear around the time of appearance of erythema nodosum and/or febrile arthropathy with BHL at the onset of sarcoidosis, there is an inverse relationship between the occurrence of erythema nodosum and the later development of the more extensive and persistent types of sarcoid infiltration of the skin. Among the 500 patients reviewed by Scadding (1972) the erythema nodosum/febrile arthropathy syndrome occurred in 69 (13.8%) of all patients, and in 12 (14.6%) of the 82 with skin infiltrations either concurrently or later. But when the skin infiltrations are separated into the persistent and the transient types, an

Table 7.4 Relationship between erythema nodosum and skin infiltrations in 500 cases of sarcoidosis (Scadding, 1972).

	Number of patients	Erythema nodosum and/or febrile arthropathy
Whole series	500	69 (13.8%)
No skin infiltration	418	57 (13.6%)
With skin infiltrations		
Lupus pernio, plaques	20 ⎫ 35	0 ⎫ 1 (2.9%)
Large nodular infiltrations	15 ⎭	1 ⎭
Small nodular infiltrations	24 ⎫	4 ⎫
Subcutaneous nodules	9 ⎬ 47	3 ⎬ 11 (23.4%)
Infiltration of scar only	14 ⎭	4 ⎭

important difference appears. Erythema nodosum was observed in only one patient out of 34 with persistent skin infiltrations, and in 11 of 48 with infiltrations of the more transient types (Table 7.4). This difference, which attains statistical significance, is to be regarded as one aspect of the generally favourable prognosis of those cases of sarcoidosis which start acutely with erythema nodosum.

TREATMENT

The skin lesions of sarcoidosis are, of themselves, not dangerous to life, and treatment of patients with skin changes will usually depend upon the associated changes, especially in the lungs. The importance of the skin changes to the patient depends upon their effect upon his appearance, which may be extremely disfiguring when the face is involved, especially with lupus pernio. The only therapeutic agents which can be relied upon to affect the course of sarcoidosis are the corticosteroids. Chloroquine and its analogues have a suppressive effect which is of slower onset and usually less impressive. The therapeutic use of these agents in sarcoidosis is discussed in Chapter 27. Only some special aspects of the treatment of sarcoids of the skin will be considered here.

The effect of corticosteroids in sarcoidosis is suppressive. Most patients with skin sarcoids, given sufficient dosage of a corticosteroid, will show clearing of the skin. With the smaller, less persistent types, this may be achieved with modest doses, and the eruption may not recur on cessation of treatment. Unfortunately, large persistent infiltrations, such as lupus pernio, may be suppressible only by large doses liable to cause serious side-effects on continued administration, necessitating reduction of dose or cessation of treatment; and the morale of a patient with a disfiguring eruption is not helped by improvement under intensive corticosteroid treatment, only to relapse on necessary reduction or cessation of treatment. Sarcoids on the trunk or limbs do not call for such treatment, apart from indications that might arise from associated visceral changes. In some circumstances, an attempt to treat disfiguring facial sarcoids, or some of the more exuberant eruptions elsewhere, is justifiable. Decision should be based upon the absence of contra-indications to corticosteroid treatment, and upon a trial to discover whether in the individual patient initial improvement, secured by full doses, was maintained by a reasonable dose of a corticosteroid. Such a decision should be made in the knowledge that treatment is likely to be required for a long time, certainly measured in years, if the skin changes are not to recur.

Occasionally, it has been observed that skin sarcoids appear for the first time shortly after cessation of corticosteroid treatment that has been given for relief of some other manifestation of sarcoidosis. This illustrates the essentially suppressive effect of corticosteroids. Scadding (1972) observed four women in whom small nodular infiltrations appeared soon after the withdrawal of corticosteroid treatment for pulmonary sarcoidosis. One of these was a West Indian, whose eruption is illustrated in Plate 7. On resumption of corticosteroid treatment both this eruption and the pulmonary infiltration, which had recurred, were suppressed. Similarly, in the case of ulcerating sarcoids of the lower legs reported by Meyers and Barsky (1978), and mentioned above, the eruption appeared shortly after cessation of corticosteroid treatment for uveitis.

Local treatment with corticosteroid topical applications has been found generally to be ineffective. Since the granulomas are beneath an intact epidermis, this is not surprising. Intralesional injections may cause regression of particularly prominent local infiltrations, but the effect is of limited duration.

The possibility that certain antimalarial drugs might be useful in the treatment of sarcoidosis was first suggested by observations of the effects on skin sarcoids of mepacrine (Shaffer *et al.* 1953; Klauder, 1953; Söderstrom, 1960), and subsequently of chloroquine (Morse *et al.*, 1961; Siltzbach and Teirstein, 1964). Mepacrine has more severe toxic effects than chloroquine, and causes yellow staining of the skin on prolonged administration, and consequently was displaced by chloroquine or hydroxychloroquine in all later studies. Siltzbach and Teirstein (1964) treated 14 patients with skin sarcoids with chloroquine; all improved, but nine relapsed during limited periods of observation after the end of treatment. The use of chloroquine in the treatment of sarcoidosis in general is discussed in Chapter 27, p. 594. The effect is temporarily suppressive, like that of corticosteroids, but appears more slowly; and possibly relapse after cessation of treatment which has led to improvement is also slower. The toxic immediate effects include anorexia, nausea and abdominal discomfort, giddiness and tremor, which may be severe enough to put a stop to treatment in 5–10% of patients; and on long-term treatment bleaching of hair and temporary photosensitivity (Dall and Keane, 1959), and some potentially serious ocular complications. These include changes in the cornea, with white or yellowish linear or punctate deposits causing blurring of vision and coloured haloes round bright lights (Hobbs and Calnan, 1958), and retinopathy causing visual field defects (Hobbs *et al.*, 1959). Because of these side-effects, and the need for ophthalmological supervision of patients on long-term treatment, the place of chloroquine in the treatment of skin sarcoidosis is evidently limited. Gilg and Brodthagen (1967) observed no effect on cutaneous sarcoidosis after treatment with up to 2 g of hydroxychloroquine for at least one year; but more favourable reports by others suggest that it may occasionally be useful in patients with disfiguring persistent infiltrations, and with contra-indications to, or severe side-effects from, long-term corticosteroid treatment.

Veien and Brodthagen (1977) treated 16 patients with disfiguring cutaneous sarcoidosis with methotrexate, 25 mg once weekly by mouth, decreasing if improvement occurred; the 'maintenance' dose in most was 10 mg. In 12, the skin lesions flattened, in eight after four months and in the others after longer periods up to 26 months. After discontinuance of treatment, the skin sarcoids generally relapsed to their former state or worse within 2–4 weeks; three experienced such relapse after longer periods, up to two years. In three of four who had uveitis, this cleared during treatment, but no effect on radiographic changes in lungs or hilar lymph-nodes was observed in six. Side-effects, usually nausea on the day of treatment occurred in ten, and led to cessation of treatment in two. Thus methotrexate appears to have a suppressive effect limited to the period of its administration on some cases of sarcoid infiltration of the skin, but indications for its use must be greatly limited by its toxic effects.

Veien (1977) found that levamisole had no effect on cutaneous sarcoidosis in an open study of 16 patients. This is in line with studies of the effects of this agent in other forms of sarcoidosis.

Chapter 8

Ocular Changes

The early history of the development of knowledge about involvement of the eye in sarcoidosis has been described briefly in Chapter 1. Uveitis is the most commonly recognized ocular change in sarcoidosis, but the eye may also be affected by infiltration of the conjunctiva, by reduced lacrimal secretion due to involvement of the lacrimal glands, causing in some cases kerato-conjunctivitis sicca, by involvement of the retina and optic nerve head, by deposition of calcium salts in the bulbar conjunctiva and in the cornea (band keratopathy) in patients with hypercalcaemia, by involvement of the lacrimal sac and duct, and by infiltration of the orbital fat causing exophthalmos.

These ocular changes in their milder grades may be symptomless and discoverable only by ophthalmological examination. Hence it is not surprising that in reported series the proportions of patients with symptoms referable to the eyes are lower, and vary less between series, than the proportions found to have objective evidence of involvement of the eyes. In an international study, the percentages of patients in whom ocular changes were a presenting feature were 10% in London, 8.5% in Paris, 7% in New York and 10% in Los Angeles; whereas the percentages in which involvement of the eye was detected at any time were 27%, 11%, 20% and 11% respectively, and 32% in Tokyo, for which city the number presenting with ocular symptoms was not stated (Siltzbach *et al.*, 1974). There are probably differences in liability to serious eye involvement between ethnic groups, series from North America including high proportions of blacks showing large numbers with such changes. Obenauf *et al.* (1978) reviewed 532 cases of sarcoidosis in North Carolina, of which three-quarters were in black patients; 19% had ocular symptoms on presentation, and 38% were found to have some sort of ocular involvement during the course of the disease, described as chronic granular uveitis in 20%. By contrast, in North Finland

Table 8.1 Frequency of diagnosed and symptomatic ocular changes in 281 cases of sarcoidosis in North Finland. Data extracted from Tables V and VI of Karma (1979), by kind permission of Dr A. Karma.

	Diagnosed		*Symptomatic*	
Uveitis	22	7.8%	17	6.0%
Fundal change				
(without evident uveitis)	3	1.1%	1	0.4%
Reduced lacrimal secretion	32	12.6%*	12	4.3%
Enlarged lacrimal gland	6	2.1%	3	1.1%
Dacryostenosis	5	1.8%	5	1.8%
Conjunctival granuloma	37	17.0%†	4	1.4%
Episcleritis	5	1.8%	5	1.8%
Band keratopathy	11	3.9%	2	0.7%

* of 254 examined   † of 218 examined

Karma (1979) carried out detailed ophthalmological examinations in 281 patients with sarcoidosis, repeatedly when indicated, and found eye changes of some sort in 28.1% (Table 8.1). The incidence of eye changes in these Finnish patients was relatively low; but this study, in which all patients were studied ophthalmologically, gives information both about the relative frequency of the various ocular changes and about the liability of each of them to cause symptoms. Most, but not all, cases of uveitis were symptomatic; whereas the two most frequent objective findings, reduced lacrimal secretion and conjunctival granulomas demonstrable by biopsy, were associated with symptoms in only a minority of cases.

UVEITIS

Uveitis is the most frequent manifestation of sarcoidosis in the eye to cause symptoms. Schumacher (1909) was the first to refer to it in a brief report of bilateral chronic irido-cyclitis in a 42 year old woman with Boeck's sarcoids on the limbs, which had erupted after the subsidence of bilateral parotid gland swellings. In the same year, Heerfordt described the syndrome of uveo-parotid fever, but had no idea that it was related to sarcoidosis; and uveitis was known to be a frequent finding in sarcoidosis before the Heerfordt syndrome was generally recognized to be a rare combination of features of that disease.

Affection of the anterior part of the uveal tract, giving rise to subacute or chronic iridocyclitis is the most prominent feature in most cases of sarcoid uveitis. The posterior part may also be affected, with choroidal and retinal changes, which are difficult to detect if they are peripherally located or in the presence of severe involvement of the anterior chamber. Crick *et al.* (1961) found evidence of uveitis in 61 (33%) of 185 patients with sarcoidosis examined ophthalmologically, the anterior part of the uveal tract being involved in 55 and the posterior in 40; in 29 (16%) eye symptoms were the presenting feature. This study, in London, resembled that of Karma (1979), in which only 7.8% of patients were found to have uveitis, in that all patients were examined by one ophthalmologist using all available methods. Different methods of referral of patients may account for part of the considerable difference in apparent incidence of uveitis. The Finnish study included all known patients with sarcoidosis in a defined area, whereas in London patients referred to specialist clinics were studied. Nevertheless, it seems likely that this difference is in part due to a lower liability of Scandinavian patients with sarcoidosis to develop uveitis. Other studies in London have shown incidences similar to that found by Crick *et al.* (1961). Of 275 patients reviewed by one of us (JGS) in 1967, 27 (10%) presented with symptomatic uveitis and another 12 developed uveitis at intervals ranging up to seven years from the apparent onset of sarcoidosis; thus 39 (14%) were found to have uveitis at some stage. Among 537 patients attending a sarcoidosis clinic, James (1974) found 107 (20%) to have anterior, and 34 (6%) posterior uveitis.

In most published series, the incidence of uveitis was higher among women than among men, both as a presenting feature and later in the course of sarcoidosis. Among Scadding's 275 patients, 16% of women and 12% of men had uveitis. James (1974) found uveitis to be twice as common in women as in men. Karma (1979) detected uveitis in 17 of 163 women and five of 118 men with sarcoidosis in North Finland.

Although uveitis is generally recognized to be a possible manifestation of sarcoidosis, only a few of the many patients attending ophthalmological clinics with uveitis of obscure cause are found to be suffering from sarcoidosis. Perkins (1958) reported that of 653 patients with uveitis investigated at the Institute of Ophthalmology, London, only 2.1% had evidence of sarcoidosis; and ten years later, when the number studied had increased to 1846, the proportion remained the same (Perkins, 1968), in spite of possibly increased awareness of sarcoidosis. In a survey of 653 patients presenting with uveitis at a hospital in northern Finland, Saari *et al.* (1975) concluded that only nine (1.4%) were due to sarcoidosis. Findings in such surveys can be interpreted only with knowledge of the source of referral of patients. Nordentoft and Møller (1970) reported the results of mediastinoscopy in 77 of 108 patients with uveitis referred from ophthalmologists; lymph-nodes showing changes characteristic of sarcoidosis were found in 14 (13%). James *et al.* (1976) described the findings in 368 patients admitted to a Medical Ophthalmology Unit for investigation of 'endogenous' uveitis; a recognized cause or associated systemic disorder was identified in 171, and there was sarcoidosis in 25 (7%).

The uveitis of sarcoidosis presents with symptoms similar to those of other forms of iridocyclitis, in some cases less severe than might be expected from the objective findings, and occasionally discovered only by routine examination. In most cases, the symptoms are watering and redness of the eye with discomfort or aching and possibly some photophobia, blurring of vision and floating specks in the field of vision. Most commonly, both eyes are affected, sometimes consecutively, but in a few cases the changes are unilateral. The objective findings are those common to all sorts of iridocyclitis, such as circumcorneal ciliary congestion, irregularity of the papillary margin and of the pattern of the iris, sluggish papillary responses, keratic precipitates in the anterior chamber and aqueous flare. Nodules are observed in the iris in only a minority of cases. Crick *et al.* (1961) found them in one-quarter of their cases, and commented that they were seen only in association with cells in the anterior chamber and keratic precipitates, and that they might also occur in non-specific uveitis.

As noted above, the proportion of cases in which the posterior part of the uveal tract has been found to be affected varies greatly between reported series; this variation is in large part due to differences in extent of investigation. Karma (1979) using three-mirror contact lens ophthalmoscopy to examine the periphery of the fundus, found that in only one of 22 cases of sarcoid uveitis was the posterior segment unaffected during an average of four and a half years' observation; she commented that in many cases fundal changes were peripheral and might not have been observed without this procedure. Vitreous haze and opacities are frequent in the active stage. Landers (1949) drew attention to discrete grey-white bodies in the lower part of the vitreous body, varying in size up to one-third or more of the disc diameter. These may be scattered or in chains; larger ones have been called 'snowball' opacities. They may lie so far in front of the retina that they cast shadows. Karma (1979) found opacities in 21 of 22 cases of sarcoid uveitis, of 'snowball' type in nine. Gould and Kaufman (1961) found that in 30% of reported cases of sarcoid involvement of the fundus, vitreous globoid bodies or 'strings of pearls' were seen. Changes that may be observed in the fundus include choroido-retinitis of non-specific appearance, and retinal nodules, exudates alongside veins (periphlebitis retinae) and masses at the optic nerve head, all probably granulomatous, papilloedema and macular oedema; these are discussed below.

Sarcoid uveitis may present acutely or insidiously. Correlations between mode of onset, initial ophthalmological findings and course are inconstant, but there seems to be a group of cases in which an acute or sub-acute irido-cyclitis without features suggestive of granulomatous changes occurs at an early stage of sarcoidosis, and runs a benign course, clearing spontaneously or after local treatment only and leaving no or insignificant sequelae (James *et al.* 1964). Clinico-pathological correlations cannot be made in such cases; but it seems possible that in them, irido-cyclitis, like the erythema nodosum and febrile arthropathy that may occur at a similar stage of the natural history of sarcoidosis, is non-granulomatous. But some cases beginning insidiously also follow a benign self-limiting course; and although many of those with a prolonged course begin without acute symptoms, uveitis with appearances suggesting granulomatous changes, and following an unfavourable course with poor response to treatment, may begin acutely. Crick *et al.* (1961) found no evidence that acuteness of onset was related to prognosis. Among 35 patients with sarcoid anterior uveitis, the onset was sub-acute in 24, of whom seven did well, ten were left with mild symptoms, and seven did badly; it was chronic in 11, of whom six did well, four continued with mild symptoms, and one did badly. Karma (1979) found a correlation between ophthalmological findings and course; among nine patients with a more or less sudden onset, remission in six months, and no recurrence, five were classified as 'non-granulomatous', because they did not show at any stage iris nodules, fatty keratic precipitates, snowball vitreous opacities, candle-wax exudates, or chorio-retinitis; among 13 with an insidious onset and prolonged course, or with prolonged remittent course, all showed one or more of these changes. There was no clear correlation between the course of the uveitis and other manifestations of sarcoidosis, either in the eye or elsewhere in the body, with the exception that hypercalcaemia and band keratopathy occurred in four of those with a chronic course, and none of those with a favourable short course.

HEERFORDT'S SYNDROME

Uveitis is one of the cardinal features of the syndrome of uveoparotid fever; but only a minority of patients with sarcoid uveitis show any of the other features of the syndrome described by Heerfordt (1909), which in its complete form is very rare. The term 'Heerfordt's syndrome' has been used in a variety of ways deviating from the original description and not always clearly stated. Its continued use can thus cause confusion, and can usually be avoided. The syndrome is of mainly historic interest. 'Febris uveo-parotidea subchronica' was described by Heerfordt (1909) as characterized by a protracted course, low fever, localization in the parotid gland and in the uveal tract, and the frequent appearance of complicating pareses of the cerebro-spinal nerves, especially the facial. Heerfordt thought that since this syndrome had some features in common with epidemic parotitis (mumps), it was very possible that it might be caused by the same or related agent. Bering (1910) seems to have been the first to describe a case in which features of this syndrome were linked with sarcoidosis; in this case, there were enlargements of parotid and submaxillary salivary glands, iridocyclitis, and skin sarcoids, and biopsy of a submaxillary gland showed infiltration with epithelioid and giant cells and lymphocytes, without necrosis or discoverable acid-fast bacilli. Garland and Thompson (1933) analysed

46 published cases and reported one of their own, and their review provides an excellent summary of the earlier literature on the subject. Nearly two-thirds of the cases they reviewed occurred in female patients, and a similar proportion in the second and third decades of life. Fever was observed in only half the patients. Parotitis, bilateral in all but two patients, and uveitis were, by definition, constant features. The submaxillary glands were involved as well as the parotids in five, and the sublingual in one. The salivary gland enlargement gradually subsided after intervals varying from two weeks to three years. Facial palsy was noted in 20 cases, and was bilateral in eight; it usually followed the parotitis at intervals of up to six months, but in a few cases preceded it. It usually persisted for only a few weeks, the longest reported duration being one year. Evidence of involvement of other cranial nerves was found in a few cases; it consisted in dysphagia in six cases, palatal paralysis in one, paralysis of the vocal cords in one, and ptosis in two. Evidence of peripheral neuropathy in the form of muscle weakness, loss of tendon reflexes, and disturbances of sensation were found in five. Involvement of lacrimal glands and of other organs and tissues, especially lymph-nodes, lungs and skin, is frequent in Heerfordt's syndrome. In the case of Garland and Thompson, the myocardium was found at necropsy to be extensively infiltrated; and Longcope and Freiman (1952) reported a black female patient (Case 16) who presented with the complete Heerfordt syndrome, BHL and sarcoid skin lesions, and developed clinical and electro-cardiographic evidence of myocardial changes.

The association of uveitis with enlargement of salivary glands, sometimes accompanied by cranial nerve palsies is a striking and memorable clinical picture. But uveitis, parotid gland enlargement and facial palsy are related only by their being possible features of sarcoidosis; each occurs mo·e frequently alone than in association with the others. Crick *et al.* (1961) commented on the rarity of Heerfordt's syndrome in their study of 61 patients with sarcoid uveitis; only two had both parotid gland enlargement and facial palsy, four having each of these without the other. Of the 275 patients with sarcoidosis reviewed by one of us (JGS) in 1967, 29 (14%) had uveitis producing symptoms; of these four had parotid gland enlargement, and two facial palsy, none having both. Stjernberg and Wiman (1974) reported 15 patients, among 299 seen in northern Sweden, as cases of Heerfordt's syndrome, defining this as 'sarcoid affection of the eyes and parotid glands'; but of these, only seven had uveitis and parotid gland enlargement, only one of these having also facial palsy, one had uveitis and facial palsy without parotid gland enlargement, and the rest had parotid gland enlargement with eye changes other than uveitis. Of 22 patients with sarcoid uveitis reported by Karma (1979), three had parotid gland enlargement and four facial palsy, but these occurred together in only one; in three of these seven patients, lacrimal glands were enlarged.

Greenburg *et al.* (1964) studied parotid gland enlàrgement in sarcoidosis. They found it in 23 (6%) of 388 patients, bilaterally in 19; only eight had uveitis.

Thus Heerfordt's syndrome can be regarded as an occasional association in one patient of a number of features of sarcoidosis, whose practical importance is that it is virtually diagnostic of sarcoidosis, in many cases widespread and persistent.

DIAGNOSIS OF SARCOID UVEITIS

That a uveitis is a manifestation of sarcoidosis is not recognizable from the local appearances alone, although it may be suspected; it depends upon the finding of other evidences of sarcoidosis, and the establishment of this diagnosis on the lines discussed in Chapter 26. In many cases, uveitis is the first clinical evidence of sarcoidosis; among 39 of the 275 patients with sarcoidosis reviewed by Scadding (1967) who at any time had uveitis, it was the presenting feature in 22 (70%). In 33, the state of the lungs at the onset of uveitis was known; BHL, with or without lung infiltration, was present in 27, and lung infiltration in the remaining six, in one of whom it was known to have been preceded by BHL. Of James's (1959a) 30 patients with sarcoid uveitis, 16 had BHL with or without lung infiltration, and four had radiographically normal lungs. Of the 22 patients with uveitis in Karma's (1979) study of ocular sarcoidosis, ten had BHL, ten had BHL and lung infiltration, and two radiographically normal lungs; four had erythema nodosum, seven sarcoids of the skin and six symptoms referable to joints. Associations with the other features of Heerfordt's syndrome, parotid gland enlargement and facial palsy are mentioned above. Thus, most patients with sarcoid uveitis show easily found evidence of sarcoidosis elsewhere. In some, other evidences of sarcoidosis in the eye are found; among her 22 cases, Karma (1979) found that five had conjunctival granulomas, ten reduced lacrimal secretion, two enlargement of lacrimal glands, and four band keratopathy. Conjunctival biopsy as a source of confirmatory histology is discussed below.

When uveitis develops in a patient already known to have sarcoidosis, it will usually be accepted as part of that disease. Occasionally doubt may arise because of the concurrence of a second possibly relevant disease. One of us (JGS) has observed a man aged 25 with concurrent sarcoidosis, with BHL followed by lung infiltration, histologically confirmed by scalene node biopsy and resolving spontaneously, and ankylosing spondylitis with characteristic clinical features and radiographic changes in sacro-iliac joints, also becoming quiescent with physiotherapy; uveitis appeared while both these processes were active, and resolved with local treatment only. This patient remained well during several years of further observation, and it was not possible to decide whether the uveitis should be related to sarcoidosis or to ankylosing spondylitis.

Weinberg and Tessler (1976) studied serum lysozyme levels in patients with uveitis; mean levels were higher in those with active sarcoid uveitis than in those with 'idiopathic irido-cyclitis', but the ranges overlapped. Low levels were found in those with inactive sarcoid uveitis. Weinreb and Kimura (1980) studied serum angiotensin-converting enzyme; in 20 patients with sarcoidosis and ocular changes and in 27 with uveitis classified on local appearances as granulomatous but without evidence of systemic sarcoidosis, levels were significantly ($P<0.001$) higher than in controls, while 17 with uveitis of other recognized sorts levels were similar to those in controls. Thus although high levels of either of these enzymes may suggest a diagnosis of sarcoidosis in a patient with unexplained uveitis, detection of manifestations of sarcoidosis elsewhere remains desirable for the establishment of this diagnosis.

PROGNOSIS

The prognosis of sarcoid uveitis is difficult to assess, because of the difficulty of observing a series of cases which represents a fair sample of all those occurring in the community. Scadding's (1967) series probably included an unduly high proportion with anterior uveitis accompanying an early stage of sarcoidosis and having a strong tendency to spontaneous resolution, and low proportion with persistent changes localized in the eyes. Of 37 patients observed long enough to permit assessment of the outcome, 30 had recovered with no impairment of vision; three no longer had active uveitis but had moderate or severe visual impairment; and four still had active uveitis requiring corticosteroid treatment. Crick et al. (1961), whose series contained a higher proportion of patients with severe ocular changes, reported that visual acuity was reduced to below 6/9 in 11 of their 61 patients; six of those left with impaired vision had had severe uveo-parotitis, and had first been treated before corticosteroids became available. The complications common to all forms of uveitis, which it is beyond the scope of this monograph to discuss, may occur. Crick et al. (1961) noted glaucoma in three of their patients. The findings of Karma (1979) in a survey of all known patients with sarcoidosis in a defined area give an indication of the general prognosis in the population studied. Changes in the posterior segment, found in 21 of the 22 patients, may have affected visual prognosis in a few; cataract and glaucoma were prominent among the causes of severe visual loss. Raised intra-ocular pressure was noted at some time in seven patients. It was attributed to corticosteroid treatment in two; in three of the others, it fell to normal as the uveitis subsided, and in two it required surgical treatment. Six patients developed cataracts; of these one required operation because of imminent capsular rupture and one proceeded to complete opacity of one lens, while the other four developed slight posterior cataract during prolonged corticosteroid-treated uveitis. One, with retinal vascular changes, suffered retinal detachment, and one developed cystoid macular oedema. Overall, during the period of observation, visual acuity of 24 eyes remained unchanged, of 12 deteriorated and of eight improved.

Discussion of the treatment of uveitis is outside the scope of this monograph, except in relation to the use of corticosteroids in sarcoidosis (Chapter 27). In general, manifestations likely to run a favourable course do not constitute indications for corticosteriod treatment. But uveitis, especially if the posterior segment is involved, may lead to impairment of vision by processes whose active stage can be suppressed by corticosteroids and will eventually come to an end. Moreover, uveitis may remain active, or become reactivated, after other evidences of sarcoidosis (in most cases intrathoracic) have regressed. It therefore should be considered a strong indication for corticosteroid treatment. Since its effect is suppressive and not curative, the duration of this treatment depends upon the unpredictable duration of activity of the disease, and cannot be decided in advance; and its intensity should be determined by the varying needs of individual patients. Some cases of anterior uveitis will respond to local instillation of corticosteroid drops, together with the usual treatment of uveitis with mydriatics. Crick *et al.* (1961) treated 20 patients in this way; five resolved and eight improved. Posterior uveitis is not affected by local corticosteroid treatment, and they therefore treated patients presenting with severe uveitis, those with posterior uveitis, and those failing to respond to local treatment with systemic corticosteroids; of 12 patients so treated, four showed resolution and eight improved. They noted that where nodules were present in the iris, systemic treatment was more effective than local. Karma (1979) treated all her 22 patients with uveitis with dexamethasone drops topically, and 14 with oral prednisolone as well. She noted that there was an initial good response in all cases, and that fresh iritic nodules might respond rapidly to local treatment; but many cases proved chronic, uveitis reactivating when treatment was discontinued or reduced to 'maintenance' level, and in nine cases, uveitis was still under treatment at the end of her study. A mild anterior uveitis should therefore be treated initially with topical corticosteroids, and in some cases will resolve without visual impairment. If this fails, or if the posterior segment is involved, systemic corticosteroid treatment is indicated.

THE OCULAR FUNDUS

It is convenient to consider together the changes that may be found in the ocular fundus, including those in the choroid, the retina and its vessels, and the optic disc. Findings in series of cases have been published by Geeraerts *et al.* (1962), Letocha *et al.* (1975) and Spalton (1979) and reviews by Gould and Kaufman (1961), Turner *et al.* (1975) and Sanders and Shilling (1976).

Choroido-retinal changes described as non-specific or as scarring were found in 40% of 66 cases reviewed by Gould and Kaufman, and in 50% of 33 reported by Spalton (1979). Changes regarded as specially suggestive of sarcoidosis include various sorts of choroido-retinal nodules, perivasculitis, and tumour-like masses in the region of the optic disc. Macular oedema and papilloedema without raised cerebro-spinal fluid pressure may also be seen.

Nodule-like changes, usually near vessels, range from small round well-defined pale spots to larger irregular-shaped areas. Franceschetti and Babel (1949) described an appearance which they likened to spots of candle-wax (taches de bougie) in a patient with sarcoidosis. One of the affected eyes became blind and painful with cataract and glaucoma and was removed; granulomas were found in choroid, retina, optic nerve and sclera. This appearance has been found to be very suggestive of sarcoidosis. Karma (1979) found taches de bougie exudates in ten of 22 cases of sarcoid uveitis. They are associated in many cases with periphlebitis, the first report of which in a patient with sarcoidosis was by von Bahr (1938), who observed well-defined sheathing of retinal vessels by grey-white infiltration in a patient with uveo-parotitis; these perivascular infiltrations resolved in six months. It seems likely that in sarcoidosis periphlebitis is an especially perivascular distribution of granulomatous change similar to that which underlies taches de bougie. Witmer (1948) found granulomas of epithelioid cells and a few Langhans giant cells distributed along retinal veins in an eye enucleated because of painful blindness due to long-standing sarcoidosis. In a review of 40 published cases of sarcoid retinopathy, Gould and Kaufman (1961) found that 20 had periphlebitis and 14 taches de bougie, 12 having both these appearances. Among ten patients presenting with retinopathy as the first manifestation of sarcoidosis, Letocha *et al.* (1975) found periphlebitis in nine and candle-wax spots which they regarded as a more florid change of the same sort in five; of these ten patients, two had no evidence of anterior uveitis, and the other eight showed only mild changes of this sort. Spalton (1979) reported perivenous sheathing in 20 of 33 patients with sarcoid retinopathy. Perivascular infiltration may result in narrowing of the lumen, and the vessel wall itself may be involved (Levitt, 1941; Gass and Olson, 1973). Rarely, venous thrombosis has been reported (Goldberg and Newell, 1944). Like other forms of periphlebitis, that of sarcoidosis may be complicated by haemorrhage. Retinal, subhyaloid and vitreous haemorrhages may be observed in sarcoid retinopathy, in some cases apparently due to periphlebitis; in others, neovascularization of old lesions is the apparent source of bleeding. Ainslie and James (1956) reported a patient with sarcoid uveitis in whom periphlebitis retinae was accompanied by recurrent vitreous haemorrhages. Only one of the 61 patients with sarcoid uveitis reported by

Crick *et al.* (1961) had a vitreous haemorrhage; there were multiple foci of choroido-retinitis, but the changes seen after the haemorrhage had cleared were not thought describable as periphlebitis. During the time of their study, these authors had observed six patients with perivasculitis retinae with no evidence of sarcoidosis. Chumbley and Kearns (1972) described 'scattered blot haemorrhages' associated with diffuse periphlebitis in one of their four patients with sarcoid retinopathy, all of whom showed periphlebitis and candle-wax spots. Among their ten patients with retinopathy as the presenting feature of sarcoidosis, Letocha *et al.* (1975) found haemorrhages in six, of both superficial flame-shaped and deep round types, the latter tending to be peripherally located; in two cases, the haemorrhages were seen to be centred on perivascular exudate, and in one the macula was involved. Flame-shaped haemorrhages were observed in sarcoid retinopathy by Quock and Donohoe (1967) and Turner *et al.* (1975).

Neovascularization may develop at the sites of taches de bougie, periphlebitic and other infiltrations and at the optic disc, and may be the source of haemorrhage. In a patient with hilar lymph-node and pulmonary sarcoidosis who developed a uveo-parotid syndrome, Algvere (1970) found on fluorescein angiography leakage from newly-formed vessels and retention of dye in perivascular exudates. Sanders and Shilling (1976) described in three cases the development of multiple areas of preretinal neovascularization leading to haemorrhage after resolution of the acute stage of sarcoid retinopathy; there was leakage from the new vessels and large areas of capillary non-perfusion. Spalton (1979) studied fluorescein angiograms from 26 patients with sarcoid retinopathy, and found evidence of neovascularization in seven, involving either the site of previous perivenous infiltration or the optic disc, where it was thought to be secondary to retinal hypoxia. Asdourian *et al.* (1975) reported the cases of three black patients with sarcoidosis in whom peripheral fan-shaped areas of neovascularization were seen on fundoscopy; one showed also periphlebitis, candle-wax spots, choroidoretinal scars, and old and new vitreous haemorrhage; one also had anterior uveitis and periphlebitis; and the third had no other ocular sign. Fluorescein angiography showed profuse leakage from the abnormal vessels and avascularity of the retina anterior to them. The similarity of this neovascularization to that seen in some other conditions, notably sickle-cell anaemia, was noted; a feature seen in the sarcoid patients, who were shown to have normal haemoglobin, that had not been observed in retinal neovascularization in other diseases, was the presence of a few vessels passing through the neovascular area into avascular retina. The problem of differential diagnosis in black patients with both sarcoidosis and homozygous sickle-cell disease who were found to have this sort of neovascularization has been discussed by Madigan *et al.* (1977) and by Raymond *et al.* (1978).

Other studies of sarcoid retinopathy by fluorescein angiography have show leakage from venules involved in periphlebitis and fluorescence of candle-wax spots (Chumbley and Kearns, 1972; Letocha *et al.*, 1975; François *et al.*, 1977). Turner *et al.* (1975) in one case found that there was no leakage from candle-wax spots; late leakage was seen from capillary dilatation in nodular areas, both in the region of the swollen optic discs and more peripherally. Kobayashi (1974) observed increased permeability of both veins and arteries on fluorescein angiography in all of 13 patients with ocular sarcoidosis. Karma (1979) found that fresh 'granulomas' of the retina and optic disc pushed vessels aside or hid them, and did not fluoresce; older ones showed intense late fluorescence; perivenous exudates and taches de bougie showed leakage of dye in the active stage. She also reported fluorescein angiographic studies of the iris in anterior uveitis; more granulomas were seen than could be seen by biomicroscopy, with leakage of dye in the active stage, usually diminishing or ceasing as the condition became inactive.

As already noted, retinopathy may occur without anterior uveitis. There was no evidence of anterior uveitis in one-third of the 40 published cases of sarcoid retinopathy reviewed by Gould and Kaufman (1961), in any of four reported by Chumbley and Kearns (1972), in two of ten by Letocha *et al.* (1975) and in eight of 33 by Spalton (1979). In her study of 281 patients with sarcoidosis, Karma (1979) observed three with fundal changes without evident uveitis.

Swelling of the optic disc has been observed as part of a sarcoid retinopathy in patients without overt evidence of intracranial sarcoidosis; e.g. by Spalton (1979) in nine of 33. In view of the frequency of concurrent involvement of the fundus oculi and the central nervous system, noted below, differential diagnosis from papilloedema due to intracranial sarcoidosis or to involvement of the optic nerve within the optic foramen, discussed in Chapter 14, p. 305, may be difficult (James *et al.*, 1967). Nodular masses, presumably of sarcoid granuloma, may be seen at the margin of or over the optic nerve head (Goldberg and Newell, 1944; Mackensen, 1952; Laties and Scheie, 1972). They follow an unpredictable course; Laties and Scheie watched the shrinkage of two such lesions in a patient with BHL and lung changes, leaving very minor 'gliosis' and no visual defect; in Case 1 of Goldberg and Newell (1944), a white mass extending three dioptres into the vitreous and associated with haemorrhage led to extensive new vessel formation. In other cases, masses at the optic nerve head have been part of more widespread ocular changes, with an unfavourable course which has resulted in a few in indications for enucleation, providing the possibility of histology which confirmed the granulomatous nature of the nodular masses (Laval, 1952; Kelley and Green, 1973). Gass and Olson (1973) reported the necropsy findings in a black man aged

41 with sarcoidosis involving lungs, hilar nodes, liver, central nervous system and eyes in whom a large white mass near the left optic disc had been part of extensive changes in the optic fundus; candle-wax perivascular exudates, preretinal and intravitreal nodules, and localized tumefactions at the optic nerve head which had been seen ophthalmoscopically were found to be due to epithelioid cell granulomas. Brownstein and Jannotta (1974) reported the case of a black man aged 17 who presented with coma due to obstructive hydrocephalus, and died after an operation at which a 'tumour' was found in anterior part of the third ventricle; at necropsy, there were granulomas in the leptomeninges and in the brain in perivascular spaces especially in the hypothalamus, tuber cinereum, the lentiform nucleus and the optic chiasma and tracts; in the left eye the retina showed a white elevated mass of sarcoid-type granuloma, and the right optic nerve was found to be infiltrated by a similar granuloma; there was no evidence of anterior uveitis. In the enucleated eye whose pathology was described by Laval (1952), granulomas in the retina and a granulomatous nodule in the optic nerve head were accompanied by papilloedema. Possibly granulomas within the optic nerve head account for some of the cases of optic disc swelling without evidence of raised intracranial pressure which have resolved spontaneously or after corticosteroid treatment (Fine and Flocks, 1953; James *et al.*, 1967; Hart and Burde, 1979).

Oedema of the macula has also been observed in active sarcoid retinopathy (Goldberg and Newell, 1944; Chumbley and Kearns, 1972, one case out of four; Letocha *et al.*, 1975; Turner *et al.*, 1975; Karma 1979, three of 21 cases with fundal changes). Fine and Flocks (1953) and Hart and Burde (1979) observed confluent swelling of the optic disc and of the macula. Of the ten cases reported by Letocha *et al.* (1975), two showed macular haemorrhage and and one macular oedema. These changes may be due to venous narrowing by periphlebitis.

In their review of published cases of sarcoid retinopathy, Gould and Kaufman (1961) found that one-third had also evident involvement of the central nervous system, as did two of the four reported by Chumbley and Kearns (1972). In the series of ten patients seen by Letocha *et al.* (1975) as out-patients, only one had signs of central nervous system involvement. The magnitude of the association between sarcoid retinopathy and symptomatic involvement of the central nervous system probably lies between the high estimate suggested by the review of published cases, likely to include many with an unfavourable course or unusual features, and the lower figure suggested by a study of out-patients. There is no evidence that patients with anterior uveitis as the predominant ocular manifestation have an unusually high incidence of intracranial sarcoidosis; the occasional association with cranial and other neuropathies is discussed above.

LACRIMAL APPARATUS

Lacrimal gland

In 1934, before Heerfordt's syndrome was generally recognized to be a manifestation of sarcoidosis, Savin reviewed 66 published cases; in nine lacrimal gland enlargement had been noted. Later, cases were reported in which painless enlargement of lacrimal glands was found by biopsy and association with other features of sarcoidosis to be a part of that disease (Rosenbaum, 1941; Sniderman, 1941; Schultz, 1945; Longcope and Freiman, 1952; Ainslie and James, 1956; Gruber et al., 1956; Crick et al., 1961; Cook et al., 1972), and granulomas have been found in lacrimal glands of normal size in patients with sarcoidosis (Crick et al., 1961; Greenburg et al., 1964). Lacrimal secretion, when tested, is frequently found to be deficient in patients with sarcoidosis, with or without evidence of other sorts of ocular involvement; it may lead to the syndrome of kerato-conjunctivitis sicca. Crick et al. (1961) noted that many of their patients with sarcoidosis complained of dryness, soreness and redness of the eyes attributed to lack of lacrimal secretion and consequent degeneration of the epithelial cells of the cornea and conjunctiva, especially in their exposed parts. Eighty-eight patients with sarcoidosis were examined by slit-lamp microscopy after the instillation of 1% rose bengal solution; staining was observed in 66% as compared with 6% of a control series. In another group of 30 patients, they estimated lacrimal secretion by Schirmer's test, and found that changes in the cornea demonstrated by rose bengal staining correlated well with deficient secretion. In two cases, one with and one without palpable swelling of lacrimal glands, biopsy of the gland showed infiltration with sarcoid tubercles. They concluded that the deficiency of tears was due to sarcoid infiltration of the lacrimal glands, which must therefore be more frequent than had been suspected. These evidences of lacrimal gland involvement were not specially correlated with uveitis or conjunctival granulomas. The incidence of kerato-conjuctivitis sicca reported by observers who have used less intensive methods for its discovery is much lower. For instance, James (1959a) observed it in seven of his 200 patients. Karma (1979) found diminished lacrimal secretion in 32 of 254 patients with sarcoidosis submitted to Schirmer's test; of these, only 12 complained of relevant symptoms. Of 22 patients with uveitis, less than half (ten) also had reduced lacrimal secretion; and of 30 with reduced lacrimal secretion submitted to conjunctival biopsy, nine (30%) showed granulomas, compared with 17% of all patients so investigated.

The kerato-conjunctivitis sicca of sarcoidosis might be confused with that of Sjögren's syndrome, especially since in this syndrome the salivary and lacrimal glands may be enlarged. The dryness of the mouth, the inflammatory and often painful nature of the salivary gland enlargement, usually with variations in size, occurrence predominantly in post-menopausal women, associated with features of connective-tissue disorders ranging from rheumatoid arthritis to atypical systemic lupus erythematosus with non-organ-specific auto-antibodies, and the absence of clinical or histological evidence of sarcoidosis should distinguish Sjögren's syndrome without undue difficulty. Usually, lacrimal gland sarcoidosis is accompanied by easily detected evidence of sarcoidosis elsewhere; very occasionally, as in Case 1 of Cook *et al.* (1972) it presents as the first evidence of sarcoidosis, diagnosis being made only by biopsy and search for sarcoidosis in other locations.

Lacrimal passages

A few cases in which sarcoidosis has involved the lacrimal sac have been recorded (Neault and Riley, 1970; Fisher *et al.*, Coleman *et al.*, 1972), some complicated by bacterial infection leading to dacryocystitis which may be suppurative and need treatment with antibiotics and possibly incision. Five female patients among the 281 studied by Karma (1979) had epiphora due to dacryostenosis; three had suffered from nasal obstruction, presumably due to involvement of nasal mucosa. Dacryorhinostomy was performed in three cases, but was successful in only one; this operation was performed also in the cases reported by Neault and Riley (1970) and by Fisher *et al.* (1971). In the case of Neault and Riley, involvement of the nasal mucosa was demonstrated, and it seems likely that in most cases obstruction of lacrimal passages is secondary to nasal sarcoidosis (Chapter 13).

CONJUNCTIVA

Lutz (1919) seems to have been the first to describe sarcoid nodules in the conjunctiva, with histological findings. Some scattered references were made subsequently to conjunctival lesions in sarcoidosis in the ophthalmological literature (e.g. Blegvad, 1931). Crick *et al.* (1955) reported that in patients with sarcoidosis examination of the conjunctiva for suspicious-looking follicles, usually in the lower fornix, and subsequent biopsy had frequently led to the finding of typical sarcoid lesions. Crick *et al.* (1961) described their extended experience with conjunctival biopsy. Of 139 patients, 79 were found to have conjunctival follicles; in 20 of these biopsy showed appearances regarded as typical sarcoidosis. All the positive biopsies were obtained from follicles in the lower fornix of the conjunctiva. Typical follicles were described as small elevations, translucent and slightly yellow in colour, and just visible to the naked eye, most frequent in the fornices, where they may be confluent, but occasionally in the bulbar conjunctiva. They may be confused with lymphoid follicles, which are frequent in the conjunctiva, and from which they can be distinguished with certainly only by biopsy and examination of serial sections. Crick *et al.* also noted that in acne rosacea small elevations may be present in the bulbar conjuctiva with the histological appearance of sarcoid tissue; but in this disease, the fornix conjunctiva appears to be unaffected. Another possible source of error has been pointed out by Zimmerman (1961). Obstruction of the Meibomian glands in the tarsal plate causes the common chalazion. Multiple small chalazia might be confused with sarcoid nodules; Blegvad (1931) described the appearances of the conjunctival sarcoidosis in his three cases as small to large chalazion-like tubercles, varying from single to many, studding the conjunctiva. Histologically the typical chalazion presents no sarcoid-like features, though occasionaly epithelioid cells and giant cells may be present, presumably as a reaction to the fatty content of the retained secretion, and the giant cells may even contain inclusion bodies of the Schaumann and asteroid types.

Bornstein *et al.* (1962) found granulomas on conjunctival biopsy in 25% of 64 patients with sarcoidosis and in none of 28 control subjects with other diseases. Conjunctival involvement was not specially related to other evidence of ocular sarcoidosis. Three of the 16 patients with positive biopsies and seven of 48 with negative biopsies had signs of intraocular sarcoidosis. A positive conjunctival bioposy was obtained in only one of 25 patients with sarcoidosis limited to the intrathoracic organs, as compared with 15 out of 39 with clinical evidence of involvement of both extrathoracic and intrathoracic organs.

Karma (1979) found granulomas in 17% of biopsies taken after careful inspection of the conjunctiva in 218 patients with sarcoidosis; 41% of 66 cases in which nodules thought suspicious of sarcoidosis had been seen, and 6.6% of 152 without such findings showed granulomas. Sarcoidosis of the conjunctiva was usually symptomless, but in four patients it caused redness and oedema, and in one, large vegetations on the conjunctiva of the lower lid and fornix, which appeared at the same time as infiltration of old scars on the skin and lung infiltration, causing discomfort. In 12 patients cutaneous sarcoids and conjunctival granulomas became evident at the same time. Granulomas were found in 35% of patients with active and in 10% with inactive sarcoidosis; and in 10% of those with BHL and clear lungs, 24% of those with BHL and prefibrotic lung infiltration, and 43% of those with chronic lung changes. In relation to other eye changes, the proportion of those with uveitis showing granulomas was 25%, only slightly higher than that for the whole series; with reduced lacrimal secretion it was 30% and with lacrimal gland enlargement 67%; and with band keratopathy 40%.

It is evident that granulomas are present in the conjunctiva of many cases of sarcoidosis, usually scanty and rarely causing symptoms. They are most likely to be numerous in the active stages of the disease and when there are widespread changes in other organs. Only exceptionally is conjunctival biopsy likely to be helpful in difficult cases where clinically evident manifestations are localized in one organ. A case of this sort has been reported by Fulton *et al.* (1976); in a patient investigated for dyspepsia, endoscopy showed polypoidal changes in the antrum of the stomach, histologically granulomatous; search for evidence of sarcoidosis elsewhere showed minute nodules in the lower fornix of the conjunctiva, biopsy of which showed granulomas of sarcoid type, no other change suggestive of sarcoidosis being found in other organs or elsewhere in the eye. In general, conjunctival biopsy is least likely to be helpful as a diagnostic procedure when it is most needed. The possibility of its successful use depends upon expert examination to discover typical-looking follicles for biopsy, followed by serial sectioning and interpretation of the sections by an observer thoroughly familiar with the histology both of sarcoidosis and of the eye. The method is therefore likely to be of more value to the ophthalmologist who can perform the minor biopsy procedure with little trouble in the course of a complete examination, than to the physician who will usually find biopsy of some other tissue not only more convenient and easier to interpret, but also more likely to be helpful in obscure cases.

The conjunctiva may also be affected by non-granulomatous changes. Kerato-conjunctivitis sicca, secondary to deficient lacrimal secretion, has been discussed above. Punctate calcification may occur as a consequence of hypercalcaemia, often with band keratopathy, discussed below. In the early acute stage of sarcoidosis, episcleritis may occur, usually with erythema nodosum. Karma (1979) observed it in five cases, coinciding with the appearance of erythema nodosum in four, and subsiding within a few months;

CORNEAL AND CONJUNCTIVAL CHANGES ASSOCIATED WITH HYPERCALCAEMIA

The hypercalcaemia that occurs in a few patients with sarcoidosis can give rise to deposition of calcium salts in the cornea and conjunctiva (Haldimann, 1941). Of the 19 patients with band keratopathy due to hypercalcaemia reported by Cogan *et al.* (1948), two had sarcoidosis. Calcium salts tend to be deposited especially in the exposed parts of the conjunctiva (Fig. 8.1) and cornea. Crick *et al.* (1961) observed such changes in seven of their 185 patients, four having both corneal and conjunctival, two corneal and one conjunctival deposits. Karma (1979) found band keratopathy, associated with white crystals in varying number in the limbal conjunctiva in 11 of 282 patients, and confirmed the association with hypercalcaemia. With very high calcium levels, acute deposition of calcium salts in the cornea and

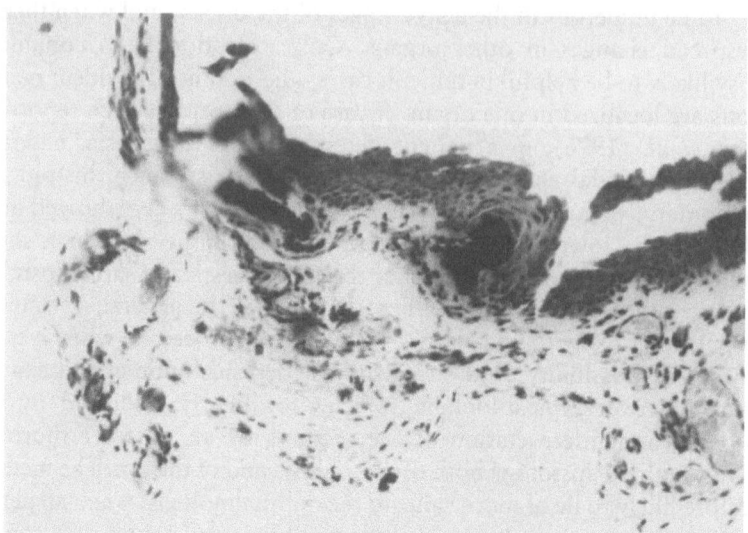

Figure 8.1   Biopsy of conjunctiva of a woman aged 35 with sarcoidosis and hypercalcaemia, showing deposits of calcium salts staining deeply with von Kossa's stain. × 170.

conjunctiva may give rise to photophobia, redness and aching in the eyes. Treatment of the hypercalcaemia (Chapter 19) leads to subsidence of these acute changes, and gradual removal of the calcium deposits.

It is probable that deficiency of lacrimal secretion is in many cases a contributory factor to the deposition of calcium salts in the conjunctiva and cornea. Karma (1979) found reduced lacrimal secretion in half her patients with band keratopathy, and hypercalcaemia in rather more than half those with reduced lacrimal secretion.

EXOPHTHALMOS DUE TO SARCOID INFILTRATION IN THE ORBIT

In 1931, Reis and Rothfeld reported the case of a girl who died at the age of 17 years. At the age of 15, she had developed sarcoid infiltration of the skin of the cheeks and later of the limbs, chiefly on the upper arms. Biopsy showed epithelioid cell tubercles without caseation, and no tubercle bacilli, either on direct examination or on guinea-pig inoculation. She also had spindle-shaped swellings of the fingers with dystrophy of the nails and radiographic changes characteristic of sarcoidosis of the metacarpals and phalanges. The skin gave no reaction to a Mantoux or a Pirquet test. She later developed headache, vomiting and loss of vision. She was found to have bilateral exophthalmos, more severe on the left; papilloedema and optic atrophy on the right side; and involvement of the whole left retina in a white tumour over which the retinal vessels were running. There was also some weakness in the right leg and extensor plantar responses on both sides. Shortly before her death one and a half years after the beginning of the illness she developed epileptic seizures. At necropsy, there was an extensive somewhat translucent yellowish infiltration over the base of the skull, extending from the cerebral peduncles to the optic chiasma, involving both temporal lobes laterally and infiltrating the floor of the third ventricle. This was found to have the same histological pattern as had been seen in the skin biopsy, consisting in epithelioid cell tubercles without giant cells or caseation. The 'tumour' involving the left optic nerve and retina had a similar histology. The authors did not discuss the cause of the exophthalmos, nor did they state whether the infiltration extended into the orbit. Their account of the case was devoted mainly to a detailed description of the pathology of the enucleated eyes. In relation to the other organs, they stated that a generalized tuberculosis was found, with the primary changes in the peribronchial lymph-nodes and in the lungs at various stages of development from fresh tubercles with very little tendency to caseation to fibrosis and calcification; no bacteriological studies were reported.

Melmon and Goldberg (1962) described the case of a 37 year old black man who noticed pain and redness of the right eye, which became protuberant. Later a small mass was noticed in the upper lid, and the left eye became protuberant. In addition to bilateral exophthalmos, a generalized superficial lymphadenopathy, hepatosplenomegaly, bilateral hilar lymph-node enlargement with lung infiltration and evidence of right-sided anterior uveitis were found. A tuberculin test with 0.005 mg PPD was negative. Biopsies of the orbital mass and of a supraclavicular lymph-node both showed sarcoidosis. The condition responded to prednisone treatment. but relapsed when it was stopped.

In these two cases, there was evidence of widespread involvement of other organs and tissues, justifying the diagnosis of sarcoidosis. A number of other cases have been recorded (King, 1939; Benedict, 1949, two cases; Knapp and Knott, 1949; Rider and Dodson, 1950; Bodian and Lasky, (1950) in which masses of sarcoid tissue in the orbit have caused exophthalmos. In these cases no incontrovertible evidence of sarcoid lesions elsewhere has been found, although King's (1939) patient had an unexplained bronchial stenosis and transient weakness and numbness in the left leg, and in the patient reported by Rider and Dodson (1950) there was a generalized adenopathy, a single biopsy showing no evidence of sarcoidosis. Local excision of a mass of sarcoid tissue was followed in some cases by no recurrence (King, 1939; Benedict, 1949, Case 1), but in others (Benedict, 1949, Case 2; Rider and Dodson, 1950) by recurrence. In the case reported by Rider and Dodson, part of the bony orbit was eroded, and the maxillary antrum invaded.

One of us (JGS) has observed a patient with exophthalmos due to sarcoid infiltration of the orbital fat, with some other features of sarcoidosis and some atypical features.

A woman, aged 54, developed swelling round both eyes, starting with subcutaneous nodules in the upper lids, and leading to progressive proptosis and left-sided ptosis. Tissue was removed from both orbits for biopsy; it showed well-defined epithelioid cell tubercles with some giant cells, and no caseation, set in loose fibrous tissue arranged in a rather whorled pattern around them. A chest radiograph at this time was normal. One year later, she had iritis for six weeks only. About this time she had pain in the left side of the chest and radiographically the left side of the diaphragm was 'tented'. After this, she remained well – apart from the ptosis and dryness of the eyes – for three years, when she developed left sciatica, shown to be due to a prolapsed intervertebral disc. While in hospital for the treatment of this, she developed fever, with left-, then right-sided pleurisy with small clear effusions, which resolved spontaneously leaving slight basal pleural thickening. One year later, she was free from symptoms apart from those of the ocular condition. The exophthalmos had diminished but was still evident; there was left ptosis, and dryness of the eyes but not of the month. The ocular movements were restricted in all directions. There was radiographic evidence of slight bilateral hilar lymph-node enlargement with some calcification on the right side. There were several small papules on the right shin and an infiltrated scar on the left shin, which appeared compatible with sarcoid infiltration, but were not submitted to biopsy. The skin reacted to 100, but not to 10 IU of tuberculin. Thirteen years from the onset, no further symptoms or signs of sarcoidosis had developed, but vision was severely impaired by ptosis, symblepharon, interference with external ocular movements, and cataracts.

In this case, the uncharacteristic intrathoracic changes, bilateral pleural effusions, and failure to demonstrate sarcoid-type granulomas elsewhere than in the orbit, must lead to doubt about categorization as sarcoidosis. The cases reported by Reis and Rothfeld (1931) and by Melmon and Goldberg (1962) certainly showed evidence of generalized sarcoidosis, and infiltration of the orbit causing exophthalmos must therefore be accepted as a possible though very rare manifestation of this disease. Some of the other cases reported suggest the possibility that an exuberant sarcoid tissue infiltration may sometimes occur in the orbit as an isolated phenomenon in response to some unknown local stimulus. Detailed study of individual cases is necessary before it can be decided whether the orbital changes are part of a generalized disease.

Chapter 9

Bones, Joints and Skeletal Muscles

BONES

The early history of the development of knowledge about the changes in the bones of the hands and feet in sarcoidosis is briefly described in Chapter 1. After the original description of the typical changes in cases of lupus pernio by Kreibich (1904), a number of accounts of one or two cases were published (e.g. Bloch, 1907; Rieder, 1910; Schaumann, 1919; Jüngling, 1920). The first detailed accounts of the radiology were those of Fleischner (1924) and Jüngling (1928). Schaumann's paper in 1919 contained a full study of the histological changes, and emphasized the location of the specific granuloma in the marrow. Although as early as 1907, Bloch had described a case in which the ulna as well as two metacarpals were affected, radiologically evident involvement is much less frequent in the long bones, the vertebrae and the skull than in the bones of the hands and feet.

Incidence

The frequency of bone changes reported in different series varies, like that of other manifestations, with the population from which the cases were drawn, the interests of the observer, and the methods of investigation. A high proportion of patients with chronic forms of skin sarcoidosis, especially lupus pernio, have changes in the bones of the hand and feet. Kissmeyer (1932) found that among 26 cases with skin sarcoids seen in Copenhagen, seven had radiographic changes in the bones of the hands and feet. Gravesen (1942) observed 112 patients in Denmark, and found that 32, all with skin sarcoids, had radiographic changes in bones of hands and feet; of these four had changes in other bones – the ulna and the tibia in one case each, and the nasal bones in the other two. Reisner (1944), in New York, found that among 35 patients, of whom 30 were black, nine had changes in the bones of the hands and feet; and in three, other bones were affected, the carpal bones in one, the ulna in one, and the tibia, fibula, radius and ulna in the third. Longcope and Freiman (1952) found that among 55 patients in Baltimore nine (15.8%) and among 45 in Boston ten (22%) had radiographic changes in the bones of the hands and feet; in one of the Boston group the radius and ulna and in one of the Baltimore group the radius, ulna, tibia and fibula were also involved. In 15 of the 19 cases skin sarcoids were also present. Stein *et al.* (1956) in Philadelphia studied a series of 175 patients. Among 81 with histological evidence, 14 (17.2%), and among 94 with clinical evidence only three (3.1%), had definite radiographic changes in bones. In six cases, carpal or tarsal bones as well as metacarpals or metatarsals and phalanges were involved. Extensive radiographic surveys of bones were made in ten patients with changes in the bones of the extremities; one was already known to have changes in radius, ulna and tibia, but no previously undetected lesions were found in this or any of the other nine cases. Unlike other observers, they were unable to detect any correlation between the bone and skin changes. Gilg (1955) studied a series of 191 patients, of whom 91% had skin lesions; among 179 of them who had radiographs of the hands and feet, 42 (23.5%) were found to have bone changes.

All the series just quoted contained high proportions either of cases with skin sarcoids, or of chronic cases with extensive organ involvement. At the other end of the scale, Löfgren (1953) described 212 early cases at the stage of bilateral hilar lymph-node enlargement, of whom more than half had erythema nodosum; in 30 of these, the hands and feet were examined radiographically soon after the disease was discovered, and two were found to have skeletal lesions. Under observation for periods of 2–16 years, only one other was observed to develop bone changes; but radiography of the extremities does not appear to have been performed routinely. Series which include a high proportion of early cases at the stage of BHL, certainly in Europe, appear to contain fewer patients with bone lesions than the series including high proportions of black patients or those derived from dermatological clinics. Mather (1957) in London found that of 120 patients, nine (7.5%) had radiographic changes in the bones of the hands or feet; of these five had skin lesions. James (1959b), also in London, in a series of 200 patients found 11 with bone lesions; there were 33 with skin sarcoids, of whom ten had bone lesions, but only one of the 167 without skin sarcoids. In a series of 275 patients, not all of whom had radiographs of the hands and feet because it was found that the incidence of bone changes among those without skin sarcoids or other manifestations of chronic sarcoidosis was low, one of us (JGS) detected bone changes in the hands or feet in ten, of whom seven had skin sarcoids, all of the lupus pernio type, and one had subcutaneous nodules in the pulps of two fingers, the bones of which were not affected. Among the seven patients with lupus pernio, the skin over the affected bones was involved prominently in four, slightly in one, and not evidently in two; the face was involved prominently in four, slightly in two, and not evidently in one. In the latter case skin changes were evident only over the affected bones, with the exception of infiltration of a scar on the knee. In two cases in which great toes were involved, there was a clear history that the changes appeared soon after an injury. Neville *et al.* (1977) reported that of 567 patients attending a sarcoidosis clinic in London, 26 had changes in the bones of the hands or feet, one in the temporal bone, one in the hard palate and three in the nasal bones in association with nasal mucosal involvement. Skin sarcoids were present in 19 (66%) of those with bone changes, and took the form of lupus pernio in 14. Erythema nodosum had occurred in only one of the 26 with bone involvement, as compared with 33% of the whole series.

Pathology

Schaumann (1919, 1926) gave a detailed account of the pathology of the changes in the small bones of the hands and feet, based upon the examination of two amputated toes. These came from a woman who had had sarcoidosis of the skin of the face and of superficial lymph-nodes, both histologically confirmed, and histologically specific changes in the tonsils removed for biopsy. Radiographic changes were found in two toes, at first without external evidence; but four years later, the toes had become swollen and were amputated though the skin still looked normal. Even in parts of the bone showing a normal radiographic pattern, tuberculoid follicles surrounded by lymphocytes replaced the marrow between normal trabeculae; in the parts showing rarefaction, the trabeculae were resorbed, leaving a space filled with a large mass of the tuberculoid granulation tissue. In the compact bone, there was irregular resorption of bone with enlargement of Haversian canals which contained a few granulomas. In a few places, especially near the ends of the phalanx, granulomatous tissue extended into the tissues around the bone; it infiltrated tendon sheaths, but did not affect tendons. Schaumann concluded that the granulomatous process may remain confined to the marrow, without producing any radiographic change; it may cause general rarefaction of bone; this rarefaction may be accentuated locally to cause the radiographic cyst-like spaces; and periosseous infiltration may occur, though tendons remain intact. Similar changes to those described by Shaumann were found by Hollister and Harrell (1941) in a toe removed at necropsy from a black man with extensive sarcoidosis; although it was not externally abnormal, a typical cyst-like rarefaction had been detected radiologically during life in its middle phalanx.

Indications for biopsy of bones of the hands or feet affected by sarcoidosis rarely arise, since the diagnosis is usually evident without it. Very occasionally, patients have presented with localized swelling of a finger, radiographic changes have been found in an underlying phalanx, and biopsy has led to the diagnosis of sarcoidosis, subsequently confirmed by other clinical features. Such cases have been described by Griffiths (1969) and Pierson *et al.* (1978). We have records of two, one of which is illustrated in Figs 9.1 and 9.2. Involvement of other bones is rarer, but causes diagnostic difficulty leading to biopsy in a higher proportion of cases. In general, the findings have been concordant with Schaumann's description of the changes in phalanges. As noted below, in a few cases there has been radiographic

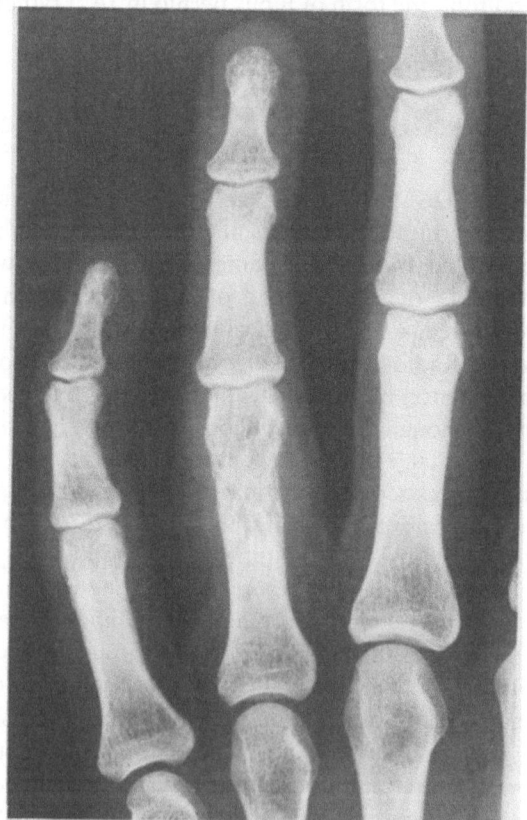

Figure 9.1   Radiograph showing sarcoidosis of proximal phalanx of ring finger in a woman aged 30. She had noticed swelling of this finger for eight months.

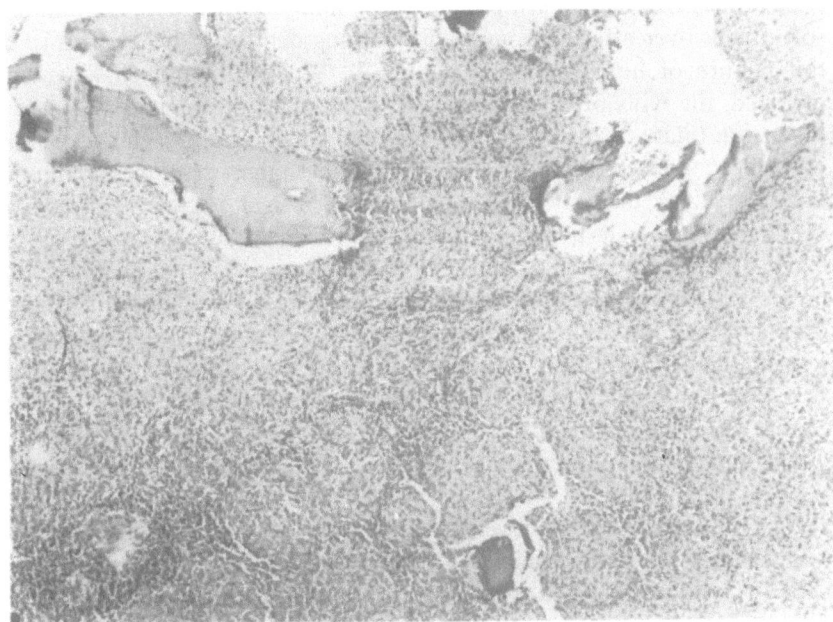

Figure 9.2 Biopsy of the affected phalanx shown in Fig. 9.1. Between the bone trabeculae there are densely packed non-caseating epithelioid cell tubercles, with here and there a narrow zone of lymphocytic infiltration between them. H & E. × 55. After this biopsy, she was found to have bilateral hilar lymph-node enlargement, and a Kveim test gave a granulomatous response.

evidence of increased bone density, and in some of these biopsy has shown thickening of bone trabeculae (Bonakdarpour *et al.*, 1971; Young and Laman, 1972). In one case, the biopsy sample from a swelling in the parieto-occipital region of the skull, where an area of bone rarefaction was found, showed fibroblasts with a few giant cells and occasional epithelioid cells, and was thought sufficiently suggestive of meningioma to be treated by wide removal of affected skull; histology of this larger specimen showed epithelioid cell granulomas, and in the presence of a symptomless radiographic infiltration of the lungs established the diagnosis of sarcoidosis (Turner and Weiss, 1969).

Hands and feet

In some cases, bone changes are found incidentally on routine radiography of the hands and feet and cause no symptoms at any time; e.g. in four of the ten with changes in these bones in 275 cases reviewed by one of us (JGS). Of the 26 patients with involvement of digits in the group reported by Neville *et al.* (1977) half had no symptoms. The commonest symptom is swelling of soft tissues over affected bones, with varying degrees of lividity, up to the full picture of lupus pernio (Chapter 7). When terminal phalanges are involved, the nails often become dystrophic, with thickening, ridging and distortion (Plate 2). Affected parts may be tender, and movement of joints adjacent to affected bones stiff and painful, but in most cases these symptoms are less severe than the degree of swelling might suggest. Tendons are very rarely involved, but in a patient under the care of one of us (JGS) the extensor tendon became detached from an affected terminal phalanx, leaving permanent weakness of extension, although the bone and skin changes eventually resolved almost completely. In very florid cases, complete resorption of parts of affected bones leads to severe deformity, sometimes made worse by pathological fractures. Neville *et al.* (1977) observed destructive changes in three of their 26 patients.

Accounts of the radiographic changes have been published by Fleischner (1924), Jüngling (1928), Nielsen (1934), Holt and Owens (1949), Stein *et al.* (1956), and Neville *et al.* (1977). Fleischner (1924) discussing bone changes in lupus pernio and Boeck's 'miliary lupoid' described a type showing sharply defined round foci of rarefaction principally in the phalanges without affection of the cortical bone, and accompanying the nodular form of Boeck's sarcoids; and a type affecting also metacarpals and metatarsals with a generalized lattice-like or honeycomb-like alteration of trabecular structure and accompanying lupus pernio or diffuse infiltrating sarcoids of the skin. Jüngling (1928) described three types of change in phalanges. In Type I, the phalanx is diffusely expanded, the compact bone is thinned, and the bone appears to consist of a number of cyst-like spaces of various sizes. In Type II, the changes consist only in localized round or oval well-defined 'punched-out' areas of featureless transradiancy. In Type III, the radiographic shadow cast by the bone has a uniform fine lattice-like structure. Jüngling thought that Type I was the early active stage, and Type II represented the stage of healing; and in one case, he observed a transition between these two types during the course of 16 years' observation, the transition from diffuse to localized changes having occurred in seven years. But in two of four cases in which one of us (JGS) observed localized cyst-like changes, principally at the ends of phalanges (Fig. 9.3), it was known that these represented an early stage of the disease. The illustrations of Jüngling's case suggest that the 'late' cyst-like spaces were surrounded by some irregular sclerosis, which is not evident in the 'early' cyst-like spaces. Neville *et al.* (1977) described 'lytic' lesions consisting of either small cortical defects in phalangeal heads or larger rounded cysts usually in the heads of middle and proximal phalanges, occasionally in metacarpal heads; they noted that in healing these lytic lesions become corticated. Thus cyst-like spaces may be an early or a late change. Jüngling's Type III seems to correspond with that

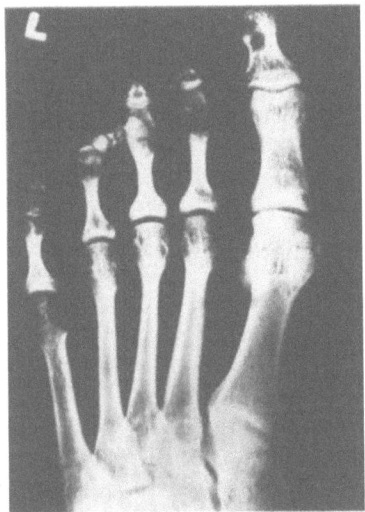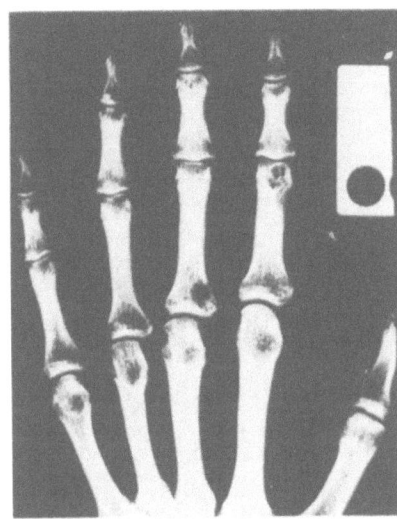

Figure 9.3 Cyst-like rarefactions in distal phalanx of left great toe, distal end of proximal phalanx of left index finger and base of proximal phalanx of left middle finger, causing no symptoms in a woman aged 22 with sarcoidosis involving also lungs, lymph-nodes and liver.

described by Neville *et al.* (1977) as 'permeative', which they observed in nine out of their 26 patients. This sort of change is commonly accompanied by evident swelling of soft tissues, and possibly by changes in the overlying skin. It is illustrated in Fig. 9.4.

With all patterns of bone change, periosteal reaction is rare; sclerosis occurs only perifocally as part of the healing process; joints are involved only when adjacent bone is destructively involved; there is no sequestration; and the process is usually very indolent, the possibility of healing being limited only by the degree of bone destruction and deformity in severe cases.

In North America, blacks seem to be more liable than whites to severe and deforming sarcoidosis of the bones of the hands. Morrison (1974), reporting 18 black South African patients with extensive skin sarcoidosis commented on the frequency and extent of involvement of bones of the hands; radiographic changes were found in ten, and in many of these cyst formation encroached on joints, in some with virtual disappearance of phalanges and gross deformity. In a comparative study in Cape Town, Benatar (1977, 1980) confirmed that changes of this sort were frequent in black and rare in white patients with sarcoidosis.

The effect of corticosteroid treatment on sarcoidosis of the bones of the hands and feet is difficult to assess. In some cases, treatment may be indicated for changes at other sites – e.g. in the lungs or the eyes; in a few, local pain, swelling and stiffness may call for relief. In general these symp-

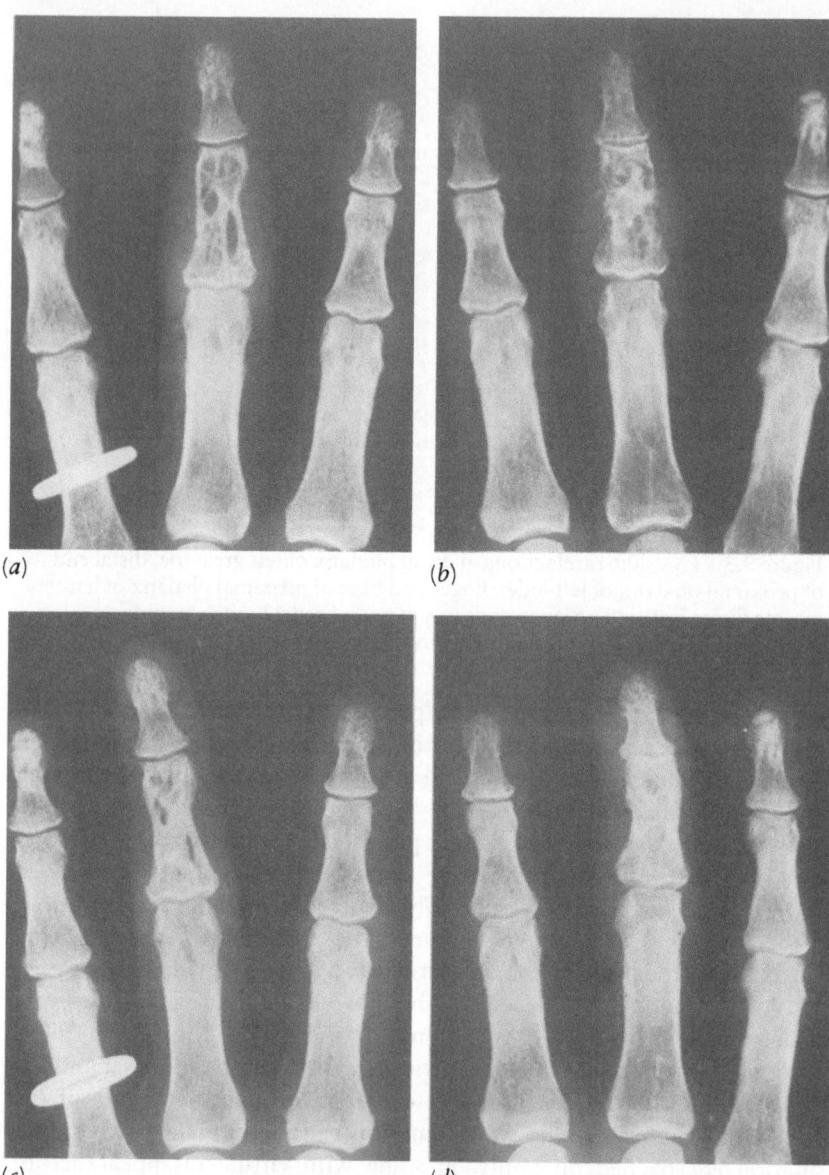

Figure 9.4 The index, middle and ring fingers of a woman aged 48 with sarcoidosis involving also the lungs and lymph-nodes. (*a*) and (*b*) Lattice-like rarefactions in the middle phalanx of the left middle finger and more irregular changes with some periosteal involvement in the corresponding phalanx on the right side. (*c*) and (*d*) Two years later, showing considerable resolution under corticosteroid treatment, undertaken for painful swelling of the right middle finger.

toms are alleviated by corticosteroids. With prolonged suppression of the activity of sarcoidosis, reparative changes may be observed in affected bones (Fig. 9.4), but it is of course impossible to say whether this might have occurred in the untreated course of the disease.

Skull

Involvement of nasal bones is well recognized in cases of lupus pernio affecting the nose (Hudelo *et al.*, 1925; Jüngling, 1928; Neville *et al.*, 1976) and of intranasal sarcoidosis (Chapter 13).

Cases of sarcoidosis in which the cranium has been involved as the only detected site of bone involvement have been reported by Teirstein *et al.* (1961), Olsen (1963), Nou (1965), Turner and Weiss (1969), Perrin-Fayolle *et al.* (1971), and Neville *et al.* (1977); and as one among several bones by Posner (1942), Franco-Saenz *et al.* (1970); Toomey and Bautista (1970, Case 1), Lin *et al.* (1973), Zimmerman and Leeds (1976), Silver *et al.* (1978) and Rohatgi (1980, Case 2). Most of these cases occurred in patients already known to have sarcoidosis, in some florid and long-standing; e.g. that of a 38 year-old black woman, reported by Teirstein *et al.* (1961), who for six months had had lacrimal gland enlargement and subcutaneous nodules both showing sarcoid changes on biopsy, hepatomegaly, BHL, and a positive Kveim test, when she developed frontal headache and swellings in this area. Three oval areas of rarefaction were found in the skull, and biopsy confirmed local sarcoid infiltration. In the case reported by Olsen (1963) multiple transradiant areas were found in the parietal bone when a woman aged 51 was investigated for persistent cervical lymph-node enlargement and a swelling in the left labium major; biopsies from these three sites all showed sarcoid-type granulomas; without treatment, all lesions resolved in 18 months. Headache which led to radiography of the skull showing many areas of rarefaction in the fronto-parietal parts of the skull was a presenting symptom in a 46 year old woman whose case was reported by Perrin-Fayolle *et al.* (1971); later BHL with fine mottling at the bases of the lungs, regressing with corticosteroid treatment, made the diagnosis of sarcoidosis probable. A swelling appearing shortly after a minor injury in the parieto-occipital region in a man aged 34 with no previous symptom was found by Turner and Weiss (1969) to overlie an area of bone rarefaction; as described above (p. 231) initial biopsy was thought suspicious of meningioma, but material provided by a wide excision of bone was histologically compatible with sarcoidosis.

In a few other cases, local soft-tissue swellings (Neville *et al*, 1977) or headache (Nou, 1965; Rohatgi, 1980), drew attention to cranial lesions in patients with sarcoidosis; bone surveys in patients found to have changes in other bones have occasionally revealed them; but in some reports, the reasons for radiography of the skull which led to their discovery are not stated. Radiographically, multiple areas of rarefaction, ranging from a few millimetres to 3 cm in diameter have been found in most cases; only three were seen in the case reported by Teirstein *et al.* (1961), and one in the unusual case of Turner and Weiss (1969). Most observers have noted the absence of reactive sclerosis; but Perrin-Fayolle *et al.* (1971) found some irregular peripheral sclerosis, and Silver *et al.* (1978) reported a case in which widespread changes in bones, including the skull, were radiographically dense.

Vertebrae

Although, as noted below, there are a number of reports of the finding of granulomas in vertebral bone-marrow at necropsies in cases of sarcoidosis, there are relatively few records of the detection of sarcoidosis of vertebrae during life. In most cases, attention has been drawn to it by back-pain in patients with sarcoidosis. Cases in which vertebrae were the only detected osseous localization of sarcoidosis have been reported by Robert (1944), Rodman *et al.* (1959), Goobar *et al.* (1961), Zenem *et al.* (1963) and Stump *et al.* (1976); and in association with evident involvement of other bones by Bloch *et al.* (1968), Young and Laman (1972), Baldwin *et al.* (1974), Brody *et al.* (1976), Zimmerman and Leeds (1976) and Cutler *et al.* (1978). The case reported by Rodman *et al.* (1959) is quoted as an example of those with vertebral involvement only.

> A 33 year old black man, three years after a diagnosis of sarcoidosis had been made because of lung changes and confirmatory cervical lymph-node biopsy, presented with low back pain and fever. There was a generalized slight enlargement of superficial lymph-nodes; hilar node enlargement and a diffuse reticular pattern in the chest radiograph; and evidence of a lytic lesion of adjacent parts of the bodies of the 11th and 12th thoracic vertebrae. At operation, a bone fusion was performed, and biopsy of tissue removed confirmed the diagnosis of sarcoidosis. Improvement followed the operation without further treatment.

The case recorded by Young and Laman (1971) provides an example of more widespread bone involvement, predominantly in the vertebrae.

> A 23 year old black man had a history of BHL, with sarcoid changes in a scalene node biopsy, which had resolved. It was noted that the left 5th rib became radio-dense anteriorly during the follow-up period. He complained of intermittent pain in the right eye, the only abnormality found being slight proptosis. Survey of bones showed areas of abnormal density with thickening of trabeculae in the right sphenoid bones, the bodies of several vertebrae (C2; C5, T6–10, L3–5, S1) and the medial parts of both iliac bones. The affected

part of the left 5th rib was removed, and showed thickening of bone trabeculae, with replacement of the marrow by cellular connective tissue with many non-caseating granulomas. A Kveim test gave a granulomatous response. A year later, there was no clinical or radiological change. The slight proptosis remained unexplained, but the changes in the sphenoid bone suggest the possibility of sarcoid infiltration of the orbital fat.

The generally sclerotic radiographic appearance of the affected bones in this case seems exceptional. In most cases, the changes have been described as lytic or destructive, in some with collapse or wedging of vertebral bodies (Bloch *et al.*, 1968; Stump *et al.*, 1976; Cutler *et al.*, 1978). Zenen *et al.* (1963) described sclerotic changes in two vertebrae, with a small rarefaction peripherally in one of them, and sclerotic margins to areas of rarefaction have been noted (Bloch *et al.*, 1968; Brody *et al.*, 1976). Paravertebral soft tissue shadows adjacent to affected vertebrae were found by Zenen *et al.* (1963), Baldwin *et al.* (1974) and Stump *et al.* (1976); Zenen *et al.* noted that this mass disappeared during an observation period of one year. Disc spaces adjacent to affected vertebrae were narrowed in several cases (Baldwin *et al.*, 1974; Brody *et al.*, 1976; Stump *et al.*, 1976; Cutler *et al.*, 1978).

In several cases, the condition of affected vertebrae improved (Zenen *et al.*, 1963; Brody *et al.*, 1976), or resolved (Berk and Brower, 1964) under observation. Baldwin *et al.* (1974) observed symptomatic improvement but not radiological change in the spine, though BHL subsided, and, as noted above, Young and Laman (1972) observed no clinical or radiological change after one year. Responses to corticosteroid treatment appeared favourable in the cases of Goobar *et al.* (1961) and Stump *et al.* (1976, Case 1), and doubtful in that of Bloch *et al.* (1968). Spinal fusion operations were performed in cases reported by Robert (1944), Rodman *et al.* (1959), and Zimmerman and Leeds (1976). The results were said to be satisfactory in the first two of these. In the case of Zimmerman and Leeds, a white woman aged 72 with 'biopsy-proved sarcoidosis', multiple lytic defects were found in the skull and later in the odontoid process of the second cervical vertebra with a pathological fracture; surgical fusion was followed by quadriplegia which later resolved; unfortunately, there is no record of the histology of the bone.

Long bones

As noted above, in several large series of cases of sarcoid involvement of the bones of the hands and feet, a few have been found to show localized rarefactions in the distal ends of the bones of the forearm and lower leg, or in carpal and tarsal bones.

Jordan and Osborne (1937) described two cases, both in black men with widespread sarcoidosis and much cyst-like rarefaction in the bones of the hands and feet; one had similar changes in all the long bones of the limbs, and the other in the head of the radius and the distal third of the ulna, confirmed in both by biopsy from an affected long bone to have the histology of sarcoidosis.

In other cases, long bones have been involved with skull or pelvis.

Posner (1942) reported the remarkable case of a two year old white girl with loss of weight, fever, general lymphadenopathy, and a hypoplastic anaemia with granulocytopenia, requiring blood transfusions. Radiography of bones showed rounded areas of rarefaction in long bones and skull. Under observation, diabetes insipidus developed. The Mantoux test was negative to 1:500 old tuberculin. At necropsy, non-caseating tubercles were found in the lungs, liver, kidney, lymph-nodes and pituitary, and were especially numerous in the spleen and bone-marrow; no acid-fast bacilli were seen in sections of the lung. In a complex case reported by Toomey and Bautista (1970, Case 1), a white girl aged 14 with sarcoidosis affecting mediastinal and peripheral lymph-nodes and eyes, with hypercalcaemia, was found to have multiple areas of rarefaction in skull, humeri, and femora, shown by biopsy of the skull to be of sarcoid histology; treatment with prednisone was followed by evidence of recalcification. In the case of sarcoidosis of the skull reported by Franco-Saenz *et al.* (1970), small rarefactions were found in both humeri; and in the case of osteosclerotic changes affecting mainly the pelvic bones reported by Bonakdarpour *et al.* (1971), the upper thirds of both femora were similarly affected.

Watson and Cahen (1973) reported the case of a black woman with sarcoidosis involving lungs, mediastinal and peripheral lymph-nodes, skin and nasal mucosa in whom localized rarefactions in both olecranon processes were observed. A fall led to fracture of the right olecranon; biopsy at an operation for internal fixation showed non-caseating granulomas; six months later because of non-union the olecranon was excised, with synoviectomy; there was granulomatous synovitis, and infiltration of bone. On continued treatment with prednisolone, there was good movement at the elbow 18 months later, but further rarefaction in the left olecranon.

Rohatgi (1980, Case 1) described the case of a woman aged 29 with fever, joint pains, mediastinal and peripheral lymphadenopathy, biopsy showing sarcoid changes both in a lymph-node and a skin lesion on the nose; skeletal survey showed widespread rarefactions in long bones and two metatarsals, with periosteal reaction over lesions at the ends of both tibiae. Radio-isotope scans showed increased uptake over areas of rarefaction, and also the femoral condyles and some phalanges not showing such changes. Treatment with prednisone led to relief of symptoms, but a repeat scan was unaltered.

Pelvic bones

Involvement of pelvic bones has been reported by Bloch *et al.* (1968), Bonakdapour *et al.* (1971), Lin *et al.* (1973) and Silver *et al.* (1978), all in black patients with extensive sarcoidosis. The patient described by Bloch *et al.* (1968) was a boy aged 15 with a uveo-parotid syndrome, hepatosplenomegaly, hilar lymph-node enlargement and maculo-papular skin lesions; he had pain in the back, cyst-like rarefactions with sclerotic margins being found in the 11th and 12th thoracic vertebral bodies, with wedging, and areas of rarefaction in the left ilium and ischial tuberosity and in some proximal phalanges, and iliac crest and conjunctival biopsies showing sarcoid granulomas. In this case, the bone changes were found at the clinical onset of sarcoidosis. In the other three, they were found six months, 13 years and 19 years after the diagnosis of sarcoidosis, and the radiographic changes consisted of areas of increased density. Biopsy of the iliac crest in one of these (Bonakdapour *et al.*) showed thick cancellous bone with little osteoblastic or osteoclastic activity, and scattered non-caseating granulomas in the haemopoietic and fatty marrow. In this case, the bone changes, found 13 years from the onset, produced no symptoms; in the pelvis they were located in the medial parts of the ilia, in the ischia and in the superior rami of the pubis, and in the lateral parts of the sacrum; other bones similarly involved were the femora in their upper thirds and one phalanx. The patient described by Silver *et al.* (1978) was a black woman who complained of lower back pain 19 years after the diagnosis of sarcoidosis, and was found to have dense areas in both iliac bones and in the skull; 99 m technetium pyrophosphate scan showed increased uptake in these areas and also in the femora and ribs; biopsy from the iliac crest showed sarcoid granulomas; treatment with prednisone led to relief of pain, but radiographic and radioisotopic findings remained the same. The patient reported by Lin *et al.* (1973) with diffuse osteosclerotic changes in the pelvis and sacrum, a black man aged 36, ^omplained of back pain six months after the diagnosis of sarcoidosis, but the lung changes were said to be fibrotic, suggesting a longer duration of the disease; biopsy of iliac crest, lymph-node and a Kveim test confirmed the diagnosis.

Ribs

Involvement of ribs was noted in conjunction with vertebral sarcoidosis in cases reported by Young and Laman (1972), Baldwin *et al.* (1974), Stump *et al.* (1976) and Cutler *et al.* (1978), and was detected by radio-isotope survey in the case of extensive bone sarcoidosis reported by Silver *et al.* (1978). Radiographically, there may be localized rarefactions (Baldwin *et al.*, 1974; Cutler *et al.* 1978), or densities (Young and Laman, 1972). Baldwin *et al.* performed an open biopsy of a rib which showed radiographically an erosion of its lower boarder with an associated pleural reaction, and found the periosteum oedematous and the rib soft, with many non-caseating granulomas. As noted above, Young and Laman (1972) on biopsy of a rib showing increased density found thickening of bone trabeculae and replacement of marrow by connective tissue and well-defined granulomas.

Bone-marrow

As noted above, it is the marrow that is principally involved in sarcoidosis of the bones. There are several reports of the finding of granulomas in bone-marrow at necropsy, without evidence of bone changes during life. Nickerson (1937) examined the vertebral bone-marrow in five cases of extensive sarcoidosis, and found typical lesions in three; they were sparse, usually in small groups in haemopoietic tissue. He found sarcoid tubercles in femoral bone-marrow in the one case in which it was examined, but none in tibial marrow in another. Hollister and Harrell (1941) found granulomas in the marrow of a vertebra and a rib; and Rubin and Pinner (1944) in a black woman who had died of miliary tuberculosis after an illness starting with uveo-parotitis, generalized lymphadenopathy and lung infiltration, with negative tuberculin test and sarcoid histology in a lymph-node biopsy, found both fibrosing and caseating granulomas.

The first reference to the diagnostic use of sternal puncture in sarcoidosis appears to have been by Dressler (1938). He described the case of a man with hilar lymph-node and lung changes and splenomegaly, in whom the material obtained by sternal puncture contained two clearly defined sarcoid tubercles. Lucia and Aggeler (1940) examined sternal marrow in three cases of sarcoidosis, and found no specific changes. Gormsen (1948) found epithelioid cell granulomas in sternal marrow obtained by puncture in ten of 39 patients with sarcoidosis, all of five with miliary tuberculosis, and 15 of 22 with brucellosis. He considered that sarcoid granulomas could not be differentiated from non-caseating tubercles, but that in most instances the granulomas of brucellosis could be distinguished from caseating or non-caseating tubercles. In 31 patients with pulmonary tuberculosis, neither miliary in type nor terminal, he found no granulomas; but among 20 who had died of pulmonary tuberculosis, examination of the sternal marrow at necropsy showed tubercles in eight.

Joints

The most frequent form of involvement of the joints in sarcoidosis is the febrile arthropathy which may occur in the early stage of bilateral hilar lymph-node enlargement, either as an accompaniment of erythema nodosum, or especially in men, without this exanthem (Chapter 5). This usually involves several joints, has the clinical characters of an inflammatory process, and usually resolves spontaneously; limited evidence available suggests that it is not granulomatous, and in the following discussion it will be called acute polyarthritis. Two sorts of more chronic arthropathy may occur at a later stage. There are involvement of joints adjacent to affected bones, especially in the hands and feet, and granulomatous infiltration, principally of synovial membranes. Both these sorts of chronic arthropathy have been reported more frequently in blacks than in other ethnic groups, in which they are rare; and are less frequent even in blacks, than the early acute polyarthritis. Gumpel *et al.* (1967) observed joint changes in 45 of 118 patients in Baltimore with sarcoidosis, most of whom were black. They recognized a transient polyarthritis at or near the onset in 29, of whom two-thirds had erythema nodosum; and a less widespread chronic arthropathy later in the course in 16. Siltzbach and Duberstein (1968) reviewed joint changes observed in 311 patients with sarcoidosis. Arthropathy thought to be unrelated to sarcoidosis occurred in four; 38 had joint changes related to sarcoidosis. In 30 of these there was an acute polyarthritis, associated with erythema nodosum in 21; in eight, the arthritis was chronic. In this series, in New York, the frequency of the erythema nodosum-acute arthropathy syndrome was highest in Puerto Rican (30%), lowest in black (6%), and intermediate (10%) in white patients. Both these series contained a high proportion of black patients; the incidence of chronic arthropathy in series consisting wholly or predominantly of white patients is much lower, joint changes tending to be exclusively of the acute transient sort. Thus, in Finland, Putkonen *et al.* (1965b) found polyarthritis of this sort in 23 of 94 patients with sarcoidosis, none having chronic sarcoid arthropathy; one had definite and one probable rheumatoid arthritis, a frequency similar to expectation.

Acute polyarthritis

The acute arthropathy that accompanies erythema nodosum in the early stages of sarcoidosis is discussed in Chapter 5. Its severity varies from case to case; it may occur without erythema nodosum, and seems to be cognate with erythema nodosum in the course of sarcoidosis. In some populations it occurs alone in a higher proportion of cases of EN-acute arthropathy-BHL in men than in women. The joints most frequently affected are the ankles, knees, small joints of the hands and feet, wrists, and elbows, though the shoulders and hips may be involved (Williams, 1961; Gumpel *et al.*, 1967). In mild cases, there may be no objective signs, pain and stiffness in the joint being the only evidence; in the more severe, swelling, tenderness and limitation of movement are found. Joints are usually affected symmetrically; various groups may be affected consecutively, but migration from one joint to another, as may occur in rheumatic fever, is rare. Painful oedematous swelling of the ankles may occur, with or without erythema nodosum, especially in patients who remain ambulant (Gumpel *et al.*, 1967). The duration of the arthropathy varies greatly; it may clear within a few weeks, but may persist for several months. The symptoms respond nearly always to non-steroidal anti-inflammatory drugs (Chapter 27); corticosteroids are rarely, if ever, required for the suppression of this sort of inflammatory arthropathy in sarcoidosis.

There is little information about the pathology of this acute self-terminating arthropathy, since there can rarely be a valid indication for biopsy. Ferguson and Paris (1958) reported a case of typical febrile arthropathy, BHL and lung infiltration with histological evidence of sarcoidosis in a scalene node biopsy and in a Kveim reaction, and eventual complete resolution; in this case biopsy of the synovial membrane of the knee showed only an infiltration of mononuclear cells around small blood-vessels and into the synovial layer, no specific changes being found. Siltzbach and Duberstein (1968) performed biopsy of the synovium of the knee in the tenth week after the onset of a typical EN-arthropathy-BHL syndrome in a 16 year old girl, and found normal synovium.

A few cases in which acute polyarthritis has recurred during the course of sarcoidosis have been reported. Moreau (1949) reported two cases, and Ridley (1957) one case with recurrent episodes of febrile arthropathy and generalized lymph-adenopathy leading eventually to the appearance of multiple sarcoids of the skin, histologically confirmed. Erythema nodosum occurred in the second episode in one, and in the first in the other of Moreau's cases, but not in Ridley's. These appear to be cognate with the rare cases of recurrent erythema nodosum (Chapter 5, p. 96).

Joint changes accompanying bone involvement

When the small bones of the hands and feet are severely affected, the intervening joints are frequently involved also. In thse circumstances, confusion with primary diseases of joints is unlikely, especially when, as is the rule, there are also changes of lupus pernio type in the overlying skin. Very occasionally, the bone changes may present an untypical appearance and if, in such cases, there are no skin changes, the clinical picture may resemble that of rheumatoid arthritis.

> Two cases reported by Moyer and Ackerman (1950) illustrate this point. In one, the diagnosis of sarcoidosis rested upon symptomless BHL with lung infiltration and histological changes in a cervical lymph-node; radiologically, the hands showed osteoporosis, narrowing of joint spaces, erosion of interphalangeal joint spaces, but no cystic rarefactions, and the possibility of coincidental rheumatoid arthritis was not excluded. In the other, there were similar but more severe radiographic changes in the hands, with gross deformity, and at first no skin changes. Concomitant cystic rarefactions in the heads of several metacarpals, and the later appearance of multiple skin sarcoids, histologically proved, especially over the affected joints, left no doubt that the joint changes were of specifically sarcoid character.

Synovitis of tendon sheaths may occur in association with lupus pernio, as in Besnier's original case (p. 1), and it is probable that granulomatous changes in tendon-sheaths and in the synovium of joints adjacent to affected bones contribute to the soft tissue swelling which occurs in some cases of sarcoidosis of the bones of the hands.

Chronic arthropathy

Chronic changes may occur in joints without evident involvement of adjacent bone, but are rare; as noted above, most of the reported cases have been in black patients. Sokoloff and Bunim (1959) reported five cases of sarcoidosis with conspicuous polyarthritis, all in young black men. In three, the joints were affected early in the clinical course, and in two about two years after other symptoms. In all the patients several other systems were involved and histological evidence of the disease was obtained from at least one site other than the joints. In three the joint symptoms had persisted for periods up to eight years, and involved large as well as small peripheral joints. Biopsies of synovial tissue from the knee (three cases) and the elbow (one case) showed non-caseating tubercles, typical in three and compatible with sarcoidosis in one. In the fifth case, with five brief episodes of polyarthritis in three years, biopsy from the wrist showed non-specific changes in the synovial tissue. One patient had, in addition to the polyarthritis, severe changes in the hands associated with lupus pernio, and another had some cystic change in phalanges of the feet; but there was no radiographic evidence, either in these or in other cases, of destruction of bone in the vicinity of the involved joints, including those from which tissue for biopsy was obtained. Serological tests for rheumatoid arthritis and search for lupus erythematosus cells were both negative. Bianchi and Keech (1964) studied 12 patients, all black, with sarcoidosis and chronic joint changes. Biopsies of synovium from affected joints were obtained in six; five of these showed sarcoid-type granulomas in addition to synovitis with hypertrophy of lining cells. Spilberg *et al.* (1969) studied seven selected patients with arthropathy appearing during the course of sarcoidosis, seven months to six years from the onset; none with persistent arthritis had erythema nodosum. They noted tenosynovitis at the wrists in two; tendon sheath biopsies showed granulomatous changes.

Grigor and Hughes (1976) reported the case of a Nigerian man, aged 34, in whom chronic symmetrical polyarthritis of the knees, ankles, interphalangeal joints and extensor tendon-sheaths at the wrists was the presenting feature; rheumatoid and anti-nuclear factors were not found; small plaques of skin infiltration appeared on the back, and old scars became infiltrated, slight enlargement of superficial lymph-nodes and of the spleen and diffuse radiographic shadowing in the lungs were found, and the diagnosis of sarcoidosis was established by the finding of granulomas in biopsies of skin, tendonsheath synovium and a Kveim test.

Bjarnason *et al.* (1973) reported the case of a black woman, aged 51, who had been treated with prednisone for one year for sarcoidosis, with BHL, lung changes and hepatosplenomegaly, when she presented with pain and stiffness in the knees; there was radiographic evidence of bone atrophy in the lateral condyles of the femora with a small sequestrum; under observation these changes progressed to extensive destruction of the epiphyses; arthroscopy showed hypertrophied synovium, and biopsies of it and of bone from the femoral condyle showed granulomas. In this case, it seems possible that corticosteroid treatment may have been a factor in the destructive changes in bone.

In a review of 154 patients with sarcoidosis in South Africa, of whom 30 were black, 27 white and 102 of mixed race, Benatar (1980) found 'deforming arthritis' in two black patients and none in the other two groups, and stated that it was recorded in 15 of 56 published cases of sarcoidosis in South African blacks. It appears, however, that this term refers to changes in the hands secondary to bone involvement as described by Morrison (1974).

Polyarthritis in children

Single cases of polyarthritis in young children with extensive sarcoidosis have been published by Burman and Mayer (1936), Zweifel (1946), Castellanos and Galan (1946), Schweizer and Kanaar (1967) and Toomey and Bautista (1970, Case 2), and six cases from several centres in the United States and Canada by North *et al.* (1970). In all these 11 cases, the disease started at a very early age, the first evidence of sarcoidosis appearing between four months and four years of age, and of arthropathy between nine months and four and a half years. All but one were reported to have skin eruptions, generally widespread, and described as confluent papules or macules, and confirmed to be granulomatous on biopsy; in two cases subsidence of this eruption, either under corticosteroid treatment (Schweizer and Kanaar, 1967) or spontaneously (North *et al.*, 1970) left slightly atrophic macules. All but two had uveitis, and salivary glands were noted to be involved in five. Hypercalcaemia was noted in two, and band keratopathy in three more; and splenomegaly in four. In only three was involvement of the lungs mentioned; Castellanos and Galan found miliary shadows in their case, and North *et al.* transient infiltration in one, and persistent lung changes with cardiac decompensation in another of their six cases. The joints most commonly affected were ankles, wrists, knees, elbows, the metacarpo-phalangeal and interphalangeal joints being also involved in a few cases. Tendon-sheaths at the wrists or the dorsum of the hands were noted to be involved in some. The diagnosis of sarcoidosis was established by biopsy from other sites in all, from multiple sites in most, and from biopsy of synovium from large joints or from tendon-sheaths in most cases. The resemblance of the clinical picture of the joint changes to that of Still's disease was remarked by several authors, but the florid signs of sarcoidosis elsewhere were unmistakable.

The case reported by Schweizer and Kanaar (1967) exemplifies this peculiar group of cases. A male child aged 18 months developed an eruption of closely-packed papules on shoulder and hip areas, extending to trunk and face, biopsy repeatedly showed sarcoid-type granulomas. Shortly afterwards both ankles and the proximal phalanges of the fingers, and later the knees and wrists became swollen. At the age of two and a half, he was found to have hypercalcaemia; biopsy of the knee capsule showed granulomatous inflammation. Treatment with prednisone led to rapid subsidence of the eruption, leaving slightly atrophic macules in the skin, and of the joint swelling, and normocalcaemia. This improvement was maintained only by continuation of lower doses, but at the age of five, bilateral iridocyclitis appeared, and was controlled by local corticosteroid treatment. Growth and development remained normal; a younger brother developed skin sarcoids about the time of the report.

The case of a Cuban child, reported by Castellanos and Galan (1946) is of interest because of its termination. This boy developed a polyarthritis resembling Still's disease at the age of three, and later a maculo-erythematous rash on the face and arms. At the age of six, he was found to have generalized lymph-node enlargement, splenomegaly and swelling and limitation of movement of large joints; miliary shadows in the chest radiograph; tuberculin test with 100 IU negative; and biopsy showed non-caseating granulomas with some hyalinization in subcutaneous tissue and skeletal muscle, and chronic inflammatory changes in synovial membrane of the knee. Four months later, a pleural effusion appeared, and tuberculosis of the dorsal spine developed, followed by death from tuberculous meningitis.

Associated arthritis of other types

It is to be expected that sarcoidosis will occasionally be associated by chance with one of the common varieties of arthritis. Davis and Crotty (1952) described the case of a 24 year old woman who had both sarcoidosis, with BHL, lung infiltration, and a histologically typical skin lesion on the forehead, and rheumatoid arthritis with characteristic joint changes and a histologically proved rheumatoid nodule on the elbow. In a patient under the care of one of us, chronic sarcoidosis was accompanied by mild arthritis of rheumatoid type, with histologically-confirmed rheumatoid nodules over the olecranon processes (Clinico-pathological Conference, 1950). In another ankylosing spondylitis and sarcoidosis co-existed (p. 213). As noted above, Putkonen *et al.* (1965b) found two patients with rheumatoid arthritis among 94 with sarcoidosis. Siltzbach and Duberstein (1968) in the series of 311 patients in which they found 38 with joint changes attributed to sarcoidosis found one with systemic lupus erythematosus, one with osteoarthritis, and two with transient arthritides, unspecified.

SKELETAL MUSCLES

The first published case of sarcoidosis of skeletal muscle appears to have been that of a 17 year old girl demonstrated at the Moscow Dermatological Society by Licharew (1908). She had lupus pernio, an enlarged spleen, and multiple nodules in muscles. Since then, many cases of sarcoidosis involving muscles have been reported. In only a few of these did the muscle involvement take the form of symptomless nodules, as in Licharew's case. In most, the clinical picture was that of a polymyositis with widespread weakness, usually with wasting, and occasionally with additional features such as fibrosis and induration, contractures, palpable nodules, and, rarely, pseudo-hypertrophy. In 1952, Myers *et al.* first reported that in cases of active sarcoidosis granulomas might be found in clinically normal muscles. Since then, it has become evident that such symptomless infiltration of muscles is probably frequent, although clinically evident muscle involvement is rare. In the following discussion, 'random muscle biopsy' refers to biopsy of a muscle showing no clinical evidence of disease.

Clinically inapparent granulomas in muscles

Myers *et al.* (1952) reported four cases of early active sarcoidosis with fever, arthralgia, erythema nodosum in three, bilateral hilar lymphadenopathy in all, and such other manifestations as uveitis, palpable enlargement of lymph-nodes, and splenomegaly each in one or more. Biopsies of gastrocnemius muscle in three of these all showed epithelioid and giant-cell granulomas of sarcoid type, although there were no symptoms specifically referable to muscles. Similar findings in random muscle biopsies in patients with active sarcoidosis were reported by Powell (1953), Maurice (1955), Lafon *et al.* (1955), and Phillips and Phillips (1956). Wallace *et al.* (1958) performed random muscle biopsies in 42 patients with sarcoidosis with histological support from biopsies from other sites in 32 and from Kveim tests in ten. Although most of the biopsies were from gastrocnemius, some were from other muscles (pectoralis, sternomastoid, platysma and other neck muscles). Twenty-three of the 42 showed sarcoid granulomas in muscle. Of six with erythema nodosum or febrile arthralgia and BHL, five had positive muscle biopsies. The more organs involved, the more likely were the muscles to be found to be infiltrated. Of 552 muscle biopsies, only one showed a sarcoid-type granuloma without clinical evidence of sarcoidosis elsewhere.

These observations suggest that symptomless infiltration of muscles with sarcoid granulomas is frequent in active sarcoidosis, and that this resolves in the great majority of cases in the natural course of the disease. In this respect, the course of events in the muscles is similar to that in the liver (p. 260).

Palpable nodules in muscles

Licharew's (1908) case has been mentioned above. There are only a few descriptions of cases in which palpable nodules were the only clinical evidence of sarcoidosis of muscles. Sundelin (1925) described the case of a man with uveitis, radiographic changes in the bones of the fingers and symptomless nodules in the muscles of the limbs, head and neck, which on biopsy showed hard tubercles, many elongated in the direction of the muscle fibres; power in the affected muscles seemed normal. Of the six cases described by Powell (1953), three, all with sarcoidosis involving hilar lymph-nodes, lungs and other organs, showed multiple nodules in muscles. More frequently, however, palpable nodules have been found in association with weakness or other symptoms referable to muscles.

Figure 9.5 shows the histology of a palpable sarcoid nodule in the triceps brachialis of a man aged 40; the only other manifestation was bilateral hilar lymph-node enlargement.

Symptomatic granulomatous polymyositis

In most of the reported cases, symptoms arising from the muscles have been the presenting feature, and in some no unequivocal evidence of granuloma-

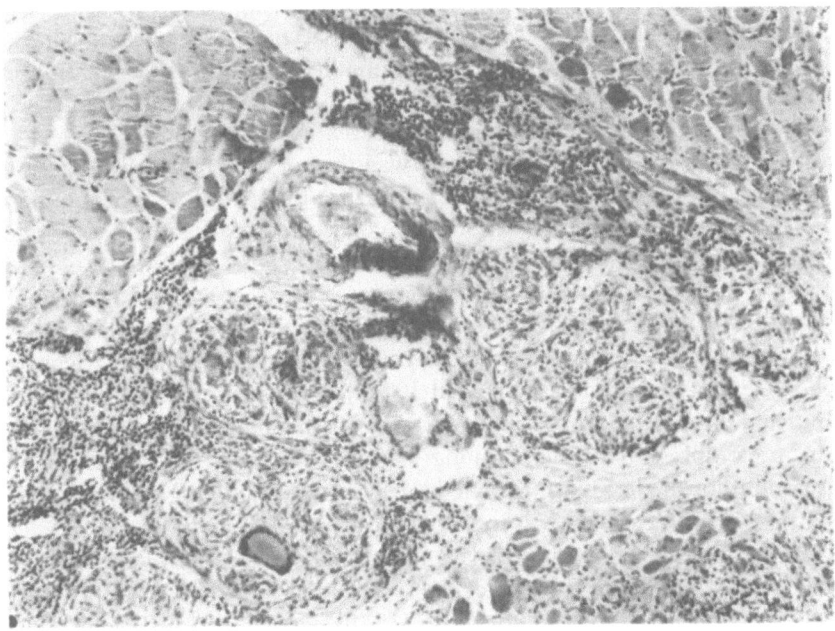

Figure 9.5   Biopsy of a palpable nodule in the triceps muscle of a man aged 40, who also had bilateral hilar lymph-node enlargement. H & E. × 100.

tous changes in other organs have been found, leaving legitimate doubt about the diagnosis of sarcoidosis. Among patients with known sarcoidosis, symptomatic granulomatous myopathy is rare, contrasting with the frequency of symptomless transient granulomatous infiltration. Silverstein and Siltzbach (1969) reviewed 800 patients with confirmed sarcoidosis; severe persistent sarcoid myopathy occurred in two; one with febrile arthropathy and BHL had muscle pain and tenderness which proved to be transient, and was found to have granulomas in the gastrocnemins muscle on biopsy; and in eight, all with extensive, active sarcoidosis, but no muscle symptoms, random muscle biopsies showed granulomas.

The muscles most frequently involved are those of the limb girdles and the proximal parts of the limbs, though any muscle may be involved. Some cases have presented with progressive wasting and weakness of muscles. Cases of this sort in patients with evidence of sarcoidosis elsewhere have been reported by Bates and Walsh (1948), Bammer (1958), Crompton and MacDermott (1961, Cases 1 and 2), Rothfeld and Folk (1962), Dyken (1962), Pauli *et al.* (1969), Dumas *et al.* (1971, Case 1) Groslambert *et al.* (1971), Powell-Jackson *et al.* (1971), Callen (1979) and Khan *et al.* (1981). The relationship of the myopathic to other manifestations varied from an established diagnosis of sarcoidosis followed years later by muscle weakness and wasting, to diagnosis of sarcoidosis only at necropsy in a patient presenting with myopathy. The patient reported by Powell-Jackson *et al.* (1971) was a woman who, seven years after sarcoidosis had been diagnosed by the finding of symptomless radiographic lung shadows and lymph-node biopsy, developed weakness and wasting of proximal shoulder and pelvic girdle muscles, biopsy showing non-caseating granulomas. Case 1 of Crompton and MacDermott (1961) was that of a woman who presented with weakness of the legs, and later the arms, thought to be attributable to polymyositis, but not responding to corticosteroid treatment; she died suddenly three and a half years from the onset, and at necropsy was found to have widespread granulomatous changes in muscles, and in lungs, lymph-nodes and spleen. In some cases, other manifestations of sarcoidosis have appeared simultaneously with the myopathy; Khan *et al.* (1981) reported the case of a West Indian man aged 30, who presented with proximal limb muscle weakness, and was found to have a harsh pulmonary systolic murmur due to compression of the pulmonary artery by an enlarged lymph-node at the hilum of the left lung. Muscle biopsy showed sarcoid granulomas, and corticosteroid treatment was followed by symptomatic improvement, fall of high creatine phosphokinase levels to normal, subsidence of the enlarged hilar node, and disappearance of the systolic murmur. In cases reported by Weinberger (1933), Bates and Walsh (1948), Powell (1953, Case 1), Coers *et al.* (1956), Garcin and Lapresle (1958), and Crompton and MacDermott (1961, Case 1), pain and tenderness in affected muscles and, in some, fever suggested a polymyositis rather than a myopathy or progressive muscular atrophy; in all of these there was evidence of systemic sarcoidosis, either clinically or at necropsy.

Cases of granulomatous myopathy without detected manifestations of sarcoidosis elsewhere have been reported by Snorasson (1947), Devic *et al.* (1955), Warburg (1955), Ammitzbøll (1956), McConkey (1958), Brun (1961), Harvey (1959), Kryger and Ronnov-Jensen (1959), Crompton and MacDermott (1961, Case 3), Hinterbuchner and Hinterbuchner (1964), Talbot (1967), Dumas *et al.* (1971, Case 2), Gardner-Thorpe (1972) and Douglas *et al.* (1973, Case 2). In most of these, the pattern of the myopathy resembled that most commonly seen in patients shown to have concurrent other manifestations of sarcoidosis, and in some there was a past history of disorders, such as uveitis, which might have been of sarcoid character. Moreover, in some of the cases with necropsy evidence, only late residues of sarcoidosis were found in other organs; e.g. in Case 2 of Crompton and MacDermott (1961), giant cells with conchoidal bodies in the lungs were the only remaining evidence of granulomatous changes apart from those in muscles. This suggests that in some cases granulomatous myopathy may be a persistent localization of active granulomas in muscles after those in other organs have become inactive or resolved in patients who have passed through the active generalized stages of sarcoidosis without obvious symptoms. A similar pattern of events is known to occur in relation to other localizations of sarcoidosis; and as in other organs, a provisional diagnosis of granulomatous myopathy is advisable in the absence of at least suggestive evidence of past or present other manifestations of sarcoidosis. The problem of differential diagnosis in such cases has been discussed by Hewlett and Brownell (1975). Gardner-Thorpe (1972) had drawn attention to the high proportion of post-menopausal women among patients presenting with chronic granulomatous myopathy. He reported six cases in women aged from 56–75 years with widespread weakness in limb and limb-girdle muscles and granulomatous inflammatory changes in the muscles on biopsy; the only evidence of other localizations of sarcoidosis were enlarged hilar shadows in one, and a single sclerotic epithelioid and giant-cell granuloma in a liver biopsy in another of these patients. As well as weakness and wasting, affected muscles may show other abnormal signs. Patients reported by Snorasson (1947), Warburg (1955) and Brun (1961) presented with a picture of indolent progressive fibrosing myositis, with nodules, contractures and knotty thickenings in the muscles. In none of these was evidence of sarcoidosis found clinically outside the muscles, the diagnosis being suggested by biopsies of affected muscles.

A few cases in which granulomatous myopathy in patients with sarcoidosis caused pseudo-hypertrophy have been recorded.

Mucha and Orzechowski (1919) reported the case of a woman, aged 30, with slowly developing difficulty in walking and myalgia, in whom the affected muscles of the legs and shoulder girdles were in part atrophic and in part pseudo-hypertrophic; she had typical skin sarcoids and the muscles showed hard tubercles on biopsy. Ozer *et al.* (1961) described the case of a black woman, aged 55, who had hard masses apparently in muscles in both groins, both thighs and one forearm; the lumbar muscles were swollen and indurated; she also had a peripheral neuropathy. Biopsies of one of the masses and of apparently unaffected gastrocnemius muscle showed a sarcoid-type granuloma. She died suddenly of a pulmonary embolism, and at necropsy sarcoid changes were found in the lungs, spleen, muscles, lymph-nodes, stomach and pancreas, and in the perineural sheaths of lumbar nerves. In Case 1 of Douglas *et al.* (1973), a woman aged 59 presented with a five month history of fever and stiffness and weakness of leg muscles; the weak muscles were swollen, simulating pseudo-hypertrophy, and biopsy showed exuberant sarcoid-type granulomas between normal-looking muscle fibres; there was proteinuria, renal biopsy showing resolving glomerulonephritis. Prednisolone treatment led to improvement with reduction in the swelling of the muscles. Two years later, she died of pulmonary embolism, and at necropsy granulomas were found in muscles, liver, spleen, lymph-nodes and bones. The remarkable case recorded by Furtado and Carvalho (1947) as 'tuberculose musculaire' in a boy aged six seems better categorized as granulomatous myopathy of sarcoid type. This boy's development had been delayed since the age of two, and he had shown increasing rigidity of the limbs from the age of four. The affected muscles of the shoulder girdle, upper arms and thighs were larger than normal and indurated. The facial muscles were contracted and the frontal muscles large and indurated. Several muscle biopsies showed elongated epithelioid and giant-cell granulomas between the muscle fibres.

In a number of cases of sarcoidosis in which skeletal muscle has been found at necropsy to be involved, myocardial sarcoidosis was also found. Bates and Walsh (1948) reported the case of a black man, aged 31, who had widespread atrophy of skeletal muscle, uveoparotitis, and BHL, and died suddenly; at necropsy, there was very widespread sarcoidosis in many organs including the skeletal muscles and the heart, in which both ventricles were extensively infiltrated. In one of the six cases of sarcoidosis of skeletal muscle reported by Powell (1953), sarcoid lesions were found in the walls of the superior vena cava and the pulmonary veins in one; and Powell stated that of seven cases then recorded in which sarcoidosis of skeletal muscle had been found at necropsy, six also had myocardial involvement.

Association of widespread muscle changes with nervous system involvement may give rise to confusing clinical pictures, as in the two cases described by de Morsier *et al.* (1954), and mentioned in Chapter 14 (p. 313). One of these mimicked amyotrophic lateral sclerosis. Krabbe (1949) reported the case of a man with peripheral neuropathy, cerebellar signs, and nodules in the limb muscles, consisting of epithelioid and giant-cell granulomas. Adams *et al.* (1962) refer briefly to a case of sarcoid infiltration of muscle combined with polyneuritis, presumably of sarcoid origin. In Case 2 of Douglas *et al.* (1973) electromyography suggested mixed myopathic and neuropathic changes.

Treatment

As would be expected in view of the differing stages of sarcoidosis at which involvement of muscles may be found, and of the varying pathology of the muscles, response to corticosteroid treatment is variable. Gardner-Thorpe (1972), reviewing published reports and his own six cases, thought that a useful response had been obtained in 20 and no benefit in six. In most of the cases in which improvement has been observed, it has been necessary to continue 'maintenance' treatment to avoid relapse, and, especially in the post-menopausal women who constitute a high proportion of those with chronic sarcoid myopathy, this is apt to have side-effects necessitating discontinuance.

Diagnostic difficulty may occasionally arise when myopathy appears in patients with sarcoidosis under treatment with corticosteroids, since corti-costeroid myopathy commonly has a proximal limb and limb-girdle distri-bution similar to that seen in many cases of sarcoid myopathy. One of us has observed a patient who developed weakness of the proximal muscles of the limbs while under treatment with triamcinolone for pulmonary sar-coidosis. Muscle biopsy showed no granulomas, and cessation of triamcino-lone was followed by return of power in the affected muscles.

In summary, the available evidence suggests that infiltration of muscle by sarcoid granulomas, causing no symptoms, is frequent in the early active phase of sarcoidosis, especially those with an acute onset with fever, arth-ralgia or erythema nodosum. Wallace *et al.* (1958) described the histological changes at this stage as consisting in sarcoid granulomas usually next to blood-vessels but also in the muscle sheaths; adjacent muscle fibres may show some atrophy and there is usually slight lymphocytic infiltration. Presumably this early infiltration resolves uneventfully in most cases. In a small minority, especially of those with progressive sarcoidosis elsewhere, the muscle infiltration remains active and extends, causing the symptoms of a polymyositis. In most cases this affects principally the proximal parts of the limbs and the limb girdles, sometimes with palpable nodules in the muscles. In an even small number, a picture of chronic painless atrophic myopathy develops, and in these the sarcoidosis may be confined, as far as clinical observations go, to the muscles. Histologically, in the progressive symptomatic types of muscle involvement the sarcoid granulomas tend to be elongated between muscle bundles; giant cells and Schaumann bodies are frequently seen; there is atrophy, fatty degeneration, and fibrosis of muscle fibres; and lymphocytic infiltration may be prominent. In the late stages, contractures may develop, and, very rarely, pseudo-hypertrophy has been reported.

Chapter 10

Superficial Lymphadenopathy

INCIDENCE

Enlargement of superficial lymph-nodes is a frequent finding during the course of sarcoidosis. As with other manifestations, the proportion of cases in which it has been reported varies from series to series, for several reasons. It seems likely that the true incidence varies with the racial composition of the series; and that the recorded incidence varies with the thoroughness and frequency of clinical examination and with the examiner's opinion of what constitutes enlargement of lymph-nodes, especially in such sites as the axilla and the groin. Series reported from the United States, and including many black patients, show a high proportion with evident superficial lymph-node enlargement; e.g. Reisner (1944) all of 35 patients, Ricker and Clark (1949) 74% of 300, Riley (1950) all of 52 cases, Longcope and Freiman (1952) 80% of 142, Israel and Sones (1958) 69% of 160, and Mayock et al. (1963) 76% of 145. In reports from Europe, the incidence has generally been lower: e.g. Nitter (1953) 31% of 90 patients, James (1956) 37% of 150, and Smellie and Hoyle (1960) 30% of 125. Cowdell (1954) reported peripheral lymphadenopathy in 82% of 90 cases, but his series included a large proportion discovered through a Lymph-Node Registry. James et al. (1976) in a survey of 3676 patients reported from 12 centres around the world found that lymphadenopathy was noted in 808 (22%). Mikhail et al. (1980) noted palpable lymph-nodes, predominantly axillary and/or cervical, in 7.7% of 401 patients presenting with sarcoidosis at a general hospital in London.

Lymph-nodes in any group may be involved, the cervical most frequently, followed by the axillary. Löfgren and Lundback (1952) found cervical nodes palpable in 55 (26%) of 212 cases of bilateral hilar lymph-node

Table 10.1   Sites of palpably enlarged superficial lymph-nodes in 85 out of 275 cases of sarcoidosis.

Neck		61
anterior triangle only	3	
posterior triangle only	43	
anterior and posterior triangles	15	
Axillae		36
Epitrochlear		18
Groins		11
Pre-auricular		1

enlargement attributed to sarcoidosis; those in the supraclavicular fossa, especially on the right side, were most frequently affected. Longcope and Freiman (1952) among 52 patients with sarcoidosis, mostly black, in Boston found cervical nodes enlarged in 28, axillary in 16, inguinal and femoral in 14, and epitrochlear in six; in the neck, nodes in the anterior triangle, below the jaw, were frequently affected. In a series of 275 patients with sarcoidosis in London, one of us (JGS) found enlarged superficial lymph-nodes in 85 (31%). In nine, all four principal groups – cervical, axillary, epitrochlear and inguinal – were affected, and in six more, nodes in three of these groups were abnormally palpable. But in most cases, nodes in only one or two groups seemed abnormal. The group most frequently involved was the cervical, followed by the axillary, the epitrochlear and the inguinal, in that order (Table 10.1).

In the neck, the nodes of the posterior triangle, and especially those just above the clavicles, were most frequently affected; when those of the anterior triangle were affected, it was usually in association with those of the posterior triangle, and in only three cases were anterior triangle nodes alone palpable. Epitrochlear nodes were enlarged in about one-fifth of the patients with palpable superficial lymph-nodes. The proportion in which inguinal nodes were recorded as enlarged was less than that reported by Longcope and Freiman (1952); this difference may be in part a reflection of difficulty in deciding whether palpable nodes in this site should be regarded as abnormally large. Another difference between the London and the Boston patients was that in London the anterior triangle of the neck was less frequently involved.

CLINICAL CHARACTERISTICS

The superficial lymphadenopathy of sarcoidosis generally gives rise to no more than slight enlargement of the affected nodes, and is found in the course of clinical examination. In some cases, the enlargement is sufficient to attract the patient's attention, or even to cause a visible swelling. They may thus constitute a presenting feature, as in ten of Scadding's 275 cases.

Sarcoid lymph-nodes are characteristically discrete, firm and elastic, mobile, not adherent to skin or to deeper structures, painless and not tender. Of the two varieties of enlarged lymph-nodes with which they are most likely to be confused, they generally resemble those of Hodgkin's disease more than those of caseating tuberculosis both in clinical characteristics and in their preferred sites; but exceptionally they may form confluent masses, partially adherent and, especially if located in the anterior triangle of the neck, resemble those of caseating tuberculosis.

Very occasionally, lymph-nodes enlarged by sarcoidosis become painful. Inguinal nodes may become large enough to cause discomfort. This may be associated with symptomatic involvement of abdominal lymph-nodes (Chapter 17, p. 377). We have seen one patient, under the care of Dr K. M. Citron, with long-standing sarcoidosis of which painful enlargement of inguinal and cervical lymph-nodes became a prominent feature. This woman's illness began with uveitis and BHL, and lymphadenopathy affecting cervical, inguinal and abdominal lymph-nodes became apparent nine years from the onset. Tenderness and pain in the superficial lymph-nodes, especially in the groins, were a troublesome feature. Control of this by corticosteroids was made difficult by diabetes; eventually, the most painful group, in the right groin, was removed surgically, with relief of symptoms. Other features of sarcoidosis in this patient were hypercalcaemia and narrowing of the right middle and apical lower bronchi.

DIFFERENTIAL DIAGNOSIS

Diagnosis rarely remains long in doubt, both because associated clinical and radiological features are likely to give a clue to it, and because removal of a node for biopsy is a simple and safe procedure. It is a possibility, though a remote one, for local sarcoid reactions in lymph-nodes (Chapter 2) to cause confusion; and histology may be equivocal between sarcoidosis and caseating tuberculosis. Zettergren (1954) in an extended study of the histology of lymph-nodes containing tuberculoid granulomas emphasized the difficulty of distinguishing between sarcoidosis and caseating tuberculosis of the chronic hyperplastic type, and found that necrobiotic changes in sarcoid granulomas were more prevalent in lymph-nodes from patients with recent acute sarcoidosis. Among lymph-nodes obtained by mediastinoscopy from 250 patients with sarcoidosis, Carlens et al. (1974) found 15 in which the degree of granular necrosis was difficult to distinguish from caseation; all came from patients with an acute febrile illness, many with erythema nodosum or arthropathy, and six with positive tuberculin tests. Thus histological findings in lymph-nodes must be supported by a compatible clinical picture and course, or by evidence of granulomas in other organs or at a Kveim test site to establish the diagnosis of sarcoidosis.

Among the ten cases in the series reviewed by one of us in which superficial lymphadenopathy was a presenting feature, the principal alternative diagnosis to be considered was caseating tuberculosis in three and Hodgkin's disease in seven.

In all three of the cases in which there was doubt whether they should be classified as sarcoidosis or caseating tuberculosis, there had been an episode of tuberculous lymphadenitis of the neck, at an interval varying from 4–7 years before the appearance of the manifestations interpreted as sarcoidosis; in one, this had been proved by the culture of tubercle bacilli from pus, in another the Mantoux test was recorded as positive, and in all the clinical course at this time was compatible with the diagnosis of caseating tuberculosis. In two, the sarcoid manifestations appeared as a generalized superficial lymphadenopathy, accompanied by a palpable spleen, low or absent tuberculin sensitivity, typical enlargement of hilar lymph-nodes and symptomless radiographic shadowing in the lungs, together with, in one, iridocyclitis and, in the other, a sarcoid skin lesion on the forehead; and lymph-nodes removed for biopsy showed typical non-caseating sarcoid tubercles. In both of these cases, spontaneous regression of the sarcoidosis, to complete disappearance in one and to slight residual inactive fibrosis in the lungs in the other, was observed. In the third patient, the initial tuberculosis adenitis of the neck responded partially to two short courses of treatment with antituberculosis drugs; but seven years from the first episode, the lymph-nodes enlarged once again, and now there was enlargement of hilar lymph-nodes and later mottling in the chest radiograph, non-caseating tubercles in the cervical lymph-node removed for biopsy, failure to respond to antimycobacterial drugs, and a typical response to corticosteroid treatment, symptoms and signs being suppressed but recurring on withdrawal of the treatment. In these patients, then, the diagnosis of sarcoidosis rather than a recurrence of caseating tuberculosis rested upon the combination of a clinical syndrome characteristic of sarcoidosis together with the finding of non-caseating tubercules in lymph-nodes removed for biopsy. The patient in whom the initial tuberculous adenitis was confirmed bacteriologically reverted several years after the 'sarcoid' episode to a frankly caseating phase, and this event is of sufficient interest to warrant a brief summary of the case.

A man, aged 22, developed tuberculous adenitis in the left side of his neck; this softened and was aspirated, tubercle bacilli being cultured from the pus. Four years later, he developed a generalized enlargement of lymph-nodes, affecting cervical, axillary, and inguinal groups; a node removed for biopsy showed non-caseating epithelioid cell tubercles. The spleen was easily palpable. A few months later, he developed iridocyclitis in the right eye. A chest radiograph showed bilateral hilar lymph-node enlargement, with diffuse fine mottling mainly in the middle zones of both lungs. A tuberculin test gave a moderate reaction to 10 IU. Over the next six months all these manifestations gradually subsided, the lymph-nodes and the spleen becoming impalpable, the eye free from inflammatory changes, and the chest radiograph clear. He remained quite well for four years, when a lymph-node swelling appeared again in the left side of the neck. The skin now reacted to 10 IU with an area of induration 20×20 mm. He was treated with isoniazid and p-aminosalicylic acid. The lymph-node softened and sterile pus was aspirated from it; after this the adenitis subsided completely, and the patient has remained well since. Culture of the pus failed to grow tubercle bacilli, but the specimen was taken after one and a half years' antibacterial treatment. Thus in this case, there was a change from caseating tuberculosis to sarcoidosis and then back again to a caseating phase.

Among the seven patients in whom initially the possibility of Hodgkin's disease had to be considered, two presented with a widespread superficial adenopathy, affecting principally the cervical group, and the spleen was palpable; the chest radiograph showed slight enlargement of hilar nodes and some mottling in the lungs; and biopsy of superficial lymph-nodes showed the typical histological pattern of sarcoidosis. In four, the adenopathy was limited to the neck; two of these had also enlarged hilar nodes and mottled shadowing in the lungs, one also with a few papular skin lesions on the face and shoulders; and two had no clinical signs apart from the cervical adeno-pathy. The diagnosis was established by biopsy of a cervical lymph-node in three and of a skin lesion in the fourth. In the remaining case of the seven, enlargement of inguinal lymph-nodes to a size sufficient to incommode the patient was accompanied by less obvious enlargement of cervical lymph-nodes and a mass in the abdomen shown at laparotomy to be due to enlargement of mesenteric lymph-nodes; diagnosis was established by two biopsies of inguinal nodes, the second resulting from surgical excision of the nodes because of their inconvenient size, and by a persistently negative reaction to intradermal tuberculin. Thus the differential diagnosis between sarcoidosis and Hodgkin's or other lymphoma was not difficult in any of these cases.

Nevertheless, occasionally much more difficulty may be met, as in the following case, where the diagnosis finally was reticulum cell sarcoma, although for a long time repeated biopsies suggested sarcoidosis.

A man, aged 21, noticed a swelling in the left side of the neck, at first without other symptoms. Five months later, he started to feel ill, and was found to be febrile, with a mass of enlarged rubbery discrete lymph-nodes in the left side of the neck, and a just palpable spleen. The chest radiograph was normal. On three occasions, nodes were removed for biopsy and showed non-caseating epithelioid cell tubercles. In the third biopsy specimen, the epithelioid cells were arranged rather diffusely, but there were some definite sarcoid-like follicles, and some hyaline connective tissue like that seen in scarred sarcoid lesions. Because of the persistent fever, prednisolone was given with relief of symptoms and considerable diminution in size of the enlarged cervical lymph-nodes. However, when the dosage was reduced, the symptoms returned.

Seventeen months from the beginning of the illness, a fourth lymph-node biopsy showed equivocal appearances, consisting of a mixture of granuloma-tous foci of sarcoid type including a few Schaumann bodies and others resembling Hodgkin's disease having eosinophils, reticulum cells and some giant cells, together with zones of old hyaline-fibrosis. The clinical picture now strongly suggested Hodgkin's disease, with increase in size of the nodes in both sides of the neck, new enlargement of inguinal nodes, and masses in the abdomen. In spite of radiotherapy, the patient died just under two years after the first enlargement of the cervical nodes had been noticed. At necropsy, there was gross enlargement of abdominal lymph-nodes, especially the para-aortic, and of mediastinal lymph-nodes, and many nodules in much enlarged liver and spleen. Histologically, the appearances were interpreted as reticulum cell sarcoma.

In this case, presumably the underlying disease throughout was the lym-phoma, and the misleading appearance of the lymph-nodes removed for biopsy was due to an unusually extensive local sarcoid reaction to this disease. It is significant that at no time was there evidence of involvement in a manner characteristic of sarcoidosis of the lungs, the skin, the eyes or any other organ except the locally affected lymph-nodes.

Cowdell (1954, Case 90) mentioned briefly a case in which sarcoid changes were found in lymph-nodes on one side of the neck, at the same time as a larger mass on the other side due to Hodgkin's disease. In a case reported by Oppenheim and Pollack (1947) and mentioned in Chapter 17, p. 368), sarcoidosis of superficial lymph-nodes was followed after some years by Hodgkin's disease. The occurrence of lymphoma in patients with, or known to have had sarcoidosis, is discussed in Chapter 24, p. 535.

BIOPSY OF SUPERFICIAL LYMPH-NODES

Palpable superficial lymph-nodes are favourable material for biopsy. The neck, especially its supra-clavicular area, and the axilla are the most fre-quently involved areas; but since enlarged nodes at any site may show granulomas in patients with sarcoidosis, careful search of all areas may be rewarding in obscure cases. Israel and Sones (1964) found that of 200 palpable lymph-nodes removed for biopsy, 86% showed confirmatory his-tological changes. Löfgren and Snellman (1964) reported that of 194 palp-able lymph-nodes removed from patients clinically suspected of sarcoidosis, 173 (89%) confirmed this diagnosis, and four gave evidence of other dis-eases. In the series of 275 patients with sarcoidosis reviewed by JGS, palpable nodes were removed for biopsy in 72, of which 66 (92%) showed sarcoid-type granulomas; four from the epitrochlear region and two from the groin all showed such changes, as did one high in the posterior triangle of the neck, just below the mastoid process, which was the only palpable lymph-node in a patient with uveitis and lung changes.

The finding of sarcoid-type tubercles in a lymph-node without evidence of changes suggestive of sarcoidosis elsewhere poses a diagnostic problem. The possibilities that this finding may be explicable either as a local sarcoid reaction to a malignant tumour in the related area, or as a non-caseating reaction peripheral to a focus of caseating tuberculosis should be considered. In such cases, if all reasonable investigation has failed to produce corroborative evidence of any of the possibilities, it may be wise to await the development of further manifestations before making a definite diagnosis.

SCALENE NODE BIOPSY

The procedure of removing the pad of fat which overlies the scalenus anticus muscle and usually contains a number of small lymph-nodes in order to obtain material for biopsy in intrathoracic disease was introduced by Daniels (1949), and became widely used as a method of seeking histological evidence in sarcoidosis and in intrathoracic diseases, especially malignant disease. It is convenient to consider this method of biopsy here, although the nodes contained in the scalene fat pad are not, strictly speaking, superficial. If they are sufficiently enlarged, of course, these nodes may become palpable. Some confusion has arisen in terminology, some authors including biopsy of palpable as well as impalpable nodes under the heading scalene node biopsy.

Carstensen *et al.* (1956) reported scalene node biopsies in 237 patients with clinical and radiographic evidence of sarcoidosis, with supporting evidence in 148 (62%), and positive evidence against this diagnosis in one, which showed Hodgkin's disease. Lillington and Jamplis (1963) in a general review of this method of biopsy tabulated the results obtained by a number of investigators; in 14 series, excluding that of Carstensen *et al.*, quoted above, 138 (83%) of proven cases of sarcoidosis showed specific changes in nodes in scalene fat pads removed from patients without palpable superficial lymph-nodes. Stjernberg *et al.* (1980) compared the results of complete removal of the scalene fat pad by a surgeon with special experience of this technique in a group of 39 patients with clinical and radiographic evidence of sarcoidosis, with those obtained in 43 patients with similar clinical findings submitted to 'scalene node biopsy', presumably by a less meticulous technique by several surgeons. Nodes with histological changes compatible with sarcoidosis were found in 82% of the first, but only 47% of the second group.

Scalene fat pad biopsy involves dissection in an area through which important and vulnerable structures run. Although most authors who have discussed it minimize its risks, several refer to such complications as haematoma and infection in the wound, transient Horner's syndrome and damage to the thoracic duct or right lymphatic duct. Berger *et al.* (1963) described three serious complications in 320 scalene node biopsies. All the complications occurred in patients with bronchial carcinoma; one had serious damage to the subclavian artery and two damage to the subclavian vein with air embolism.

Mediastinoscopy, which provides a means of obtaining lymph-nodes from the superior mediastinum, entails no greater risk than scalene node biopsy, and is now generally regarded as a preferable procedure where differential diagnosis of mediastinal lymphadenopathy is in question, and no superficial lymph-nodes are palpable. It is considered in Chapter 26.

Chapter 11

The Liver

Few patients with sarcoidosis show clinically evident involvement of the liver, although both biopsy and necropsy studies show that in many the liver contains granulomas. In most cases, these cause no symptoms and resolve uneventfully, though tests of liver function may show transient abnormalities. In a very few, they progress to cause varying combinations of portal hypertension, jaundice and hepato-cellular failure. Especially if these occur in patients in whom the diagnosis of sarcoidosis is not readily evident from involvement of other organs, a wide range of diseases in which granulomatous changes may be found in the liver must be considered in differential diagnosis.

INCIDENCE OF HISTOLOGICAL INVOLVEMENT OF THE LIVER

Branson and Park (1954) reviewed 117 reported necropsies in sarcoidosis, and found that in 78 (66.5%) the liver was stated to be involved, while in 31 (26.5%) there was a definite statement that it was not involved.

The best available evidence of the frequency of symptomless granulomas in the liver in sarcoidosis comes from studies made when aspiration liver biopsy was widely used to obtain histological support for the diagnosis of sarcoidosis. In 1943, Van Beek and Haex were the first to report the use of aspiration liver biopsy in sarcoidosis; they found typical non-caseating tubercles in biopsies from 2 of 4 cases with clinical features of sarcoidosis, although there was no other evidence of liver involvement. Van Buchem (1946) found specific changes in liver biopsies in all of 14 cases of sarcoidosis. Scadding and Sherlock (1948) found sarcoid granulomas in the liver in all of three cases, and in addition reported that in one patient, with no clinical evidence of either sarcoidosis or tuberculosis, liver biopsy unexpectedly showed two non-caseating tubercles. Granulomas of sarcoid type were found in liver biopsies in 16 of 21 cases in which the diagnosis of sarcoidosis seemed likely on other grounds by Shay *et al.* (1951). Mather *et al.* (1955) studied 93 patients with sarcoidosis, of whom 59 (63%) showed tuberculoid granulomas on liver biopsy; 11 had had erythema nodosum, and of these ten showed specific changes. Among patients with intrathoracic changes, the liver showed granulomas in a higher proportion (75%) of those with hilar lymph-node enlargement, with or without lung infiltration, than in those with lung infiltration only (38%). In a series of 275 patients under the care of one of us (JGS) with a final diagnosis of sarcoidosis, liver biopsy was performed to help in diagnosis in 73; granulomas were found in 48 (66%) of these, more frequently in the earlier stages of the disease. Of the biopsies done when the intrathoracic changes consisted in hilar lymph-node enlargement only, 87% were positive; when there was also an infiltration of

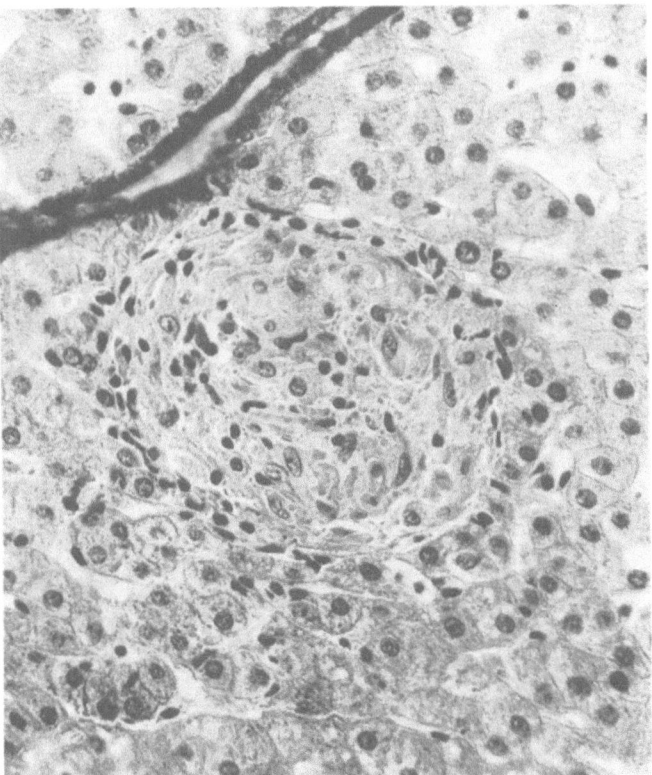

Figure 11.1 A small typical sarcoid tubercle in a liver biopsy from a woman aged 22 with symptomless infiltration of the lungs, the cystic changes in phalanges shown in Fig. 9.3, and non-caseating granulomas in a cervical lymph-node removed for biopsy. H & E. × 344.

the lungs, 67% were positive; and when there was infiltration of the lungs without hilar node enlargement, 59% were positive. A lower incidence of hepatic granulomas was reported in Finland by Lehmuskallio *et al.* (1977). Needle biopsies in 121 patients with sarcoidosis showed granulomas in only 29 (21%), and in patients with BHL only the proportion (16%) was lower than in those with lung infiltration (30%).

In biopsy samples from the liver in patients with sarcoidosis, granulomas may be situated either within the lobule or in the portal zone. They are rounded or oval in shape, and of very variable size, the lower limit being set by the need to have sufficient cells in recognizable arrangement to give a specific appearance (Fig. 11.1), and the upper for a non-confluent lesion being about 1 mm. They are clearly demarcated from the liver cells, and there is no cellular reaction around them. Sherlock (1958) pointed out that in a glycogen-stained section they stand out very clearly from the surround-

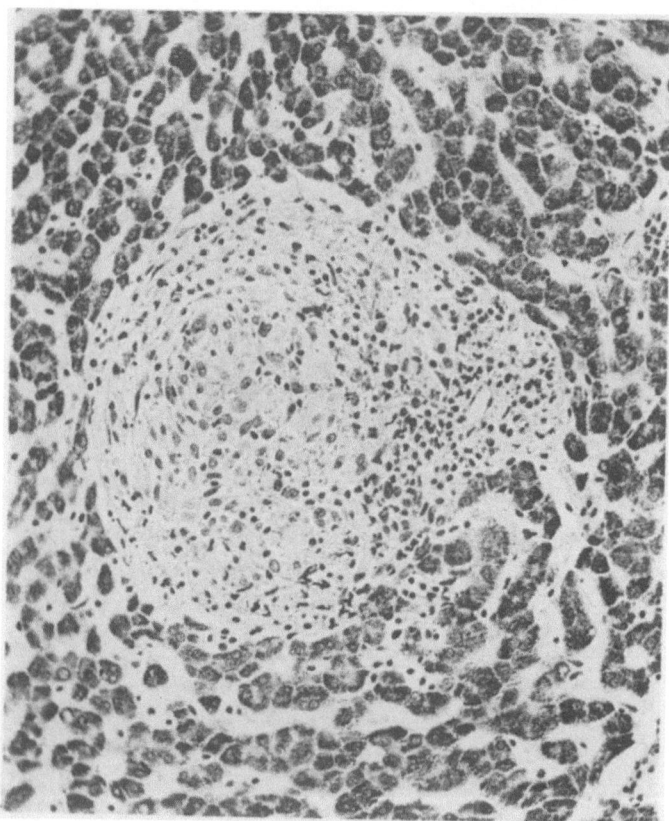

Figure 11.2 A sarcoid tubercle in the liver, showing the contrast with liver cells in a section stained for glycogen. Best's carmine. × 176.

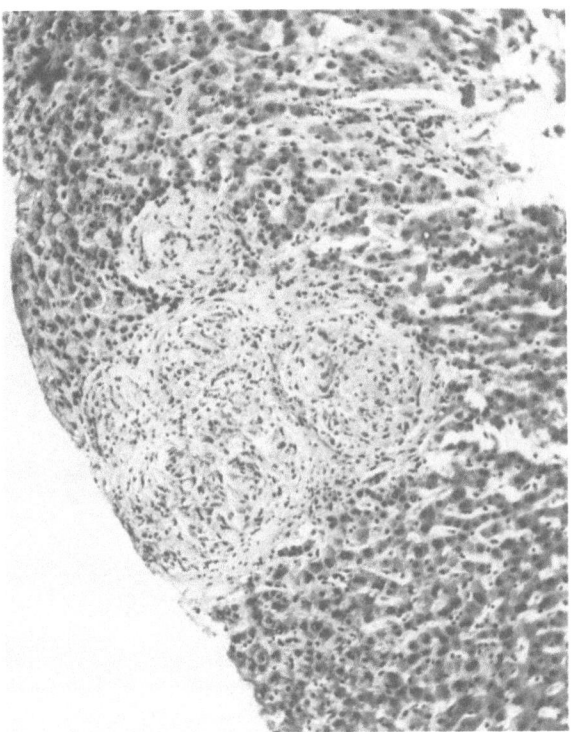

Figure 11.3   A confluent group of sarcoid tubercles in a liver biopsy from a woman aged 35 with sarcoidosis of four years' duration, showing commencing hyalinization. H & E. × 104.

ing liver cells (Fig. 11.2). They have the usual structure of a non-caseating epithelioid cell tubercle; there may be a few lymphocytes especially at the periphery, and the number of giant cells is very variable. Asteroids are only occasionally and Schaumann bodies very rarely seen in the liver. In older lesions, there is a variable amount of hyaline fibrosis and the number of epithelioid cells decreases and of lymphocytes increases (Fig. 11.3); and sometimes groups of hyalinizing tubercles become confluent, in extreme instances giving rise to extensive fibrosis (Fig. 11.4). Mather *et al.* (1955) found an average of three (range 1–25) tubercles in biopsy specimens which they estimated to represent on an average about 1/50 000 part of the liver; this would suggest between 50 000 and 1 250 000 in the whole liver. In spite of the large number of tubercles which may be present, it is essential to section the biopsy specimen serially, both to ensure that a single tubercle is not missed, and also to follow an equivocal abnormality into adjacent sections.

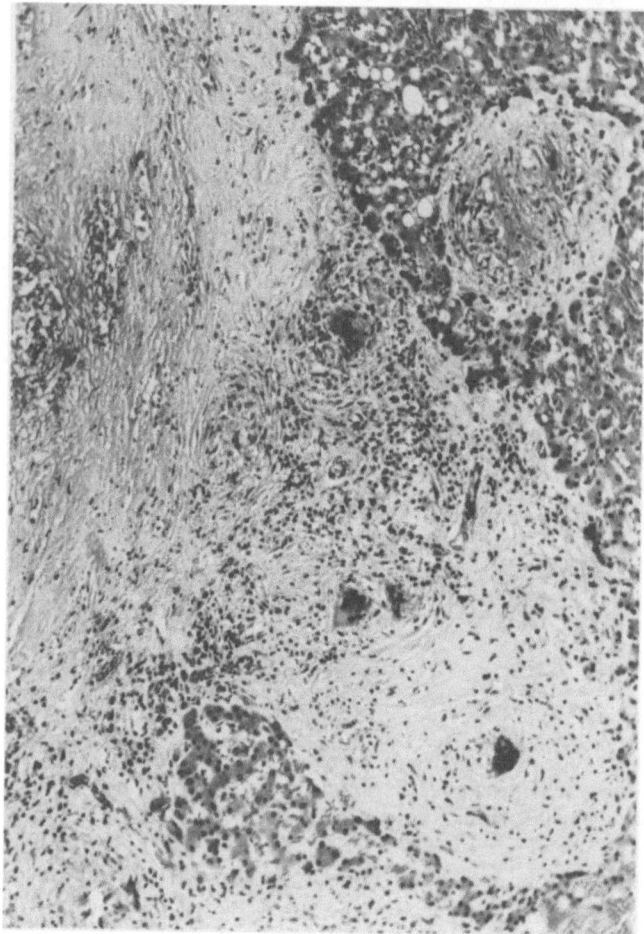

Figure 11.4 Extensive fibrosis in the liver, with hyalinized sarcoid granulomas and some giant cells, found at necropsy in a woman who died at the age of 42 with long-standing fibrotic pulmonary sarcoidosis. H & E. × 80.

Hepatic granulomas

The contribution to the diagnosis of sarcoidosis of the finding of granulomas in a liver biopsy must be considered in relation to the total clinical picture, like that of other biopsy procedures (Chapter 26), and is limited by the frequency of granulomatous changes in the liver in a variety of other local and systemic diseases. Such changes may be a response to a wide variety of infective agents, parasitic infestations, and drugs and toxic substances, may occur in systemic granulomatous diseases of unknown cause, or may be a feature of disease affecting predominantly the liver (Holdstock *et al.*, 1979). A few cases remain which after full investigation cannot be placed in any of these categories.

Among infective agents, those causing predominantly granulomatous inflammation, notably *M. tuberculosis*, and in endemic areas histoplasma and coccidioides, are most likely to cause hepatic granulomas resembling those of sarcoidosis.

Van Beek *et al.* (1948, 1949) found tubercles in liver biopsies from seven often patients with erythema nodosum attributed to primary tuberculosis, and from all of seven with acute haematogenous tuberculosis. Klatskin and Yesner (1950) found tuberculoid granulomas in liver biopsies from seven of 18 patients with tuberculosis; only one of these showed caseation. Mather *et al.* (1955) investigated 32 patients with various forms of tuberculosis. All of three with miliary tuberculosis, four of ten with active primary tuberculosis, and only one of 19 with other forms of tuberculosis showed tubercles in the liver. The tubercles were indistinguishable from those of sarcoidosis, and no tubercle bacilli were demonstrated in them. The same authors surveyed 34 necropsies in cases of tuberculosis and found that of 12 with tubercles in the liver all had miliary or meningeal tuberculosis. They classified the results of liver biopsy from several published series according to the type of tuberculosis, and found that all of 13 with miliary tuberculosis, 16 of 25 with primary tuberculosis, and only 16 of 152 with other forms of tuberculosis had been reported to show tubercles. Korn *et al.* (1959) in a study of the liver in extrapulmonary tuberculosis performed biopsies in 30 patients, mainly with peritoneal and lymph-node involvement, but some with miliary or meningeal tuberculosis; 24 showed granulomas. Bowry *et al.* (1970) found granulomas in eight of 32 patients with pulmonary tuberculosis; of five who also had extrapulmonary, including miliary, disease, four had hepatic granulomas. Klatskin (1976) found granulomas in liver biopsies in 43% of 164 patients with tuberculosis; 94% of those with miliary tuberculosis, 71% with both pulmonary and extrapulmonary disease, 31% with active pulmonary and only 10% of those with inactive pulmonary disease had hepatic granulomas. Acid-fast bacilli were seen in granulomas in three of 18 patients with miliary tuberculosis, in three of five with 'primary' hepatic tuberculosis, in one of six with tuberculous lymphadenitis, but in none of 33 with pulmonary or of eight with other forms of tuberculosis.

Granulomas may be found in the liver in a number of other infectious diseases, such as brucellosis (Spink *et al.*, 1949; Barrett and Rickards, 1953), histoplasmosis (Pinkerton and Iverson, 1952), blastomycosis (Martin and Smith, 1939) and tularaemia (Bernstein, 1935). Klatskin and Yesner (1950) also found granulomas in the liver in infectious mononucleosis, in influenza

B, in unidentified viral infection and in actinomycosis, but the granulomas were small and atypical. In general, the granulomas in the liver in these diseases tend to be less well-defined than those of sarcoidosis, and to be accompanied by non-granulomatous inflammation. For instance, Barrett and Rickards found granulomas in liver biopsies in ten of 12 patients with chronic brucellosis; most of them were well-defined though without a clear limiting sheath, but some merged indefinitely into the surrounding liver, and there appeared to be more inflammatory cell infiltration than is found in sarcoidosis. In the remaining two patients, there were focal lymphocytic infiltrations in the portal tracts.

In chronic beryllium disease (Chapter 22) there may be granulomas in the liver. In Agate's (1948) patient epithelioid cell granulomas were found in a liver biopsy, and Hardy (1951) referred to similar findings without saying anything about their frequency. In necropsy material, Chesner (1950) found granulomas in the liver in two of three cases, but Martland *et al.* (1948) found none in four cases. Klatskin and Yesner (1950) found none in a liver biopsy from one patient, but later (1976) Klatskin stated that granulomas were present in biopsies from all of four with 'berylliosis'.

Among parasitic infestations, schistosomiasis is especially liable to cause widespread granulomatous changes in the liver; the ova that incite the formation of granulomas may be demonstrable.

As in other organs, granulomas in the liver may be a response to malignant or inflammatory disease. Of 72 patients with liver biopsies showing granulomas not attributable to any systemic or local hepatic disease reported by Klatskin (1976), ten were associated with intra-abdominal lymphoma, five with carcinoma, and four with inflammatory bowel disease. Bagley *et al.* (1972) studied liver biopsies in Hodgkin's disease, and found non-caseating granulomas in five of 89 untreated patients; none of those with granulomas had evidence of Hodgkin's disease in the liver.

Granulomatous elements may be found in the histology of many of the commoner categories of liver disease, but in most are insignificant and cause no diagnostic difficulty. In primary biliary cirrhosis (chronic non-suppurative destructive cholangitis) granulomas are frequent, being found in 42% of one series (Fox *et al.*, 1969); and there may be problems of differentiation from sarcoidosis discussed below. The large series of liver biopsies reported by Klatskin (1976) provides an indication of the proportions of cases of the commoner categories of liver disease in which granulomatous elements can be found in the histopathology: 40% of 148 cases of biliary cirrhosis, and 5% of 1051 cases of other sorts of cirrhosis; 2% of 632 cases of viral hepatitis and 7% of 191 cases of toxic and drug-induced hepatitis, and 12% of 34 cases of chronic active hepatitis showed such changes.

CLINICAL EVIDENCES OF SARCOIDOSIS OF THE LIVER

At the time when liver biopsy was used in some centres to help in the diagnosis of sarcoidosis, it was the common experience that most patients found in this way to have granulomas in the liver had no clinical evidence of liver dysfunction. The proportion of patients in unselected series of cases of sarcoidosis reported to show enlargement of the liver varies greatly; probably differing criteria of what constitutes enlargement are in part responsible for this variability, but differences in severity of sarcoidosis in populations studied and in selection of cases for study are also likely to be important. Mayock *et al.* (1963) in a series of 145 patients in Philadelphia of whom 70% were black, found the liver palpable in 43%, though only four had evident liver disease. They reviewed a number of published series, in which the proportion with palpable livers ranged from 7–21%. One of us (JGS) in a series of 275 patients in London found the liver palpable more than one finger's breadth below the costal margin in only four, adopting this criterion as indicating unequivocal enlargement; in all four the spleen was also palpable, and in two hepatosplenomegaly was initially gross. Lehmuskallio *et al.* (1977) found the liver palpable 1 cm below the costal margin in 11.4% of 325 patients in Helsinki.

The proportions of patients in unselected series showing abnormalities in biochemical tests of liver function vary similarly. In a series of 500 patients with sarcoidosis in Baltimore, of whom a large majority were black, Maddrey *et al.* (1970) reported that 20 (4%) had both granulomas in liver biopsies and biochemical and clinical evidence of liver dysfunction; an unstated number had granulomas in the liver without other evidence of liver disease. Of the 20 with liver dysfunction, 18 were black, one Indian, and one white: nine had unequivocal evidence of hepato-cellular disease with or without portal hypertension. In a series of 325 patients in Helsinki, all white, Lehmuskallio *et al.* (1977) found elevation of alkaline phosphatase in only 1.3%, of aspartate aminotransferase in three of 61 examined, and of bromsulphthalein retention in 8%. These abnormalities were found principally in patients with erythema nodosum, and a comparative group of patients with erythema nodosum not associated with sarcoidosis showed similar proportions with abnormal results for these tests. Only two showed slightly elevated bilirubin levels, and in both these returned to normal. Among the 121 submitted to liver biopsy, abnormal enzyme levels were found in a higher proportion of those with than of those without detected granulomas, but the presence of granulomas was not correlated with palpability of the liver. These Finnish patients had less severe and extensive sarcoidosis than those in Baltimore; none had portal hypertension or liver failure.

In those cases in which involvement of the liver in sarcoidosis has caused overt symptoms, various combinations of portal hypertension, jaundice and hepato-cellular failure have been observed. Since many cases have presented with one of these as the predominant feature, it is convenient to discuss them under these headings, although, of course, they overlap. In some cases, it is difficult to decide whether such factors as viral infection, alcoholism, and malnutrition may have played a part in the causation of changes in the liver which include non-granulomatous inflammation and fibrosis, as well as granulomas, especially if these are scanty or undergoing hyalinization. An idea of the relative frequency of clinical syndromes of liver disease associated with granulomas in the liver in patients with sarcoidosis can be obtained from the series reported by Maddrey *et al.* (1970). Of their nine such cases, five were shown to have portal hypertension and in four of these it was the principal cause of symptoms, giving rise to bleeding from oesophageal varices in two; hepato-cellular dysfunction was the principal feature of five; serum bilirubin was raised in six, and jaundice with obstructive features was observed in two; three deaths of patients with severe liver disease were reported, one after an operation for portal-systemic shunt, and two from the combined effects of hepatic and pulmonary sarcoidosis.

Portal hypertension

Cases in which portal hypertension was an important feature of hepatic sarcoidosis have been reported by Mino *et al.* (1948), Dunlap and Hallenbeck (1952), Klatskin (1976), Fraimow and Myerson (1957), Cheitlin *et al.* (1960), Porter (1961), Mistilis *et al.* (1964), Nelson and Schwabe (1966), Maddrey *et al.* (1970), Vilinskas *et al.* (1970) and Rosenberg (1971). Bleeding from oesophageal varices causing haematemesis and melaena was an important symptom in about half these cases: ascites was noted in five of them; in a few the diagnosis of portal hypertension was established in patients without either of these indicants by the finding of oesophageal varices, and in some confirmed by measurement of splenic pulp or wedged hepatic vein pressure. In most, both liver and spleen were enlarged, usually grossly. Enlargement was slight or not noted in a few, e.g. those of Dunlap *et al.* (1952), Fraimow *et al.* (1957), and Case IV A of Maddrey *et al.* (1970). Portal hypertension may occur both with pre-fibrotic granulomatous infiltration and at a later stage with extensive fibrosis. Vilinskas *et al.* (1970) reported the case of a black man aged 19 who presented with haematemesis and gross splenomegaly known to have been present a year earlier; oesophageal varices were found, and the hepatic vein wedge pressure was 31 mm Hg and the splenic pulp pressure 370 mm saline; a liver biopsy showed non-caseating granulomas without fibrosis. Eighteen months later, splenectomy and spleno-renal shunt were performed: the portal vein pressure was 390 mm, the liver was normal in size but cirrhotic, having a hobnail appearance, and histologically showed disruption of the lobular pattern by bands of connective tissue with lymphocytic infiltration but no granulomas, and the spleen, weighing 1220 g contained many epithelioid and giant-cell granulomas, as did an adjacent lymph-node. In this case, as in several others with gross splenomegaly (e.g. Dunlap and Hallenbeck, 1952; Lebacq *et al.*, 1956a; Cheitlin *et al.*, 1961), there was pancytopenia, which was relieved after splenectomy; and less degrees of hypersplenism have been noted in other cases.

Maddrey *et al.* (1970) and Valinskas *et al.* (1970) discussed the mechanisms of portal hypertension in hepatic sarcoidosis. In most cases in which both wedged hepatic pressure and splenic pulp pressure have been measured, both were raised, as is observed in most forms of cirrhotic portal hypertension. Mistilis *et al.* (1964) described a case in which the wedged hepatic vein pressure was normal, with an intrasplenic pressure of 460 mm, suggesting presinusoidal obstruction by granulomas in the portal areas, though it seems that granulomas so located would need to be more profuse than has been observed in some patients with portal hypertension in the absence of extensive fibrosis. In cases where there is fibrosis amounting to cirrhosis the mechanisms concerned in other forms of fibrosis probably operate. Other possible factors include raised splenic blood flow in patients with grossly enlarged spleens; in Case IV 4 of Maddrey *et al.* (1970) wedged hepatic venous pressure fell from 25 to 8 mm Hg after removal of a spleen that extended 20 cm below the costal margin.

Corticosteroid treatment has in general been found to be ineffective in reducing raised portal venous pressure, although manifestations of sarcoidosis in other organs, the size of the spleen, pancytopenia, biochemical evidence of hepato-cellular dysfunction and constitutional symptoms may improve. Portal-systemic shunt with (Mino *et al.*, 1948; Dunlap and Hallenbeck, 1952; Fraimow and Myerson, 1957; Vilinskas *et al.*, 1970) or without (Klatskin, 1976; Maddrey *et al.*, 1970; Rosenberg, 1971) splenectomy has in most cases given satisfactory results, and appears to be indicated in patients with portal hypertension due to sarcoidosis without serious hepato-cellular dysfunction; in those with enlarged spleens and hypersplenism, splenectomy and spleno-renal shunt may be the operation of choice.

Jaundice and hepato-cellular failure

Cases of sarcoidosis of the liver in which jaundice and/or hepato-cellular failure were leading features have been reported by Goeckerman (1928), Klatskin *et al.* (1950), Shay *et al.* (1951), Dagradi *et al.* (1952), Wagoner *et al.* (1953), Branson and Park (1954), Kelley and McHardy (1955), Porter (1961), Nelson and Sears (1968), Maddrey *et al.*, (1970), Rudzki *et al.*

(1975) and Bass *et al.* (1982). Several of these – e.g. Cases III 4 and 5 of Maddrey *et al.* – showed evidence of portal hypertension also; and some which presented with bleeding from oesophageal varices – e.g. that of Nelson and Schwabe (1966) – proceeded to jaundice and hepatic coma.

Jaundice may be due to intrahepatic cholestatis, resulting in a clinical and biochemical picture resembling that of primary biliary cirrhosis. Foxworthy and Freeman (1952) reported briefly the case of a young black man with jaundice, hepatosplenomegaly, cutaneous xanthomas and high serum lipids and granulomas in liver and lymph-nodes; all these features improved on treatment with ACTH and cortisone. Rudski *et al.* (1975) reported five young black men with sarcoidosis, the diagnosis being established in all by involvement of several organs and histology, who either presented with or developed hepatomegaly and cholestatic jaundice, with pruritus and eleva- tion of serum alkaline phosphatase and cholesterol levels. In one, skin xanthomas appeared. In three ascites and oesophageal varices developed late in the course, death in one being due to bleeding from varices. One died, ten years after the first evidence of sarcoidosis and six years after the appearance of jaundice, from renal failure, cause unspecified; three died from the effects of the liver disease nine, 11 and 18 years from its onset, and one was surviving at 16 years. Histologically, the livers showed granulo- mas, intrahepatic cholestatis, diminishing numbers of interlobular bile ducts, periportal fibrosis leading to micronodular cirrhosis, and high copper levels in hepatocytes. None of the patients had been exposed to known hepatotoxic drugs or environmental factors, and tests for antibodies to mitochondria, nuclei and smooth muscle were negative in all. Response to corticosteroid treatment was limited to temporary reduction in bilirubin levels in two patients and relief of pruritus in one. Bass *et al.* (1982) reported two similar cases in West Indians in London. In both the diagnosis of sarcoidosis was based on compatible clinical features, granulomatous re- sponses to Kveim tests, and the finding of granulomas in tissues, including the liver. In both, bile ducts were reduced, and portal hypertension de- veloped; one progressed to biliary cirrhosis and the other suffered variceal haemorrhage; mitochondrial antibody tests were negative in both.

Cases with features leading to combined diagnoses of sarcoidosis and primary biliary cirrhosis have been reported by Holtzman (1961) and Karlish *et al.* (1969).

Obstructive jaundice was due to narrowing of the common bile duct by granulomatous infiltration of its wall and involvement in a mass of sur- rounding granulomatous lymph-nodes in a black woman aged 29 whose case was reported by Bloom *et al.* (1978); she presented initially with broncho-pulmonary and hilar lymph-node sarcoidosis and 18 months later with jaundice. Corticosteroid treatment after temporary biliary drainage by T-tube led to relief of jaundice.

In some reported cases of liver disease in patients with sarcoidosis, the evidence available leaves doubt whether the liver changes were pathogenetically part of the generalized sarcoidosis, or partly or wholly due to some other factor, and thus to be regarded as indicative of another disease. It seems possible that in patients with sarcoidosis exposure to pathogenetic factors potentially damaging to the liver may determine the development of granulomas in the liver, producing complex clinico-pathological pictures. There is no evidence that sarcoidosis patients have any special liability to hepatitis. Sharma *et al.* (1970) tested the sera of 45 patients in Los Angeles for Australia antigen, with negative results; Fouts *et al.* (1970) tested 130 in Philadelphia and found only two positive, in both of whom there were explanations for the carrier state.

DIAGNOSIS OF LIVER DISEASE WITH GRANULOMATOUS FEATURES

Although a few present diagnostic difficulties, most patients with granulomas in the liver present a total clinical picture and other histological features in the liver which permit appropriate categorization with little difficulty. In a survey of 2813 liver biopsies in the practice of a general hospital, Iversen *et al.* (1970) found 19 with epithelioid cell granulomas; the final diagnosis was sarcoidosis in six, miliary tuberculosis in one, acute hepatitis in three, cirrhosis of the liver in two, chronic alcoholism in three, fatty liver in one, hepatomegaly (not further categorized) in one, fever of unknown origin in one, and malignant pleurisy in one. Two others with less well formed 'lipogranulomas' were suffering from mononucleosis and acute hepatitis. The authors emphasized that if epithelioid cell granulomas are found in an otherwise normal or nearly normal liver, the probable diagnosis is either sarcoidosis or tuberculosis. This conclusion might need to be modified in an area with differing prevalences of infectious diseases.

The recognition of mycobacterial infection as the cause of a granulomatous hepatitis may be difficult if the liver is the only evidently involved organ. Acid-fast bacilli are found only in very few cases. A positive tuberculin test favours but does not establish a diagnosis of tuberculosis. If the tuberculin test is positive, and the general clinical picture is suggestive of this diagnosis, a therapeutic trial of antimycobacterial chemotherapy is advisable. Unequivocal response to such treatment was observed in a case reported by Frank and Raffensperger (1965) and in two by Fitzgerald *et al.* (1971), supporting the provisional diagnosis of tuberculosis.

Differential diagnosis between primary biliary cirrhosis and hepatic sarcoidosis causing hepato-cellular dysfunction with or without cholestatic jaundice may be difficult both clinically and histologically. In primary biliary cirrhosis, granulomas are part of the histological pattern in many cases, usually in relation to characteristically abnormal bile-ducts; occasionally they can be found in lymph-nodes at the hepatic hilum. The disease most commonly affects middle-aged women, and the serum contains antibodies to mitochondria in nearly all cases. As in sarcoidosis, impairment of Type IV hypersensitivity reactions is commonly found (Fox *et al.*, 1969). Stanley *et al.* (1972) reported two otherwise typical cases in which at necropsy granulomas were found in lymph-nodes in the abdomen and mediastinum, and in the spleen in one, and in the lungs, where during life they had caused radiographic mottling and dyspnoea. Many of the cases of cholestatic jaundice attributable to sarcoidosis have been in men (Foxworthy and Freeman, 1952, Karlish *et al.*, 1969; Maddrey *et al.*, 1970, Case III 2; Rudzki *et al.*, 1975; Bass *et al.*, 1982, Case 2). Points of differential value are clinical and other evidence of granulomatous changes in other organs, of uveitis, of erythema nodosum in the past, or of hypercalcaemia, favour a diagnosis of sarcoidosis. Pruritus and xanthomas are common in primary biliary cirrhosis, but may occur in sarcoidosis. Antibodies to mitochondria are an expected finding in primary biliary cirrhosis, and not in sarcoidosis. A granulomatous response to a Kveim test is evidence in favour of sarcoidosis, but can be expected only in a minority of patients with predominantly hepatic involvement. A report by Fagan *et al.* (1983) of four middle-aged women with hepatic granulomas, lung changes, and high titres of mitochondrial antibody illustrates the difficulties of diagnostic categorization. All had hepatomegaly, and other histological changes compatible with biliary cirrhosis; one had cholestatic jaundice and one died of fulminant hepatic failure. All had pulmonary infiltrations causing symptoms and signs, and shown in three to be granulomatous. Kveim tests were performed in three, with a granulomatous response in one, and negative responses in the other two, who were receiving corticosteroid treatment. One also had features of systemic sclerosis, and one coeliac disease; both of these had antinuclear antibody. Evidently it is not possible to fit such cases into current diagnostic categories.

The case of sarcoid splenomegaly with thrombocytopenia, treated by splenectomy, with persistent equivocal histological changes in the liver, described in Chapter 12, p. 285, illustrates the simulation of biliary cirrhosis by a condition which seems to be appropriately categorized as sarcoidosis.

Diagnostic problems of patients presenting with granulomatous hepatitis have been discussed by Israel and Goldstein (1973) and Simon and Wolfe (1973). Israel and Goldstein studied 30 patients with granulomas in liver biopsies and normal chest radiographs. In 16 there was clinical and/or biopsy evidence of changes in other organs justifying a diagnosis of sarcoidosis; Kveim tests were performed in 15 of these, but only one was positive, indicating that this test has no value in excluding a diagnosis of sarcoidosis; four improved spontaneously and ten on corticosteroid treatment, one died of an unrelated cause, and in one the outcome was unknown. Of 14 with no evidence, direct or indirect, of granulomas in other organs, one was found at necropsy to have Hodgkin's disease, and the liver granulomas were thought to be a response to this. One had positive reactions both to tuberculin, 5 IU of PPD, and to a Kveim test, and there was no response to two years of anti-mycobacterial chemotherapy. This, and the other 12 cases, in which there was no evidence of any recognized systemic disease or infection, were left with no final diagnosis, beyond granulomatous hepatitis; seven recovered spontaneously, three after tetracycline given on an unsubstantiated suspicion of Q fever. Simon and Wolfe (1973) analysed 13, among 200 patients investigated for prolonged fever, who were found to have granulomas in liver biopsies. Of these, one had had bilateral hilar lymph-node enlargement, and in spite of some central necrosis in the granulomas was thought to have sarcoidosis; one responded to anti-mycobacterial chemotherapy, and in one the final diagnosis was Hodgkin's disease. In the remaining ten, the changes in the liver could not be associated with any systemic disease or causal factor. Evidently, there are cases in which diagnostic categorization can be carried no further than granulomatous hepatitis, a category which should be regarded, at least initially, as provisional.

Gall bladder

Lloyd-Davies and Forbes (1965) reported the case of a man who at the age of 21 presented with a history of vomiting and pain in the right hypochondrium. An adherent fibrotic gall-bladder was removed; non-caseating granulomas of epithelioid cells and a few giant cells were present in the fibrotic wall and mucosa of the gall-bladder, and in the adherent liver. No other evidence of sarcoidosis was found, and a Kveim test was negative; but two years earlier, he had had unexplained transient enlargement of submandibular glands, and the Mantoux test was negative both then and later. Although the evidence is incomplete, it seems likely that this was a case of sarcoidosis with localization in the gall-bladder.

In the case of obstructive jaundice due to involvement of the common bile duct reported by Bloom *et al.* (1978) and mentioned above (p.270), the gall-bladder was removed and found to be infiltrated with sarcoid granulomas.

Chapter 12

The Spleen and the Blood

THE SPLEEN

Involvement of the spleen at necropsy in cases of sarcoidosis has been reported with variable frequency, ranging from 17 of the 22 reported by Ricker and Clark (1949) and 31 of the 40 reports collected from the literature by Longcope and Freiman (1952) to only ten of the 26 spleens from their own necropsy cases examined microscopically by the latter authors. Selroos (1976) performed aspiration biopsies of the spleen in 77

Table 12.1   Palpability of spleen in sarcoidosis.

Author	Location	No. of patients	Spleen recorded as palpable	
			No.	%
Reisner (1944)	New York	35	8	23
Ricker and Clark (1949)	United States	195	16	8
Riley (1950)	New York	52	21	40
Robinson and Pound (1950)	Australia	30	6	20
Longcope and Freiman (1952)	Baltimore	90	22	24
	Boston	52	22	42
Nitter (1953)	Copenhagen	90	5	6
Kimbrell (1957)	Virginia	80	13	16
Israel and Sones (1958)	Philadelphia	160	24	15
James (1959)	London	200	27	13.5
Smellie and Hoyle (1960)	London	125	28	22
Mayock et al. (1963)	United States	145	43	30
Scadding (1967)	London	275	31	11
Siltzbach et al. (1974)	London	537	62	12
	New York	311	57	18
	Los Angeles	150	20	13
	Paris	329	22	6.7
	Tokyo	282	4	1.4

patients with sarcoidosis; in six of these the spleen was judged radiographically to be enlarged, but in only one was it palpable. Groups of epithelioid cells were found in the splenic aspirate in 53% of all cases, and in five of the six with enlarged spleens. The proportion varied little with the extent of intrathoracic changes, or with the presence of overt extrathoracic changes. In clinical series, the proportion reported to have palpable spleens varies greatly (Table 12.1).

Clinical features of splenic involvement

In sarcoidosis, enlargement of the spleen rendering it no more than palpable a few centimetres below the costal margin causes no identifiable symptoms, apart from the rare cases, discussed below, in which it is associated with thrombocytopenia or, more doubtfully, haemolytic anaemia; nor does it seem to be indicative of generally extensive disease or an unfavourable prognosis. On the other hand, a grossly enlarged spleen is in many cases a part of chronic and extensive sarcoidosis, and tends to be accompanied by important involvement of the liver, and by depression of some or all aspects of haemopoeisis; and it may cause local symptoms by its size. In a series of 275 patients followed for periods up to 20 years, one of us (JGS) recorded the spleen as palpable in 31. In five of these it was grossly enlarged, and in all of these lung changes became fibrotic; in four the liver was at some time enlarged, in three as much as a hand's breadth below the costal margin. On the other hand, milder degrees of splenic enlargement had no special prognostic significance. Kataria and Whitcomb (1980) found that of 233 patients with sarcoidosis, 32 had enlarged spleens. Of these, 69% had hepatomegaly compared with only 3% of a matched group with impalpable spleens. The proportion with skin sarcoids was 38%, compared with 19% among those with impalpable spleens, but pulmonary involvement was similar in the two groups.

The association of hepatic and splenic involvement may lead to complicated clinical pictures, with various combinations of gross splenomegaly, hepatomegaly, thrombocytopenia, purpura, bleeding from oesophageal varices and hepatic failure. These are discussed in Chapter 11.

In a few cases reported as sarcoidosis of the spleen, the only detected site of granulomas was a surgically removed spleen, and in these it is legitimate to doubt whether the criteria for the diagnosis of sarcoidosis were satisfied. But in others, otherwise similar, evidence of sarcoid lesions in other organs and tissues has been available, leaving no doubt of this diagnosis. As has been noted previously, a similar situation exists in relation to involvement of certain other organs – e.g. the lungs and the central nervous system – where in a proportion of cases the clinically evident disease appears to be confined to one organ or system. In the case of the spleen, however, if the liver has been investigated, it has generally been found to be infiltrated as well, even though no evidence of involvement of other organs is available.

Several cases reported in the past as tuberculosis of the spleen probably belong rather to the category sarcoidosis, e.g. the two reported by Hickling (1938) and probably two of the four reported by Engelbreth-Holm (1938).

Among the symptoms attributed to sarcoidosis of the spleen are local pain, discomfort, anorexia and vomiting (Culligan and Snoddy, 1945; Hickling, 1938, Case 2; Kay, 1950, Cases 1, 2 and 3; Partenheimer and Meredith, 1950); and general ill-health and weakness (Culligan and Snoddy, 1945; Hickling, 1938, Cases 1 and 2; Kay, 1950, Case 1).

Young and Mouney (1968) reported the case of a man aged 41 with a short history of tiredness and left abdominal pain relieved by lying on the right side, who was found to have gross splenectomy and generalized enlargement of superficial lymph-nodes; the spleen, weighing 1933 g, was removed, and both it and an axillary lymph-node contained sarcoid-type granulomas; relief of symptoms followed, and the lymph-node enlargement slowly subsided.

In many cases in which an enlarged spleen has been removed surgically, the surgery was undertaken principally for haematological reasons; these are reviewed below. In some, gross enlargement with or without local symptoms seems to have been an additional or the principal indication.

Kay (1950) reported the case of a black male, aged 33, with extensive sarcoidosis, from whom an infiltrated spleen weighing 4800 g was removed, partly because of pancytopenia. Jackson (1957) reported the removal of a spleen weighing 2400 g and densely infiltrated with sarcoid granulomas from a woman, aged 39, in whom it was causing no special symptoms, although she had a hypochromic anaemia which improved afterwards; an abdominal lymph-node removed at the same time showed similar histological changes, and radiographic changes were present in the lungs. Case 2 of Bertino and Myerson (1960) was that of a black man, aged 29, with abdominal enlargement due to gross hepatosplenomegaly, the liver being 12 cm below the costal margin. The spleen, weighing 1820 g, was removed. It was found to be infiltrated with granulomas including occasional Schaumann bodies, and biopsy of the liver showed both granulomas and cirrhotic changes. The operation was followed by relief of symptoms. In the complex case observed by us over many years, and reviewed on p. 515, an infiltrated spleen weighing 3600 g was removed because it was causing abdominal discomfort. Splenectomy was performed in ten of 12 selected patients with gross splenomegaly reported by Webb et al. (1980), the indications being abdominal discomfort in six, infarction in one, rupture in one, and haematological in two.

Even a very large spleen may diminish either spontaneously or under corticosteroid treatment.

Two patients observed by us illustrated this. One, a woman aged 33, sought advice because she had felt a lump in the abdomen, and denied other symptoms. She was found to have an enlarged firm spleen extending to the umbilicus, widespread mottling in the chest radiograph, and sarcoid-type granulomas in a scalene lymph-node. Under observation, the spleen gradually receded, becoming impalpable in four years, and the lung infiltration largely resolved, leaving some residual fibrosis but no disability. The other, a woman aged 24, presented with symptomless bilateral hilar lymphadenopathy; the spleen was found to be palpable. Two years later, the spleen had increased greatly, so that the patient herself noticed it, and it extended to the umbilicus; the BHL had subsided but there was a widespread fine mottling in the chest radiograph. Under prednisolone treatment, both the splenomegaly and the pulmonary shadowing diminished, so that after one year the spleen was only just palpable. Burt and Kuhl (1971) reported the case of a woman who at the age of 43 was found to have enlargement of cervical lymph-nodes and of the left parotid gland, biopsy of which showed sarcoid-type granulomas. Four years later, the spleen was found to be palpable. Two years later, the spleen had increased greatly, so that the patient herself noticed it, and it extended to the umbilicus; the BHL had subsided but there was a widespread fine mottling in the chest radiograph. Under prednisolone treatment, both the splenomegaly and the pulmonary costeroids, six showed reduction in spleen size during treatment, but this was not maintained when treatment was withdrawn.

It is probable that if splenomegaly is due to sarcoid infiltration it will respond to the suppressive effects of corticosteroids; but, as in other organs, hyalinization and changes secondary to it, and enlargement attributable to portal hypertension from sarcoid involvement of the liver (Chapter 11) which frequently accompanies splenic involvement cannot be expected to respond.

Traumatic rupture of the spleen in a patient known to have sarcoidosis was reported by Roberts and Rang (1958).

A boy aged 13 presented with epigastric pain, vomiting and low fever; the liver and spleen were palpable, and liver biopsy showed epithelioid and giant-cell granulomas. A short period of prednisone treatment led to relief of symptoms and diminution in the size of the liver and spleen. A year later, a fall from his bicycle in which he hit his left side on the handlebars was followed by severe abdominal pain. At laparotomy, the spleen weighing 370 g was removed; there was a transverse tear extending from the hilum, and sarcoid tubercles similar to those in the liver were found in the splenic substance. No evidence of sarcoidosis elsewhere than in the liver and spleen was found, even after 18 months' further observation. Sharma (1967) reported the case of a woman aged 28 who developed left upper abdominal pain after a blow on the left side. A ruptured spleen which showed multiple non-caseating granulomas was removed. A Kveim test was reported as 'positive', and although the chest radiograph was normal, lung volumes, carbon monoxide transfer factor and compliance were slightly reduced.

Apparently spontaneous rupture of spleens infiltrated by sarcoid tubercles has been described by James and Wilson (1945) and by Philips and Luchette (1952).

In the first of these cases, a man, aged 49, suffered spontaneous rupture of a normal-sized spleen; it was removed, and found to be infiltrated with sarcoid tubercles. There was no evidence of sarcoidosis elsewhere, but the Mantoux test was negative to 1:100 OT, and was not converted to positive by vole bacillus vaccination. The second was that of a man aged 21; at laparotomy a spleen weighing 306 g was found to have a linear tear on its convex surface and was removed; it was found to contain scattered epithelioid cell tubercles with occasional giant cells, but no caseation or acid-fast bacilli. The skin gave no reaction to 1:100 OT, but no evidence of sarcoidosis elsewhere was found.

The macroscopic appearance of sarcoidosis in the spleen varies from small pale foci difficult to distinguish from germinal centres to large grossly evident nodules. Histologically, there may be discrete or confluent well-formed non-caseating epithelioid cell tubercles; but in some reported cases epithelioid cell aggregations have been less clearly defined. The number of giant cells also varies greatly. The presence of many asteroid bodies in affected spleens has been reported by Friedman (1944) and by Kay (1950).

BLOOD CELL CHANGES

Lymphopenia

Apart from the pancytopenia, thrombocytopenia and possibly haemolytic anaemia that occur in a few cases, usually in asscociation with splenomegaly, and are discussed below, the only feature of the peripheral blood count that is generally agreed to be a feature of sarcoidosis is lymphopenia in the active stages. Early observers (Snapper and Pompen, 1938; Harrell, 1940; Reisner, 1944; McCort *et al.*, 1947; Leitner, 1950; Longcope and Freiman, 1952) reported a variety of changes in varying proportions of cases; these included low total leucocyte counts, monocytosis and eosinophilia, but, apart from the association of splenomegaly with leucopenia, could not be correlated with clinical features or course.

The lymphopenia of active sarcoidosis was first described by Hoffbrand (1968), and has been confirmed by subsequent authors. It has immunological implications, and is discussed in Chapter 20, p. 428.

Selroos and Koivunen (1979) investigated the prognostic significance of the initial white cell count in 140 patients, of whom 22 later developed chronic sarcoidosis. There was no correlation between initial granulocyte count and clinical course; low lymphocyte counts were observed especially in those patients over 40 years of age, with negative tuberculin tests, and found to require corticosteroid treatment. Those with low initial lymphocyte count were especially liable to develop chronic disease. Those with initial erythema nodosum had high monocyte counts.

Pancytopenia: 'hypersplenism'

Like other forms of splenomegaly, splenic enlargement in sarcoidosis may be associated with low erythrocyte, granulocyte or thrombocyte counts in the peripheral blood; and, as noted above, the causal relationship may be confirmed if there is a clinical indication for splenectomy, which is usually followed by return of counts to normal. Millbourne (1950) reported the case of a 53 year old woman with anaemia, reticulocytosis, leucopenia and thrombocytopenia, hepatomegaly and splenomegaly; a spleen weighing 2100 g was removed; it and a lymph-node both contained discrete and confluent non-caseating tubercles; no other evidence of sarcoidosis was found, though the Mantoux test was negative to 1:100 OT; post-operatively the blood count became normal. Pancytopenia was found accompanying very large spleens in Case 2 of Hickling (1938), in the case described by Meira, Ferreira and Jamra (1949), in the four cases described by Kimbrell (1957), and in Case 13 of Ferguson and Paris (1958). Of the 32 patients with enlarged spleens reviewed by Kataria and Whitcomb (1980) seven, all of whom had very large spleens, showed such evidence of 'hypersplenism': three had pancytopenia, one anaemia and leukopenia, one leukopenia and thrombocytopenia, one anaemia and one thrombocytopenia.

Hess *et al.* (1971) reviewed 14 patients with 'dilutional anaemia of splenomegaly' in whom splenectomy was performed; in only one of these was sarcoidosis the cause of the splenomegaly.

Nilsson *et al.* (1978) reported a case of sarcoidosis with splenomegaly, anaemia and hypercalcaemia; anaemia remitted after splenomegaly, but hypercalcaemia persisted and required continued corticosteroid treatment. A man aged 25 presented with symptomless BHL, followed by pulmonary infiltration, the diagnosis of sarcoidosis being confirmed by mediastinoscopy and by a granulomatous response to a Kveim test. Four years later, he was found to have a moderately enlarged spleen, with a normochromic normocytic anaemia, without evidence of haemolysis, and hypercalcaemia. Removal of a 720 g spleen was followed by relief of the anaemia, but hypercalcaemia persisted; it was noted that the granulomas in the spleen showed some central necrosis, whereas those in the liver and abdominal lymph-nodes removed at splenectomy showed sclerosis, suggesting that the splenic granulomatosis was more recent and acute.

We have observed over many years the course of a patient with chronic sarcoidosis in whom increasing splenomegaly was associated with pancytopenia, which remitted after splenectomy, though granulomatous hepatitis remained active and became fibrotic.

A man aged 27 was found at a routine examination to have widespread mottling in a chest radiograph, maximal in the upper halves of the lungs. The skin gave no reaction to 100 IU. Kveim test, scalene node and liver biopsies were all negative. Cultures for tubercle bacilli were negative, but in view of the distribution of the radiographic shadowing, treatment with PAS and isoniazid, initially accompanied by streptomycin, was given for two years. He returned to work as a road patrolman, and remained symptom-free, with little change in radiographic appearance. After nine years, at the age of 36, he developed a cough, lost some weight, and was found to have a slightly elevated sedimentation rate. Bronchoscopy and bronchial mucosal biopsy showed no abnormality. Shortly after this, a superficial abscess appeared on the right forearm, just below the flexure of the elbow. It was incised, and biopsy of its wall showed granulomatous changes with some necrosis suggestive of tuberculosis; culture of the pus produced both *Staph. aureus* and, later, *M. tuberculosis*, sensitive to streptomycin, PAS and isoniazid. He was treated with isoniazid and PAS and the abscess healed. At this time the spleen was noted to be palpable. Over the next two years, he continued at work, but did not feel well; the spleen was observed to be increasing in size and the liver became palpable. At the age of 39, 12 years after the initial abnormal radiograph, he was fully investigated. The spleen was palpable 6 cm below the costal margin, and was very firm, and the liver 4 cm and soft. There was no change in the chest radiograph. The haemoglobin level was 12.0 g dl^{-1}, leucocytes 2000 and platelets 81 000 mm^{-3}; the bone marrow showed normal numbers of haemopoietic cells, but few mature. Urinary calcium excretion was elevated at 777 and 612 mg/day, and serum calcium on the high side at 10.6 mg 100 ml^{-1}. Transaminase and alkaline phosphatase levels were elevated. Needle biopsy of the liver showed some lymphocytic infiltration focally and in portal tracts. A tuberculin test with 100 IU gave a 10 mm reaction. A Kveim test gave a granulomatous response. Splenectomy was performed, the spleen being noted to be very large. Enlarged lymph-nodes were seen around the splenic pedicle and along the pancreas; the spleen, lymph-nodes and a sample of liver removed for biopsy all showed many sarcoid-type granulomas. After an initial excessive rise in platelet count, the cell-counts in peripheral blood returned to normal, and serum calcium was recorded at 9.4 mg 100 ml^{-1}. Two years after splenectomy, he had renal colic, with passage of two small stones, and the following year a spontaneous pneumothorax, which required pleurectomy to secure re-expansion. Hepatomegaly with elevated liver enzymes persisted, and four years after splenectomy, at the age of 45, he had haematemesis and melaena, with evidence of oesophageal varices and portal hypertension; at this time, liver biopsy showed hyalinization of many granulomas with surrounding inflammatory cell infiltration.

Thrombocytopenia and purpura

In most reported instances of the association of thrombocytopenic purpura with sarcoidosis, purpura has appeared in patients known to have sarcoidosis; in some, purpura has been the presenting feature, the diagnosis of sarcoidosis having been made in a few from the histology of tissues removed at splenectomy, or at necropsy; and in a very few cases, purpura has preceded the appearance of clinical evidence of sarcoidosis. Most of the early reports concerned either fatal cases, or patients treated by splenectomy.

Among the early reports is that of Jersild (1938) who described the case of a man with uveo-parotid fever and lung changes who also had thrombocytopenia, varying from 16 000–57 000 mm^{-3}, and purpura. Berblinger (1939) reported the case of a man, aged 35, who, having had iridocyclitis and fever five months previously, developed purpura and haematuria with almost completely absent platelets and died from cerebral haemorrhage; at necropsy 'atypical tuberculosis' was found in lymph-nodes, spleen, liver and lungs. The patient reported by Kraus (1942) with hypopituitarism due to sarcoidosis had been anaemic for ten years, had been known to have thrombocytopenia, and died of epistaxis; at necropsy the spleen weighed 500 g and contained many sarcoid nodules. Case 2 of Cattell and Wilson (1951) was that of a 19 year old man with splenomegaly and thrombocytopenia but no purpura; the spleen removed weighed 1460 g, and it and a piece of liver removed for biopsy were found to be infiltrated with sarcoid tubercles. Edwards *et al.* (1952) reported the case of a 15 year old white girl who had had iritis leading to impairment of vision for three years, a generalized lymphadenopathy, shown histologically to be sarcoid, hilar lymph-node enlargement, and a moderately enlarged spleen; she developed purpura with epistaxis, with no platelets visible in the peripheral blood, and died of a massive cerebral haemorrhage. At necropsy extensive sarcoidosis was found, involving the lymph-nodes, spleen, liver, kidneys, lungs and stomach, but the spleen was only slightly enlarged, weighing 210 g.

Before the introduction of corticosteroid treatment, splenectomy was the principal therapeutic procedure, and in most cases was found to lead to remission of symptoms, though the period of observation after operation in some was brief.

Nordland *et al.* (1946) described the case of a woman whose spleen was removed for thrombocytopenic purpura in the sixth month of pregnancy. She had had hilar node tuberculosis with later development of calcification in childhood; the Mantoux test was then recorded as positive, but when she was 24 it had become negative. At the age of 25, she first had multiple petechiae in the skin with a low platelet count. A year later, at the fifth month of pregancy, the purpura and low platelet count recurred, and in spite of transfusions, haematuria developed. The spleen removed weighed 275 g, and showed replacement of malpighian bodies by non-caseating epithelioid and giant-cell tubercles. There was no further purpura, and a normal delivery at term. Ribaudo *et al.* (1949, Case 2) reported a good symptomatic response to splenectomy in a woman, aged 23, who had had recurrent purpura for seven years. The platelet count was 110 000 mm^{-3} and the bone-marrow showed 'hyperplasia of megakaryocytes'. The spleen removed was slightly enlarged and histologically was infiltrated with sarcoid tubercles. Bruschi and Howe (1950) recorded the case of a man, aged 37, who had been ill for four years with nausea, vomiting, jaundice, anaemia, splenomegaly and miliary shadows in the chest radiograph, when he developed purpura, epistaxis and bleeding from the gums. The platelets numbered 36 000 mm^{-3}. After removal of a spleen weighing 680 g, he made a good recovery, and was well 15 months later. Both the spleen and an abdominal lymph-node showed sarcoidosis histologically. The case described by Kunkel and Yesner (1950) was that of a man, aged 55, who had had purpura for six weeks and suffered a subarachnoid haemorrhage. No platelets were seen in the peripheral blood, but many megakaryocytes in the marrow. The spleen, weighing 210 g, and several accessories were removed with disappearance of the purpura and return of the platelet count to normal. The skin failed to react to 250 TU of PPD. A chest radiograph was said to show changes consistent with diffuse sarcoidosis. The spleen removed showed rounded sub-capsular nodules, and histologically epithelioid cell granulomas of varied size; no granulomas were seen in a liver biopsy. Case 1 of Cattell and Wilson (1951) was that of a ten year old girl who had had purpura for several years. A platelet count was 58 000 mm^{-3}. Removal of a spleen, weighing 135 g, and infiltrated with sarcoid-type tubercles, was followed by remission. Ehrlich and Schwartz (1951) in a discussion of 110 cases of thrombocytopenic purpura mentioned one in a girl aged 16, which appears to have been described previously by Schwartz (1945). She had had purpura and menorrhagia for one month. She had a large spleen, a low platelet count (15 000 mm^{-3}) and anaemia (haemoglobin 6 g dl^{-1}); diffuse shadows were seen in a chest radiograph. The spleen, weighing 507 g and infiltrated with sarcoid nodules up to 0.4 cm in diameter, was removed. In spite of a prompt rise of platelet count, she developed a subarachnoid haemorrhage four days after the operation, from which she nevertheless made a good recovery. Wright *et al.* (1951) referred briefly to the case of a boy aged four years, in whom a spleen removed for thrombocytopenic purpura and a specimen of liver removed at the same time for biopsy both showed evidence of sarcoidosis. Elliott and Turner (1951) reviewed splenectomy for purpura haemorrhagica; of ten cases associated with systemic diseases, three, all in young women, showed histological changes interpreted as sarcoidosis in the spleen, though no evidence of sarcoidosis was found elsewhere; all improved after splenectomy. The case described by Klein and Lehotan (1952) was that of a woman, aged 33, who developed severe purpura with a platelet count of 4000; a large hard spleen with many accessory spleens was removed and showed miliary tubercles without caseation or acid-fast bacilli; the Mantoux test was negative to 1:500 OT; radiographic changes were found in the lungs and in a metacarpal bone; and splenectomy was followed by remission of the purpura and rise in platelet count. Schrijver and Schillings (1952) reported the case of a girl, aged 16, with bleeding from the gums, purpura, no platelets detectable in the blood and bilateral hilar lymph-node enlargement; after initial treatment with blood transfusion and corticotrophin, a spleen weighing 95 g and densely infiltrated with epithelioid cell granulomas was removed, with remission of the purpura.

Treatment with corticosteroids has generally been reported to lead to improvement or remission of thrombocytopenia, though in some cases the follow-up period has been brief. In a few cases, response to corticosteroids has been unsatisfactory, and in some of these, splenectomy has been followed by remission.

Dickerman *et al.* (1972) reported two cases, both in black boys: the first was aged 13 when he presented with purpura, and was found to have enlarged cervical and axillary lymph-nodes, a spleen palpable 2 cm below the costal margin, a platelet count of 7000 mm^{-3}, many young megakaryocytes in the bone marrow, and sarcoid-type granulomas in a cervical lymph-node removed for biopsy. There was a prompt response to treatment with prednisone, platelets rising to 164 000 mm^{-3}; a year later the platelet count remained normal, but active bilateral uveitis had appeared. The second had been known to be suffering from sarcoidosis involving liver and lungs since the age of 11 years: when he was aged 14 the cessation of prednisone treatment was followed by uveitis and after three months by purpura, epistaxis and haematuria. There was hepatosplenomegaly, and platelets were much reduced. The platelet count rose and bleeding ceased on treatment with platelet infusions and methylprednisone, and was maintained during a follow-up period of two months. In the case described by Semple (1975) thrombocytopenic purpura and haemolytic anaemia, both responding to prednisolone, preceded the appearance of clinical evidence of sarcoidosis by a year. A man aged 25 presented with thrombocytopenic purpura, responding to prednisolone; seven weeks later, he was found to have a Coombs test positive haemolytic anaemia, with haemoglobin 10.3 g dl^{-1} and reticulocyte count of 19%. This also responded to prednisolone, which was discontinued without relapse. One year later, a soft tissue swelling over the left shoulder showed sarcoid-type granulomas on biopsy, a Mantoux test with 100 IU was negative, a Kveim test gave a granulomatous response, and a chest radiograph showed BHL. Eighteen months later, uveitis and enlargement of the parotid glands and of a cervical lymph-node appeared, with no recurrence of either thrombocytopenia or anaemia. Kremer *et al.* (1975) reported the case of a man aged 17 who presented with purpura, with a platelet count of 41 000, falling to 1200 mm^{-3}. BHL was found radiographically, and a lymphangiogram showed enlarged intra-abdominal lymph-nodes. The bone-marrow contained a 'high normal' number of megakaryocytes. Treatment with fluocortolone 90 mg daily, was followed by gradual improvement, the platelet count reaching 150 000 mm^{-3} by the 19th day. At this time, mediastinoscopy was performed, and a lymph-node removed showed sarcoid-type tubercles. Winter (1976) described briefly the case of a man who at the age of 23 presented with thrombocytopepic purpura responding to corticosteroid treatment; two years later recurrent bleeding led to splenectomy which was followed by remission, maintained during eight years' observation; the spleen showed histological changes of sarcoidosis. A clinico-pathological conference in 1978 (Case 39–1978), discussed the case of a woman aged 24 who presented with purpura and a platelet count of 6000 mm^{-3}. BHL was demonstrated radiographically. The bone-marrow showed plentiful megakaryocytes. Prednisone at a maximal dose of 100 mg/day led to gradual increase in numbers of platelets, reaching 475 000 on the 23rd day, and relief of purpura. A mediastinal lymph-node removed by mediastinoscopy showed the histology of sarcoidosis. Two months later, the platelet-count remained high, at 400 000 mm^{-3}. A maternal aunt and cousin of this patient had sarcoidosis.

Thrombocytopenic purpura in patients with sarcoidosis may be rapidly fatal, and may fail to respond to corticosteroids or splenectomy.

Otero *et al.* (1967) described the case of a woman aged 30 who presented with purpura and menorrhagia, with splenomegaly and enlarged superficial lymphnodes. She died of massive gastro-intestinal haemorrhage; generalized sarcoidosis was found at necropsy. Knodel and Bechman (1980) reported a case of thrombocytopenic purpura in a woman aged 23 which failed to respond to platelet infusions and dexamethasone. At necropsy, the immediate cause of death was found to be massive cerebral haemorrhage; epithelioid cell granulomas were found in the much enlarged spleen and in liver, lung, pleura and lymph-nodes, some of those in the lung showing central necrosis.

We have observed four patients with sarcoidosis in whom thrombocytopenia remitted after removal of infiltrated spleens. In the first three, purpura developed 2–6 years after the first clinical evidence of sarcoidosis. In the third, abdominal discomfort due to the very large spleen was an additional indication for surgery. In the fourth case, splenomegaly later found to be associated with thrombocytopenia was the first clinical feature, the diagnosis of sarcoidosis being established only after splenectomy; and persistent granulomatous and chronic inflammatory changes in the liver gave rise to a differential diagnostic problem (see Chapter 11, p. 271).

(1)   A woman aged 23 was found to have a widespread pulmonary infiltration, with a tuberculin test positive to 10 IU, negative cultures for tubercle bacilli, and a palpable supraclavicular lymph-node biopsy of which showed non-caseating epithelioid cell tubercles. Antimycobacterial chemotherapy had no effect on the infiltration, but prednisolone 20 mg daily led to slow resolution, which was maintained when it was reduced to 7.5 mg. After nearly two years, prednisolone was gradually withdrawn. Three months later, purpura appeared on the lower limbs, the shoulders and the buccal mucosa, the platelet count was reduced to 41 000 mm^{-3}, and the bone-marrow was found to contain many immature megakaryocytes. The spleen, weighing 400 g, was removed it was studded with pale nodules, which histologically consisted of epithelioid and giant-cell tubercles, many with central hyalinization. There were enlarged lymph-nodes along the lesser curve of the stomach and in the porta hepatis, and the liver was enlarged; biopsy of one of the nodes and of the liver showed widespread sarcoid-type tubercles but without hyalinization. The post-operative course was uneventful, and the patient became symptom-free, with normal platelet count. Shortly afterwards, small skin infiltrations, confirmed histologically to be sarcoids, appeared and slowly increased in size, and the pulmonary infiltration became denser. Two years after the splenectomy, prednisolone treatment was re-instituted. There was no recurrence of the thrombocytopenia. Nearly three years later, a pregnancy ended in still-birth at the 8th month; three months after this she died, at the age of 31, apparently of pulmonary thrombo-embolic disease, not directly related to sarcoidosis. There was no necropsy.

(2)   A woman aged 26 was found to have symptomless BHL; scalene node biopsy showed sarcoid-type tubercles. Over the next few years, BHL slowly subsided and widespread mottled shadows appeared in the lungs, without symptoms. When she was aged 31, the platelet count was found to be low, ranging between 28 000 and 48 000 mm^{-3}, the blood count being otherwise normal, but it was not until two years later that she first noticed spontaneous bruising. The spleen-tip was just palpable on deep inspiration. The platelet count was between 20 000 and 41 000 mm^{-3}, the only other abnormality in the blood count being a leucocyte count between 3000 and 5000 with a relative lymphopenia. The bone-marrow showed many immature megakaryocytes and the half-life of radio-labelled platelets was reduced to 30 min (normal 5–7 days). In spite of the widespread radiographic mottling, tests of lung ventilatory function and gas transfer were within normal limits. The spleen was removed. It was about twice normal size and contained clusters of yellowish nodules up to 2 mm in diameter, as well as Malpighian follicles 1mm in diameter; the nodules consisted of well-defined epithelioid granulomas with a few giant cells, many showing fibrosis and a few central fibrinoid

necrosis. The post-operative course was uneventful, with a rise in platelets to a maximum of 706 000 mm^{-3}, which settled to and remained at normal levels. The pulmonary infiltration slowly cleared. Seven years after splenectomy, she remained free from further manifestations of sarcoidosis.

(3)   A man aged 44 was found at a routine examination to have slight BHL and light mottling in the lung-fields. The tuberculin test was negative. Although he was symptom-free, he was treated at various times with prednisolone, hydroxychloroquine and oxyphenbutazone. Six years later, when he was receiving 5 mg prednisolone daily, spontaneous bruising appeared and the platelet count was found to range between 54 000 and 90 000 mm^{-3}. The bruising ceased spontaneously, but splenomegaly was noted for the first time, and a Kveim test gave a granulomatous response; slight hypercalciuria was found. A year later, now aged 61, he complained of nausea and upper abdominal discomfort. The spleen was found to be further enlarged, firm and non-tender, about 8 cm below the costal margin. The liver was palpable 2 cm below the costal margin. The platelet count was 78 000 mm^{-3}, the blood count showing no other abnormality. The bone-marrow was normal; a platelet survival test showed destruction in the spleen. The serum calcium level was normal, and urinary calcium excretion between 260 and 320 mg daily, with normal creatinine clearance. Chest radiography showed fine not very dense mottling, little changed over the previous few years. A tuberculin test with 100 IU was negative. Liver enzyme levels were normal. In view of the thrombocytopenia with platelet destruction in the spleen, and the possibility that the splenomegaly might be at least in part responsible for the abdominal pain and nausea, splenectomy was performed. The spleen was very large and contained many sarcoid-type tubercles; a sample of liver and an abdominal lymph-node contained similar tubercles. Post-operatively, the platelet count rose to 600 000 mm^{-3} and then settled and remained at normal levels. Followed for five years after the splenectomy, he has shown no further manifestations of sarcoidosis; slight middle zone fibrosis has developed in the lungs without disability.

(4)   Splenomegaly was noted in a woman aged 23 during a pregnancy. Three years later, the spleen was palpable to the umbilicus and firm, and the liver 2 cm below the costal margin. Platelets ranged between 96 000 and 128 000 mm^{-3}. Leucocytes numbered 2300 mm^{-3}, of which only 16% were lymphocytes, and the haemoglobin was 11.2 g dl. The chest radiograph was normal. Lymphangiography showed enlarged para-aortic nodes. The Heaf tuberculin test was negative. A Kveim test was negative. The spleen, weighing 990 g, was removed, together with a lymph-node and a biopsy sample of liver. These all showed many epithelioid and giant-cell granulomas, with slight central necrosis in places; the liver also showed lymphocytic infiltration of portal tracts with widening and distortion of interlobular pattern. Post-operative course was uneventful, the platelet count after an initial rise to 498 000 returning to normal levels. Followed eight years after the splenectomy, she has remained free from further manifestations of sarcoidosis, or symptoms referable to liver disease; but the liver remained palpable, and for several years liver enzyme levels were variably and slightly raised. Serial liver biopsies up to five years after the splenectomy continued to show inflammatory cell infiltrations of portal tracts with some focal collections of lymphocytes, epithelioid cells and occasional giant cells. This gave rise to suspicion of primary biliary cirrhosis,

but there was no evidence of developing cirrhosis, tests for antimitochondrial and other auto-antibodies were negative, and enzyme levels eventually became normal.

Death from haemorrhage after splenectomy was reported by Enzer (1946).

His case was that of a 32 year old man who had had purpura, anaemia, thrombocytopenia and leucopenia for eight months; there were radiographic changes in the lungs and a negative tuberculin test; at necropsy the lungs and lymph-nodes but not the bone-marrow were infiltrated with sarcoid granulomas as was the removed spleen.

Haemorrhagic tendency not shown to be related to thrombocytopenia has been recorded by several authors.

Of the 22 necropsy cases reported by Ricker and Clark (1949), one had had severe epistaxis and died with subarachnoid haemorrhage; there was extensive sarcoidosis and petechiae in all organs. In Case 1 of Ribaudo *et al.* (1949), the single platelet count recorded was 570 000 mm^{-3}, but the clinical picture was that of severe purpura; the patient was an 18 year old black man with recent purpura and bilateral hilar lymph-node enlargement who died of cerebral haemorrhage; at necropsy the spleen was of normal size, but it, the lungs, the lymph-nodes and the myocardium were infiltrated with sarcoid granulomas. Case 2 of Engelbreth-Holm (1938), reported as tuberculous splenomegaly, was that of a 44 year old woman who had had several episodes of jaundice, purpura, haematemesis, anaemia and ascites; a spleen 30 cm long and infiltrated with non-caseating tubercles was removed, with remission of symptoms. Blum and Mitchell (1952) recorded the case of a man, aged 50, who had had enlarged cervical and hilar lymph-node enlargement, and splenomegaly for several months, and died with persistent gastro-intestinal bleeding for which no source was found at laparotomy or at necropsy; extensive sarcoidosis was found in the lungs, spleen, liver and lymph-nodes.

In general, in the treatment of thrombocytopenia and purpura in patients with sarcoidosis, corticosteroids lead to improvement in most, and to remission in some, cases; splenectomy nearly always leads to permanent remission of the thrombocytopenia, though it has no effect on the evolution of the other manifestations of sarcoidosis, especially in the liver.

Haemolytic anaemia

Although fewer cases of haemolytic anaemia than of thrombocytopenia have been reported in patients with sarcoidosis, the number is sufficient to suggest that it occurs rather more frequently than would be expected by chance. The relative importance of factors concerned in the pathogenesis of haemolytic anaemia and of the immunological abnormalities of sarcoidosis remains a matter for speculation. The Coombs test in cases in which it has been reported has been found positive in most, though negative in a few. Response to treatment has been variable. Corticosteroid treatment has led to improvement in some cases, in a few amounting to remission, though the folow-up in many has been brief; but a few have shown no response. Similarly, splenectomy may or may not be followed by remission; and haemolytic anaemia has appeared after removal of the spleen for pancytopenia or thrombocytopenia (Lebacq *et al.*, 1956b; Thudani *et al.*, 1975).

Case 4 of Englebreth-Holm (1938), reported as tuberculous splenomegaly, was that of a 57 year old woman who had anaemia with a haemoglobin concentration of 45%, and a reticulocytosis of 26%; she died after removal of a spleen weighing 400 g, which was infiltrated with non-caseating tubercles, as was the liver. Stats *et al.* (1947, Case 1) described the case of a black girl who had long-standing haemolytic anaemia, with a haemoglobin of 43% and reticulocytosis of 15%, without sickling, spherocytosis or abnormal fragility of erythrocytes; iridocyclitis, generalized lymphadenopathy, and splenomegaly; a lymph-node biopsy showed sarcoid changes and the Mantoux test was negative. Bruschi and Howe (1950) referred briefly to the case of a black woman, aged 45, who had severe haemolytic anaemia; a spleen weighing 500 g was removed, and showed sarcoid changes with many giant cells, as did the liver and a lymph-node removed for biopsy. Improvement was said to have followed the splenectomy. Schubothe (1952) mentioned the case of a 12 year old boy known to have pulmonary sarcoidosis for several years who developed Coombs test positive haemolytic anaemia remitting after corticosteroid treatment. Davis *et al.* (1954) recorded the case of a black man, aged 34, who had been known to have an abnormal chest radiograph for two years, and presented with a haemolytic anaemia (haemoglobin 6.3 g 100 ml^{-1}, reticulocytes 25%, iron turn-over five times normal) and fever; a cervical lymph-node biopsy showed sarcoid changes; after a temporary response to cortisone, a spleen wieghing 450 g with three accessory spleens was removed; the spleen showed grey nodules 3 mm in diameter with sarcoid histology; only temporary improvement was observed after splenectomy, and further cortisone treatment was required. Lebacq *et al.* (1956) described the case of a woman aged 23, whose sister had died after removal of a granulomatous spleen, no other details being available. She presented with anaemia, leucopenia and splenomegaly; on a diagnosis of Banti's syndrome, the spleen weighing 1100 g was removed, and was found to contain many large nodules of epithelioid and giant cell granulomas. The anaemia improved after the operation. Six months later, anaemia recurred with jaundice, and was found to be of haemolytic type with positive direct Coombs test. Treatment with corticotrophin followed by hydrocortisone led to improvement. Biopsies of an enlarged lacrimal gland and of a pre-auricular lymph-node showed sarcoid changes. A relapse of haemolytic anaemia, haemoglobin falling to 32%, responded to transfusion and further corticotrophin treatment. Six months later she died, apparently of a generalized infection on a visit abroad. Michon *et al.* (1957) reported a coal-miner aged 52 who presented with Coombs test positive haemolytic anaemia with warm haemagglutinins; he had enlargement of hilar and paratracheal lymph-nodes radiographically, and palpable supraclavicular nodes, biopsy of which showed sarcoid-type granulomas. The anaemia improved on corticosteroid treatment, relapsed when it was withdrawn, and improved again when it was re-instituted. Johansson (1958) reported the case of a 53 year old woman with severe haemolytic anaemia, Coombs test positive, and BHL with pulmonary infiltration, in whom haemolysis persisted in spite of both corticosteroid treatment and splenectomy and led to death. The patient described by Garcia *et al.* (1959) was a man aged 31 who had had generalized lymphadenopathy with the histology of sarcoidosis for three years. He developed haemolytic anaemia, haemoglobin 76%, reticulocytes 23%, and hypercalcaemia. Removal of the spleen, weighing 430 g and containing sarcoid granulomas was followed by remission of haemolysis. The case reported by West (1959) was that of a 32 year old woman with a six week history of weakness, dyspnoea and, later, jaundice; the anaemia was of haemolytic type with a negative Coombs test (haemoglobin 6 g, bilirubin 2.9 mg 100 ml^{-1}, reticulocytes 29.8%); biopsy of an enlarged paratracheal lymph-node removed by thoracotomy showed sarcoid changes; the spleen, weighing 530 g, was removed and it and the liver also showed histological evidence of sarcoidosis; some improvement was observed during seven months' observation after splenectomy. Wyss *et al.* (1967) reported the case of a man aged 35 who had been known to have sarcoidosis involving hilar nodes and lungs for five years, when he developed haemolytic anaemia, the haemoglobin falling to 48%; direct Coombs test was negative; the spleen was enlarged. Removal of the spleen weighing 630 g and containing many granulomas, was followed by remission of the anaemia during five months of further observation: liver biopsy showed no granulomas. Thudani *et al.* (1975) reported the case of a man aged 53 who presented with hepato-splenomegaly and pancytopenia; the spleen weighing 1250 g was removed and showed replacement of Malpighian corpuscles by groups of epithelioid cells and some pulp fibrosis, and liver biopsy showed many sarcoid-type granulomas, The haemoglobin and blood-count stabilized at normal levels after the operation. A Kveim test was negative. One year later, he developed Coombs test positive haemolytic anaemia, and died in an acute haemolytic crisis before treatment could be started. At necropsy, granulomas were found in liver, kidneys and bone-marrow. The patient described by Semple (1975) in whom thrombocytopenia, followed by haemolytic anaemia, both responding to corticosteroid treatment, preceded the appearance of overt sarcoidosis, has been mentioned above (p. 283).

In some reported cases, it seems likely that sarcoidosis and haemolytic anaemia though occurring in the same patient were pathogenetically unrelated.

In several, the spleen removed for haemolytic anaemia in patients with sarcoidosis has been found to show no specific changes.

Crane and Zetlin (1945) reported the case of a woman, aged 46, from whom a spleen weighing 485 g and showing no tuberculoid granulomas was removed for haemolytic anaemia, with only temporary improvement; two months later, the anaemia recurred with fever and in spite of repeated transfusions the patient died. At necropsy, the lymph-nodes and the sternal marrow showed multiple small epithelioid cell granulomata with a few giant cells; there were foci of erythropoiesis in the lungs, kidneys, liver and lymph-nodes; but the lungs and liver were not invaded by the granulomas. McCort *et al.* (1947) described the case of a 58 year old man who had been known for two years to have enlarged mediastinal lymph-nodes, reported on biopsy to show 'tuberculoma', when he was found to have a haemolytic anaemia and splenomegaly; the spleen removed showed no sarcoid lesions. Eight months later the hilar lymph-nodes were larger and radiographs of the hands showed 'cysts' in the bones of the finger. Cox and Donald (1964) described the case of a man aged 29, who had been known to have sarcoidosis involving superficial lymph-nodes since the age of 14, with pulmonary infiltration, and developed Coombs test negative haemolytic anaemia, which failed to respond to corticosteroid treatment: the spleen weighing 1200 g and stated not to show sarcoid changes was removed, but haemolysis continued.

Palazzo *et al.* (1972) described the case of a woman who at the age of 41 developed haemolytic anaemia with a high cold agglutinin titre; three and a half years later she was found to have BHL with sarcoid-type granulomas in a bronchial mucosal biopsy and a positive Kveim test, which subsided without treatment, some pulmonary infiltration appearing. In this case, it seems unlikely the cold-agglutinin disease and the sarcoidosis were pathogenetically related.

Chapter 13

The Upper Respiratory Tract

As early as 1905, Boeck recorded infiltration of the nasal mucosa in a case of multiple benign sarcoid, and in 1908 Kreibich and Kraus described a case of sarcoids of the skin of the nose and forehead with nasal symptoms, due to thickening of the mucosa, though the mucosa was not examined histologically. Schaumann in 1914 reported that in two out of three cases of lupus pernio the tonsils showed specific histological changes. Subsequently many reports of changes in the upper respiratory tract (URT) have appeared, but relatively few studies of their incidence in unselected series of cases of sarcoidosis presenting in other ways.

Incidence

The great variation in reported incidence of URT involvement, as of other manifestations in a specialist field of interest, is probably determined in large part by selection. Barmwater (1936) stated that among 42 patients studied at the Finsen Institute, Copenhagen, 13 had mucosal lesions of the URT, and of these only two had no skin lesions. Gravesen (1942) in a series of 112 cases collected from a number of Danish hospitals, and apparently including at least some of those reported by Barmwater, found that the URT was involved in 39, of whom 32 had skin changes, most of them including the face; among the 39, the nasal mucosa was involved in 37, the mouth and pharynx in 14 and the larynx and trachea in six. The very high incidence is probably related to the high proportion of patients with florid generalized sarcoidosis in these series. Even in a series such as that of Reisner (1944) including a high proportion of North American blacks, a group especially liable to florid forms of sarcoidosis, the incidence was lower; in a series of 35 patients in New York, of whom 30 were black, he reported that two showed involvement of nasal mucosa, confirmed by biopsy in one, and two extensive infiltration of the larynx, epiglottis and pharynx. Kämpfer (1964) studied 277 patients with sarcoidosis, and found evidence of granulomatous changes in nasal mucosa in nine, in the lingual tonsil in one, and in the larynx in one. Neville *et al.* (1976) submitted 100 successive patients attending a sarcoidosis clinic to special studies for evidence of URT involvement, and found such evidence in six, of whom three had lupus pernio. Selroos and Niemistö (1977) found a comparable incidence of URT involvement, but no special association with skin changes. In a study of 192 patients with sarcoidosis, they found that 14 had nasal symptoms, and 11 of these had granulomas in nasal mucosa; only one patient, with florid nasal polypoid granulomatous changes had skin sarcoids, and these were maculo-papular and not of the lupus pernio type.

Among reported cases of URT sarcoidosis, the nasal mucosa, especially of the inferior turbinates and adjacent part of the septum is the most frequently involved site, the nasal sinuses, pharynx, soft palate, epiglottis and larynx being less frequently involved. In studies of unselected cases of sarcoidosis, the nasal mucosa is by far the most frequent site within the URT to be affected: of the 11 with nasal granulomas found by Selroos and Niemistö (1977) in their survey of 192 consecutive patients, none had changes elsewhere in the URT. On the other hand, studies of patients selected because they have URT sarcoidosis tend to include a high proportion with extensive involvement. Lindsay and Perlman (1951) reported nine cases, all with nasal mucosal changes, with involvement also of the nasopharynx in two, the pharynx in three, the epiglottis in four, the glottis in one, and the trachea in three; McKelvie *et al.* (1968) reported 14, the nose being involved in 11 and the larynx in five, both being involved in two; and of the 17 reported by Neville *et al.* (1976), all with nasal mucosal granulomas, five also had laryngeal involvement. Nevertheless, for convenience the principal sites of involvement will be considered separately.

The nose

We have reviewed 116 recorded cases of generalized sarcoidosis in which granulomas were found clinically in the nasal cavities and histologically confirmed (Ulrich, 1918; Allison and Mikell, 1932; Novy, 1936; Kistner and Robertson, 1938; Seifert, 1939; Poe, 1940 a and b, 1942, the same case being reported later by Poe and Seager, 1950; Bordley and Proctor, 1942; Wille, 1946; Rubin and Kling, 1948; Robinson and Pound, 1950, Case 13; Larsson, 1951, Cases 7, 8, 9 and 10; Lindsay and Perlman, 1951, nine cases; Livingstone, 1956; Ferguson and Paris, 1958, Case 5; Weiss, 1960, three cases; Creston and Dibble, 1961; Arova, 1963; Siltzbach and Blaugrund, 1963, six cases; Kämpfer, 1964, ten cases; Dowie, 1964, three cases;

Black, 1966; Scadding, 1967, three cases; McKelvie *et al.*, 1968, 11 cases; Page and Seth, 1969; Di Benedetto and Lefrak, 1970; Carosso, 1974; Wright *et al.*, 1974, two cases; Gordon *et al.*, 1976, three cases; Kirschner *et al.*, 1976; Neville *et al.*, 1976, 17 cases; Delaney, 1977, Case 1; Selroos and Niemistö, 1977, 11 cases; Maillard and Goepfert, 1978; Allen, 1979; Som and Krespi, 1979; Coup and Hopper, 1980; Hammond and Kataria, 1980). Of the cases in which the sex of the patient was mentioned, 73 were in women and 25 in men; the excess of women is much greater than the usual slight excess of women in large unselected series of cases of sarcoidosis, and suggests that involvement of the URT is relatively more frequent in women. Forty-two were stated to be in blacks, of whom 28 were women. Although Selroos and Niemistö (1977) found skin sarcoids in only one of the 11 cases of nasal involvement they found in their survey of 192 consecutive patients with sarcoidosis, others have commented on the frequency of association between nasal mucosal involvement and skin sarcoids, especially of the lupus pernio type. Thus, Neville *et al.* (1976), reviewing the records of a sarcoidosis clinic, found 34 patients with involvement of the URT and/or the skin of the nose, 26 having skin changes of lupus pernio type and 17 URT sarcoidosis, these features co-existing in nine; of six who presented with nasal mucosal changes, six later developed lupus pernio. Of six patients with nasal mucosal granulomas reported by Siltzbach and Blaugrund (1963) all had skin sarcoids, the skin near the nostrils being involved in four. It is probable that involvement of the vestibule of the nose and of the nasal mucosa occurs in many cases of lupus pernio involving the nose, but has not been specifically recorded because not thought remarkable. In view of the association between persistent skin infiltrations and changes in the bones of the hands and feet (Chapters 7 and 9), it is not surprising that such changes have been found in a proportion of cases of URT sarcoidosis. Neville *et al.* (1976) found them in two of eight patients with involvement of the URT without lupus pernio, and in three of nine with lupus pernio.

The symptoms of nasal sarcoidosis are those to be expected from thickening of the mucosa, sometimes with polyp formation (Lindsay and Perlman, 1951; McKelvie *et al.*, 1968; Neville *et al.*, 1976). The most frequent symptom is nasal obstruction; other common symptoms include nasal discharge and crusting, and epistaxis or blood-staining of the discharge may occur. The most frequent finding on examination is thickening of the mucosa, sometimes extensive, but tending to affect predominantly the inferior turbinates and the adjacent part of the septum. Minute yellowish nodules may be visible in or under the mucosal surface, which may be obscured by pus or muco-pus with or without crusting. Polypoidal granulomatous masses may develop, and may be large (Selroos and Niemistö, 1977). Perforation of the septum may occur. In several cases, it has been reported after surgical procedures, notably submucous resection of the septum (Allison and Mikell, 1932; Neville *et al.* 1976, two cases; Hammond and Kataria, 1980). In a few cases, surgical procedures on the septum, with or without inferior turbinectomy, have been undertaken for relief of obstruction without this complication (Wright *et al.*, 1974; Maillard and Goepfert, 1978); and perforation may occur in patients treated conservatively (Barmwater, 1936; Neville *et al.*, 1976, one case). Association with lupus pernio and with infiltration of the vestibule of the nose and the adjacent upper lip and nostril has already been noted. The bridge of the nose may be swollen, without evident involvement of the skin (Dowie, 1964, Case 2; Black, 1966; McKelvie *et al.*, 1968, Case 19). Rarefaction of nasal bones may be evident radiologically (Curtis, 1964; Neville *et al.*, 1976). Collapse of the bridge of the nose from destruction of cartilage and bone has been reported (Di Benedetto and Lefrak, 1970; Allen, 1979).

In their survey of nasal involvement in a series of patients with sarcoidosis, Selroos and Niemistö (1977) found three with symptoms and an abnormal-looking mucosa but no granulomas on mucosal biopsy. In view of the frequency of non-specific nasal symptoms, this is hardly surprising. Symptomless sarcoid infiltration of the nasal mucosa appears to be rare. Random biopsies from the inferior turbinates in patients with sarcoidosis without symptom or sign of nasal involvement showed granulomas in only one of six cases reported by Weiss (1960) and in none of seven by Siltzbach and Blaugrund (1963).

Nasal sinuses

The diagnosis of sarcoidosis involving nasal sinuses may be suggested by radiographs showing thickening of their mucosal lining in patients known to have granulomatous infiltration of nasal mucosa (Lindsay and Perlman, 1951, in three of nine cases; Gordon *et al.*, 1976, Case 2), and occasionally, polypoid granulomatous masses may be seen protruding from antral openings (Lindsay and Perlman, 1951). Loss of transradiancy of the antra with negative proof puncture in such patients has also been accepted as evidence of antral involvement (Dowie, 1964). Histological confirmation of granulomatous infiltration of the mucosa lining nasal sinuses has been obtained from tissue removed at antrostomy or ethmoidectomy (Bordley and Proctor, 1942; Robinson and Pound, 1950; Livingstone 1956; Page and Seth, 1969; Maillard *et al.* 1978). In a case of massive sarcoid infiltration of the orbit causing exophthalmos, recorded by Rider and Dodson (1950) and mentioned in Chapter 8, the maxillary antra were also involved.

Two patients whom we have had under prolonged observation illustrate the frequent association of sarcoidosis of the nasal mucosa with sarcoids of the skin, especially of the nose, and its variable but sometimes prolonged course.

The first is a West Indian, aged 40, who first noticed a nodule in the left nostril and several small superficial nodules on the upper lip (Chapter 7, Fig. 7.16). Biopsy of the nodule in the nasal vestibule showed infiltration with an epithelioid cell granuloma. There was a generalized slight enlargement of superficial lymph-nodes and the spleen was palpable. The chest radiograph showed faint mottling in the middle zones of the right lung, with slight hilar enlargement. The Mantoux test was negative to 1:100 OT. Under treatment with cortisone, all the manifestations subsided, and did not recur when it was withdrawn after only four weeks. Last seen six years later, he remained free from evidence of disease.

The second is a woman who at the age of 36 first developed scattered nodular sarcoids of the skin, eventually involving the legs, the buttocks, the upper arms and the forehead, scars on the knees also being infiltrated. Biopsy of a skin lesion confirmed the diagnosis. There was scattered irregular infiltration of the lungs radiographically. Three years from the onset, she developed gradually increasing nasal obstruction with mucoid discharge. At the age of 43, she was found to have thickening and granularity of the mucosa over the middle turbinate, which on biopsy showed typical non-caseating epithelioid cell tubercles. The antra were opaque, but puncture produced nothing, and it was inferred that the mucosa was probably thickened by the sarcoid granuloma. Treatment with prednisolone, starting with 30 mg daily led to rapid improvement in the skin sarcoids, and relief of nasal obstruction. Under observation for a further 14 years, she has continued to require prednisolone in variable dosage to control activity of sarcoidosis, manifested mainly in the skin. Nasal obstruction has not recurred, and the lungs have shown gradual development of typical fibrotic changes, now non-progressive, and with mild to moderate functional deficit.

Olfactory disorders

Changes in the olfactory nerves and their connections are the most frequent causes of disorder of the sense of smell in sarcoidosis, and are considered in Chapter 14. Delaney *et al.* (1977) reported five cases with disorders of taste or smell; in one of these, with granulomatous nasal and laryngeal changes and no evidence of involvement of the nervous system, decrease in ability to detect or recognize vapours at the primary olfactory area was attributed to nasal sarcoidosis.

Nasopharynx

In several of the reported cases of nasal mucosal sarcoidosis, the nasopharynx has been noted to be involved. Larsson (1951) reported ten cases of generalized sarcoidosis in which enlargement of the lymphadenoid tissue in the nasopharynx gave rise to masses detectable radiologically as polypoid soft tissue shadows and proved by biopsy to be due to sarcoid infiltration. Four of these also had nasal mucosal infiltrations. In six, the nasopharyngeal mass simulated hypertrophy of the normal lymphadenoid tissue, in one it affected principally the right side, in one it was ulcerated, and in one it presented as a lobulated tumour, obstructing the Eustachian tube in one. Fishman and Canalis (1979) reported the case of a black woman aged 26, complaining of hearing loss, in whom this was found to be due to serous otitis media caused by obstruction of the Eustachian tubes by a smooth mass in the vault of the nasopharynx; this on biopsy showed non-caseating granulomas, and gallium scans showed increased uptake in lungs and parotid glands, though the chest radiograph was normal; and serum angiotensin-converting enzyme levels were high. These findings, together with a good response to small doses of prednisone, made the diagnosis of sarcoidosis probable.

Tonsils

Schaumann in his 1914 paper drew attention to the presence of sarcoid tubercles in apparently normal tonsils, and in 1936 he stated that in all of 21 active cases of sarcoidosis in which tonsils had been removed for biopsy, specific changes were found. Gravesen (1942) found infiltration of the tonsils in 64% of 70 cases. Others have found a considerably lower incidence. Weiss (1960) reported that of five patients with proved sarcoid lesions elsewhere, biopsy of apparently unaffected tonsils showed specific changes in only one, while of a total of 22 tonsillar biopsies in known or suspected cases of sarcoidosis, only two were positive. Reisner (1944) examined the tonsils in two established cases, and found specific histological changes in one. Barmwater (1936) reported that in some cases in which he took small biopsies from both tonsils, he found changes in one but not in the other. It is not surprising that there are few reports of large series of routine removals of tonsils for biopsy; most of the references are to no more than a few incidental findings. Larsson (1951) obtained positive biopsies from tonsils in ten cases with other nasopharyngeal lesions. Macroscopically evident abnormalities of the tonsils have very rarely been recorded. Barmwater (1936) mentioned one case in which nodules were visible in the upper poles of the tonsils. Lindsay and Perlman (1951) refer to one case in which there was a granuloma of the left tonsil, and Siltzbach and Blaugrund (1963) described the tonsils in two cases in which they were found histologically to be infiltrated with sarcoid tubercles as 'large, pale and cryptic'.

Palate

Localized sarcoid infiltration of the palate was an incidental finding in two young women with skin sarcoids and extensive involvement of the upper respiratory tract reported by Ulrich (1918). Infiltration of either the hard or the soft palate, generally without symptoms and not ulcerated, has been reported also in association with other upper respiratory tract localizations of sarcoidosis by Barmwater (1936, two cases), Poe (1942), Weiss (1960, Cases 1, 4, 8 and 9), Creston and Dibble (1961), Carasso (1974) and Kirschner and Holinger (1976). In a case of very extensive and chronic nasal sarcoidosis reported by Allen (1979), the palate was 'thickened and ulcerated', and biopsy showed an epthelioid and giant cell reaction.

Differential diagnosis of naso-pharyngeal granulomas

Many systemic and local diseases may give rise to naso-pharyngeal granulomatous changes, and among them sarcoidosis is relatively infrequent. In a review of 19 unselected cases in which nasal biopsies showed granulomatous changes, Coup and Hopper (1980) found that the final diagnosis was sarcoidosis in only one; it was tuberculosis in two, leprosy in one, Wegener's granuloma in three, cholesterol granuloma in four, unusual malignant neoplasms in two, and in six 'idiopathic granuloma'. In the latter group, of which three involved the post-nasal space, no evidence of generalized granulomatosis was found, and the local condition resolved or improved under observation. The categorization as sarcoidosis of granulomas in the nose, as in other locations, depends not only upon their histology but also upon acceptable evidence that they are part of a widespread non-caseating epithelioid cell granulomatosis (Chapter 26).

Larynx

Among reported cases of sarcoidosis of the larynx which we have reviewed and in which the sex of the patient was stated, 31 were female, and 12 male. There is thus an excess of women, as for patients with nasal involvement without laryngeal changes.

The first description of laryngeal sarcoidosis appears to have been by Ulrich (1918), in whose two cases of URT sarcoidosis the epiglottis and ary-epiglottic folds were infiltrated. Only a few cases of sarcoidosis in which the larynx was affected but the nose was stated to be uninvolved (McKelvie *et al.*, 1968, Cases 12, 13 and 14; Vico and Larsen, 1979) or not mentioned (Firooznia *et al.*, 1970, three cases) have been reported.

All parts of the larynx may be involved, but the epiglottis, the ary-epiglottic folds, the false vocal cords and the ventricles are affected more frequently that the true vocal cords, which may be unaffected in the presence of extensive supraglottic and sometimes subglottic changes (Neville *et al.*, 1976). When the vocal cords are affected, it is usually as part of widespread changes in the larynx and the URT generally (Reisner, 1944; Poe and Seager, 1950, Ferguson and Paris, 1958, Case 5; McKelvie *et al.*, 1968, Case 10; Firooznia *et al.*, 1970, Case 1; Weisman *et al.*, 1980, Cases 3 and 4), though in a few cases they were the principally involved part (Rosedale, 1945; Siltzbach and Blaugrund, 1963). Sparing of the cords in the presence of extensive changes elsewhere was noted by Carasso (1974), in whose patient the true cords appeared normal although the epiglottis, the ary-epiglottic folds and the false cords were extensively involved causing stridor, and by Kirschner and Holinger (1976) in a 14 year old black male with very extensive sarcoidosis involving epiglottis, arytenoids and ary-epiglottic folds, both false vocal cords and the sub-glottic region, but whose true cords showed erythema only. The epiglottis is very frequently affected, either as the only evidently involved part (Barmwater, 1936, two cases; Seifert, 1939, Lindsay and Perlman, 1951, four cases; Weiss, 1960, Cases 1 and 6; Weisman *et al.*, 1980, Case 1), or with the arytenoids or ary-epiglottic folds (Allison and Mikell, 1932; Kämpfer, 1964, Case 5; Devine, 1965; Di Benedetto and Lefrak, 1970; Firooznia *et al.*, 1970, Case 2; Som and Krespi, 1979). Airflow may be obstructed by general thickening of mucosa by widespread granulomatous infiltration or by local polypoid masses; in active stages, the appearances may suggest some oedema, and in the later stages, fibrosis may narrow and distort the laryngeal airway. Polypoidal masses may develop, usually above the vocal cords, and most commonly on the epiglottis, the arytenoid region, the ary-epiglottic folds, the false cords, or in the laryngeal ventricles (Trible, 1958; Devine, 1965; Di Benedetto and Lefrak, 1970; Carasso, 1974). Involvement of the sub-glottic region and the trachea (see below) may contribute to obstruction (Barmwater, 1936; Poe and Seager, 1950; Devine, 1965; Firooznia *et al.*, 1970, Case 1; Kirschner and Holinger, 1970; Weisman *et al.*, 1980, Case 2).

In many of the reported cases, the laryngeal changes have been accompanied by extensive sarcoidosis elsewhere, especially in lungs, lymph-nodes and skin. If the larynx is the only clinically evident site of granulomatous changes, the diagnosis may remain doubtful (Chapter 26). For instance, Nickol (1961) reported the case of a woman with healed apical pulmonary tuberculosis in whom dyspnoea was due to tumour-like swelling of both ary-epiglottic folds; on the strength of a biopsy this was regarded as sarcoid, but there was no evidence of sarcoid changes elsewhere, nor was the tuberculin test reported. And in Devine's (1965) report of eight cases, only one showed unquivocal evidence of generalized sarcoidosis; in five, characteristic macroscopic appearances of the laryngeal changes, with demonstration of granulomas on at least one occasion and a compatible long-term clinical course made the diagnosis of sarcoidosis acceptable, while in the remaining two, the diagnosis remains in doubt.

Even extensive granulomatous changes in the larynx, as elsewhere, may show complete or substantial resolution, as in two cases briefly mentioned by Reisner (1944) and Cases 1 and 2 of Weisman *et al.* (1980). But especially when the larynx is involved as part of extensive and chronic sarcoidosis, the laryngeal changes tend to be persistent or recrudescent, and to cause obstruction to airflow, giving rise to stridor and dyspnoea; changes in the voice may occur, but are less frequent. This is illustrated by the patient whose course over ten years was described by Poe (1940 a and b, 1942), and by Poe and Seager (1950).

A black woman with sarcoidosis of the skin of the face, the nose and the external ear, hilar lymph-nodes and the bones of the hands and feet was found to have extensive changes in the URT. There was infiltration of the mucosa of the nasal septum and inferior turbinates, of the hard palate, of the epiglottis, ary-epiglottic folds and arytenoids, spreading to involve the cords and the trachea. Local removals of exuberant tissue from the larynx and trachea on several occasions having failed to relieve obstruction, tracheostomy became necessary; obstruction recurred after the tracheostomy was allowed to close, and at this time the whole larynx was described as a mass of granuloma but with intact mucosa, and the condition was treated by thyrotomy and piecemeal removal of the exuberant tissue which was histologically confirmed as sarcoid.

A patient the earlier part of whose case was reported by McKelvie *et al.* (1968, Case 10) and has been observed by us for 18 years similarly illustrates the chronic course of sarcoidosis affecting the larynx and the nose.

A previously healthy woman first noticed epiphora from obstruction of the right lacrimal duct at the age of 28 years. Six months later, she complained of nasal obstruction, followed by slight swelling of the bridge of the nose. Two years from the onset of symptoms, she was found to have granulomatous masses in the ethmoid region obstructing the airway, and biopsy showed epithelioid cell tubercles; a Kveim test showed a granulomatous response. Radiography of the nose showed rarefaction of the nasal bone (Fig. 13.1) and of the chest enlargement of lymph-nodes at the hilar especially the left, and in the right paratracheal region, with clear lung-fields. Under treatment with prednisolone, the intrathoracic lymph-nodes subsided, and initially nasal obstruction and the swelling of the bridge of the nose diminished; but two years later, when prednisolone had been reduced to 7.5 mg daily, nasal obstruction and epiphora gradually recurred, although the chest radiograph showed persistently clear lung-fields, and no recurrence of the lymph-node enlargement. Throughout the subsequent course, the chest radiograph remained normal. At this stage, granulomatous masses were removed from the nose, and a series of local injections into the affected areas of a depot preparation of methylprednisolone were given. This was followed by subsidence of the intranasal granuloma, leaving a persistent atrophic rhinitis. One year later, slight stridor was noted; indirect laryngoscopy showed diffuse chronic inflammation, and biopsy showed no granulomas. The stridor gradually increased, with huskiness of the voice, and some dyspnoea. Increase in prednisolone dosage to 30 mg daily led to lessening of dyspnoea, but little change in the stridor. At this stage there was evident supraglottic swelling, and at laryngofissure the inlet was enlarged by excision of part of the false vocal cords; the tissue removed showed principally submucous fibrous thickening, in which one epithelioid-cell granuloma was seen. Depot methylprednisolone was injected into the area from which the exuberant tissue had been removed.

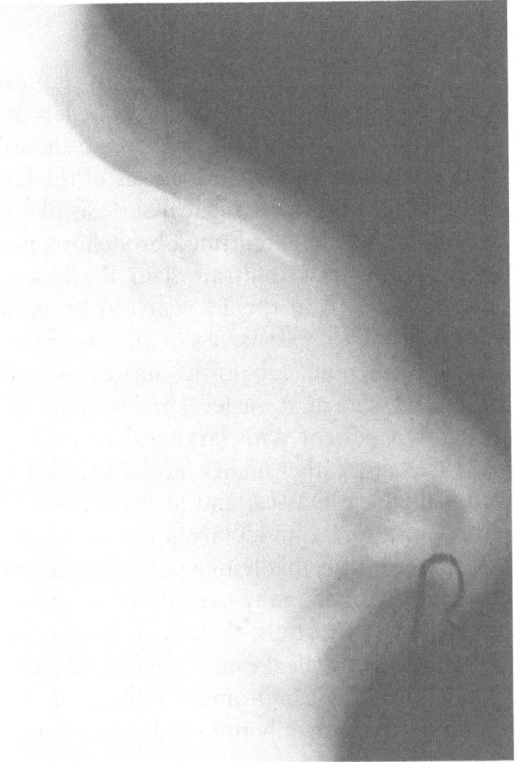

Figure 13.1   Radiograph showing rarefaction of nasal bones in a woman aged 30 who had extensive sarcoidosis of the upper respiratory tract.

After this procedure, there was considerable diminution in stridor and dyspnoea. The oral prednisolone was very gradually withdrawn over the next 18 months. The patient became pregnant two years after the end of prednisolone treatment. At the 7th month she developed stridor after a respiratory infection, and at laryngoscopy it appeared that the scarred remnant of the epiglottis was causing intermittent inspiratory obstruction which was relieved if the tongue was pulled forward. In spite of this, she successfully completed the pregnancy. Paroxysmal cough recurred a month later; there was no change in the laryngoscopic appearance; biopsy of tissue from the anterior commissure showed chronic fibrosis only, with no granulomas. There was no radiological evidence of subglottic disease. The paroxysmal cough was controllable only by morphine; reinstitution of prednisolone treatment had no effect on it, and tracheostomy was therefore performed, with complete relief of cough. One year later, at the age of 39, she had the first episode of paraesthesiae in the limbs, ataxia and transient visual disturbance which after full investigation and further observation for more than eight years proved to be due to multiple sclerosis, which has followed a typical course. There has been no further evidence of activity of sarcoidosis in the nose, the larynx or elsewhere; the tracheostomy was closed after four years without recurrence of the symptoms for which it was performed.

Trachea

In rare cases, the trachea has been involved with the larynx. Barmwater (1936) mentioned a case in which infiltration of the larynx extended down the trachea to its bifurcation, as it did in the case described by Poe and Seager (1950) and mentioned above. Sarcoidosis of the larynx was accompanied by radiographic evidence of tracheal sterosis above the carina and narrowing of both main bronchi confirmed bronchoscopically with biopsy confirmation of granulomatous infiltration in the case described by Di Benedetto and Lefrak (1972). In the 14 year old black male reported by Kirschner and Holinger (1976) extensive sarcoidosis of the nose and larynx was accompanied by polypoid subglottic masses and narrowing of the trachea radiographically evident at the level of C6 and 7. Similar evidence of tracheal narrowing in a patient with laryngeal sarcoidosis was noted by Vico and Larsen (1979) at a rather higher level. In Case 2 of Weisman *et al.* (1980) there were subglottic masses, and at bronchoscopy a similar mass was seen at the carina. Spencer and Warren (1938) reported the necropsy findings in a case of sarcoidosis involving many organs, including the heart, in which the treachea contained many irregularly arranged submucosal foci with fibrosis causing local distortion; there was no note whether the larynx was involved. Whether the tracheal mucosa tends, like that of the bronchi (Chapter 6), to be involved by symptomless infiltration in the active stages of sarcoidosis of the intrathoracic lymph-nodes and lungs is unknown.

Treatment

Because of the relative infrequency of URT sarcoidosis, and of the urgent indications for treatment which some cases present, no systematic study of its treatment has been made. Corticosteroids should be considered as the first line of treatment for patients with troublesome symptoms due to this, as to other localizations of sarcoidosis (Chapter 27).

A few case-reports have stated that nasal (Dowie, 1964; McKelvie *et al.*, 1968, Cases 3, 7 and 9) or laryngeal (McKelvie *et al.*, 1968, Case 10; Som and Krespi, 1979) sarcoidosis did not respond to systemic corticosteroid treatment, but it is doubtful whether dosage and duration of treatment was optimal. In most cases, corticosteroid treatment in sufficient dosage has led to at least some shrinkage of swollen mucosa and relief of obstruction in both nose and larynx, and in a few, to disappearance of large polypoidal masses from the nose (Selroos and Niemistö, 1977; Fishman and Canalis, 1979). Local treatment of nasal sarcoidosis by corticosteroid sprays has been found helpful by some (Wright *et al.*, 1974, Case 1; Maillard and Goepfert, 1976; Hammond and Kataria, 1980), but ineffective by others, and seems likely to be frustrated by severe obstruction. The local injection into thickened tissue of corticosteroids, usually in a depot formulation, has been found effective both in the nose (McKelvie *et al.*, 1968, Cases 7, 8 and 10; Maillard and Goepfert, 1976, Case 1) and in the larynx (Devine, 1965, Case 3; McKelvie *et al.*, 1968, Cases 10, 11, 12 and 14; Som and Krespi, 1979), in some cases after removal of thickened or polypoidal tissue (McKelvie *et al* 1965, Case 10). As in other locations, sarcoid granulomas may recur with relapse of symptoms after cessation of corticosteroid treatment, and the attainment of long-term remission depends upon the end of the active phase of sarcoidosis. Atrophic rhinitis and atrophic changes in laryngeal mucosa may develop, and persist after resolution of granulomatous changes, possibly aggravated by local corticosteroid treatment (McKelvie *et al.*, 1968).

Surgical treatment of nasal obstruction by removal of exuberantly swollen inferior turbinals or polypoidal masses appears to be safe, but unnecessary if response to corticosteroid treatment is satisfactory. Although in a few reported cases other procedures such as submucous resection of the septum, ethmoidectomy and Caldwell-Luc and intranasal antrostomy have been undertaken without ill-effect (Page and Seth, 1969; Wright *et al.*, 1974; Maillard and Goepfert, 1978), in others operations on the nasal septum have been followed by perforation (Neville *et al.*, 1976; Hammond and Kataria, 1980); and it appears that such operations are generally unnecessary and should be avoided.

In a few patients with urgent laryngeal obstruction, response to corticosteroids may not be rapid or complete enough to avoid the need for temporary tracheostomy (Trible, 1958; Devine, 1965, Cases 1, 2 and 6; McKelvie *et al.*, 1968, Case 10; Vico and Larsen, 1979; Weisman *et al.*, 1980, Case 2); and persistently active sarcoidosis of the larynx or fibrotic narrowing and distortion that may persist after the active stage in severe cases may necessitate permanent tracheostomy (Rosedale, 1945; Poe and Seager, 1950; Di Benedetto and Lefrak, 1970). Local removal of obstructing tissue, either endosopically or by laryngotomy may be helpful (Poe and Seager, 1950; Devine, 1965, Cases 2 and 6; McKelvie *et al.*, 1968, Case 10). In a black woman with a long history of widespread sarcoidosis, Carasso (1976) treated laryngeal obstruction by large masses of granulomatous tissue which had not responded to 40 mg prednisone daily by radiotherapy to the larynx, with immediate improvement and no recurrence of laryngeal obstruction in five years' later observation.

In summary, the active granulomatous stage of sarcoidosis of the URT may be expected to respond to the suppressive effect of corticosteroids. But even at this stage relief of symptoms from severe narrowing of airways, especially by polypoid masses, may be slow; and later, fibrotic narrowing and distortion of structure may be irreversible. Thus in a few cases, surgical procedures, either the removal of obstructing tissue, or, for laryngeal obstruction, tracheostomy may be required.

Chapter 14

The Nervous System

Sarcoidosis of the nervous system may be considered for convenience under two headings; neuropathies and infiltrations of the central nervous system. Both cranial and peripheral nerves may be affected, and the changes in them may be either granulomatous or non-granulomatous. In the central nervous system, granulomatous infiltration of the meninges and diffuse and focal granulomatosis of the brain or more rarely the spinal cord may occur. There are some relatively frequent patterns of involvement; e.g. facial and other cranial nerve palsies in the uveo-parotid syndrome, and within the central nervous system, granulomatous infiltration of the meninges at the base of the brain and in the adjacent hypothalamus causing neuro-endocrine and visual disturbances. But any part of the nervous system may be affected, and the great variety of possible combinations of pathological changes can give rise to bizarre clinical features. Diagnostic difficulty may be increased by occasional association with sarcoid myopathy (Chapter 9) or with the neuro-psychiatric effects of corticosteroid treatment or of hypercalcaemia (Chapter 19).

In a number of large reported series, the proportion of patients with sarcoidosis found to have nervous system involvement has been about 5% (Siltzbach *et al.*, 1974; Delaney, 1977). Transient neuropathy, especially of the facial nerve, has been the most frequently reported manifestation. Granulomatous changes in the central nervous system, which tend to be more persistent and may be life-threatening, probably figure unduly prominently among published cases. Many of these have been in North American blacks, among whom involvement of the central nervous system seems to be more frequent than among white patients with sarcoidosis. Delaney (1977) reported from Washington, DC, that of 77 patients seen in five years with a diagnosis of sarcoidosis, five (7%) had evidence of central nervous system involvement; all were black. Douglas (1974) in Edinburgh among over 500 cases of sarcoidosis observed only six (1.2%) with such evidence. In a review of the material of the US Armed Forces Institute of Pathology, Ricker and Clark (1949) found that among 195 cases with a histologically confirmed diagnosis of generalized sarcoidosis, the incidence of brain and meningeal lesions was 2.6% among blacks. No case was recorded among white persons who constituted about 40% of the total series; of 22 fatal cases with necropsy reports three, all blacks, had central nervous system changes. Among patients under observation with an established diagnosis of sarcoidosis, the proportion developing clinically evident central nervous system involvement is low. Silverstein *et al.* (1965) in New York found such evidence in six of 450 patients. Of 275 patients followed by one of us (JGS) in London for periods up to 20 years, three developed evidence of central nervous system involvement. It seems likely that in at least some patients with sarcoidosis granulomas are disseminated in the central nervous system during the active stage and resolve spontaneously without causing symptoms, as is known to occur in liver, lungs and skeletal muscles; but the proportion in which this occurs is unknown.

NEUROPATHIES

The neuropathies that occur in the course of sarcoidosis range from transient facial palsy to widespread involvement of peripheral nerves. Usually, they take the form of variable and remittent involvement of one or a few nerves; and in most cases either cranial or spinal nerves are predominantly or apparently exclusively affected, although in a few both these groups are involved. Transient, sometimes fluctuating, palsies of cranial nerves are the most frequent manifestation.

Facial nerve

Of the cranial nerves, the facial is the most frequently involved, characteristically by a transient palsy of lower motor neurone type. Rarely, an upper motor neurone paralysis may be observed, usually as a part of a hemiplegia caused by a deposit in the brain, as in Cases 2 and 9 of Höök (1954) and Case 4 of Jefferson (1957). The following discussion concerns only the common lower motor neurone palsy, which is probably the most frequent clinical evidence of involvement of the nervous system in sarcoidosis. Colover (1948) found that the facial nerve was involved in about half the reported cases of sarcoidosis affecting the nervous system. James and Sharma (1967) reported that among 38 patients with nervous system involvement the facial nerve was affected in 25, bilaterally in seven; by contrast, other cranial nerves were affected in only four. Facial palsy is one of the features of Heerfordt's uveo-parotid syndrome (p. 211). Its association in this syndrome with enlargement of the parotid gland suggests the possibility that the nerve may be involved as it traverses the infiltrated gland; but the complete Heerfordt syndrome is rare, and the facial nerve is affected far more frequently without than with parotid gland enlargement. Facial palsy often occurs without either of the other features of the syndrome; and of them, it is uveitis rather than parotid gland enlargement that accompanies facial palsy more frequently in incomplete forms of the syndrome. Silverstein *et al.* (1965), reporting 18 cases of nervous system involvement in 450 cases of sarcoidosis, stated that facial palsy was observed in 12, as the sole lesion in the nervous system in six; it was accompanied by uveitis in eight and by parotid gland enlargement in only two. As with other forms of lower motor neurone facial palsy, if the lesion is above the level of the chorda tympani, disturbance or loss of taste (ageusia) may accompany, and very occasionally precedes, the palsy. In most cases, the palsy proves transient, recovering even though the activity of other manifestations of sarcoidosis may continue, or fresh manifestations appear. Very rarely recovery is incomplete (Macbride, 1923; Rothfeld, 1930; Matthews, 1959). The palsy usually starts unilaterally, but in about one-third of the cases the second side is involved usually after a variable interval but sometimes simultaneously. Transient facial palsy affecting the two sides of the face in this way should direct attention to the possibility of sarcoidosis.

Knowledge of the causation of the facial palsy is surprisingly incomplete. The facial nerve traverses two sites in which the surrounding tissue may become infiltrated with sarcoid granulomas, the parotid gland and the subarachnoid space at the base of the brain; and in the facial canal pressure by a few granulomas or inflammatory changes may have disproportionate functional effects. But only in a minority of cases is there associated parotid gland enlargement, and in even fewer basal arachnoiditis; and the fairly rapid recovery of many patients suggests that in them the nerve is affected by non-granulomatous inflammation.

Olfactory nerves

A few cases in which impairment of the sense of smell has been a symptom of sarcoidosis have been recorded, in some as a presenting symptom (Levin, 1935; Colover, 1948; Widerholt and Sickert, 1965; Delaney *et al.* 1977). Delaney *et al.* (1977) point out that, as in one of their cases, anosmia may be due to granulomatous changes in the nasal mucosa, but suggest that olfactory impairment of neural origin probably occurs more frequently than the scanty records suggest. In most of the reported cases, it has been accompanied by symptoms and signs of changes at the base of the brain, such as meningeal involvement, and affection of other cranial nerves, especially the second, seventh and eighth, and of the hypothalamus and pituitary gland. Thus, Levin (1935) observed anosmia, worse on the left side, impairment of vestibular function and hearing, and loss of sensation in the middle of the face, in a patient with uveoparotitis who also developed diabetes insipidus; and Matthews (1959) reported loss of smell in two patients who also had facial palsy with ageusia, and sternomastoid muscle weakness. All four of the patients with anosmia of neural origin reported by Delaney *et al.* (1977) had multiple changes of these sorts, as did two of the three reported by Wiederholt and Sickert (1965), the remaining one having facial palsy only. Involvement of the olfactory bulbs and tracts in granulomatous changes at the base of the brain and basal meninges was found at necropsy in cases reported by Lenartowicz and Rothfeld (1930), Longcope and Freiman (1952), Wiederholt and Sickert (1965) and Delaney *et al.* (1977).

Optic nerve

The optic nerve may be affected in any part of its course. Changes in the retina are considered in Chapter 8. Papilloedema may occur, and in most cases is due to raised intracranial pressure caused by granulomatous infiltration of basal meninges, or within the cerebrum obstructing interventricular foramina or simulating cerebral tumours. James *et al.* (1967) reviewed 422 patients with sarcoidosis, of whom 112 had evidence of ocular and 31 of nervous system involvement, and found papilloedema in four.

Although granulomatous infiltration of the optic nerve is usually bilateral, and part of widespread changes at the base of the brain, in a few cases unilateral swelling of the optic disc has been shown by surgical exploration to be due to local infiltration of the optic nerve within the optic foramen (Statton *et al.*, 1964; Barbolini and Mastronardi, 1967), or thought to be so caused because of subsidence after corticosteroid treatment (Blain *et al.*, 1965, Cases 2 and 3; Kirkham, 1973, Case 1). In the cases reported by Statton *et al.* (1964), by Anderson *et al.* (1966) and by Kirkham (1973, Case 3) the optic foramen on the affected side was shown radiographically to be enlarged. In cases described by Ingestad and Stigmar (1971) and by Jampol *et al.* (1974), localized swellings with sharp margins at the optic nerve head in patients with sarcoidosis resolved on corticosteroid treatment.

In Case 2 of Morax (1956), loss of vision in the left eye, starting with a temporal field defect, was found at craniotomy to be due to a tumour-like mass over the optic nerve near the chiasma; histologically this showed sarcoid-type granulomas. A year later, similar loss of vision started in the right eye, and improved rapidly on corticotrophin treatment. There were similar findings at craniotomy in a patient seen by one of us, and reported as Case 4 by Kirkham (1973). A man aged 30 awoke with severe headache and loss of vision in the left eye, followed by impairment in the right. Vision in the left eye was reduced to perception of hand movements, and the visual field of the right eye was restricted in the upper nasal and both temporal quadrants. At craniotomy, the leptomeninges in the chiasmatic cistern were thickened, and there was a white mass adherent to the medial side of the right optic nerve, biopsy of which showed fibrous tissue with foci of round cells and degenerate macrophages, some giant cells and collections of epithelioid cells with some necrosis. Post-operatively, dexamethasone was given. The chest radiograph showed no abnormality. A Kveim test gave a florid granulomatous response with some necrosis. Treatment was continued with prednisolone, and, in a view of the strongly positive response to a tuberculin test with 1 IU, isoniazid and para-aminosalicylic acid. Visual acuity returned to normal, although ophthalmoscopic signs of left optic atrophy persisted. Treatment was continued for 18 months, and three and a half years from the onset the patient was well with normal visual acuity.

Widespread involvement of optic pathways is a frequent feature of basal meningeal and cerebral sarcoidosis. It is exemplified in its most exuberant form by the case reported by Lenartowicz and Rothfeld (1930) and Reis and Rothfeld (1931), in which there was infiltration of the right optic nerve and the chiasma, replacement of the right retina with a tumour-like mass of sarcoid tissue, and nodules of sarcoid granuloma over the base of the brain, the medulla and the cerebellum; there was also exophthalmos, discussed in Chapter 8 (p. 224). Other cases with widespread involvement of various parts of the optic pathways, including the retina, have been reported by Alajouanine *et al.* (1958), Brownstein and Jannotta (1974) and Urich (1976). After reviewing published cases of sarcoidosis involving the optic pathway, Urich concluded that the intraocular, intraorbital and intracranial parts may be affected independently. The intraorbital part of the nerve and the nerve-head may be unilaterally affected, sometimes as an apparently isolated finding, but the intracranial part of the pathway is usually affected bilaterally, though not necessarily symmetrically, as part of more widespread changes in the central nervous system.

Oculomotor nerves

The oculomotor nerves are rarely affected. In view of the widespread changes in many cases of central nervous system sarcoidosis, this low incidence is remarkable.

Colover (1948), reviewing 118 recorded cases of sarcoidosis with involvement of the nervous system, was able to find records of only three patients with third nerve palsy, one with sixth nerve palsy and one with fourth nerve palsy. In Case 2 of Pennell (1951), mentioned below, there was unilateral abducens palsy. In Case 1 of Dickinson (1971) meningo-cerebral sarcoidosis initially causing diabetes insipidus and hypothalmic signs later led to hearing loss and visual disturbances, and eventually to external ophthalmoplegia with non-reacting pupils, which appeared to be attributable to extensive involvement of the mid-brain among other sites found at necropsy. Henkind and Gottlieb

(1973) reviewed the few recorded cases of sarcoidosis of the central nervous system in which internal ophthalmoplegia was a feature, and reported the case of a black woman aged 40 with fever, uveitis, bilateral hilar lymph-node enlargement, peripheral neuropathy and sarcoid-type granulomas in a muscle biopsy, in whom internal ophthalmoplegia was attributed after neuro-pharmacological investigation to a mid-brain lesion.

The trigeminal nerve

The trigeminal nerve is affected more often in its sensory than in its motor functions, usually unilaterally and with other cranial nerves. Among the 118 cases collected by Colover (1948) there were five with loss of sensation on the face, and three with diminution of corneal reflexes, but only two with weakness of the muscles of mastication. Engberg and Jepsen (1936, Case 4) found numbness of the upper lip and left cheek and diminution of corneal sensation in a patient with iridocyclitis, facial palsy, partial loss of hearing and vestibular function, and signs of pyramidal tract involvement. Sensory loss in the trigeminal area were found in three of the 23 cases reported by Delaney (1977), associated with anosmia in two and with facial palsy in one.

The eighth cranial nerve

The eighth cranial nerve is relatively frequently affected. In the series of 118 cases of CNS sarcoidosis reviewed by Colover (1948), there were eight with nerve deafness and four with vestibular nerve damage.

In Case 2 of Pennell (1951) deafness on one side developed under observation in a man with skin sarcoidosis, headache, vomiting, abducens palsy on the opposite side, and pleocytosis in the cerebro-spinal fluid (CSF). In Höök's (1954) Case 7, iridocyclitis, facial palsy, mental deterioration, and lung changes were accompanied by nerve deafness and sluggish response to caloric tests. Gristwood (1958) reported the case of a woman in whom uveitis, left facial palsy and ataxia preceded sudden deafness; there was bilateral hilar lymph-node enlargement, and the diagnosis of sarcoidosis was confirmed by biopsy of a cervical lymph-node; investigation showed nerve deafness and depressed caloric responses; the condition improved spontaneously at first and further when prednisone was given. Engberg and Jepsen (1963) studied four patients with sarcoidosis at an early stage as shown by BHL in the chest radiograph, and confirmed by histology from biopsy of lymph-nodes in three and muscle in one. All had uveitis and all but one facial palsy. All had nerve deafness, confirmed by audiometry, and two had tinnitus. Two complained of dizziness, and all four showed depression or loss of caloric responses. This report suggests that routine study of auditory and vestibular function in patients with active sarcoidosis might reveal a higher proportion with eighth nerve involvement than the scattered reports in the literature indicate, and that sarcoidosis may affect the labyrinth itself. One of the patients reported by Silverstein *et al.* (1965) with uveitis, generalized lymphadenopathy, and hepatomegaly, the diagnosis of sarcoidosis being confirmed both by lymph-node biopsy and Kveim test, developed tinnitus and rapid hearing loss, together with loss of caloric responses on one side; cortisone treatment produced no improvement in the hearing. Hooper and Holden (1970) reported audiological studies in two women who developed hearing loss and vestibular · disturbance shortly after erythema nodosum; both also developed uveitis, in one with BHL and a positive Kveim test and in the other with enlarged axillary lymph-nodes showing sarcoid-type granulomas on biopsy. In both, deafness and vertigo fluctuated, but during limited periods of observation showed general improvement. Among the 23 cases of sarcoidosis involving the nervous system reviewed by Delaney (1977), deafness was noted in three, all with extensive granulomatous infiltration of meninges and structures at the base of the brain, found at craniotomy in one and at necropsy in two.

These reports suggest that, like other cranial nerves, the eighth in both its divisions may be affected early in the course of sarcoidosis by reversible changes the pathology of which is not established, and later by involvement in persistent, usually widespread, granulomatous changes at the base of the brain.

The glossopharyngeal and vagus

These nerves are also relatively frequently affected. Dysphagia due to paralysis of pharyngeal and palatal muscles was reported in 29 and paralysis of one or both vocal cords in nine of the 118 cases reviewed by Colover (1948). These changes are often accompanied by other cranial nerve palsies or by uveitis; e.g. in Case 8 of Höök (1954) by facial palsy, uveitis, and left hemiparesis and partial hemianaesthesia, and in Cases 1 and 3 of Matthews (1959) by uveitis and involvement of the facial and other cranial nerves. Singh and Fitzpatrick (1964) reported a case in which six months after the diagnosis of sarcoidosis in a patient with BHL confirmed by scalene node and liver biopsies, dysphagia developed and was shown to be due to paresis of hypopharyngeal muscles; prednisone treatment led to rapid improvement, with resolution of the slight pleocytosis in the CSF which had been found in the acute stage.

The spinal accessory nerve

This nerve is rarely affected. Colover (1948) was able to find only one other case besides one of his own with weakness of sternomastoid and trapezius muscles.

The hypoglossal nerve

This was affected in seven of the cases reviewed by Colover, with impaired movement of the tongue, usually with deviation to one side on protrusion; in one case fibrillation was observed.

Peripheral neuropathy

In the syndrome of uveo-parotid fever, peripheral as well as cranial nerves may be affected, as in one of Heerfordt's (1909) original cases. But peripheral neuropathy has been reported, with or without involvement of cranial nerves, in patients with a variety of other manifestations of sarcoidosis. Colover (1948) summarized 21 published cases of sarcoidosis with polyneuropathy. In 14, cranial as well as peripheral nerves were involved; the facial nerve was among those affected in 12, and in eight two or more cranial nerves were affected. The affection of the spinal nerves was in most instances of patchy distribution, but in a few was widespread, all four limbs being involved. The symptoms and signs consisted in varying combinations of sensory and motor disturbance, paraesthesiae, analgesia and sometimes hyperaesthesia, flaccid weakness of muscles, sometimes wasting, and depression or absence of tendon reflexes. In four cases, there was intercostal neuritis, with sensory disturbance in the relevant dermatomes and loss of the corresponding abdominal reflexes. Matthews (1959) described three cases of sarcoidosis with facial palsy in all and with other cranial nerve palsies in two; all of them had evidence of peripheral neuropathy, consisting in weakness and patchy hypaethesia in the legs in one, analgesia over the skin of the abdomen in one, and sensory changes in the left hand and round the lower ribs in one.

Silverstein *et al.* (1965) found evidence of peripheral neuropathy in four of their 18 cases of nervous system involvement in sarcoidosis. Three of these also had facial palsy; the neuropathy was exclusively motor in two, and motor and sensory in two. The CSF was examined in three; the protein was raised in two and the cell count was normal in all. All improved, two without and one before the beginning of corticosteroid treatment.

All types of neuropathy, ranging from mononeuritis to widespread sensory and motor involvement simulating the Guillain-Barré syndrome, may occur. In a case of the latter sort, reported by Strickland and Moser (1967), a woman aged 27, who developed first sensory changes, then motor weakness in all four limbs two years after the onset of sarcoidosis with BHL, improved rapidly on treatment with prednisone, improvement being maintained on reduced dosage during 18 months' observation.

There are few reports of the pathology of neuropathies in sarcoidosis, and of these only a minority have shown granulomatous changes. Winkler (1905) described perineural inflammatory changes in the form of small cell infiltration with sparse epithelioid cells in a man with multiple cutaneous and subcutaneous sarcoids.

Mazza's (1908) Case 1 had a very extensive eruption of histologically typical skin sarcoids with sensory changes in the hands and forearms; the patient died from an unrelated cause, and at necropsy there were spindle-shaped swellings of the median, radial and ulnar nerves, caused by infiltration between the fibres of granulomas composed of epithelioid and giant cells, lymphocytes, and plasma cells. Oh (1979) reported the case of a woman aged 58 who presented with polyneuropathy affecting principally the legs, biopsy of the sural nerve showing showing sarcoid-type granulomas in the epineurium and perineurium, angiitis and axonal degeneration; other localizations of sarcoidosis were sought, but the only evidences found were radiological changes in the hands said to be compatible and impairment of ventilatory capacity of the lungs with a normal chest radiograph. There was rapid improvement on treatment with prednisone. This case differs from most of those with polyneuropathy occurring in the course of sarcoidosis, in which the sarcoidosis has been extensive or in an acute, possibly febrile, phase. In some such cases, no granulomatous changes have been found in nerves involved in peripheral neuropathy. Garland and Thompson (1953) reported that at necropsy in a patient with uveoparotitis, with weakness and hypotonia in the limbs and slight sensory ataxia, the brain, spinal cord, meninges, and the median and sciatic nerves showed no pathological change; and Kömpf *et al.* (1976) found no granulomatous or inflammatory change in a nerve biopsy from a patient who developed mononeuritis multiplex two months after the onset of sarcoidosis with febrile bilateral hilar lymphadenopathy; unfortunately treatment of this had included the antituberculosis drugs ethambutol and isoniazid, a possible though in view of the short period of administration unlikely cause of neuritis.

It must be recognized that nerve biopsy is subject to large sampling errors in a search for granulomas that may be sparsely distributed, but clinical evidence is compatible with the possibility that some of the transient neuropathies in the early stage of sarcoidosis may be non-granulomatous, and cognate with other non-granulomatous inflammatory changes, such as erythema nodosum, febrile arthropathy, and transient anterior uveitis, that may occur at this time.

Matthews (1975), discussing pathogenesis in a review of sarcoid neuropathy, noted that while both involvement of cranial nerves and spinal nerve roots in granulomatous meningitis has been recorded in a few cases, as has granulomatous infiltration of peripheral nerves, it is difficult to account for all cases of sarcoid neuropathy, especially of spinal nerves, in these ways; demyelination as a remote effect of the disease process is an alternative explanation, although as yet there is little support for this possibility from histological or nerve conduction studies.

SARCOIDOSIS OF THE BRAIN, SPINAL CORD AND MENINGES

Sarcoidosis may affect both the meninges and the substance of the brain and spinal cord. The distribution varies greatly from case to case; in general, the meninges tend to be involved more extensively, and the brain is more frequently affected than the spinal cord. The meninges generally show diffuse thickening as well as granulomatous nodules, with cellular infiltration accompanying granulomas both in this meningeal thickening and around blood-vessels in affected parts of the brain. The pathology of sarcoidosis of the central nervous system has been reviewed by Herring and Urich (1969), and with special reference to meningeal changes by Meyer *et al.* (1953).

Infiltration of the leptomeninges is usually most prominent at the base of the brain, sometimes extending in the sulci over the brain and cerebellum. At the base of the brain, it may surround and involve the optic nerve, chiasm and tracts, the seventh and eighth nerves, and the olfactory nerve, the floor of the third ventricle and the pituitary gland; local confluence of granulomas gives rise to tumour-like masses in some cases. Even where the gross changes are evident only in the meninges, microscopic granulomas may be found extending locally into the brain along the Virchow-Robin spaces. In a few cases, local infiltrations of the brain, and more rarely cerebellum, develop into well-circumscribed tumour-like masses, which may cause focal symptoms and signs. Although these may occur in any part of the brain, the hypothalamus and the brain-stem, especially the pons, are common sites for them. In a few cases, local tumour-like masses of sarcoid granuloma have been the principal feature, with little or no meningeal involvement.

Pathologically, diagnosis presents no problem when non-caseating granulomatous changes in the central nervous system occur in a patient with similar changes elsewhere, or with acceptable clinical evidence of their previous presence. Difficulty has arisen chiefly in two circumstances. In some cases, there is prominent involvement of vessels in the nervous system, possibly with more non-granulomatous inflammatory change than is regarded as characteristic for sarcoidosis; and in some there is no convincing evidence of granulomatosis elsewhere.

In cases acceptable as sarcoidosis of the central nervous system, the adventitia of blood-vessels frequently contains granulomas; in a few the media and even the intima are involved. The prominence of these changes varies greatly; cases in which they were especially prominent have been reported by Camp and Friersen (1962) and Aronson and Perl (1973). Cases of giant-cell granulomatous angiitis of the central nervous system, involving both arteries and veins, without granulomatous but some with vasculitic changes in other organs, have been reported (Cavioto and Feigin, 1959; Kolodny *et al.*, 1968; Nurick *et al.*, 1972), and it is likely that some, at least, of these are unrelated to sarcoidosis. Differential diagnosis in cases of this sort has been discussed by Reske-Nielsen and Harmsen (1962) and Urich (1977). There remains after full investigation a small group of cases which can at present be categorized only as granulomatous angiitis of the central nervous system; and this label should carry no necessary implication about pathogenetic relationships to sarcoidosis or other systemic disease.

Failure to find granulomatous changes in other organs does not controvert a diagnosis of sarcoidosis if histological changes in the central nervous system are characteristic, and are distributed in a pattern known to occur in patients with an established diagnosis of sarcoidosis. Sarcoidosis of the central nervous system presenting as an apparently localized disease probably results from locally persistent activity of a generalized disease whose manifestations elsewhere have resolved or regressed to an inactive residue, as is the case with clinically localized sarcoidosis of other organs. In a number of cases of extensive intracranial sarcoidosis coming to necropsy – e.g. those of Robert (1962), Dickinson (1971) and Snyder *et al.* (1976) – sclerosing changes in lymph-nodes were the only other evidence of past or present granulomatosis.

Clinical features of intracranial sarcoidosis

Patients with sarcoidosis of the central nervous system usually have manifestations of sarcoidosis outside the nervous system, of sorts that would be discoverable clinically if sought; and in some cases these are obvious. But in many cases, the changes in the nervous system cause the first symptoms; and, as already noted, there is good evidence that in some such cases they are a persistent localized manifestation of a disease whose early stages in other organs have resolved or reached an inactive stage without giving rise to symptoms.

In order to obtain some idea of the relative frequency of various features, we have reviewed publications over the past 20 years giving information about 102 cases of intracranial sarcoidosis, with histological evidence from biopsy or necropsy or highly probable on grounds short of this. This group is, of course, likely to include high proportions of patients with extensive disease, with localizations giving rise to obvious or medically interesting symptoms, with indications for surgical intervention, or dying and submitted to necropsy; and relatively few known to have sarcoidosis and developing symptoms and signs suggestive of central nervous system involvement but not submitted to definitive local biopsy procedures, and improving spontaneously. Two-thirds of these published cases presented as neurological (or neuro-endocrinological) problems without concurrent clinical evidence or past history of sarcoidosis, the histological diagnosis being made from tissue removed at craniotomy or lesser biopsy procedure, or, in a substantial minority of cases, at necropsy. In the other one-third, there were clinically evident manifestations of sarcoidosis outside the central nervous system, in some cases florid, when the symptoms referable to the nervous system appeared. The large majority of patients were in the age-range 15–60 years at this time.

> The youngest recorded case (Naumann, 1938) presented unusually florid and rapidly progressive changes. The patient, a girl aged three months, died after an illness of six weeks' duration, with skin sarcoids, hepatosplenomegaly, convulsions, neck rigidity and pleocytosis in the CSF; at necropsy, sarcoid infiltration was found in the skin, lymph-nodes, kidneys and in the meninges, both pia-arachnoid and dura, the region of the falx, the tentorium cerebelli and the cranial sutures being specially affected. At the other end of the age-range, a woman aged 72, reported by de Tribolet and Zander (1978), showed unusual localization, simulating a sub-dural haematoma, no evidence of other concurrent localizations of sarcoidosis, and an indolent course.

The great variety of possible clinical presentations of sarcoidosis of the central nervous system could be described completely only by citing individual cases. Features suggesting infiltration of basal meninges and adjacent neural structures, sometimes accompanied by symptoms referable to other parts of the central nervous system, are especially suggestive of sarcoidosis. This complexity is illustrated by a review of 14 cases of granulomatous meningitis by Meyer *et al.* (1953). In these, there were meningeal signs and raised intracranial pressure in six; visual disturbances from involvement of optic pathways in five; other cranial nerve affections in two; convulsive attacks in five, described as focal in one; pyramidal tract signs in three; cerebellar signs in one; polydipsia in two; and obesity and mental dullness in one. Five had skin sarcoids, recognized as such before the nervous system changes in three; in the remaining nine, the diagnosis of sarcoidosis was made only at surgical exploration or at necropsy. A patient reported by Zollinger (1941) presented a syndrome suggesting atypical multiple sclerosis for one year before death at the age of 21, and at necropsy was found to have sarcoid granulomas in the leptomeninges and scattered in the brain, and also in hilar and paratracheal lymph-nodes. Association with peripheral neuropathy or with sarcoid myopathy (Chapter 9) may further complicate the picture, as in Case 2 of De Morsier *et al.* (1954), a man aged 68 who presented with widespread weakness and muscle pain, mental confusion and agitation and sometimes aggressiveness; at necropsy there was granulomatous infiltration of muscles, and of meninges and scattered in the brain and cerebellum in relation to blood-vessels. On the other hand, in some cases the clinical picture suggests a localized lesion, for instance, with focal epilepsy, evidence of raised intracranial pressure and localizing signs simulating cerebral tumour.

It is convenient to consider possible clinical features individually, recognizing that they often occur in complex combinations, in which involvement of the visual pathways, the fifth, sixth and seventh cranial nerves and hypothalamus are frequent elements.

Raised intracranial pressure

This may be caused by granulomatous obliteration of the subarachnoid space at the base of the brain or obstructing the outflow from the fourth ventricle (Lukin *et al.*, 1975), by granulomatous infiltration of the ependyma of the ventricles and the subjacent brain, especially in the region of the aqueduct (Kumpe *et al.*, 1979), and by the space-occupying effect of granulomatous masses, both above and below the tentorium, discussed below (p. 317).

Hypothalamic syndromes

Symptoms such as a rapid gain of weight, somnolence, polydipsia and polyuria, loss of libido, disturbances of temperature regulation and hypoventilation may occur, either as elements in a complex picture, or as the leading features. Specifically endocrine aspects of these are considered in Chapter 16, together with the effects of involvement of the pituitary gland.

In two black men with extensive sarcoidosis, Daum *et al.* (1965) found evidence of diabetes insipidus and also of alveolar hypoventilation manifested by a high arterial P_{CO2} which could readily be reduced by voluntary respiratory effort; they suggested that this was attributable to involvement of the mid-brain. Salm (1969) reported the case of a man who at the age of 25 developed erythema nodosum with BHL, a lymph-node biopsy showing sarcoid-type granulomas, and later generalized enlargement of superficial lymph-nodes and nasal obstruction shown on biopsy to be due to granulomatous infiltration. Two years later, he began to have episodes of unsteadiness, headache and diplopia, with occasional drowsiness and mental confusion; these symptoms continued in spite of treatment with prednisolone. At this time, the hilar lymphadenopathy had subsided, and radiologically the lungs appeared normal. The cerebro-spinal fluid (CSF) contained 35–450 mg dl^{-1} of protein on repeated examinations with no excess of cells. Polyuria was noted, and was investigated by a water deprivation test; this resulted in 15 hours of unconsciousness, from which the patient recovered on intensive corticosteroid treatment. There were no localizing neurological signs. He was referred to one of us at this stage. On maintenance prednisolone treatment, 30 mg daily, the only abnormality found was alveolar hypoventilation; with normal ventilatory and gas transfer function of the lungs, the mixed venous P_{CO2} was found to range up to 58 mm, and was readily reduced by voluntary hyperventilation. This suggested that central alveolar hyperventilation was at least a factor in causation of the drowsy episodes. These continued, and six months later he was admitted to hospital comatose and died. At necropsy, the brain showed dilatation of both lateral ventricles, with many small nodules in the ependyma and choroid plexuses, and of the third ventricle, the aqueduct of Sylvius being almost occluded by subependymal nodules. Histologically, these nodules were found to consist of confluent granulomas, and granulomas were also seen in the leptomeninges at the base of the brain, and around the spinal cord and in posterior nerve roots, although all these structures looked normal macroscopically; none were seen in the pituitary gland. Granulomas were found microscopically in the lungs, in the respiratory mucosa, and subcarinal and paratracheal lymph-nodes; the latter were largely fibrotic; none were found in other organs examined.

Hyperthermia was observed in patients with widespread granulomatous changes in the basal meninges and hypothalamus reported by Robert (1962) and by Delaney (1977, Cases 9, 14 and 17).

Convulsive attacks
Convulsive attacks may be the presenting symptom, or part of a complex clinical picture. They occurred in five of 14 cases of granulomatous meningitis reported by Meyer *et al.* (1953), as already noted, and in five of 23 cases of sarcoidosis of the central nervous system reported by Delaney (1977). They may be focal or generalized.

Everts' (1947) case presented with right homonymous hemianopia and occasional focal epilepsy starting in the right leg; at craniotomy a large occipital lobe 'tumour' was removed and proved to be a sarcoid deposit. In Aszkenazy's (1952) Case 4, left-sided Jacksonian epilepsy, followed by hemiparesis, was found at craniotomy to be associated with cortical scars in the arm area and a histologically evident infiltration of the leptomeninges with granulomas. In Jefferson's (1957) Case 4, epilepsy starting in the left side of the face and the left arm was found to be associated with a localized induration at the lower end of the motor cortex with overlying adhesions; this had the histological structure of sarcoidosis, and a history of two earlier attacks of uveitis was elicited. Ross (1955) reported the case of a man who had had uveitis with parotid gland enlargement and BHL at the age of 24; six years later he developed headache and generalized fits, and was found to have papilloedema, right homonymous upper quadrant visual loss, and slight right-sided pyramidal signs; craniotomy showed an avascular tumour in the left temporal lobe, which proved to be a mass of non-caseating tubercles; 14 years later, at the age of 44, he died after a fit; at necropsy, sarcoid tubercles were found in the brain in the neighbourhood of the old left temporal lobectomy and in the right occipital cortex, with histological evidence of calcification in the left temporal lesions; a few foci of sarcoidosis were found in the liver; and there was patchy calcification in the enlarged hilar nodes. This is one of the earliest references to dystrophic calcification in long-standing sarcoidosis. Thompson's (1961) patient had had attacks of focal epilepsy, starting in the left side of the face; at necropsy widespread discrete or confluent sarcoid granulomas, some active and some hyalinized, were found in the meninges and cortex, but the most striking localized lesion, in the inferior part of the left frontal lobe, with meningeal adhesions and involvement of the olfactory nerve, was clearly not responsible for the focal epilepsy. Convulsions were prominent features in the cases reported by Douglas and Maloney (1973), Griggs *et al.* (1973), Ho *et al.* (1979) and Kumpe *et al.* (1979).

Fine *et al.* (1963) reported the case of a man aged 28 in whom headache and generalized convulsions preceded by nausea and epigastric discomfort and visual hallucinations of dazzling yellow-white light were the presenting symptoms; the only abnormality on examination was left homonymous hemianopia; CSF was under high pressure and contained excess cells and protein; ventriculogram showed dilatation of both lateral and the third ventricles with a filling defect posteriorly in the right lateral ventricle; at craniotomy a tough mass was found extending from the island of Riel to the temporal horn of the ventricle, and was partially removed. Histologically it showed dense relatively acellular collagen centrally with peripheral granulomatous follicles extending into brain tissue. A history of erythema nodosum at the age of 11 was obtained; a tuberculin test with 1:1000 OT was negative; the serum calcium was elevated, three estimations ranging from 11.5 to 12.2 mg dl⁻¹. No other evidence of sarcoidosis elsewhere was obtained, radiographs of the chest and hands being normal. Left hemiparesis developed after the operation; there was no record of corticosteroid treatment, and deterioration led to a further operation for drainage of the right lateral ventricle into the cisterna magna, in which the leptomeninges were found to be infiltrated with sarcoid granulomas. Some months later, the patient was found dead in bed; there was no necropsy.

In a patient under the care of one of us (JGS), visual 'fits' with dyslexia and occasional generalized convulsions developed in a woman with long-standing lupus pernio and pulmonary sarcoidosis. At the age of 18, this right-handed patient developed lupus pernio on the nose and cheeks. Over the next ten years, small and large nodular sarcoids appeared on the limbs and trunk. Biopsy of one of these showed the typical histological picture. When she was aged 31, the skin lesions had ceased to spread and some of them had actually regressed, when she experienced the first of a series of attacks of a visual disturbance. These consisted of unformed hallucinations in the right half of the visual field, at first lines of white light falling like sleet, and later waves or flashes of coloured light, lasting usually up to one hour but sometimes longer. These tended to occur about ten days before the menstrual period. During the attack, she noticed difficulty in reading because she failed to understand the meaning of written words, but none with speaking or understanding spoken words. On only three occasions in the following nine years, these symptoms were followed by loss of consciousness and falling to the ground. When she was aged 37, swellings over the middle phalanges of the second, third and fourth fingers of the right hand appeared, and the nails of the third and fourth fingers became white, opaque and dystrophic. When she was aged 40, there was florid lupus pernio of the face and fingers and scattered large and small sarcoid infiltrations of the skin and subcutaneous tissues on the limbs and trunk (Plates 1 and 2). Radiographs of the chest showed mottling predominantly in the middle zones of the lungs, with hypertransradiancy of the upper zones, suggesting some fibrosis in the more densely infiltrated parts; and of the hands and feet, multiple areas of rarefaction in the proximal and middle phalanges of the third and fourth fingers and of some of the terminal phalanges on the right, and in the proximal phalanges of both great toes. The mental state was normal. There was a right upper quadrantic hemianopia and the tendon reflexes were difficult to elicit in the lower limbs, but apart from this, clinical examination of the nervous system showed no abnormality. The cerebro-spinal fluid was under normal pressure, clear, with 4 cells mm⁻³, and increased protein, 120 mg dl⁻¹. The Mantoux test with 100 IU was negative. Electro-encephalography showed unstable alpha rhythm of 8 sec⁻¹, disturbed by runs and bursts at 5–7 and 22–24 sec⁻¹, the changes being generalized from both hemispheres with no evidence of a focal abnormality. It seemed likely that there were sarcoid deposits in the left occipital and parietal lobes, but there seemed to be no justification for surgical exploration which alone could prove this. Cortisone treatment was tried, with unsatisfactory results. Although at first some improvement in the skin changes was observed, there was little effect on the 'attacks', and in view of this and the excessive gain in weight and oedema caused by the cortisone, the treatment was discontinued at the patient's request. During the next 12 years, the attacks gradually diminished in duration and severity, so that when she was aged 52, they lasted only half an hour, and occurred not more frequently than once a month; the skin lesions had slowly faded, leaving remarkably little residual change, though there was some atrophy of the tips of the worst affected fingers. The concurrent improvement in the skin sarcoids and the nervous system symptoms in this case is compatible with the latter being due to cerebral sarcoidosis, especially in view of their rather bizarre character.

In another patient under the care of one of us, focal epilepsy originating in the upper part of the right Rolandic area developed in a man aged 29 who two years earlier had been found to have pulmonary and lymph-node sarcoidosis, confirmed by biopsy of a peripheral lymph-node. Treatment with corticosteroids and anticonvulsants led to diminution in the frequency and severity of convulsive episodes; it appeared that anticonvulsants were more effective in this respect than corticosteroids. These episodes ceased when he was aged 40, but progressive pulmonary fibrosis, leading to pulmonary hypertension led to his death at the age of 53. At necropsy, the lungs were grossly fibrotic with bullous emphysema, but no granulomas were seen histologically in them; some granulomas persisted in a normal-sized spleen; the brain was examined only macroscopically, and no abnormality was reported. We are grateful to Dr A. T. Hendry for information about the latter part of the course of this case.

Simulation of cerebral tumour

In some of the cases mentioned above, the onset of convulsive attacks with focal neurological signs initially suggested a diagnosis of cerebral tumour. Localized masses of sarcoid granuloma may cause other syndromes suggestive of cerebral tumour.

In Jefferson's (1957) Case 5, excessive gain of weight, polydipsia, loss of libido, headache and somnolence and the macroscopic findings at necropsy suggested a hypothalamic tumour; but histologically the diagnosis of sarcoidosis affecting the hypothalamus, hilar lymph-nodes, lungs and liver was established. Géraud et al. (1965) described the case of a man aged 33 in whom investigation of episodic intracranial hypertension led to a diagnosis of tumour encroaching on the third ventricle; at craniotomy this was found to be composed of sarcoid granulomas, and subsequently a scalene lymph-node biopsy showed similar granulomas. The patient developed right hemiplegia and aphasia, and died 16 months later, in spite of corticosteroid treatment.

Saltzman (1958) reported briefly the case of a boy aged 16 who presented with signs of increased intracranial pressure, and was found on pneumoencephalography to have hydrocephalus with a large mass in the pineal area; this was confirmed at craniotomy, part of the mass being removed and found to have the histological pattern of sarcoidosis. Schaeffer et al. (1977) reported a similar case in a 13 year old boy, with a brief history of headache and disturbance of vision, from whom a localized, apparently encapsulated tumour was removed from the pineal region, and was found to consist of granulomas with many giant cells, containing both crystalline and Schaumann inclusion bodies, and with much sclerosis. In both these cases, there was radiological evidence of calcification in the region of the tumours;

no other localization of sarcoidosis was found; post-operative progress was satisfactory; and during follow-up periods of seven years and one year, no other evidence of sarcoidosis became apparent. The question whether the changes in the pineal gland represented the residue of an originally generalized sarcoidosis, or were an entirely localized condition must be left open.

That sarcoidosis of the central nervous system may be or become localized is illustrated by a case reported by Popper *et al.* (1960).

A black man aged 23 developed BHL, and 18 months later became weak and dizzy with cerebellar signs and an abnormal CSF with high protein content. Symptoms improved at first on corticosteroid treatment but recurred, with fluctuating levels of consciousness, papilloedema and extensor plantar responses. Ventriculography showed dilatation of the ventricles with a mass in the posterior part of the fourth ventricle. At suboccipital craniotomy a firm mass in the inferior vermis, invading both cerebellar hemispheres, and herniation of the cerebellar tonsils through the foramen magnum were found. The patient died post-operatively, and at necropsy, there was extensive sarcoid infiltration of the cerebellum, with focal calcification, but none was found in the brain above the tentorium; granulomas were found in the lymph-nodes, liver, spleen and kidneys. Skillicorn and Garrity (1955) and Goodman and Margulies (1959) reported cases in which the clinical syndrome and findings at craniotomy suggested meningioma at the base of the brain, but the tissue removed was shown histologically to be granulomatous. No other clinical manifestation of sarcoidosis was found in either case, but in that of Goodman and Margulies a Kveim test gave a granulomatous response. The diagnostic difficulty that may arise from the occurrence of a cerebral tumour in a patient with sarcoidosis is illustrated by the case reported by Rosen and Wang (1965); a 41 year old woman was investigated after a single episode of clonic movements of the left arm, followed by unconsciousness; she was found to have enlargement of hilar and right paratracheal lymph-nodes, and scalene node biopsy showed sarcoid granulomas; brain scans showed increased uptake in the right parietal region. On a provisional diagnosis of cerebral sarcoidosis, treatment with prednisone was begun, and was followed by improvement in the brain scan; but after a year free from symptoms, the patient had a generalized seizure, and at craniotomy was found to have a meningioma.

Pyramidal tract signs

Such signs may appear, usually as part of a complex neurological picture. Of the 23 cases reviewed by Delaney (1977), four, all with extensive involvement of the nervous system, developed hemiparesis. In a few cases, hemiparesis has been an early finding.

Saltzman's (1958) Case 4 was that of a man aged 49 who developed left hemiplegia one year after sarcoidosis had been diagnosed by lymph-node biopsy; carotid angiography showed a poorly vascularized expanding lesion in the right temporal region. At craniotomy, a large mass was found extending into the temporal horn of the right lateral ventricle, and was partially removed. The patient was said to be well two years later. In a woman aged 36 whose case was reported by Robert (1962) drowsiness, headache and oligomenorrhoea after childbirth were accompanied by right hemiparesis; she became hyperthermic and comatose and died after a needle biopsy, and at necropsy was found to have widespread granulomatous changes in the cerebral meninges, the hypothalamus, the caudate nucleus, corpus callosum and septum pellucidum, perivascular spaces and the walls of large veins being notably involved. The only evidence of sarcoidosis outside the nervous system was found in the hilar lymph-nodes, which were fibrotic centrally with peripheral epithelioid and giant cells. Griggs *et al.* (1973) described the case of a black man aged 18 who after a few months of difficulty with speech, impaired vision and incoordination had a focal seizure starting in the right arm, followed by right hemiplegia and aphasia. Investigations showed a mass in the left temporo-parietal area, confirmed at craniotomy; biopsy showed granulomatous infiltration of the brain and meninges. No other localization of sarcoidosis was detected. There was some improvement on corticosteroid treatment; two and a half years later, further seizures were followed by left-sided hemiparesis, and a new avascular mass was found in the right hemisphere on brain scanning and angiography. Intensive corticosteroid treatment was followed by improvement, but continued treatment was required to maintain freedom from further seizures. Norwood and Kelly (1974) reported the case of a woman aged 59 who developed frontal headache and episodes of numbness and weakness in the right leg, then in the right arm and face and finally in the left leg, leading in three months to inability to walk. She was found to have left hemiparesis and paresis of the right leg, right optic atrophy with vision reduced to perception of light; brain scan and arteriography showed bilateral posterior parietal avascular masses. At craniotomy, the right-sided mass was partially removed, and found to consist of non-caseating granuloma of the brain and leptomeninges. Post-operatively, there was a flaccid left hemiplegia, which improved on treatment with prednisone. No other localization of sarcoidosis was detected; the only possible relevant finding was a past history of sudden loss of vision in the right eye 20 years earlier.

Dementia

As is to be expected, impairment of intellectual function may be observed as part of the clinical picture in patients with cerebral sarcoidosis. Delaney (1977) noted dementia in six of the 23 cases he reviewed. Very rarely, it is an early and prominent symptom, as in a case reported by Gaines *et al.* (1979).

A 60 year old woman had a seven year history of increasing dementia, with memory loss and episodes of confusion, and early morning nausea and vomiting and disturbance of gait. She was found to be dysarthric with left homonymous hemianopia, left facial weakness, increased tone in the limbs and grasp reflexes; hydrocephalus due to obstruction of outflow from the fourth ventricle was treated by ventriculo-atrial shunt, with improvement; no concurrent evidence of sarcoidosis in other organs was found, but there was a granulomatous response to a Kveim test and review of the histology of an enlarged lymph-node removed at earlier cholecystectomy showed non-caseating granulomas. The earliest symptom in a man aged 50 whose case was reported by Höök (1954) was mental deterioration for one year. He was found to have generalized lymphadenopathy, including BHL, and hepatomegaly, and developed a left hemiplegia; at craniotomy, a mass of sarcoid tissue was found in the temporal horn of the right lateral ventricle, arising from the choroid plexus; two years later he was improved, but still mentally dull and with pleocytosis and raised protein in the CSF.

Spinal cord

Granulomas have been found incidentally in the spinal cord or its meninges at necropsy in some cases with symptom-producing sarcoidosis of the brain and its meninges (e.g., Erickson *et al.*, 1942; Walker, 1961, Case 1; Camp and Friersen, 1962; Herring and Urich, 1969, Cases 3 and 5). A number of cases in which histologically confirmed sarcoidosis within the spinal theca has been the principal or only involvement of the central nervous system have been reported.

In Aszkenazy's (1952) Case 1, the lesion was at T 1 level; at necropsy there was thickening of the meninges ventrally, and the affected part of the cord was atrophic and infiltrated with sarcoid granulomas, associated especially with blood-vessels. In the case described by de Morsier *et al.* (1954), a woman aged 61 presented with weakness in all four limbs and extensor plantar responses. The clinical picture resembled that of amyotrophic lateral sclerosis, but electromyography suggested an affection of the muscles. At necropsy nine years later, extensive sarcoid lesions were found in the muscles, and in the liver, spleen, lungs, heart and lymph-nodes; and the meninges and the spinal cord were infiltrated. Jefferson's (1957) case was that of a 66 year old woman who had had left-sided focal fits, diminished in frequency by treatment with phenobarbitone, for three and a half years when she gradually developed a left spastic hemiparesis sparing the face, diminished postural, touch and pain sensation in the left limbs, and a left Horner's syndrome; at laminectomy five years from the onset she was found to have a tumour of the cervical cord, which proved to be a sarcoid granuloma; she died a week later, and at necropsy, sarcoid lesions were found in the cord and the pia-arachnoid in the cervical region, in the lungs, lymph-nodes and liver, but not in the brain. Wood and Bream (1959) described the case of a man, aged 24, with signs of cord compression at T 10 level. He had an abnormal chest radiograph and a positive Kveim test. Laminectomy showed thickening of the arachnoid, which was infiltrated with aggregates of epithelioid cells and scattered lymphocytes. The monozygotic twin of this patient had lymph-node and pulmonary sarcoidosis, but no evidence of nervous system changes. In the case described by Banerjee and Hunt (1972) a black woman aged 36 presented with a four month history of symptoms and signs suggestive of a cervical cord tumour, a myelogram showing narrowing of the spinal canal at C 6–7 level, with widening of the cord; at laminectomy a gelatinous tumour was seen to this site, and as much as possible of it was removed and found to consist of granulomas with some central necrosis; there was some deterioration postoperatively and limited improvement on subsequent treatment with prednisone; outside the nervous system, other evidences of sarcoidosis were BHL and enlargement of lacrimal glands. Semins *et al.* (1972) reported the case of a woman aged 68 with paraparesis shown by myelography to be due to an intramedullary lesion at D 6–9 level; at laminectomy, a mass of tissue was found within the cord and partially removed, and found to contain scattered granulomatous foci with many giant cells, some containing Schaumann bodies, separated by dense astrocytosis; no unequivocal evidence of sarcoidosis elsewhere was found, but there was a recent history of malaise, joint and muscle pain and erythema nodosum, and a tuberculin test was negative; some improvement occurred after corticosteroid treatment. Snyder *et al.* (1976) reported the case of a woman aged 43 with an intramedullary mass in the cord at C 4–5 level, which was partially removed and found to be granulomatous; in spite of some initial improvement on treatment with prednisone, she deteriorated, and died of intercurrent osteomyelitis and septic arthritis of the hip six years from the onset of symptoms; at necropsy, the leptomeninges in the lower cervical and upper thoracic segments were fibrotic and adherent, and the cord enlarged and replaced by firm gelatinous tissue resembling glioma, found histologically to be 'inactive fibrotic granulomas'; no granulomas were found elsewhere in the cord or brain, and the only evidence of sarcoidosis outside the nervous system consisted of enlarged mainly fibrotic hilar lymph-nodes with some peripheral granulomas. Nathan *et al.* (1976) described the cases of two black patients. The first, a woman aged 43, died suddenly of pulmonary embolism after several months of increasing paraplegia; at necropsy, the cervical part of the cord was swollen by 'severe granulomatous panmyelitis and meningitis', with patchy changes of similar sort elsewhere in the cord, a few granulomas only in the hippocampal region of the brain, and granulomas in lungs, liver, spleen, lymph-nodes and kidneys. The second, a man aged 19 with established sarcoidosis, developed paraplegia with a sensory level at T 10, where myelography showed a block; the course was remittent, with a response to prednisone in the fourth episode. Baruah *et al.* (1978) described the case of a black man aged 25 with weakness and numbness of the right arm and both legs who was found at laminectomy at C 3–5 level to have a thick adherent arachnoid with an extramedullary mass antero-lateral to the right side of the cord, histologically showing granulomatous infiltration surrounded by fibrous tissue; other evidence of sarcoidosis was sought, and BHL found radiographically, and granulomas on bronchoscopic lung biopsy; considerable improvement followed corticosteroid treatment. Case 1 of Day and Sypert (1977) was that of a man aged 33 known to have sarcoidosis with BHL and confirmatory biopsy of a lymph-node, when spastic weakness of the left leg which he had noticed for six months was found to be due to an intradural mass adherent to the cord at the level of the T 8–9 intervertebral space; it was partially removed and found to consist of noncaseating granulomas with many giant cells; improvement followed prednisone treatment. Their Case 2 occurred in a black man aged 43 with weakness and numbness in both legs for 12 months, later involving the right arm; BHL was found in the chest radiograph, and liver biopsy showed granulomas; myelography showed an intramedullary mass causing partial block at C 5–6; this was removed as much as possible, and showed histology compatible with sarcoidosis; post-operatively he was quadriplegic, but this gradually improved, so that nine years later, he was quadriparetic but his condition was regarded as stable; response to prednisone treatment was thought to be doubtful. Bernstein and Rival (1978) reported the case of a black man aged 31 in whom pain with hyperaesthesia over the left side of the thorax was found to be due to intramedullary granulomatous infiltration, of which they described only the biopsy findings; a liver biopsy also showed granulomas. Delgado *et al.* (1981) described a case in which the region of the foramen magnum was involved: a black woman aged 37 with a three week history of weakness and numbness in all four limbs was found to have a spastic paraparesis, with a block at C 4–5 on myelography; laminectomy at C 1–4 level showed a firm mass, outside and within the cord extending through and above the cisterna magna; this was removed piecemeal and shown to be a non-caseating epithelioid and giant-cell granuloma; no other localization of sarcoidosis was mentioned.

A number of cases have been reported in which clinical evidence of a spinal cord lesion in a patient with sarcoidosis elsewhere, with improvement either spontaneously or after corticosteroid treatment, has justified a diagnosis of sarcoidosis involving the spinal cord.

Moldover's (1958) case was that of a 24 year old man with symptoms and signs of a spinal lesion in the lower thoracic and upper lumbar segmental level, and a generalized lymphadenopathy, histologically sarcoid; after prolonged intermittent cortisone treatment, the earlier part of which was characterized by suppression of symptoms during treatment with recrudescence on its withdrawal, the neurological signs cleared up. Cases of probable involvement of the spinal cord in sarcoidosis have been reported briefly by Zeman (1951); Siltzbach (1952); Reisner (1944), further information about this case being given by Moldover (1958); and Walker (1961, Case 6). Reisner's patient improved without treatment, and Siltzbach's showed some response to cortisone but relapsed. In a woman aged 33 observed by one of us (JGS), symptoms and signs of spinal myelitis at mid-thoracic segmental level were accompanied by radiographic mottling in the lungs, maximal in the middle zones, and hilar lymph-node enlargement, the skin giving no reaction to 1:10 old tuberculin; both the nervous system symptoms and the lung infiltration improved spontaneously during 18 months' observation. Case 3 of Day and Sypert (1977) was that of a black woman aged 49 with sarcoidosis involving eyes and hilar lymph-nodes, confirmed by lymph-node biopsy, in whom quadriparesis developed; the CSF contained excess protein and lymphocytes, but myelography showed no abormality; the quadriplegia improved rapidly on prednisone treatment, with no residual weakness, and reversion of plantar respones to flexor.

Mixed and anomalous syndromes

In view of the wide range of possible sites of infiltration of sarcoid granuloma in the central nervous system, and of cranial and peripheral nerve involvement, it is not surprising that a great variety of clinical pictures may be produced in this disease. Cases mimicking multiple sclerosis (Zollinger, 1941) and amyotrophic lateral sclerosis (de Morsier *et al.*, 1954)have already been mentioned. In the presence of evidence of sarcoidosis elsewhere, the presumption that a bizarre neurological picture is due to the same disease is high. If the course is favourable, this supports the presumptive diagnosis but removes the possibility of objective proof.

Kahan (1952) reported such a case with left facial weakness, pyramidal signs suggesting a right cerebral hemisphere or brain stem lesion, and sensory changes in the arms suggesting a cervical cord lesion. Howell's (1954) case was thought to have deposits involving the left optic tract and the pyramidal tract in the spinal cord. In Jefferson's (1957) Case 3, lower motor neurone facial palsy and impairment of trigeminal sensory function, both on the right side, severe cerebellar ataxia and papilloedema recovered within a year. In Walker's (1961) Case 7, a man, aged 34, complained of blurring of vision, dysphasia, dizziness and pain in the legs; he was lethargic and somnolent, and showed left ptosis, right facial weakness, brisk tendon reflexes on the right side, and pleocytosis and high protein content in the CSF; and recovered spontaneously. In Höök's (1954) Case 5, dizziness was accompanied by absence of the right ankle jerk and irregular pupils fixed to light and reacting sluggishly to accommodation. Internal ophthalmoplegia and peripheral neuropathy were associated in the cases reported by MacKay (1921), by Critchley and Philips (1924) and by Henkind and Gottlieb (1973). A woman under the care of one of us (JGS) was found to have symptomless hilar lymph-node and pulmonary sarcoidosis at the age of 55; later the lung changes led to some breathlessness, and she complained of headaches and mental slowing; at the age of 63, she was found to have unequal and irregular pupils, the right being larger than the left, reacting poorly to light and briskly to accommodation, and predominantly right-sided Parkinsonian signs, with general immobility of posture and no swing of the right arm on walking. The CSF contained less than one cell mm^{-3} and 56 mg protein dl^{-1}..Because the tuberculin test, initially negative, now gave a brisk response to 10 IU, treatment with antituberculosis drugs was given. One year later, Parkinsonian features were no longer evident; and two years later still, she was noted to be more active mentally, with only occasional headaches, and the shadowing in the chest radiograph had diminished.

Concomitant disease of the central nervous system

It is to be expected that in a few cases of sarcoidosis with its possibly prolonged course unrelated disease of the nervous system will occur. The diagnostic difficulty caused by the occurrence of cerebral tumour in a patient with sarcoidosis is illustrated by the case of concomitant meningioma reported by Rosen and Wang (1965) and mentioned above (p. 318).

A patient with sarcoidosis mainly affecting the upper respiratory tract who late in its course developed multiple sclerosis is reported in Chapter 13 (p. 298).

Wells (1967) referred briefly to a patient who died of motor neurone disease, having had the diagnosis of sarcoidosis confirmed by biopsy 16 years earlier; at necropsy, granulomas were found in lungs and lymph-nodes, but not in the central nervous system.

Progressive multifocal leuco-encephalopathy, a rare disorder, most cases of which have been terminal events in patients with malignant lymphoma or leukaemia (Richardson, 1961), and thought to be due to a viral infection in a host with depressed immune responses, has been reported in a few patients with sarcoidosis. Two of the 22 cases reviewed by Richardson (1961) occurred in patients with sarcoidosis. Javitt and Daniels (1959) reported the complex case of a woman aged 46 who three years from the onset of myasthenia gravis, at first involving principally the eyes with some general weakness and later causing dysphagia, developed erythema nodosum, fever, and pain and swelling of the joints of the hands. She was found to have granulomas in biopsies of the liver, skeletal muscle, and a Kveim test site. Chest radiography showed only evidence of healed apical tuberculosis, and a tuberculin test with 1 IU was positive. Treatment with prednisone was followed by cessation of the need for pyridostigmine which had been required to control the myasthenia, but the period of observation was only a few weeks. Simpson (1960) mentioned that among 440 patients with myasthenia gravis, one 'had sarcoid at the onset'; and Wolf *et al.* (1966) referred to a woman who developed ocular myasthenia gravis at the age of 31, and ten years later was found to have symptomless BHL and pulmonary infiltration, biopsy of a skin lesion showing granulomas. Fiechtner *et al.* (1978) referred briefly to a patient with myasthenia gravis and another with oculocraniosomatic myopathy who were found to have sarcoidosis with BHL and biopsy confirmation.

The significance of these rare associations is doubtful.

Infections of the central nervous system and meninges by known agents – e.g. mycobacteria, cryptococcus – in patients with sarcoidosis are discussed in Chapter 23.

Diagnostic procedures

The diagnosis of the anatomical location and functional effects of changes within the central nervous system follows neurological practice. Here only some special features that have been reported in cases in which changes are attributable to sarcoidosis will be considered.

Cerebro-spinal fluid

Changes in cell count, protein content and pressure of the CSF are in general in accordance with expectations from knowledge of the site and nature of the lesion. The following summary is based on a review of pre-1967 publications reporting findings in the CSF. In patients with infiltration of the cerebral meninges, usually at the base of the brain, with or without intracerebral deposits, the range of values for protein content of the CSF was 90–560 mg dl^{-1}, and for the cell content 6–250 mm^{-3} with a single exceptional value of 6000. Where the lesion took the form predominantly of a local deposit in the brain, the CSF was less abnormal; the protein content in eight such cases ranged up to 120 mg dl^{-1} and the cell-count up to 13 mm^{-3}.

When the spinal cord was affected, the CSF changes depended principally upon the degree of spinal block; in Walker's (1961) Case 6, the protein content ranged up to 2360 mg dl^{-1}, with a normal cell content; Moldover (1958) found protein 128 mg dl^{-1} and 4 cells mm^3; and Jefferson (1957, Case 7) found protein 128 mg dl^{-1} and 66 mm^{-3} cells. In nine patients with predominantly cranial nerve palsies the findings ranged from normal figures for both protein and cells to 140 mg dl^{-1} and 68 mm^{-3} respectively. Among four with polyneuritis, the protein tended to be higher, ranging up to 720 mg dl^{-1}, and the cell content about the same, ranging up to 52 mm^{-3}. It is possible, of course, that in some of these meningeal infiltration may have been an additional factor.

Gaines *et al.* (1970) reviewed 57 patients with sarcoidosis of the central nervous system, and found that 72% had raised cell counts, 70% high protein content, and 18% low glucose content in the CSF. In their patient with hydrocephalus due to obstruction to outflow from the fourth ventricle, presumably due to meningeal infiltration (see above, p. 314) the glucose content of the CSF was 25 mg dl^{-1}, the level in the blood being 84 mg. In 20 patients reported by Delaney (1977), 10 had pleocytosis, with cell counts ranging from 8–300 mm^{-3}, 14 had high protein levels, ranging from 50–1000 mg dl^{-1}, and four low glucose content; in six levels of all three were normal. Opening pressure at lumbar puncture was raised in five.

Radiological findings
Radiological findings in sarcoidosis of the central nervous system have been discussed by Saltzman (1958), Lawrence *et al.* (1974), Lukin *et al.* (1975) and Bahr *et al.* (1978). Case 3 of Lawrence *et al.* is of interest in that carotid angiography showed multiple short narrowings with intervening dilatation in the anterior and middle cerebral arteries, suggesting granulomatous angiitis. Radio-isotope scanning has been used to demonstrate enhanced uptake at areas of sarcoid granulomatosis (Schwartz and Baum, 1968; Vitye *et al.*, 1969; McCartney *et al.*, 1979). The use of computer assisted tomography has been described by Bahr *et al.* (1978), Babu *et al.* (1979), Brooks *et al.* (1979), Decker *et al.* (1979), Ho *et al.* (1979) and Kumpe *et al.* (1979). In general, granulomatous masses appear as areas of high attenuation enhancing after intravenous contrast medium injection. Diminution in size of such areas after corticosteroid treatment has been reported, and regarded as confirmatory of the diagnosis of sarcoidosis (Bahr *et al.*, 1978, Case 1; Brooks *et al.*, 1979; Ho *et al.*, 1979). In the case of meningioma in a patient with sarcoidosis reported by Rosen and Wang (1965) diminution in the area of enhanced radio-isotope uptake after corticosteroid treatment was misleading, suggesting the erroneous initial diagnosis of basal meningeal sarcoidosis.

Electro-encephalography (EEG)

Reported EEG changes in sarcoidosis of the CNS have been concordant with the anatomical distribution of lesions. Niitu *et al.* (1974a) reported the results of EEG in 28 patients with intrathoracic sarcoidosis, of whom all but one had BHL. Although no patient had clinical evidence of CNS involvement, nine EEG records were regarded as abnormal; of six with abnormal records who were followed for periods up to two years, abnormalities disappeared in three and diminished in two. These findings were compatible with the anatomical distribution of lesions. Niitu *et al.* (1974a) reported the lessly disseminated in the CNS in a proportion of patients, and subsequently resolve spontaneously in the majority of those affected.

Treatment

The effect of treatment is difficult to assess, in view of the variable and unpredictable natural course. It is useful to distinguish among patients with sarcoidosis involving the nervous system between those at a labile stage, capable of resolution, and often accompanied by changes with similar characteristics in other organs, and those belonging to a generally later stage of the disease when the clinically important changes tend to be localized in one organ, to include irreversible fibrotic elements incapable of resolution, and to be liable to continued activity. Patients with cranial and peripheral neuropathies as the principal feature generally fall into the first group; it is possible that in some of them the nerves are not infiltrated by granulomas; and there is a strong tendency to spontaneous recovery and to respond to the suppressive effects of corticosteroid treatment. In other cases, with meningeal, cerebral or spinal granulomatous infiltrations, associated features may suggest the probability of their belonging to one or other of those prognostic groups, but only observation of the natural course or of response to corticosteroid treatment justifies a conclusion on this point.

Difficulty in assessing the results of treatment applies especially to surgery, which has been undertaken in some cases to establish diagnosis where it remains in doubt after less invasive investigation, and in others to relieve symptoms arising from obstructive hydrocephelus or from tumour-like masses involving the brain or spinal cord. Many of the cases in which surgery has been undertaken have been prognostically unfavourable, and few reports give information about long-term results. Of the 102 published cases of intracranial sarcoidosis which we have reviewed (p.312), 46 were explored surgically. In 11 of these, only biopsy was performed, with three post-operative deaths. In 27 removal of granulomatous masses, inevitably partial but usually stated to be as complete as possible, was undertaken; among these there were five post-operative deaths, improvement was noted after the operation in ten, in one marked, and there was no improvement after operation in 12 surviving patients; six later deaths were recorded. In eight cases, shunt operations for relief of hydrocephalus were performed, with three post-operative and two later deaths; and improvement was noted in only four. Of four cases submitted only to needle biopsy of the brain, two died after the procedure. It must be remembered that these published cases include a high proportion in which the diagnosis was not established, or in some suspected, pre-operatively.

Sarcoidosis within the spinal theca presents an even more intractable problem for the surgeon, with diffuse infiltration of the leptomeninges, sometimes forming localized masses, usually adherent to the cord and surrounding nerve-roots, and infiltration of the cord causing enlargement and sometimes more or less localized masses. We have reviewed 11 published cases in which laminectomy was performed; piecemeal removal was attempted in ten, biopsy only being undertaken in one. In three there was deterioration post-operatively, with increase in extent and degree of paresis. In those in which improvement was observed, corticosteroid treatment was given post-operatively.

It seems that for most patients with a strong presumption of sarcoidosis of the central nervous system surgery has little to offer, and that if a surgical procedure appears to be indicated – e.g. for the relief of hydrocephalus or the removal of a mass producing local epileptic or other symptoms – the possible benefits of corticosteroid treatment should be explored before it is undertaken.

The effect of corticosteroid treatment is suppressive, and confined to still active granulomas and associated cellular reactions, whatever tissue is involved (Chapter 27). Review of published reports and scattered personal experience suggests that more cases of sarcoidosis of the central nervous system than of other organs respond poorly or not at all to corticosteroid treatment; and in view of the pathological features and location of the lesions in some cases, this is not surprising. Whether the response will be favourable can be determined only by trial. If it is favourable, with relief of symptoms, treatment must be continued as long as activity of the disease persists; and this also can be determined only by trial. Of the 102 reports of intracranial sarcoidosis we have reviewed, information about response to corticosteroid treatment is given in 27, unfortunately only about short-term response in most. Useful long-term improvement was noted in eight, there was no response in six, and initial improvement, either transient or during a limited period of observation, in 13; among these 27 cases, there were 11 later recorded deaths. Of 13 reports in which response of sarcoidosis of the spinal cord or its meninges was mentioned, useful long-term response with substantial restoration of function was observed in two, and with some improvement in three; some improvement during limited periods of observation in seven; and no response in one; two later deaths were recorded.

In view of the unpredictable natural course of sarcoidosis, it is probable that those patients with involvement of the central nervous system who do not relapse after an initial good response to corticosteroid treatment are those who would have experienced a natural remission even without previous suppression of the activity of the disease. A trial of corticosteroid treatment is indicated if symptoms are persistent and severe; if they are relieved or improved, the duration of treatment can be determined only by occasional trial of withdrawal; and if response is partial, the benefits of continued treatment must be balanced against the side-effects of long-term corticosteroid treatment.

Chapter 15

The Heart

Sarcoidosis may affect the heart either directly by granulomatous infiltration of the myocardium, the conducting tissues, and more rarely the pericardium, or secondarily to involvement of the lungs, leading to pulmonary hypertension, right venticular hypertrophy, strain and eventual failure. The latter presents a clinical and functional picture similar to that occurring with other sorts of chronic lung disease and, apart from a few cases with extensive granulomatous changes in pulmonary arteries, requires only brief discussion in the present context. Direct involvement of the heart causes symptoms in only a small minority of patients known to have sarcoidosis, but in these it may present remarkable features, including a disturbing liability to sudden death; and sarcoidosis of the heart without evident involvement of other organs may present clinically with arrhythmias, conduction defects, congestive heart failure of obscure cause, or a picture suggesting myocardial infarction, or to the pathologist as sudden death in a previously symptom-free individual. Many published reports are of single or a few cases presenting in one of these remarkable ways. Reports of larger numbers of personally studied cases, with reviews, have been published by Fleming (1974), Roberts *et al.* (1977) and Silverman *et al.* (1978).

Frequency of cardiac involvement

It is probable that in many cases of sarcoidosis at least a few granulomas are present in the myocardium in the active stage without causing symptoms, as in skeletal muscle and many other tissues, but the proportion is unknown. If so, these granulomas presumably resolve spontaneously in most cases; and the only evidence of their presence likely to be obtained clinically is that provided by electrocardiography (ECG). Mikhail *et al.* (1974) studied 147 cases routinely and found 14 with ECG abnormalities. In three, these were thought to be due to unrelated cardiac disease. In ten, there were no symptoms related to the heart; all had various combinations of T wave and ST interval changes, and seven prolongation of PR interval in the acute stage, all of which resolved later. Only one had symptoms referable to sarcoidosis of the heart, developing ventricular tachycardia ten months after the diagnosis of hilar lymph-node and pulmonary sarcoidosis, soon after the start of corticosteroid treatment for deterioration in the pulmonary infiltration. The tachycardia was controlled by practolol, with continuation of the corticosteroid, and did not recur during one year's further observation. Stein *et al.* (1973) surveyed 80 patients aged under 40 years attending a sarcoidosis clinic, with no history or present clinical evidence of cardiac disease or hypertension. ECG was regarded as abnormal in 41; disturbances of rhythm and conduction were observed in 15, the most frequent being prologation beyond 0.2 sec of the PR interval, and minor repolarization abnormalities in 26. These changes could not be correlated with ethnic group, sex, duration of sarcoidosis, radiographic grouping of lung changes, or treatment.

In unselected clinical series of patients with sarcoidosis, the number showing clinical evidence of granulomatous changes in the heart is small. In 500 consecutive patients under the care of one of us (JGS), four showed such evidence. In three of these, the diagnosis of cardiac sarcoidosis was presumptive, consisting in the development of otherwise unexplained complete heart block in a man aged 21 with pulmonary, lymph-node and splenic involvement; unexplained congestive cardiac failure in a woman aged 47 with chronic pulmonary, bronchial mucosal and lymph-node sarcoidosis; and cardiomegaly with persistent but initially variable T wave changes in leads $V_4 - V_6$ of the ECG in a man with sarcoid BHL. The fourth, a man who developed ventricular arrhythmia and bundle branch block six years after the symptomless onset of intrathoracic sarcoidosis, and died suddenly eight years later, is described more fully below.

In necropsy studies of sarcoidosis, the proportion of cases with granulomas in the heart is much higher than the proportion of known cases of sarcoidosis with symptoms caused by cardiac involvement during life. This is not only because of the incidental finding of granulomas in the heart in patients dying from other manifestations of sarcoidosis, but also because of the inclusion of cases in which sudden death was the first evidence of disease of any sort, or of cardiac involvement in patients with sarcoidosis. Longcope and Freiman (1952) found the myocardium involved in four of their 30 fatal cases, and in 18 of 92 necropsies in cases of sarcoidosis reported by others. Of 50 cases of cardiac sarcoidosis occurring in the United Kingdom, reviewed by Fleming (1974), 20 were fatal; in 14 of these the diagnosis of sarcoidosis had not been made in life. Matsui *et al.* (1976) studied material from 72 cases reported as sarcoid or giant-cell myocarditis in Japan, and finally diagnosed 42 as myocardial sarcoidosis; in only five of these had the diagnosis of sarcoidosis been made during life, and death had been sudden in 16. Roberts *et al.* (1977) reviewed 113 necropsy cases of cardiac sarcoidosis, 35 personally studied at the US National Institutes of Heath, and 78 reported by others. In 24 of these 113 cases, myocardial involvement found at necropsy was not thought to have been a cause of death; among the 89 in which it was the cause of death, the diagnosis of sarcoidosis had been made during life in only 24, and death had been sudden in 60. Silverman *et al.* (1978) reviewed 84 consecutive necropsies on patients with sarcoidosis at the Johns Hopkins Hospital, including 12 of those previously reported by Longcope and Freiman (1952); they found myocardial involvement in 23. A more general perspective is given in the report by Abelen (1975) based upon 2950 consecutive necropsies at a general hospital in Oslo. Sarcoidosis was found in 13; the heart was involved in two of these, and in neither had the diagnosis of sarcoidosis been made during life.

PATHOLOGY

Review of published descriptions of pathology of sarcoidosis of the heart suggests that a useful distinction can be made between cases in which the changes are evident only microscopically and those in which they are visible to the naked eye. Scattered microscopic granulomas have been found most frequently in patients with sarcoidosis who have died from involvement of other organs or from unrelated diseases. When local confluence of granulomas has led to massive replacement of myocardium visible to the naked eye, this involvement of the heart has generally been the cause of death. Of the 35 cases of cardiac sarcoidosis studied by Roberts *et al.* (1977), 26 had shown symptoms attributable to this finding; in all 26 there were grossly visible changes in the heart, consisting in pale areas of granulomatous replacement of myocardium in 25 and transmural scars without coronary artery disease in one. In the remaining nine with scattered discrete granulomas only, this cardiac involvement was not thought to be a cause of death, although extensive pulmonary sarcoidosis had led to cor pulmonale in four, and three had other forms of heart disease. Silverman *et al.* (1978) classified the pathological findings in their 23 cases as mild in 19 and severe with grossly visible changes in four. In all four classified as severe, death had been sudden and was attributed to cardiac sarcoidosis; in those with mild changes, there had been a high incidence of cardiac arrhythmias, and death was attributed in some to cor pulmonale and in some to non-sarcoid heart disease, but in none was sarcoid involvement of the heart thought to be the cause of death.

Sites of cardiac involvement

The myocardium, especially of the ventricles and interventricular septum, is the common site of cardiac granulomas. The epicardium and endocardium are rarely involved except by extension from the myocardium, though a very few cases of pericardial effusion have been recorded. The valves are very rarely directly involved, though mitral incompetence due to papillary muscle involvement may occur. Exceptionally, the great vessels may show granulomatous changes; pulmonary hypertension may result from such changes in pulmonary arteries.

In the myocardium, the parts most often affected by grossly visible changes are the left ventricular free wall, the interventricular septum and the papillary muscles, especially on the left side; the right ventricular wall is rather less often, and the atria relatively rarely, involved. Reviewing the distribution of visible changes in the heart in 69 cases in which cardiac sarcoidosis had caused dysfunction, 25 personally observed and 44 reported with sufficiently detailed necropsy findings, Roberts *et al.* (1977) found the left ventricle affected in 94%, the interventricular septum in 75%, the right ventricle in 40%, the papillary muscles in 42%, the right atrium in 16% and the left atrium in 13%. In nine personally studied cases in which they found granulomas microscopically only, without naked-eye changes, the left ventricle was affected in all, the septum in two, the right ventricle in five and the atria in none.

Parts of the heart infiltrated by confluent granulomas appear to the naked eye as pale areas of varying size and usually irregular outline, contrasting sharply with adjacent normal myocardium, both on its epicardial and endocardial surfaces and in cut sections. In the ventricles they tend to extend through a considerable part of the thickness of myocardium, and may replace the whole of it. Such massive replacement may be accompanied by scattered smaller areas elsewhere. The upper part of the interventricular septum is more often affected than its lower apical part; this correlates with the frequency of disturbances of conduction. Several necropsy cases of aneurysmal dilatation of the ventricles at the site of extensive sarcoid replacement have been reported, most of them involving the left ventricle (Hines and Sancetta, 1963; Duvernoy and Garcia, 1971; Morales *et al.*, 1974; Chun *et al.*, 1975; James, 1977, Case 2; Roberts *et al.*, 1977, two cases); the right ventricle may become similarly thinned and dilated (Clark and Blount, 1966; Harthorne and Freiman, 1975). The aneurysmal wall may consist of no more than a thin layer of connective tissue, all granulomas having undergone fibrosis; some residual granulomas are found in most cases.

The atria are less frequently affected than the ventricles, and when they are, generally show small scattered infiltrations rather than massive confluence of granulomas.

Sarcoid granulomas in the heart appear to undergo a similar evolution to those elsewhere, from a fresh epithelioid and giant-cell non-caseating tubercle to hyaline fibrosis in which the typical appearances are lost; but survey of the recorded cases suggests that the appearances are more frequently atypical in the myocardium than elsewhere. This can perhaps be attributed to modification by the rhythmic contractile activity of the myocardium. In several cases, the myocardium has presented either an unspecific granuloma or a patchy hyaline fibrosis with little remnant of the characteristic granuloma, although other organs contained better-defined sarcoid tubercles (Spencer and Warren, 1938; Jonas, 1939; Güthert and Hübner, 1944; Kulka, 1950; Adickes *et al.*, 1951; Oille *et al.*, 1953; Stephen, 1954; Porter, 1960). In one of the cases studied by Roberts *et al.* (1977) transmural myocardial scars without coronary artery disease were accepted as the end-result of earlier granulomatous replacement. Matsui *et al.* (1976) in their study of 42 fatal cases commented that in myocardial sarcoidosis the granuloma is less well defined than in other organs, and found fibrotic changes in most of their cases; lymphocytic infiltration and oedema might be prominent, and was the principal change in one case; granulomas without fibrosis were seen in six, and with fibrosis in 21; and in 11 cases, the principal change was fibro-hyaline.

Ferrans *et al.* (1965) described histochemical and electron-microscopic studies of the myocardium in a black man who died at the age of 25 from intractable cardiac failure with ventricular arrhythmias and varying atrioventricular block. At necropsy, sarcoid granulomas were found in lungs and hilar lymph-nodes, and in confluent areas in the heart, in the interventricular septum, both ventricles and the left atrium. Myocardium not involved by granulomas showed degenerative changes in myofilaments, mitochondrial swelling and disruption of some mitochondria, and loss of mitochondrial enzymes, with many mast cells in the zone adjacent to granulomas; lipid droplets and increase in pinocytotic vesicles were seen in some capillaries. Some of these changes were thought to be irreversible; intensive corticosteroid treatment had been given, and complicated the interpretation of these findings.

Valves

The most frequently observed valve dysfunction is mitral incompetence, from weakness of affected papillary muscles. This is discussed below.

Direct involvement of cardiac valves appears to be very rare. Of the few reports suggestive of such changes, most are inconclusive.

Cotter (1939) reported the case of a black man, aged 18, who died of right ventricular failure after a brief illness. At necropsy, extensive sarcoidosis involving lungs, heart, liver, spleen, testis, gut and subcutaneous tissue was found. The myocardium of the left ventricle showed many irregular areas of confluent sarcoid infiltration; on the contact surface of the aortic cusp of the mitral valve were several greyish nodules, the histology of which was not described. Simkins (1951) described the necropsy findings in a woman who died in a Stokes-Adams attack at the age of 50; there was extensive myocardial sarcoidosis, with thickening of the endocardium just below the aortic valve and a few vegetations in the valve with irregular thickening of the cusps of aortic and mitral valves; no details of the histology of the valves was given, but an illustration shows fibrosing granulomas at the base of the aortic valve. Deneberg (1965) reported the case of a black man who died at the age of 51 after a five month illness characterized by arrhythmias, principally atrial flutter, initial fever, loss of weight and dry cough, and terminal thrombo-embolic disease with renal infarction. At necropsy, extensive sarcoidosis, with fibrosis, was found in the lungs and hilar lymph-nodes, and some granulomas in the liver; there were pericardial adhesions, and many areas of fibrosis in the myocardium of the left ventricle and septum, and thickening of one cusp of the mitral valve, with thrombus on the edge of the valve and in the left atrial appendage. Histologically, the myocardial changes were found to be granulomatous; the aorta showed minimal atherosclerosis; there were many granulomas in the adventitia, partly involving the media. Sales (1953) found the aortic valve stenosed in a black man aged 20 who died of severe myocardial sarcoidosis, but did not report the histology of the valve. Laroche *et al.* (1955) described the case of a man who died at the age of 40 after an illness lasting three years, with relapsing febrile polyarthritis, hepatosplenomegaly, tachycardia and terminal cardiac failure; lymph-node and tonsillar biopsies showed non-caseating epithelioid and giant-cell tubercles. At necropsy the heart weighed 620 g; the pericardium was adherent; the cusps of the mitral valve were ulcerated with irregular vegetations, the tricuspid showed a few vegetations, and the aortic and pulmonary valves were normal. Histologically the vegetations were fibrinous; the endocardium was thickened with fibrosis, leucocytic infiltrations, and a few epithelioid nodules, and similar nodules were seen in myocardium and pericardium. Faivre *et al.* (1956) reported the case of a man, aged 42, who after a three year illness with low fever, enlargement of lymph-nodes, histologically sarcoid, joint pains and dyspnoea, died in cardiac failure with mitral and aortic valve disease. At necropsy, there was a mitral and aortic endocarditis characterized by firm nodular thickening of the edges of the valves. Histologically, the aortic valve vegetations consisted of a deeper zone of vascular connective tissue with lymphocytes, some plasma cells and fibroblasts, and a more superficial zone formed of a background of hyalinized fibrin with a few fibroblasts enmeshing large histiocytes; no micro-organisms were seen. The myocardium showed unspecific changes, and the histology of other organs was not described.

In the absence of unequivocal histological evidence, it must remain doubtful whether the changes found in the heart at necropsy in the latter three cases were attributable to sarcoidosis. The occasional coincidence of sarcoidosis with heart disease of unrelated cause is to be expected, especially since it is known that many cases of asymptomatic sarcoidosis coming to light as a result of screening procedures resolve spontaneously; and several cases in which evidence of sarcoidosis was found in patients with unrelated heart disease have been recorded.

Thorbjarnarson and Glenn (1956) reported the case of a man, aged 48, with mitral stenosis. A valvotomy was performed; two much enlarged lymph-nodes were found at the aortic arch; the mitral valve, less than 1 cm^2 in cross-section was split, but the patient died from cardiac arrest. At necropsy, the diagnosis of rheumatic heart disease was confirmed, Aschoff bodies being found in the left auricle, the left ventricle and the interventricular septum; there were also many non-caseating epithelioid and giant-cell granulomas in the mediastinal and pancreatic lymph-nodes and a few in the myocardium and epicardium; the lung showed 'marked fibrosis and arteriolar sclerosis'. Botti and Young (1959) found both sarcoid and rheumatic changes in the heart at necropsy in a woman, aged 32, who presented with complete heart block causing Stokes-Adams attacks, and aortic valve disease. She died in asystole 60 hours after aortic valvotomy. At necropsy there was rheumatic mitral stenosis, aortic stenosis and tricuspid valvulitis, and a few Aschoff bodies were found in the myocardium. The atrioventricular node and bundle were destroyed by infiltration with sarcoid granulomas, some including asteroids; and similar granulomas were found in the lungs, liver, spleen and lymph-nodes. Tice *et al.* (1967) recorded the case of a black woman, aged 18, with tetralogy of Fallot, in whom enlarged hilar shadows were found to be due in part to large lymph-nodes, and scalene node biopsy showed non-caseating granulomas; at operation for complete repair, myocardial biopsy showed 'collections of lymphocytes, epithelial histiocytes and giant cells' and scattered zones of relatively acellular fibrosis. The report does not mention the operative appearance of the hilar nodes. Case 6 of Ghosh *et al.* (1972) was that of a man aged 38, known to have had aortic valve disease for many years; the tissue removed at aortic valve replacement contained granulomas; he died six months later from subacute bacterial endocarditis, and at necropsy, similar granulomas were found in the liver and the spleen. One of us (JGS) was consulted about a man aged 50 about to undergo valve replacement for calcific aortic stenosis, in whom the chest radiograph had shown a widespread pulmonary mottling. Biopsy of the lung at the operation showed a mainly pre-fibrotic sarcoid infiltration. The post-operative course was uneventful, and the infiltration spontaneously resolved.

Roberts *et al.* (1977) found calcium deposits in the mitral valve ring in one of their patients, aged 34, with cardiac sarcoidosis, and mentioned another with sarcoidosis and heavy calcification in the mitral ring but without granulomas or scars in the myocardium; both had had severe hypercalcaemia and had been treated with corticosteroids.

Great vessels

Involvement of the adventitia of the aorta in a patient with extensive myocardial sarcoidosis reported by Deneberg (1965) has been mentioned above. Sarcoid tubercles were found in the aorta in Case 1 of Jonas (1939) and Case 4 of Powell (1954), and in the superior vena cava and pulmonary veins in Case 1 of Powell (1954). Matsui *et al.* (1976) in their review of 42 fatal cases of cardiac sarcoidosis noted that the adventitia of the aorta was involved in four, and the pulmonary artery in three. In rare cases widespread involvement of small pulmonary arteries causes pulmonary hypertension (p. 346 below; Chapter 6, p. 107 and p. 163).

Pericardium

Although sparse granulomas in both visceral and parietal pericardium have been recorded in a number of cases as part of more widespread cardiac sarcoidosis, gross changes in the pericardium are rare. Pericardial effusion (see below) has been recorded during life (Schiff *et al.*, 1969; Gozo *et al.*, 1971). Matsui *et al.* (1976) in their 41 necropsy cases noted that visible nodules were frequent in the epicardium, but were seen in the pericardium in only three cases, haemorrhagic pericardial effusion being present in one. Two of the 35 necropsy patients studied by Roberts *et al.* (1977) had had recurrent pericardial effusion; both were found to have sarcoid granulomas in the parietal pericardium and in the left ventricular myocardium.

Conducting tissues

The liability of the upper part of the interventricular septum to be the site of heavy granulomatous infiltration is likely to be a factor in determining the frequency of atrioventricular and bundle-branch block. Morales *et al.* (1974) made special studies of the conducting tissues in four cases in which sarcoidosis of the heart had led to sudden death, preceded by observed ventricular tachycardia in one and supraventricular tachycardia followed by ventricular fibrillation in one. Large parts of the conducting tissues were affected, granulomas with lymphocytic infiltration and fibrosis being observed in two and fibrosis and lymphocytic infiltration in two. Roberts *et al.* (1977) studied serial sections of the atrioventricular node and bundle in one of their patients with complete heart block, and found complete destruction of the node with disruption of the bundle branches from their origin. James (1977) found, in the heart of a black woman aged 30 who had died suddenly after two years of syncopal attacks from ventricular arrhythmia, a left ventricular aneurysm whose wall showed both granulomas and fibrosis; there were foci of sarcoid granulomas in the sino-atrial and atrioventricular nodes, and fatty change in the bundle of His; additionally, while large coronary arteries were normal, small branches were narrowed by sarcoid granulomas. Abeler (1979) studied the myocardium in the region of the pace-making and conducting tissues in nine patients who had died of or with sarcoidosis. In a woman who had died suddenly at the age of 52, sarcoid granulomas were found in heart, lungs, liver, spleen, lymph-nodes and bone-marrow; in the sinus node region, confluent granulomas replaced pacemaker fibres, and in the septum, subendocardial granulomas interrupted the left bundle branch. In a woman aged 71 who died of aortic valve stenosis and myocardial ischaemia, widespread sarcoid granulomas, mostly hyalinized, were an incidental finding; there were some in the interventricular septum near to but not involving the conducting tissues. No cardiac granulomas were seen in the other seven patients.

Association with sarcoidosis of other organs

When sarcoidosis involves the heart extensively, cardiac symptoms tend to dominate the clinical picture. Pathologically, gross cardiac sarcoidosis may or may not be accompanied by obvious changes in other organs. In some cases, myocardial sarcoidosis is part of florid granulomatosis involving many organs, including the central nervous system (Vogt, 1949; Clinicopathological Conference, 1957; Poon and Forbus, 1959). Longcope and Freiman (1952) noted the frequency with which the heart had been found to be infiltrated by sarcoid in the recorded necropsies on patients with uveoparotid fever (Souter, 1929; Garland and Thompson, 1933; Granström *et al.*, 1946; Bates and Walsh, 1948; van Rijssel, 1947, Case 1; Adickes *et al.*, 1951; Yesner and Silver, 1951; Longcope and Freiman, 1952, Case 16). On the other hand, others (Fleming, 1974; Roberts *et al.*, 1977; Virmani *et al.*, 1980) have commented on the rarity of clinically evident cardiac involvement in patients with symptomatic sarcoidosis of other organs. This variable relationship to changes in other organs is not peculiar to the heart. Sarcoidosis of the lungs, the skin, the eyes or the lymph-nodes may similarly present with predominant involvement of one involved site or as part of an evidently widespread disease; and in liver and skeletal muscle, granulomatous infiltration is known to be frequent in generalized sarcoidosis but rarely causes symptoms, and when it does tends to produce obvious symptoms and signs which may or may not be accompanied by others referable to other organs.

At necropsy, granulomatous changes in the heart, especially if they are partly hyalinized, cannot be categorized with certainty unless they are accompanied by granulomas of sarcoid type in other organs, or there is a history of recognized manifestations of sarcoidosis in the past, preferably with histological confirmation.

Giant-cell myocarditis

The number of giant cells found in sarcoidosis in the myocardium, as elsewhere, is very variable. Several reports have emphasized the large numbers that were present – e.g. Garland and Thompson (1933), Cotter (1939), Adickes *et al.* (1951), Forbes and Usher (1962). Giant cells have been seen in the hearts of patients with infective endocarditis, rheumatoid arthritis,

Takayasu's arteritis and Wegener's granulomatosis (Roberts *et al.*, 1977), but form only a small element in a generally recognizable clinico-pathological picture. Granulomatous giant-cell myocarditis, in which the granulomatous process is found only in the heart, or predominantly in the heart, with minor changes in one or a few other organs, has been described. In some of these, not only has the distribution of the granulomatous inflammation in the heart been similar to that observed in undoubted cases of sarcoidosis with cardiac involvement, but granulomas have been found in one or more other sites (Gentzen, 1937; Hirayama, 1939; Didion, 1943); Long, 1961; one of 11 cases reported by Davies *et al.*, 1975; in such cases, there is little reason to question correctness of categorization as sarcoidosis. In Case 3 of Lindvall *et al.* (1978) giant-cell myocarditis localized in the upper part of the interventricular septum was accompanied by a similar giant-cell granuloma in the hypophysis, which is another organ in which localized giant- cell granulomas have been reported (Chapter 16). In a case reported by Kean and Koekenga (1952), giant-cell myocarditis of similar distribution to that seen in sarcoidosis was accompanied by caseation in broncho-pulmonary lymph-nodes in which no micro-organisms were found. In some cases, such as those reported by Tesluk (1956), Dilling (1956), Collyns (1959), Rab *et al.* (1978), most of those of Davies *et al.* (1975) and cases 1 and 2 of Lindvall *et al.*, (1978) the organs commonly affected in sarcoidosis have been shown to contain no granulomas, and in the heart the principal changes has been inflammatory fibrosis with destruction of myocardial cells and many giant cells, and only poorly-formed tuberculoid granulomas. In such cases, there may be changes in other organs suggesting a systemic disease known to include a granulo-matous element; if not, the possibility that the inflammatory changes in the heart are a peculiar reaction to a localized, possibly infective, cause cannot be excluded.

CLINICAL FEATURES

Although the presence of sarcoid granulomas in the heart cannot usually be proved during life, the occurrence of symptoms and signs suggestive of an infiltrative process in the myocardium in a patient with active sarcoidosis and without evidence of any other disease which might account for the cardiac changes is generally sufficient to justify a clinical diagnosis of cardiac sarcoidosis. Discussion of the clinical features of cardiac sarcoidosis must therefore be based upon studies in which these criteria have been met, as well as those in which direct histological examination of the heart itself has been possible. As already noted, in clinical series of patients with sarcoidosis, either as far as possible unselected or selected for involvement of another organ, the number with evident cardiac involvement is very low.

Table 15.1 Numbers of cases of cardiac sarcoidosis in two reported series showing various clinical features. Fleming (1980): mostly clinically diagnosed, 33% confirmed or first diagnosed at necropsy. Roberts *et al.* (1977): all diagnosed at necropsy, about one-quarter during life.

	Fleming (1980)		Roberts et al. (1977)	
Number of cases	163		89	
	No.	%	No.	%
Diagnosis of sarcoidosis				
during life		[>72, <84]	24	27
Necropsies	53	33	all	
Complete heart block	31	19	25	28
Partial, including bundle branch				
block	56	34	35	39
Ventricular premature beats or				
tachycardia	64	39	52	58
Supraventricular tachycardia	35	21	15	17
Congestive heart failure			35	39
Myocardial disease	34	21 }27		
Simulating myocardial infarction	10	6 }27		
Valve involvement	3	2		
Pericardial involvement	2	1	3	3
Dead at time of report	70	43	89	100
Sudden deaths				
without previous illness	26	37* }64*	10	11 }67
with previous illness	19	27* }64*	50	56 }67
Death in road traffic accident	3	4*		

*Percentage of fatal cases

The principal clinical features in two published series of cases of symptomatic cardiac sarcoidosis are summarized in Table 15.1. Fleming's (1980) series consists of cases seen by him in East Anglia and those reported to him from other parts of the United Kingdom; cardiac sarcoidosis was confirmed or first diagnosed at necropsy in 53 and based upon clinical findings in the other 110. From the review by Roberts *et al.* (1977), the 89 cases in which cardiac sarcoidosis confirmed or found at necropsy was thought to have caused symptoms during life have been selected; 26 of these were studied by Roberts *et al.*, and 63 compiled from previous publications. In spite of the different ways in which these two series were collected, and reliance upon clinical diagnosis in many cases in one of them, the proportions showing during life disturbances of conduction, impulse formation and rhythm and evidence of myocardial disease, if 'congestive cardiac failure' is accepted as cognate with this, are strikingly similar, as are the proportions of deaths that were sudden.

The ages of the patients with symptomatic cardiac sarcoidosis in these two series was similar, ranging from 18–77 years (mean 45) in Fleming's, and 18–76 in that of Roberts *et al.* In both series the numbers of men and women were approximately equal. Among the 24 patients reviewed by Roberts *et al.* with cardiac sarcoidosis not causing dysfunction and discovered at necropsy, on the other hand, 16 were men and only eight women.

This age-range, throughout adult life, is extended by a few cases reported in children. The youngest appears to have been a black girl who died at the age of six years (Taussig and Oppenheimer, 1936; Jonas, 1939, Case 2).

At the age of five, she was found to have sickle-cell anaemia with a haemoglobin level of 35%, and cervical lymphadenitis. She was treated by blood transfusions, one of which unfortunely transmitted syphilis to her; for this she received appropriate treatment. At the age of six, she was found to have a generalized papular rash, generalized superficial lymphadenopathy, a very large spleen and enlargement of the heart with a systolic murmur. She died of cardiac failure. Tubercle-like lesions were found in the lungs, bronchial and abdominal lymph-nodes; in the heart there was macroscopically diffuse yellow mottling, and microscopically dense infiltration with monocytes, some destruction of muscle, and some collections of epithelioid and a few giant cells. Although some of the tubercles showed some central necrosis, no acid-fast bacilli were found. Serwer *et al.* (1978) reported the case of a black girl aged 12 who presented with ventricular tachycardia and congestive heart failure; cervical and inguinal lymph-nodes were enlarged and biopsy showed sarcoid-type granulomas. Treatment with quinidine and diuretics relieved symptoms; prednisone initially was followed by multiple ventricular premature beats, and was discontinued. Eighteen months later, she developed uveitis and skin nodules shown on biopsy to be sarcoids. Prednisone led to resolution of these without recurrence of premature beats.

At the other extreme of life is a case recorded by Pascoe (1964), in a white man aged 83, who had had occasional chest pain and some shortness of breath for several years when he was admitted to hospital because of weakness and confusion for four days. He was found to have some peripheral oedema, enlargement of the liver and cardiac irregularity thought to be due to atrial fibrillation; the morning after admission, he was found dead in bed. At necropsy, the coronary arteries showed moderate atheroma, but were patent throughout. The myocardium appeared normal, but microscopically many granulomas were found near vessels in the myocardium, and also in lung, mediastinal lymph-nodes, liver and spleen.

Sudden death

In about one-third of published cases of sudden death attributable to sarcoidosis of the heart there had been no illness preceding the fatal event, neither sarcoidosis nor cardiac disease being recognized during life. The lower proportion without recognized previous illness in the series of Roberts *et al.* (1977) may have been due to its including fewer patients who died outside hospital than Fleming's. Fleming drew attention to the fact that three in his series died in road traffic accidents, and speculated whether in at least one of these (Fleming, 1974, Case 7) the accident may have been a consequence of the arrhythmia which was the probable immediate cause of death. In most of the two-thirds with preceding illness, including those occurring in patients known to be suffering from sarcoidosis, premonitory cardiac symptoms, such as rhythm disturbances, syncope, anginal pain or congestive heart failure, have been noted before death for periods ranging from a few days to several years. As already noted, grossly visible changes are usually found in the heart in patients who have died suddenly from cardiac sarcoidosis; massive confluent fibrosing infiltrations in the ventricular and septal myocardium in most, and extensive focal deposits of similar character in the rest. The following case, whose earlier course was observed by one of us, illustrates these points:

A man aged 33 was found by routine radiography to have bilateral hilar lymph-node enlargement with some mottling in the middle zones of the lungs. Four years later, the lung shadows had become rather denser, but he remained symptom-free, and tests both of ventilatory function and of pulmonary gas transfer were normal. Two years later, at the age of 37, he had several brief episodes of palpitations one day, and the following night vomited. ECG showed right bundle branch block, inverted T waves in leads $V_1 - V_4$, and ST segment depression in leads I, II and V_6. Enzyme levels were found to be normal; a provisional diagnosis of myocardial sarcoidosis was made, and prednisolone 15 mg daily was given. No further episodes of palpitation occurred, but ECG abnormalities persisted. Further investigated nine months later, he was found to have similar ECG changes, now with ventricular premature beats; the pulmonary shadowing had diminished. Coronary angiography showed normal coronary arteries and left ventricular function. Prednisolone was continued, 10 mg daily; it was gradually withdrawn after two years. He remained symptom-free, leading an active life. Three years later, 12 years after the first evidence of sarcoidosis and six years after the first cardiac symptom, he suddenly collapsed and died with irreversible ventricular arrhythmia in spite of prompt and vigorous resuscitatory treatment. At necropsy, large areas of fibrosing confluent sarcoid infiltrations were found in the basal part of the posterior wall of the left ventricle and the adjacent septum, and separately in the septum itself; the right ventricular wall was in places reduced to a thin layer of fibrous tissue, and one tricuspid papillary muscle was fibrotic; there was atheromatous narrowing of the right coronary artery by 30% and of a branch of the left anterior descending artery by 75%; in the upper lobe of the left lung there was an area of fibrosing sarcoidosis, and elsewhere in the lungs perivascular and peribronchial granulomas; other organs were grossly unremarkable but in the liver a collection of lymphocytes and epithelioid cells was seen in one portal area.

Conduction and rhythm disturbances

In view of the possibility of widespread changes in the myocardium, sometimes confluent in the upper part of the interventricular septum, and in many cases irregularly scattered in all four chambers of the heart, it is not surprising that all grades of heart block and varieties of arrhythmia have been reported both in studies of large series of cases (Fleming, 1974;

Roberts *et al.*, 1978), and in surveys of published cases (Gozo *et al.*, 1971).

The high incidence of complete atrio-ventricular block is notable. In many instances it has been observed to be preceded by, or to alternate with, prolongation of PR interval or the Wenckebach type. Stokes-Adams attacks are a feature in many cases, and may be the initial symptom. Bundle-branch block is also frequent, with or without atrio-ventricular conduction defects. Of the 89 cases reviewed by Roberts *et al.* (1978), it was reported in 23; the block affected the right bundle-branch in 13, the left in five and was indeterminate in five.

Both ventricular and atrial rhythm disturbances are frequent, those arising in the ventricles being more frequent. Ventricular tachycardia was observed in 19 of the 89 cases reviewed by Roberts *et al.* (1977), and was associated with extensive myocardial infiltration or fibrosis. Ventricular premature beats are probably the most frequent rhythm change, and are usually multifocal in origin. Complete heart block and varying tachyarrhythmias may alternate. Atrial arrhythmias, ranging from premature beats to rather rare instances of fibrillation or flutter, seem to be less certainly attributable directly to granulomas in the atrial walls; Roberts *et al.* (1977) noted atrial arrhythmias in 15 of the cases they reviewed but granulomas were reported in atrial walls in only two of these.

Myocardial failure

Congestive heart failure may appear in patients with extensive myocardial sarcoidosis, often in combination with disturbances of rhythm or conduction; it was noted in 35 of the 89 of Roberts *et al.* (1977). The overall clinical picture may mimic that of a cardiomyopathy. Anginal pain may occur, and in combination with ECG changes, may suggest a diagnosis of myocardial infarction, as in ten of the 163 reviewed by Fleming (1980). The possible development of ventricular aneurysms at sites of extensive myocardial sarcoidosis, noted in the discussion of pathology, may add to the possibility of confusion with myocardial infarction. The diagnosis has been confirmed during life by angiocardiography (Duvernoy and Garcia, 1971; James, 1977; Lull *et al.*, 1972; Ahmed *et al.*, 1977).

Mitral incompetence

As noted above, direct granulomatous involvement of valves has very rarely been reported at necropsy. Mitral incompetence due to malfunction of infiltrated papillary muscles has been diagnosed clinically in a few cases. The early part of the course of one of these was observed by one of us (JGS).

This patient was a West Indian woman, aged 26, whose case was reported by Raftery *et al.* (1966, Case 9). Her illness started with uveitis, BHL and superficial lymphadenopathy, the diagnosis of sarcoidosis being confirmed by a Kveim test. About three months from the onset of the ocular symptoms she suddenly developed mitral incompetence causing pulmonary oedema. Treatment with prednisolone controlled the activity of the sarcoidosis, but mitral valve replacement was required to control the mitral incompetence. At this operation, performed by Professor H. H. Bentall, the valve cusps were found to be normal and mobile, but the papillary muscles presented a white glazed appearance and were so slack that the permitted inversion of the valves. histologically, the papillary muscle showed fibrosis between the muscle fibres with focal collections of lymphocytes, plasma cells and histiocytes, and the valve cusps some fibrous thickening but no specific changes. The non-specificity of the histological changes may have been due in part to the prolonged prednisolone treatment, and in part to the frequently atypical appearance and were so slack that they permitted inversion of the valves. Histologically, the papillary muscle showed fibrosis between the muscle fibres control of non-cardiac manifestations, but died suddenly five years after the operation. At necropsy, the free wall of the left ventricle and the interventricular septum were extensively infiltrated, and some granulomas were seen in the atria; lungs, liver, spleen and mediastinal lymph-nodes were also involved (Fleming, 1974). Zoneraich *et al.* (1974) described the case of a black woman, aged 29, who presented with palpitations, congestive heart failure, acute mitral insufficiency and multiple ventricular premature beats, and died of ventricular tachycardia; at necropsy there was extensive fibrosing sarcoidosis in the left ventricular and septal myocardium including the papillary muscles. Roberts *et al.* (1977) mentioned briefly two patients with severe heart failure, who had had loud apical systolic murmurs, and were found at necropsy to have extensive granulomatous infiltration of the left papillary muscles.

Pericardial effusion

A very few cases of recurrent pericardial effusion attributable to sarcoid infiltration of the pericardium have been reported. In the one reported by Schiff *et al.* (1969), a black woman, aged 31, who had had hilar lymph-node and pulmonary sarcoidosis for six months, a large pericardial effusion developed; it resolved during prednisolone treatment, but recurred when this was stopped. At this stage, partial pericardiectomy was performed: both the pericardium and a biopsy sample of lung showed sarcoid-type granulomas. Gozo *et al.* (1971, Case 1) described the case of a black woman, aged 27, who presented with congestive heart failure, atrioventicular block of Wenckebach type, and a large pericardial effusion. She died during thoracotomy, at which a large blood-stained pericardial effusion was found. At necropsy, very extensive sarcoidosis was found in the myocardium of all chambers of the heart and in the pericardium, in lymph-nodes, in liver and in gastric mucosa; in the lungs they were less numerous and found especially around arteries and veins near the hila. Roberts *et al.* (1977) mentioned three cases in which large pericardial effusions, causing tamponade in two, were shown at necropsy to be associated with epicardial sarcoid granulomas. Bailey (1966) reported the case of a 59 year old woman who presented with acute pericarditis with effusion. In the course of investigation she was found to have enlarged hilar lymph-nodes, and a scalene node biopsy showed sarcoid-type granulomas. A left pleural effusion appeared. Under treatment with 15 mg daily of prednisone, both effusions slowly resolved, but only 14 weeks' observation was recorded. In this case, doubt must remain whether the pericarditis and pleurisy were pathogenetically related to sarcoidosis, especially as the patient had suffered from rheumatoid arthritis for ten years, said to have been inactive for four years.

DIAGNOSIS

The difficulty of diagnosis of cardiac sarcoidosis varies with the circumstances of the individual case. The cause of sudden death in a person who has had no occasion to seek medical advice can be established only by necropsy. In a patient in whom the clinical diagnosis of sarcoidosis is already or can be established, the appearance of heart block of any degree or a ventricular arrhythmia is presumptive evidence of cardiac involvement, certainly in the absence of evidence of other forms of heart disease. The problem is more difficult when the symptoms and signs are those of myocardial disease in a patient known to be suffering from sarcoidosis. These may range from no more than T wave and ST interval changes in the ECG to congestive heart failure or an acute illness suggestive of myocardial infarction. If coronary artery disease seems a likely alternative diagnosis, coronary angiography may provide direct evidence of such disease, though it cannot exclude co-existing cardiac sarcoidosis. Still more difficult are cases where the possibility of sarcoidosis is considered for the first time in a patient presenting with symptoms and signs of cardiac disease, which cannot be placed in one of the commoner categories. In such cases, the first step is the establishment of the diagnosis of sarcoidosis (Chapter 26).

Myocardial scanning with ^{201}thallium has been used to detect sites of sarcoid infiltration by Bulkley *et al.* (1977) and Kinney *et al.* (1980). In five patients with known sarcoidosis and cardiac dysfunction, Bulkley *et al.* found that two with impaired pulmonary function had high uptake over the right ventricle, and three with unexplained congestive failure, mitral regurgitation or arrhythmias showed defects in left ventricular uptake, confirmed to be due to sarcoid infiltration in one at operation for mitral valve replacement and in one at necropsy. Kinney *et al.* studied 44 patients with established sarcoidosis and found defects in the left ventricle images in 14 and in the right in four, but the attribution of these to myocardial sarcoidosis remained presumptive. The role of this expensive form of investigation remains to be assessed.

Endomyocardial biopsy is a possible method of obtaining histological confirmation of cardiac sarcoidosis (Sekiguchi *et al.*, 1967); but in view of the patchy distribution of the lesions can be expected to show granulomas in only a proportion of cases. Numao *et al.* (1980) stated that among 1000 myocardial biopsies in Japan, two had shown sarcoid granulomas; in two others in which the biopsy showed no granulomas, the diagnosis of cardiac sarcoidosis was made at necropsy.

In most cases, the diagnosis of cardiac sarcoidosis during life depends upon inference from clinical findings, and remains without direct histological confirmation.

RIGHT VENTRICULAR HYPERTROPHY AND FAILURE (COR PULMONALE)

Right ventricular hypertrophy, and ultimately failure, may occur in the late stages of fibrotic pulmonary sarcoidosis, as of other forms of chronic lung dissease; but in most patients who die with progressive pulmonary fibrosis consequent upon sarcoidosis, death is due to respiratory failure, perhaps precipitated by a terminal acute infection, without clinical signs of right ventricular failure or pulmonary hypertension. Thirteen patients of 275 reviewed by Scadding (1967) were known to have died of the late effects of pulmonary sarcoidosis; only three of these showed evidence of right ventricular failure, with oedema and raised jugular venous pressure. One other, whose course had been complicated by chronic airflow limitation, presumably mainly cigarette-induced, ECG evidence of right ventricular hypertrophy, which was confirmed at necropsy, but no oedema or raised venous pressure. In two patients who died after several years of almost complete disability from dyspnoea, necropsies showed no suggestion of right ventricular hypertrophy. Battesti *et al.* (1978) studied 21 patients with chronic pulmonary sarcoidosis and radiographic evidence of fibrotic changes not responsive to corticosteroid treatment; they found ECG changes suggestive of right ventricular hypertrophy in six, with 'clinical right heart failure' (criteria not stated) in four.

In a few patients with extensive active pulmonary sarcoidosis, right ventricular changes, presumably due to pulmonary hypertension, have regressed when the pulmonary disease has improved, either spontaneously or in response to corticosteroid treatment. A case of this sort was reported by Moyer and Ackerman (1950).

A man, aged 25, was found to have evidence of enlargement of the right side of the heart, and depression of ST in lead I and inversion of T in leads II and III of the ECG at the time when he had a dense sarcoid infiltration in the lungs; these changes returned towards normal as the infiltration regressed. It is possible that in such cases granulomas in and around pulmonary arteries and veins that have been found in patients with pulmonary sarcoidosis, both by biopsy in the earlier stages and at necropsy (Chapter 6, p. 107), may contribute to pulmonary hypertension. Levine *et al.* (1971) reported the case of a man with a history of pulmonary sarcoidosis causing few symptoms for 25 years, who developed increasing dyspnoea leading after two months to orthopnoea and ankle oedema with clinical and electrocardiographic evidence of right ventricular failure and pulmonary hypertension, suggesting pulmonary embolism. He died despite appropriate treatment for this. At necropsy there was no evidence of pulmonary embolism; the lungs showed non-caseating granulomas with fibrosis distributed predominantly around small pulmonary arteries and veins, the alveoli being relatively little affected.

Granulomatous changes in pulmonary vessels might be expected to be suppressible by corticosteroid treatment, leading to relief of pulmonary hypertension, but there are few recorded cases in which this has been documented.

McClement *et al.* (1953) found that in ten patients with pulmonary hypertension associated with pulmonary sarcoidosis, the pulmonary artery pressure did not fall after corticosteroid treatment. Davies *et al.* (1982) reported the case of a 33 year old Ghanian who became acutely breathless during a transatlantic flight, having noticed slight dyspnoea on exertion, weight loss and dry cough for four months. He had clinical signs of pulmonary hypertension, a palpable spleen, and superficial lymph-node enlargement. There was extensive mottling in the lung-fields and BHL in the chest radiograph. Biopsy of a lymph-node showed non-caseating granulomas. Cardiac catheterization showed a pulmonary artery pressure of 70/35 mm Hg, falling slightly on breathing 50% oxygen to 50/25. Corticosteroid treatment led to rapid relief of symptoms, diminution in density of lung shadows, and improvement in a previously severe restrictive ventilatory defect. The pulmonary artery pressure fell after three months' treatment to 40/18 breathing air, changing only to 38/13 on oxygen. Symptomatic improvement was maintained, and corticosteroid treatment was stopped. Reviewed six years later, he remained symptom-free, with some residual lung shadowing and a slight restrictive ventilatory defect; the pulmonary artery pressure had fallen to 28/10.

In spite of the high proportion of cases in which granulomas can be found in blood-vessels if specially sought in open lung biopsies from patients with active pulmonary sarcoidosis, it is evident that these have functional effects in only a very small minority, and that in the majority they resolve completely or with insignificant residual scarring without ever giving rise to symptoms. But in exceptional cases, the possibility that pulmonary hypertension may be related to unusually prominent granulomatous vasculitis, responsive to corticosteroid treatment, should be considered.

Rarely, sarcoid enlargement of lymph-nodes may cause functionally important compression of pulmonary arteries. Battesti *et al.* (1978) reported the case of a white woman aged 49 with chronic pulmonary sarcoidosis, who developed right heart failure. Angiography showed obstruction of the pulmonary artery to the left upper lobe and narrowing of the branches to the right lower and upper lobes. Necropsy showed that these were due to compression by many calcified lymph-nodes. There were extensive fibrotic and granulomatous changes in broncho-vascular sheaths, in bronchial and vascular walls, and in lungs. The lymph-nodes were hyalinized. The changes in many vessels had led to narrowing, with evidence of old thrombosis and recanalization. Cases in which sarcoid hilar lymphadenopathy in an active stage caused narrowing of pulmonary arteries demonstrated by angiography with corresponding defects in perfusion scans but without clinically evident haemodynamic effects have been reported by Westcott and de Graff (1973), Fannce *et al.* (1976) and Hietala *et al.* (1977).

TREATMENT

The transient ECG changes without symptoms or signs of cardiac dysfunction which have been reported in a small minority of patients in the early active stages of sarcoidosis do not seem to indicate a special liability to subsequent symptomatic cardiac sarcoidosis, and call for no special treatment. The following discussion concerns patients with cardiac dysfunction attributable to granulomatous infiltration.

The treatment of arrhythmias, conduction defects, and heart failure should follow established cardiological practice. Arrhythmias may be relatively resistant to anti-arrhythmic drugs, and improved response after corticosteroid treatment has been reported (Nissen and Berte, 1964, Case 4; Gozo *et al.*, 1971; Serwer *et al.*, 1978; Walsh, 1978). Valve replacement for mitral incompetence due to papillary muscle involvement was successful in relieving this functional defect in a case reported by Raftery *et al.* (1966) and mentioned on p. 342. Successful excision of a large ventricular aneurysm due to fibrosing sarcoidosis, together with prednisolone treatment, was followed by at least short-term improvement with cessation of ventricular arrhthymia, in a case reported by Lull *et al.* (1972).

The effects of corticosteroid treatment on the lesions of cardiac sarcoidosis are probably similar to those on sarcoidosis elsewhere: suppression, partial or complete, of active granulomas with little effect on established fibrosis (Chapter 27). Published reports suggest that diminution in numbers of premature beats and of episodes of tachycardia and easier control of these arrhythmias follows corticosteroid treatment in many cases; improvement in conduction defects may occur, but is less frequent (Stein *et al.*, 1976; Lash *et al.*, 1979; Yamamato *et al.*, 1980). The danger of sudden death may be diminished, but remains.

In patients with evidence of myocardial failure, which is frequently due to massive infiltration by confluent granulomas with considerable fibrosis, resulting in replacement of parts of the myocardium by tissue without contractile function, the lost tissue cannot be replaced, and the best that can be hoped for is suppression of still cellular granulomas and further fibrosis. Roberts *et al.* (1977) expressed concern that corticosteroid treatment might encourage the development of ventricular aneurysm, since they found that of eight reported patients with aneurysms, all but one had received such treatment, but more prolonged survival because of the treatment allowing more time for the development of aneurysmal dilatation is an alternative explanation of this observation.

In practice, it seems sensible to institute corticosteroid treatment in any case with an established clinical diagnosis of cardiac sarcoidosis, and to be guided as to its continuance by the general signs of activity of sarcoidosis (Chapter 27) and by the response of the cardiac symptoms and signs; at the same time, the various elements in cardiac dysfunction should be treated appropriately. If the available evidence suggests extensive myocardial granulomatous changes, and corticosteroid treatment has led to significant improvement, decision about the duration of treatment is difficult. In view of experience of cases in which sudden death has occurred after initial favourable responses, in some after cessation of treatment, it seems that all available indices of continued activity should be used in making this decision; and a case could be made out for indefinitely prolonged treatment, certainly in the absence of serious side-effects.

Chapter 16

The Endocrine Glands

Among the endocrine glands, the pituitary is the most frequently affected in a manner giving rise to functional effects. The tendency of sarcoidosis to involve the meninges and neural structures at the base of the brain has been noted in Chapter 14. The variability of distribution and localization of hypothalamic-pituitary changes gives rise to a wide range of clinical syndromes. These include secondary effects on other endocrine glands, which do not appear to be specially liable to persistent granulomatous invasion in sarcoidosis. In some reported cases, granulomas have been found in thyroid, parathyroids or pancreas with no evident functional effects; and when endocrine dysfunction has been observed, it has been arguable in most cases whether this is a direct effect of sarcoid infiltration, indirectly linked to sarcoidosis through unidentified common immunological factors, or simply coincidental with and aetiologically unrelated to sarcoidosis. Sarcoid granulomas have very rarely been found in the adrenal glands.

PITUITARY GLAND

Since the pituitary gland is not readily accessible for biopsy, it is not surprising that in most of the recorded cases of sarcoidosis of this gland the diagnosis depended upon clinical evidence of pituitary dysfunction in patients with sarcoidosis elsewhere. In a minority of cases, the diagnosis has been proved by histology of the gland, either at craniotomy or at necropsy. In a very few, the pituitary has been found to be infiltrated with sarcoid tubercles at necropsy, although there was no record of symptoms of pituitary dysfunction during life (Ricker and Clark, 1949, Case 20; Kulka, 1950; Bleisch and Robbins, 1952, Cases 3 and 4). Cowdell (1954) reported briefly the somewhat paradoxical case of a woman who died at the age of 29 with hypertensive heart failure associated with Cushing's syndrome; and at necropsy was found to have generalized sarcoidosis with extensive involvement of the anterior lobe of the pituitary, the Cushing's syndrome being attributable to adrenal cortical hyperplasia.

As is to be expected from the widespread but patchy distribution of granulomas that may be found in the hypothalamic-pituitary area, a great variety of disorders of pituitary function may occur in patients with sarcoidosis; and these have been found to be due to varying combinations of deficiencies of pituitary hormones and hypothalamic releasing factors (Stuart *et al.*, 1978). Nevertheless, syndromes related to deficiency of one aspect of pituitary function predominate in many cases.

Diabetes insipidus and thirst disorders

The most frequently reported disorder of pituitary function in sarcoidosis has been diabetes insipidus. In only a few of the recorded cases has morbid anatomical confirmation of sarcoid infiltration of the neurophypophysis or hypothalamus been available. In the cases reported by Tillgren (1935), Wahlgren (1936), Posner (1942) and Longcope and Freiman (1952, Case 15), extensive sarcoidosis was associated with polyuria and polydipsia, and the pituitary was found at necropsy to be infiltrated. The cases described by Aszkenazy (1952, Case 2) and Jefferson (1957, Case 5), in which a syndrome including diabetes insipidus was due to sarcoid infiltration of the hypothalamus without significant infiltration of the pituitary, have already been mentioned in connection with sarcoidosis of the nervous system (p. 314).

In most of the reported cases of diabetes insipidus in sarcoidosis the diagnosis has been based upon extreme polydipsia and polyuria in patients with sarcoidosis and without evidence of renal disease. The earliest was one of Heerfordt's original cases of uveo-parotid fever (Heerfordt, 1909, Case 3), a man, aged 27, who developed polydipsia and polyuria, up to 5 litres daily, one month after the onset of parotid gland enlargement with uveitis and multiple cranial nerve palsies. The frequency with which polyuria and polydipsia has been reported subsequently in association with the uveo-parotid syndrome (Gjessing, 1916; Merrill and Oaks, 1931; Garland and Thompson, 1933; Levin, 1935; Folger, 1936; Arbuse and Madonick, 1938, Case 1; Jersild, 1939; Harrell, 1940, Case 1; Appelmans and van Horenbeeck, 1941; Franceschetti and de Morsier, 1941, Case 1; Spillane, 1953, Case 1; Höök, 1954, Case 3) suggests that this syndrome may be especially liable to be accompanied by hypothalamic-hypophyseal disturbances. But diabetes insipidus also occurs with other sorts of sarcoidosis. Occasionally this is of limited extent, as in cases reported by Lemming

(1940b) and Boman (1952) in which polyuria, transient or persistent, occurred with sarcoidosis clinically manifest only in the lymph-nodes and lungs. But in most cases, the sarcoidosis has been florid and extensive. Lesné *et al.* (1935) described the case of a boy, aged ten, with lupus pernio, extensive changes in the bones of the hands, subcutaneous nodules having a sarcoid histology, and polyuria controlled by pituitary posterior lobe extract. Other cases in which sarcoidosis with multiple clinical manifestations has been accompanied by clinical evidence of diabetes insipidus have been reported by Flandin *et al.* (1936), Snapper and Pompen (1938), Walsh (1939, Case 6), Terpstra (1944), Cameron and Dawson (1942), Rey *et al.* (1947) and Shealy *et al.* (1961, Cases 1 and 4); and, as would be expected, signs of central nervous system involvement and diabetes insipidus not infrequently occur together (Jefferson, 1957; Matthews, 1965; Morgan *et al.*, 1965; Silverstein *et al.*, 1965; Wiederholt and Sickert, 1965). Signs of involvement of the hypothalamus and structures at the base of the brain are especially frequent; e.g. anosmia (Levin, 1935), left optic atrophy with right upper temporal quadrantic visual field defect (Walsh, 1939), obesity and somnolence (Franceschetti and de Morsier, 1941); bitemporal hemianopia with changes in the cerebro-spinal fluid (Terpstra, 1944), and deafness and vertigo (Höök, 1954, Case 3).

Case 1 of Shealy *et al.* (1961) was that of a black man aged 44, with sarcoids of the skin of the face, polyuria of 6–10 litres daily controlled by pitressin, and impotence; the visual fields were normal, but the cerebro-spinal fluid showed a high protein level; corticosteroid treatment led to cessation of the polydipsia, but had no effect on the impotence. In their Case 4, a girl, aged 13, presented with amenorrhoea for three months, polydipsia for one month, and loss of vision in the left eye for three weeks; the loss of vision was due to a vitreous haemorrhage and there was papilloedema with a constricted visual field on the right side; the diagnosis of diabetes insipidus was supported by the responses to water deprivation, to hypertonic saline infusion and to pitressin, and of sarcoidosis by scalene node biopsy.

Although diabetes inspidus has been reported relatively frequently in patients with central nervous system sarcoidosis, only a very small proportion of all patients with sarcoidosis show evidence of it. Only 0.5% of 2416 reviewed by Silverstein *et al.* (1965) were so affected. Similarly, sarcoidosis is infrequent as a cause of diabetes insipidus; it was found in only one of 65 patients with diabetes insipidus by Thomas (1957).

The diagnosis of diabetes insipidus is generally suggested by the clinical syndrome of polydipsia and polyuria, the urine being of low specific gravity, but otherwise normal, and failing to concentrate after water deprivation; absence of evidence of renal disease; and the relief of polyuria by vasopressin or pituitary posterior lobe extracts. Stuart *et al.* (1980) investigated the endocrine diagnostic problems of polyuria and polydipsia in 11 patients with sarcoidosis and evidence of hypothalamic-pituitary involvement; five had polyuria and polydipsia, but of these only two had anti-diuretic hormone (ADH) deficiency. The other three had excessive thirst with adequate reserve of ADH. Excessive water-drinking was tentatively attributed to resetting of the osmotic thresholds for thirst and ADH release, presumably of central hypothalamic origin.

Discussion of the diagnostic problems of thirst disorders is outside the scope of this monograph. It may be noted, however, that in sarcoidosis polyuria is probably more often due to hypercalcaemia and the nephropathy associated with it than to hypothalamic-pituitary disorders; and Panitz and Shinaberger (1965) reported a case of granulomatous infiltration of the kidney in which polyuria was controlled by corticosteroid treatment (Chapter 19).

Another differential diagnostic problem of importance in relation to sarcoidosis arises from the fact that in histiocytosis X (p. 171), widespread lung changes, presenting radiologically first as generalized mottling in the lung fields and later becoming transformed into 'honeycombing' may be accompanied by diabetes insipidus. Thus both sarcoidosis and histiocytosis X may give rise to the combination of diffuse infiltration of the lungs and diabetes insipidus (Spillane, 1952). The differential diagnosis may be difficult, and in the absence of histological evidence from a more accessible site lung biopsy may be necessary to establish a diagnosis in a case of this sort. In Case 1 of Pennell (1951), for instance, diabetes insipidus was accompanied by a diffuse pulmonary infiltration, a cervical lymph-node biopsy showed only 'chronic lymphadenitis' and Kveim test was negative; although the case was included as one of sarcoidosis, histiocytosis X seems an equally tenable diagnosis on the evidence available.

Hypopituitarism

Deficient anterior pituitary function has been recorded in sarcoidosis rather less frequently than polydipsia of hypothalamic-pituitary origin, and in many cases these two types of disorder have been associated. Varied combinations of features attributable to deficiencies in anterior pituitary hormones and in hypothalamic releasing hormones and neuro-regulatory function may be observed.

Kraus (1942) described the necropsy findings in a woman, aged 41, who had had anaemia, thrombocytopenia, genital hypoplasia with amenorrhoea since the age of 17, and polyuria; there was generalized sarcoidosis involving lymph-nodes, lungs and spleen, and infiltrating the infundibulum, stalk and body of the pituitary gland. In Case 1 of Bleisch and Robbins (1952), a woman who died at the age of 33 had suffered from polydipsia for many years, amenorrhoea for seven years, loss of weight, and loss of body hair; she had a low basal metabolic rate (BMR) and low urinary ketosteroid excretion; at necropsy, sarcoid granulomas were found in lungs and lymph-nodes, and replacing 85% of the anterior and 50% of the posterior lobe of the pituitary, with much fibrosis and many giant cells containing Schaumann bodies.

Jackson and Hood (1958) reported the case of a man who had erythema nodosum and bilateral hilar lymph-node enlargement at the age of 32; later he developed sparse body hair, gynaecomastia, dry skin, and hepatospleno-megaly, and lymph-node biopsy confirmed the diagnosis of sarcoidosis; at the age of 43, he was found to have polyuria of 6–8 litres daily, controlled by pitressin, a low BMR, low excretion of FSH and a low uptake of ^{131}I in the thyroid, increased after thyrotrophic hormone. Nora *et al.* (1959) described the case of a black man aged 38, in whom the diagnosis of sarcoidosis was established by lymph-node and liver biopsies; he suffered from lassitude, loss of libido, and loss of body hair; on treatment with cortisone, the urine volume which had been 3–4 litres daily increased to 11 and 12 litres, and this polyuria was controlled by pitressin; he had a low BMR, low ^{131}I uptake in the thyroid gland, increased by thyrotrophic hormone, and low urinary gonadotrophin output. This case illustrated well the fact that the polyuria of diabetes insipidus can be manifested only in the presence of sufficient anterior pituitary function to maintain adrenocortical function. It may be contrasted with Case 1 of Shealy *et al.* (1961), in which diabetes insipidus associated with sarcoidosis was improved by corticosteroid treatment; presumably in this case some anterior pituitary function remained, and the improvement was due to suppression of the sarcoid granuloma in the neurophypophysis or hypothalamus. In Case 3 of Shealy *et al.* loss of body hair, testicular atrophy, and impotence, together with low blood pressure, low BMR and low ^{131}I uptake in the thyroid suggested hypopituitarism, and polyuria was controlled by pitressin; the diagnosis of sarcoidosis was supported by biopsy of an epitrochlear lymph-node and the cerebrospinal fluid contained 26 cells/mm^3 and 164 mg of protein/100 ml. Plair and Perry (1962) reported the necropsy findings in a black man aged 29, who had suffered from loss of vision, loss of libido and polydipsia; there was infiltration with fibrosing sarcoid granulomas in lepto-meninges in the inter-peduncular fossa and the lower ends of the Sylvian fissures, involving also the adjacent parts of the brain, including the floor and lateral walls of the third ventricle and the frontal lobes in the region of the optic nerves; about two thirds of the pituitary gland was infiltrated, the posterior lobe more than the anterior; and sarcoid tubercles were found in the spleen and mediastinal lymph-nodes, though only one in the lung. Vesely *et al.* (1977) reported the case of a man who was investigated at the age of 17 for delayed puberty and short stature, with a bone age of 12–13 years; he was found to have BHL, and lymph-node biopsy showed sarcoid-type granulomas. At the age of 20, there were diffuse lung changes with restricted ventilatory function, and osteolytic lesions were found radiologically in the skull; plasma levels of testosterone were normal, and of growth hormone low and not increased after insulin-induced hypoglycaemia. Treatment with prednisone led to improvement in respiratory symptoms and in the osteolytic skull lesions, and growth of 2.5 cm in height in six months.

Cases in which sarcoid infiltration at the base of the brain caused such symptoms as somnolence, impotence and amenorrhoea have been mentioned above in connection with sarcoidosis of the nervous system (p. 314). Similar changes may occur without overt neurological signs.

Gjersøe and Kjerulf-Jensen (1950) reported the case of a woman who died at the age of 29; she had had sarcoidosis since the age of 17, starting with uveitis leading to blindness, the diagnosis being established by examination of enucleated eyes; for two years before death she had become moody and somnolent and developed polydipsia and polyuria; at necropsy, there was infiltration of the hypothalamic region with fibrosing epithelioid and giant-cell tubercles. Selenkow *et al.* (1959) described the case of a woman who died at the age of 27; at the age of 20, a large spleen was removed, no pathological details being available; at the age of 25, she rapidly gained weight, became tired and slow and ceased menstruating, and skin lesions, histologically sarcoid, appeared; at craniotomy later, thickening of the arachnoid at the base of the brain, histologically granulomatous and consistent with sarcoidosis, was found; in spite of replacement therapy she died six months later; at necropsy, extensive infiltration of the meninges at the base of the brain was found, but the pars anterior of the pituitary was normal and the pars posterior reported to be condensed and 'hyper-nuclear', with only a few sarcoid granulomas at the superior margin of the gland; the floor and walls of the third ventricle were involved in the sarcoid infiltration, which filled the infundibular part of its cavity; elsewhere in the body, sarcoidosis was found in lymph-nodes, lungs, liver, peritoneum and vertebral bone-marrow. Bast *et al.* (1964) reported the necropsy findings in a man who had failed to develop secondary sex characters and had been found to have BHL at the age of 15, and died at the age of 29; there was granulomatous infiltration of the meninges at the base of the brain, the hypothalamus, and the optic chiasma and hypophysis, and granulomatous arteritis leading to aneurysmal dilation of both frontal rami of the circle of Willis.

Similar hypothalamic-pituitary syndromes, without necropsy evidence, have been reported by Doub and Menagh (1929, two cases), Barber (1945) and Magnus (1956). All these four cases were in males with widespread sarcoidosis, the skin being involved in three, and the evidence of pituitary insufficiency consisted in loss of body hair and loss of sexual function in all four, accompanied in some by such symptoms as obesity, somnolence, weakness and changes in mentality. Toulant and Morard (1936) reported the case of a boy, aged 17, with the uveo-parotid syndrome whose development was retarded and corresponded with an age of 12–13 years; Haas and Joseph (1908) reported what appears to be a similar case as one of infantilism with Miculicz syndrome and iridochoroiditis.

Owen and Henneman (1953) reported the remarkable case of a man who died at the age of 52 with hypertension and uraemia, after 15 years of ill-health with tiredness and weakness, and loss of body hair and libido. Sarcoid tubercles, some hyalinized, were found in lung, liver, spleen and lymph-nodes, and a few in the myocardium. The sella turcica was empty, no pituitary gland being discoverable; the adrenals and testes were atrophic. Section of the infundibular stalk and adjacent hypothalamus showed no sarcoid granuloma. The cause of death was a glomerulonephritis, with some granular debris and an occasional calcium deposit in the tubules; there was no record of the serum calcium level. The relationship of the complete pituitary atrophy in this case to the sarcoidosis must remain a matter for speculation.

Recent endocrinological studies suggest that in patients with sarcoidosis of the central nervous system who have symptoms and signs of deficiency of pituitary hormones the functional defect is principally hypothalamic. Stuart *et al.* (1978) studied ten patients with generalized sarcoidosis and hypopituitarism. Most had evidence of nervous system involvement: six had visual field defects, three olfactory loss, two trigeminal sensory changes, and one sensorineural hearing loss, and three had had seizures; and the CSF showed pleocytosis and raised protein content in five. All showed evidence of diminished gonadal function, with diminished libido, impotence or amenorrhoea, and low testosterone or oestrogen levels in the serum. Three of the seven women had galactorrhoea. Mild hypothyroidism with normal thyroid stimulating hormone (TSH) levels was found in three, and severe hypothyroidism with raised TSH in one; all nine tested with thyrotrophin-releasing hormone (TRH) showed increases in TSH. In all patients, deficiencies of at least two anterior pituitary hormones were found; but tests with releasing hormones and with clomiphene and chlorpromazine indicated that the pituitary remained capable of response. Similar conclusions were reached by Caro *et al.* (1980), who studied responses of growth (GH) and luteinizing (LH) hormones to stimulation by luteinizing hormone releasing hormone (LHRH) in 22 patients with sarcoidosis, of whom seven had central nervous system involvement. Of those with CNS changes, one had amenorrhoea, absent secondary sex characteristics, hypothyroidism and diabetes insipidus, one hypothyroidism, one transient diabetes insipidus, and one was excessively somnolent. Six of the seven had impaired responses, three showing no response to the standard test; but these three on further testing after prolonged LHRH infusion showed responses, suggesting a hypothalamic rather than a pituitary defect.

Galactorrhoea occurs in a few women with sarcoidosis. Turkington and MacIndoe (1972) studied four women aged 29 to 38 years with sarcoidosis referred to an endocrine clinic because of galactorrhoea and amenorrhoea, and 30 patients, ten men and 20 women, with pulmonary and extra-pulmonary sarcoidosis. Serum prolactin levels were raised (5–100 ng ml^{-1}, controls <2 ng) in the four with galactorrhoea and seven others. Eighteen patients with pulmonary tuberculosis showed normal levels. Among the sarcoidosis patients with high prolactin levels, only the four with galactorrhoea-amenorrhoea had low urinary gonadotrophin levels. Treatment with L-dopa for two months led to fall in serum prolactin and rise in urinary gonadotrophin levels in three of these four patients, with relief of galactorrhoea and amenorrhoea. Shortly after the study, the male patient with the highest prolactin level died suddenly; at necropsy, granulomas were scattered throughout the hypothalamus and median eminence, and some were found in the meninges, but none in the pituitary gland. In the study of ten patients with sarcoidosis and hypopituitarism by Stuart *et al.* (1978), three of the seven women had galactorrhoea, and all had amenorrhoea. Serum prolactin levels were raised in six, including the three with galactorrhoea. In all ten patients, serum prolactin levels were increased by TRH indicating that the prolactin-secreting system of the pituitary was intact. All three women with galactorrhoea had evidence of central nervous system involvement. Among the patients with CNS sarcoidosis whose endocrine function was studied by Caro *et al.* (1980), none had galactorrhoea; they also studied five with galactorrhoea found among 300 women attending a sarcoidosis clinic. Prolactin levels were raised in four of the seven patients with CNS sarcoidosis and in three of the five with galactorrhoea. Prolactin responses of L-dopa and TRH were normal; to chlorpromazine they were absent in those with galactorrhoea and low in those with CNS involvement. According to Tolis *et al.* (1973) the combination of response to TRH and no response to chlorpromazine suggests a functioning pituitary with failure of hypothalamic control. This is concordant with the limited morbid-anatomical evidence in sarcoidosis. Granulomatous changes in the hypothalamus presumably result in deficiency of prolactin secretion inhibitory factors, and consequent excess of pituitary prolactin secretion; but it is evident that some additional factor is required to induce galactorrhoea, since some women with galactorrhoea have been found to have normal prolactin levels, and hyperprolactinaemia is found more frequently than galactorrhoea.

Turkington and MacIndoe (1972) suggested that some cases of 'idiopathic' galactorrhoea and amenorrhoea may be related to sarcoidosis. A case reported by Fromantin *et al.* (1975) is relevant to this suggestion. A woman aged 23 developed amenorrhoea and three months later hyperthyroidism, followed by erythema nodosum, arthropathy and fever, and galactorrhoea. She was found to have BHL and a negative tuberculin test. Corticosteroid and carbimazole led to subsidence of the BHL, return to an euthyroid state and reappearance of menses, but galactorrhoea continued. However, among 222 women with galactorrhoea studied by Kleinberg *et al.* (1977) only three had sarcoidosis; all three also had amenorrhoea.

Serum prolactin levels were studied in series of cases of sarcoidosis by Malarkey and Kataria (1974) and Munt *et al.* (1975). In both studies, raised levels were rare and were not correlated with evidence of hypothalamic or other nervous system involvement. Munt *et al.* found normal levels in two women with galactorrhoea. They suggested that differences in assay methods might account in part for differences between their findings and those of Turkington and MacIndoe (1972).

Brun *et al.* (1964, 1965) investigated pituitary function in sarcoidosis by the metyrapone test of Liddle *et al.* (1959). They found that there was an abnormally large increase in urinary excretion of 17-hydroxycorticoids and of compound S after metyrapone in patients with active intrathoracic sarcoidosis, especially those in the early stage of BHL, indicating abnormal responsiveness of the pituitary gland to the stimulus of a reduced blood cortisol level. Patients with 'completely stabilized' sarcoidosis, with tuberculosis and with pneumoconioses gave normal responses. Israel and Goldstein (1968) and Nielsen (1968) could not confirm these findings; though some patients with active sarcoidosis showed rather higher increases than normal subjects or patients with other pulmonary diseases, the differences between groups were not statistically significant.

Other granulomas of the pituitary gland

The diagnosis of sarcoidosis of the pituitary gland can be made with confidence only if there is acceptable evidence that non-caseating epithelioid cell granulomas are present both in the pituitary and in other organs. Other granulomas that may involve the pituitary are those of tuberculosis and of syphilis, and histiocytosis X. In addition, cases have been described in which a giant-cell granuloma has involved, and, in some, destroyed the pituitary without convincing evidence of relationship to any known infective granuloma, to sarcoidosis or to histiocytosis X.

Simmonds (1917) described the finding at necropsy in five elderly women, who had died of unrelated causes, of infiltration of the pituitary gland with foci of lymphocytes, epithelioid cells and giant cells; they closely resembled miliary tubercles, but Simmonds thought they were not due to either tuberculosis or syphilis, and speculated whether they might be the cause of a secretory anomaly. Other cases probably belonging to the same group have been published by Boller and Goedel (1935), Sheehan and Summers (1949), Oelbaum and Wainwright (1950), Doniach and Wright (1951), and Rickards and Harvey (1954). The features that distinguish these cases from sarcoidosis, according to Rickards and Harvey, are the older age group, the greater frequency in the female sex, and the fact that whereas, as has been noted above, the great majority of the acceptable cases of sarcoidosis of the pituitary have been associated with diabetes insipidus and only a minority with hypopituitarism, the lesion described as giant-cell granuloma of the pituitary has either been associated with panhypopituitarism or has been an incidental necropsy finding. Moreover, although granulomas may be found in other organs, their distribution is less wide than, and different from, that usually found in sarcoidosis. The lungs and lymph-nodes are generally not involved; the liver may be; and the adrenals have been reported to be involved in some cases (Oelbaum and Wainwright, 1950; Doniach and Wright, 1951; Rickards and Barrett, 1954); whereas, as noted above, the adrenal is notably free from liability to invasion in sarcoidosis.

In the present state of knowledge about the pathogenesis and aetiology of sarcoidosis, it is not possible to come to a definite conclusion about the relationship of the so-called giant cell granuloma of the pituitary to sarcoidosis. In cases in which the pituitary alone is involved the possibility that the granuloma is a reaction to some primary disease of the pituitary and analogous to a local sarcoid reaction elsewhere cannot be excluded, since such reactions to a variety of pathological processes are well recognized. Where other organs are involved, the question whether the syndrome is one of the many which can properly be included in the nosological group sarcoidosis cannot at present be answered definitely.

Although some cases in which there can be no doubt of the diagnosis of tuberculosis of the pituitary have been described – e.g. by Von Hann (1913) and Kirshbaum and Levy (1941) – the pituitary seems rarely to be involved in cases of extensive tuberculosis. Kirshbaum and Levy stated that in no case among 368 of tuberculous meningitis was the pituitary affected. In some of the reported cases, the evidence available seems insufficient to permit a definite opinion whether tuberculosis or sarcoidosis is the more appropriate diagnostic category.

> Haushalter and Lucien (1908) recorded the case of a six and a half year old girl whose mother had died of tuberculosis; she developed symptoms of diabetes insipidus and died in coma; a massive non-caseating tuberculoid granuloma was found at the base of the brain, involving the pituitary; no acid-fast bacilli were found in it, but on the other hand there was a fibrotic nodule at the apex of the right lung and a caseous paratracheal lymph-node, undoubtedly a primary complex of tuberculosis. Coleman and Meredith (1940) described the case of a woman, aged 57, who presented with neurological evidence of a pituitary tumour, and at operation was found to have a large intrasellar mass which was removed and reported histologically to consist of diffuse non-caseous tuberculosis; she made a good recovery and was well more than three years later; no information about involvement of other organs is available, and it is impossible therefore to attempt to categorize this case. Glass and Davis (1944) reported the case of a man, aged 54, who had had a pleurisy diagnosed as tuberculous at the age of 35; he was suffering from a refractory macrocytic anaemia, weakness, headaches, loss of vision in the right eye, and loss of body hair and of libido; he had a low BMR and low urinary hormone excretion; the Mantoux test was strongly positive, and acid-fast bacilli were seen in gastric lavage specimens on two occasions. At necropsy, a caseous nodule was found in the right lung, and an infiltration at the right hilum which histologically was a granuloma with much fibrosis and some caseation; about nine-tenths of the pituitary was replaced by dense scar tissue with some calcification and even in places bone formation; no acid-fast bacilli were seen in appropriately stained sections.

There seems to be good reason to categorize this case as one of indolent caseating tuberculosis, though Rickards and Harvey group it as one of sarcoidosis of the pituitary. In the cases of diabetes insipidus associated with sarcoidosis reported by Wahlgren (1936) and by Rey *et al.* (1947) and mentioned above, terminal caseating tuberculous lesions developed and were found at necropsy together with older-standing sarcoid lesions.

THYROID GLAND

The incidence of symptomless involvement of the thyroid gland in sarcoidosis is unknown. A few necropsy reports have mentioned the presence of granulomas in the gland, usually in cases with extensive organ involvement. Granulomas were stated to be present in the thyroid in five of the 117 necropsy reports reviewed by Branson and Park (1954). Cowdell (1954) found granulomas in the thyroid in three of seven necropsies in cases of sarcoidosis; in none had there been clinical evidence of thyroid dysfunction. Several reports of fatal myocardial sarcoidosis have mentioned the incidental finding of granulomas in the thyroid gland (Jonas, 1939; Yesner and Silver, 1951; Powell, 1954).

An unequivocal diagnosis of sarcoidosis of the thyroid during life is possible only if occasion arises for surgical removal or biopsy of the gland in a patient with sarcoidosis. A few cases in which nodules in the thyroid were found to be confluent sarcoid granulomas have been recorded. In a black woman who died at the age of 53 with very extensive sarcoidosis, reported by Arkless *et al.* (1958), a nodule found in the thyroid two years before death was excised and shown to consist of sarcoid granulomas. Buckle (1963) reported the case of a woman, aged 48, with bilateral uveitis, hilar node enlargement and lung shadows, and a nodule in the thyroid unaccompanied by clinical evidence of thyroid dysfunction, though the blood level of protein-bound iodine was low and of cholesterol high. The skin gave no reaction to 1:100 OT. Biopsy of the thyroid nodule showed a mass of non-caseating epithelioid and giant-cell tubercles; and a cutaneous nodule on the thumb showed similar histology.

An exceptional case in which the thyroid was generally enlarged by sarcoid granulomas was reported by Hemmings and McLean (1971).

A white girl aged ten who had had a recurrent erythematous rash for four years presented with fever, generalized lymphadenopathy, hepatosplenomegaly, slight thyroid enlargement, and retarded growth. Granulomas were found in a liver biopsy, but a Kveim test was negative. The following year, the thyroid was larger; biopsy of it showed granulomas; a Kveim test was again negative. Anterior uveitis appeared and changes were found in the lungs radiographically. The generally enlarged thyroid was partially removed, the volume removed from the left lobe being 4×3×2 cm and from the right 6×4×1 cm. The thyroid tissue was reported to be replaced by granuloma. After this, thyroid replacement therapy was maintained. At the age of 13, she was again febrile, weak and dyspnoeic, the radiographic changes in the lungs were worse, and BHL was evident, and hypercalcaemia was found. At this stage she was treated for the first time with prednisone with 'dramatic improvement', including increased growth-rate.

In other recorded cases, hyperthyroidism has been the indication for thyroidectomy in patients with sarcoidosis. In some, granulomas have been found in the gland. In Oldberg's (1943) case, hyperthyroidism with general thyroid enlargement and a nodule in the isthmus was accompanied by long-standing redness of the eyes and by fine mottling in the lungs radiographically; biopsies of both the thyroid and a lacrimal gland showed sarcoid tubercles, the thyroid also showing small empty vesicles typical of hyperthyroidism. This case was complicated by the finding of a single acid-fast rod in one of the thyroid tubercles. Rywlin (1952) reported the case of a woman, aged 58, whose thyroid was removed for an adenomatous toxic goitre. At the periphery of the adenomas, epithelioid and giant-cell tubercles were seen, and lymph-nodes showed similar tubercles. The case reported by Stark (1963) seems to be best interpreted as sarcoidosis developing in a patient already suffering from hyperthyroidism.

A woman, aged 49, was treated for iron-deficiency anaemia and was found to have firm enlargement of the thyroid gland, biopsy of which showed changes suggesting a primary toxic goitre and no granulomas. In the next few months, she developed evidence of hyperthyroidism and, radiographically, of hilar lymph-node enlargement, not present previously. Thyroidectomy was performed, and now, in addition to the changes previously noted, there were non-caseating tubercles with a few giant cells, and similar granulomas were seen in a scalene lymph-node. Cases 1 and 2 of Karlish and MacGregor (1970) occurred in women aged 32 and 50 who nine months and 18 months after the detection of BHL, accompanied in one by pulmonary mottling, and confirmed as sarcoid by scalene node and bronchial biopsy respectively, developed hyperthyroidism; both were treated by thyroidectomy, scattered granulomas being found in the glands removed. Selroos and Liewendahl (1972) reported the case of a woman who had had a partial thyroidectomy for hyperthyroidism at the age of 50; at the age of 70 she developed erythema nodosum with BHL, and at the same time moderate hyperthyroidism. A Kveim test gave a granulomatous response. Biopsy from the right lobe of the thyroid, which had been shown to be active on scanning showed high follicular epithelium, many lymphocytes, and epithelioid and giant-cell granulomas in interfollicular connective tissue.

Several cases have been reported in which hyperthyroidism and sarcoidosis co-existed, and histology of the gland showed no granulomas.

Case 6 of Karlish and MacGregor (1970) was that of a man aged 57 who presented with hyperthyroidism; six months later BHL was found, a Kveim test being negative but scalene node biopsy showing granulomas; biopsy of the thyroid isthmus showed no granulomas. Selroos and Liewendahl (1972) referred briefly to the case of a woman aged 37 with a non-toxic goitre who developed acute sarcoidosis which resolved in two years; one year later she developed hyperthyroidism, treated by carbimazole and subtotal thyroidectomy; the gland showed the changes of toxic nodular goitre without granulomas. Leppard (1971) reported the case of a man aged 57 who developed hyperthyroidism with slight thyroid enlargement and was found to have BHL; the Kveim test was twice negative, but scalene node biopsy showed granulomas. Biopsy of the thyroid showed focal lymphocytic infiltration but no granulomas.

Cases in which hyperthyroidism occurred during the active stages of sarcoidosis, but no information about the histology of the thyroid was available, have been reported by Harvier *et al.* (1950), Karlish and MacGregor (1970, Cases 3, 4 and 5), Selroos and Liewendahl (1972), Cohen and Clarke (1974) and Fromantin *et al.* (1975).

In a case reported by Cummins *et al.* (1951) partial thyroidectomy was performed for hyperthyroidism after preliminary treatment with propylthiouracil; the gland showed changes compatible with this diagnosis, together with epithelioid and giant-cell tubercles, some with slight central necrosis, but no evidence of sarcoid changes outside the thyroid gland was recorded. Thompson *et al.* (1973) reported two cases, both in young women, in which firm smooth goitres were accompanied by hyperthyroidism; after treatment with carbimazole, subtotal thyroidectomy was performed, the glands showing the histological changes of treated hyperthyroidism, together with occasional sarcoid-type granulomas; Kveim tests were reported to be positive, but no other evidence of sarcoidosis was found.

Reported associations between sarcoidosis and hyperthyroidism have thus included all possible combinations, and their number is too small to suggest any important causal relationship. When granulomas have been found in the gland, they have usually been too few to be likely to affect function, and in some cases in which they have been extensive, there has been no evident disturbance of thyroid function. For instance, Turiaf *et al.* (1950) reported the case of a woman with extensive lung and bronchial sarcoidosis and a nodule in the thyroid isthmus, without thyroid functional disturbance; partial thyroidectomy showed sarcoid infiltration of the gland with a well defined cystic adenoma.

There are a few reports of various forms of thyroiditis in patients with sarcoidosis. Mayock *et al.* (1963) mentioned briefly the occurrence of the clinical picture of thyroiditis during the acute stage in three of a series of 145 patients with sarcoidosis. Karlish and MacGregor (1970) reported five patients, all middle-aged women, with both sarcoidosis and Hashimoto's thyroiditis, proved histologically in three and presumed from antibody studies in two. In one, there was also evidence of Addison's disease, and this is discussed below (p. 364). In one of the other four, generalized lymphadenopathy was shown to be due to sarcoidosis by biopsy; 15 years previously goitre had been found and thyroidectomy was said to show adenoma; the diagnosis of immune thyroiditis rested upon auto-antibody studies. The remaining three all had BHL, with erythema nodosum in two and lung infiltration in one; thyroid enlargement was noted at the same time in two, though the diagnosis of Hashimoto's thyroiditis was not made until later, and five years after BHL in one. Selroos and Liewendahl (1972) mentioned briefly a woman aged 55 with pulmonary sarcoidosis who was found to have thyroiditis with a high anti-thyroglobulin titre; initially hyperthyroid, she became hypothyroid. In spite of treatment with prednisone, hypothyroidism persisted and needed replacement therapy. Leader and Dollberg (1974) reported that at necropsy in a woman aged 59 who died of post-operative pulmonary embolism they found clinically unsuspected sarcoidosis in lung and lymph-nodes together with Hashimoto's thyroiditis. Stallard and Tait (1939) and Ustvedt (1939) recorded cases, both in women, in which myxoedema and extensive sarcoidosis were associated. Brun *et al.* (1959) reported the case of a woman who at the age of 56 was found to be suffering from myxoedema, and was treated with thyroid extract. At the age of 59, she became dyspnoeic, and the chest radiograph, previously clear, showed a diffuse infiltration. Biopsy of the thyroid gland showed dense sclerosis with some lymphoid islets and rare thyroid vesicles; there were also some non-caseating epithelioid cell tubercles and giant cells, but a cervical lymph-node showed no granulomas. In these cases it seems likely that myxoedema was probably due to Hashimoto's thyroiditis, especially in the case reported by Brun *et al.* (1959) in which the histology of the thyroid gland was compatible with this diagnosis, and antedated the appearance of sarcoidosis. A case of De Quervain's thyroiditis in which there was equivocal evidence of sarcoidosis was reported by Birchall (1966). A woman aged 65 presented with an irregular firm swelling in the right lobe of the thyroid; thyroidectomy showed the changes of De Quervain's thyroiditis (Meachim *et al.*, 1963); three months later there was transient painless swelling of both parotids, a history of recurrent iritis in the past was obtained, and a Kveim test gave a small granulomatous response.

The occasional cases in which sarcoidosis has been associated with various sorts of thyroiditis, and those in which BHL with constitutional symptoms, with or without erythema nodosum, and hyperthyroidism have appeared and subsided together, have led to speculation whether the disturbance of function of the immune system in active sarcoidosis in some way favours auto-immune changes in the thyroid. It is uncertain whether sarcoidosis and disease of the thyroid gland, apart from granulomatous infiltration, occur together more often than would be expected by chance; and no common causal factor, immunological or other, between sarcoidosis and such disease has yet been identified.

Hypothyroidism may result from sarcoidosis involving the hypothalamus; as noted above. Jawali et al. (1980) investigated four patients with presumed hypothalamic-pituitary sarcoidosis, and found hypothala-mic hypothyroidism in three. Campbell *et al.* (1980) reported in detail two patients with hypothalamic sarcoidosis in whom hypothyroidism was an important feature.

PARATHYROID GLANDS

Involvement of the parathyroid glands in sarcoidosis is rare. It is discussed in relation to calcium metabolism in Chapter 19.

ADRENAL GLANDS

There are remarkably few reports of the finding of granulomas in the adrenal glands at necropsy in patients with sarcoidosis. Kulka (1950) in a patient who had died suddenly with myocardial sarcoidosis mentioned 'a few characteristic nodes in gastric mucosa, liver, kidneys, thyroid, adrenals and pituitary gland'. A few cases in which sclerotic changes which might have been the fibrotic end-result of sarcoid granulomas were found in the adrenals have been recorded. Teilum (1951) found hyalinization with a few remnants of granulomas in the thickened capsules of the adrenal and pituitary glands of a woman aged 49 who had died with long-standing and extensive sarcoidosis; the secretory part of the glands was normal, and there had been no evidence of adrenal insufficiency. The only recorded case in which possibly sarcoid changes in the adrenals seemed to be the cause of Addison's disease is one briefly mentioned by Mayock *et al.* (1963); at necropsy in a patient who had died in an Addisonian crisis, there were sarcoid granulomas in lungs, liver, spleen and bone-marrow; most of the cortex of the adrenals had been replaced by dense fibrous tissue with a whorled appearance, no granulomas being found, and the medulla largely spared.

Horton *et al.* (1939) and Riley (1950) reported cases with concurrent sarcoidosis and mycobacterial tuberculosis in which caseating and non-caseating granulomas were found in the adrenals. Ricker and Clark (1949, Cases 10 and 11) recorded two cases in which sarcoidosis was accompanied by caseous changes in the adrenal gland which caused death from Addison's disease. In both, typical sarcoid changes were found scattered through many organs and caseous lesions resembling old tuberculosis in the adrenal glands; no acid-fast bacilli were found in the caseous glands or elsewhere, except that in one of the two cases two acid-fast bacilli were found in a section from the apex of the right lung. Pinkerton and Iverson (1952) later re-examined the material from these two cases and found structures resembling *Histoplasma capsulatum* in the caseous parts of the adrenal glands (p. 522). A patient with chronic sarcoidosis under the care of one of us died of malignant lymphoma (p. 535); at necropsy the right adrenal contained an encapsulated nodule of caseation, in which no bacteria or fungi were found.

The extreme rarity of non-caseating granulomas in the adrenals is striking in view of the frequency with which caseating changes in these glands occur in mycobacterial tuberculosis, and of the importance of tuberculosis as a cause of Addison's disease in populations with a high incidence of tuberculosis.

> Karlish and MacGregor (1970, Case 11) reported the case of a woman, aged 47, who presented with myxoedema, treated with thyroxine; nine months later she developed Addison's disease with skin pigmentation and low blood pressure, and confirmed by hormone assays; adrenal antibody tests were strongly positive. She was found to have BHL and fine pulmonary infiltration, sarcoid-type granulomas in a scalene node biopsy and a granulomatous response to a Kveim test. Thyroid biopsy confirmed Hashimoto's thyroiditis. Hormone replacement therapy relieved her symptoms, and BHL and lung changes resolved. In this case, adrenal failure, presumably auto-immune, and Hashimoto's thyroiditis and active sarcoidosis were concurrent. One of us has observed a patient with concurrent Addison's disease and resolving active sarcoidosis. This patient, under the care of Dr H. Kopelman, was found to have Addison's disease, with skin pigmentation and low blood pressure, at the age of 29. At the same time, BHL, splenomegaly, and infiltration of old tattoos on the arms were found, and scalene node and Kveim test biopsies both showed granulomas. Adrenal antibody tests were negative initially, but later became positive. An uncle of the patient was said to have died of Addison's disease. The sarcoid manifestations subsided spontaneously, and the patient was known to be well on hormone replacement therapy ten years later. Although the concurrence of sarcoidosis and auto-immune Addison's disease raises the possibility of some common pathogenetic factor, its extreme rarity gives no support to this idea.

The case of a woman who was found to have an adrenal phaeochromocytoma seven years after the onset of sarcoidosis of hilar lymph-nodes and lungs was reported by Leophante *et al.* (1972). There is no reason to suppose that this was more than a chance association.

PANCREAS

The pancreas has been reported to contain a few sarcoid granulomas in several cases of extensive sarcoidosis at necropsy; e.g. by Nickerson (1937), Ricker and Clark (1939), Leitner (1949), Longcope and Freiman (1952) and Powell (1954). Involvement sufficient to cause symptoms or disturbance of either exocrine or endocrine function is extremely rare. Ryrie (1954) reported briefly the case of a woman with sarcoidosis in whom a nodule was found in the pancreas at laparotomy for obstructive jaundice; unfortunately, no histology of the pancreatic nodule was available. This patient developed diabetes mellitus. In the case of extensive sarcoidosis involving muscles reported by Ozer *et al.* (1961), a nodule of sarcoid histology, 1.5 cm in diameter, was found at necropsy in the pancreas (p. 250). Curran and Curran (1950) reported the case of a woman, aged 48, who underwent laparotomy for upper abdominal pain and vomiting; a firm nodular pancreas enlarged to twice the normal thickness was found, and biopsy showed infiltration with sarcoid tubercles; the patient was stated to be well one and a half years after the laparotomy, but no special search seems to have been made for other manifestations of sarcoidosis.

Chapter 17

The Gastro-intestinal tract

It is probable that in a proportion of patients in the active stage of sarcoidosis granulomas are present in the gastro-intestinal tract without causing symptoms, but this proportion is unknown. Infiltration causing symptoms because of its extent or local severity is rare. Among recorded cases which can be accepted as sarcoidosis of the alimentary tract causing symptoms, the majority have involved the stomach. If the gut is the principal or the only clinically evident site of granulomatous disease, unequivocal diagnostic categorization may be difficult or impossible. In the small gut, a special difficulty arises in relation to Crohn's disease, because of the granulomatous component in the histopathology of many cases and of some immunological features which it shares with sarcoidosis.

STOMACH

The incidental finding, at necropsies in cases of generalized sarcoidosis, of sarcoid tubercles in the stomach was mentioned by Schaumann (1936, Case 3), Naumann (1938) and Kulka (1950); and in the intestine by Lenartowicz and Rothfeld (1930), Cotter (1939) and Ricker and Clark (1949, Case 16).

Lorber et al. (1954) reported routine radiological studies, by barium meal and enema, of 21 cases of sarcoidosis, many extensive. No abnormality attributable to sarcoidosis was found, though three patients were found to have unsuspected duodenal ulcers.

Palmer (1958) investigated the stomach by gastroscopy and gastric mucosal biopsy in 60 men with otherwise diagnosed sarcoidosis. At gastroscopy the mucosa lookeed normal in 54, and changes interpreted as gastritis were found in six. None of those with abnormal gastroscopic appearances showed sarcoid changes histologically, but among the other 54, six showed granulomas in the biopsy specimens. Most of the granulomas were midway between the muscularis mucosae and the surface of the mucosa. In the six showing granulomas, repeated biopsies up to one and a half years after the first generally showed persistent granulomas. Oesophagoscopy in 33 patients showed no abnormalities.

Associated peptic ulcer

Peptic ulcer may be expected to occur by chance in a few individuals with symptomless sarcoid infiltration of the stomach. Löfgren (1953) mentioned a case in which a gastrectomy was performed for peptic ulcer three years after erythema nodosum with bilateral hilar lymph-node enlargement, and the removed specimen showed infiltration of the mucosa with sarcoid tubercles. Cases in which peptic ulceration developed in patients with established sarcoidosis, gastrectomy was performed, and the resected specimen showed both ulceration and the presence of granulomas in the gastric mucosa have been reported by Pearce and Ehrlich (1955), Nathan *et al.* (1960) and Kremer and Williams (1970); and others in which after granulomas had been found in stomach-wall and neighbouring lymph-nodes at gastrectomy for peptic ulcer, further investigation showed evidence of sarcoidosis in liver, lungs, peripheral lymph-nodes or other commonly-affected sites by Ramirez *et al.* (1964), Bennington *et al.* (1968), Fung *et al.* (1975), and Ito *et al.* (1977). Haematemesis and pyloric narrowing complicated the ulcer in the case described by Nathan *et al.* (1960); and in the case reported by Kremer and Williams (1970), cirrhotic changes in the liver, presumably secondary to sarcoidosis, and increasing pulmonary fibrosis were important features. Jessing (1943), Guibert (1947), Wadina and Melamed (1966), and Kater and Stening (1967) described cases in which non-caseating tubercles were found in the mucosa and submucosa, in some in adjacent lymph-nodes also, but no evidence of similar changes elsewhere was found in subsequent investigation; in the last-mentioned, a Kveim test was negative. In view of the possibility of localized granulomatous reactions in the stomach, as in other sites (Sherman and Moran, 1954; Present *et al.*, 1966), judgment about cases of this latter sort should be reserved; a diagnosis of sarcoidosis is a possibility, but should not be accepted unless evidence of more widespread granulomatosis appears during further observation.

In the case described by Bennington *et al.* (1968), cytology of gastric aspirate was thought to be suggestive of adenocarcinoma, and together with enlargement of the liver, led to partial gastrectomy in a woman aged 44 with radiological evidence of an ulcer on the lesser curvature of the stomach. The stomach removed showed an ulcer in an area of oedematous thickening with granulomas both in the ulcerated and the more normal parts, and granulomas were found in the spleen removed with the stomach and in lymph-nodes and a wedge biopsy of the liver. Re-examination of the cytology led to the conclusion that the abnormal cells were multinucleated giant cells with bizarre nuclei.

Oppenheim and Pollack (1947) described the case of a woman, aged 50, with sarcoidosis of superficial lymph-nodes, confirmed by biopsy on two occasions, in whom partial gastrectomy for ulcer showed sarcoid infiltration of the stomach, and a liver biopsy at the same time showed similar changes. Four years later, and ten years from the first appearance of the superficial lymphadenopathy, the inguinal nodes enlarged again, and now showed the histological picture of Hodgkin's disease; the association of sarcoidosis with lymphomas is discussed on p. 534.

Several of the descriptions of peptic ulceration in stomachs infiltrated by sarcoid tubercles mentioned greater numbers of granulomas in the vicinity of the ulcer, but there is no reason to suspect that the gastric mucosa lightly infiltrated with sarcoid tubercles is specially liable to peptic ulceration; certainly patients with sarcoidosis do not seem to suffer an undue frequency of gastric or duodenal ulcers.

Symptomatic gastric sarcoidosis

Review of reported cases suggests that gastric sarcoidosis may produce symptoms either by diffuse infiltration, or by massive local infiltration simulating carcinoma.

Diffuse infiltration, with or without ulceration, may cause dyspepsia or bleeding, although it may be impossible to exclude other causes of these symptoms, either unrelated to sarcoidosis, or in some cases related to sarcoid infiltration of liver, spleen or abdominal lymph-nodes.

In Case 1 of Scott *et al.* (1953), a 20 year old black man complained of intermittent abdominal pain; an enlarged lacrimal gland had shown sarcoid tubercles in biopsy; the free and total acid content of the gastric juice was low; gastroscopy on two occasions at an interval of ten months showed a normal-looking mucosa, which on biopsy was found to be infiltrated with sarcoid tubercles. In Case 1 of Debray *et al.* (1967), a 65 year old man complained of dyspepsia, diarrhoea and loss of weight, and was found to have a pulmonary infiltration and enlarged superficial lymph-nodes, biopsy of which showed sarcoid-type granulomas, and gastric and rectal mucosal biopsies showed granulomas; symptoms responded to corticosteroid treatment. In their Case 3, a man aged 63 with extensive sarcoidosis, starting with Heerfordt's syndrome and later developing skin sarcoids, was found to have histamine-fast achlorhydria and gastroscopic appearances interpreted as 'superficial conges- tive gastritis', two epithelioid-cell follicles being seen in the biopsy; in this case, the relationship of the gastritis to sarcoidosis is arguable. Miyamoto *et al.* (1972) reported the necropsy findings in a Japanese woman who had had an illness characterized by weakness, loss of weight, oedema and hypoalbuminaemia and died at the age of 61 of intracranial haemorrhage, probably traumatic; non-caseating granulomas were found in great numbers in stomach and intestine, and scattered in liver and spleen, but not in lung. Gould *et al.* (1973) reported the case of a Jamaican, aged 29, who presented with BHL and lung infiltration, a lymph-node removed from the mediastinum showing sarcoid tubercles. Later, he developed poorly localized abdominal pain; the liver and spleen were enlarged, and the alkaline phosphatase found to be 198 KA units; barium meal showed irregularity of the gastric mucosa, especially on the greater curvature, and gastroscopy showed gastritis without ulceration, with giant-cell granulomas on biopsy. Although the rectal mucosa looked normal at proctoscopy, a granuloma was seen in a biopsy sample of mucosa. Blackstone *et al.* (1976) reported the case of a black woman aged 64 who had been known to be suffering from sarcoidosis for five years, involving hilar lymphnodes, lungs, liver and bone-marrow, with biopsy evidence from the two latter sites, and who complained of recurrent retrosternal pain and fullness after food; gastroscopy showed thickened antral folds, biopsy of which showed granulomas. Mora (1980) and Konda *et al.* (1980) both described the case of a black man aged 32 with extensive sarcoidosis of the skin and superficial lymph-nodes and granulomatous hepatitis, who was investigated for nausea, vomiting and severe loss of weight. Endoscopically, the gastric mucosa showed a cobblestoned appearance and on biopsy was found to be infiltrated with granulomas, and the rectal mucosa appeared friable with punctate bleeding and also contained granulomas. Corticosteroid treatment led to improvement.

In cases described by Scott *et al.* (1953, Case 2), McKusick *et al.* (1953, Case 2) and Obitisch-Mayer *et al.* (1958) upper gastro-intestinal bleeding was associated with granulomatous infiltration and superficial ulceration of gastric mucosa, but no evidence of granulomas elsewhere was found.

Many of the cases reported as sarcoidosis of the stomach have presented the clinical syndrome of pyloric obstruction, and have been thought radiologically and even at operation to be examples of carcinoma of the stomach, usually of the linitis plastica variety, until the histological character of the lesion was established.

Orie *et al.* (1950) described the case of a 53 year old woman who had had an infiltration in the lungs with negative tuberculin test for many years, and complained of anorexia, vomiting and epigastric pain for one year; radiologically there was persistent narrowing of the pyloric antrum, occult blood was present in the faeces, and there was a histamine-fast achlorhydria; at laparotomy there was diffuse thickening of the gastric wall, especially towards the pylorus, and lymph-nodes along the lesser curvature were enlarged; a gastrectomy was performed; histologically, there were many tubercles with giant cells and some Schaumann bodies in the basal layer of the mucosa and submucosa, and some between the muscle and the serosa, and also in the enlarged lymph-nodes, but an operative liver biopsy showed no abnormality. Sirak (1954) described similar changes in the stomach, simulating linitis plastica both radiologically and at laparotomy in a 27 year old white man, who also had generalized lymphadenopathy, parotid gland enlargement and uveitis; biopsy of stomach, adjacent lymph-nodes and liver showed epithelioid and giant-cell granulomas. He was treated with corticosteroids; De Lor (1962) reported that eight years later he was still receiving prednisone for relief of symptoms, but had developed severe hypertension, and the condition of the stomach remained similar. Similar changes found in the stomach at laparotomy and causing a similar syndrome, though there was no pre-operative indication of generalized sarcoidosis, have been reported by García Morán (1948), Allen *et al.* (1956), McLaughlin *et al.* (1961), and Thomas *et al.* (1972) in cases in which there was evidence of involvement of at least one organ besides the stomach and regional nodes; by Gore and McCarthy (1944), McKusick (1953, Case 1) and Eckstein and Parker (1958), Kossmann (1959), Fahimi *et al.* (1963, three cases), Negus (1966), and Galvin (1967, Case 2) in cases where the only discovered changes were in the stomach and the regional lymph-nodes; and by Appell *et al.* (1951), who described only the changes in the stomach itself. In García Morán's (1948) case, the whole stomach was found at laparotomy to be thickened, and nothing was done except removal of a lymph-node for biopsy, which showed non-caseating tubercles; the patient developed bilateral parotid gland enlargement and 'conjunctivitis' of which no details were given. Allen *et al.* (1956) found granulomas not only in the stomach, whose distal third was thickened, narrowed and without peristalsis, but also in lymph-nodes and in liver; and their patient, a woman aged 26, also showed radiological evidence of contraction and loss of mucosal pattern in the caecum and electrocardiographic changes suggestive of some myocardial damage. In the case reported by Negus (1966) a tuberculin test with 1 IU was positive, and in a lymph-node some caseation was reported; unfortunately the tissues were fixed without culture or guinea-pig inoculation, but no acid-fast bacilli were seen. In eight of the patients with symptoms of pyloric obstruction, achlorhydria was found (Gore and McCarthy, 1944; García Morán, 1948; Orie *et al.*, 1950; Appell *et al.*, 1951; McKusick, 1953; Kossmann, 1959; Fahimi *et al.*, 1963, Case 1; Negus, 1966), adding to the suspicion of gastric carcinoma.

Bauer (1951) reported the finding of sarcoid-type tubercles in a stomach removed surgically for carcinoma; they were found in the gastric mucosa and among the cells of the carcinoma, and also in small lymph-nodes. There was no record of findings, clinical or histological, in other organs.

OESOPHAGUS

Very few cases that can be accepted as localizations of sarcoidosis in the oesophagus causing dysphagia have been reported.

Polachek and Matre (1964) reported the case of a man aged 65 who complained of loss of weight and epigastric pain for 18 months. He had hepatosplenomegaly, fine mottling in the chest radiograph, and in a barium meal examination irregularity of the distal part of the oesophagus. Biopsies of the liver, lung and an axillary lymph-node showed the histology of sarcoidosis and the skin gave no reaction to 250 IU of PPD. Biopsy from the abnormal part of the oesophagus showed sarcoid tubercles, mostly subepithelial in position. Prednisolone treatment led to great improvement. Hardy *et al.* (1967) reported another patient with narrowing of the distal oesophagus by granulomatous infiltration. A 31 year old woman was found to have an enlarged right hilar shadow in a routine chest radiograph, and shortly afterwards lost her appetite, became dizzy, and had difficulty in swallowing and in phonation; tracheostomy was required to avoid aspiration of secretions; at thoracotomy enlarged lymph-nodes around the right main bronchus and the oesophagus, and thickening and narrowing of the distal oesophagus were found; biopsies of oesophagus, lymph-nodes and lung showed sarcoid-type granulomas; corticosteroid treatment led to improvement in swallowing and phonation.

In a case described by Davies (1972) it seems likely that localization of sarcoidosis in the oesophageal wall and in abdominal lymph-nodes caused dysphagia and abdominal pain. A man was found at the age of 46 to have symptomless shadowing in the upper part of the right lung, and two years later, bilateral hilar and right paratracheal lymph-node enlargement; these subsided spontaneously. He later experienced increasing difficulty in swallowing, shown to be associated with loss of peristaltic activity in the oesophagus. At the age of 54, he was shown by oesophagoscopy and surgical exploration to have a tumour-like swelling in the wall of the upper third of the oesophagus; on biopsy this showed non-caseating granulomas with patchy degeneration of muscle. Skeletal muscle biopsy showed no abnormality. When he was aged 60, a normal appendix was removed because of abdominal pain; skeletal muscle biopsy was again normal. Two years later, he still had severe abdominal pain and dysphagia, though his general condition remained good. Laparotomy showed enlarged lymph-nodes around the coeliac axis and behind the first part of the duodenum; biopsy of several of these showed extensive replacement by non-caseating granulomas. No other localization of sarcoid granulomas was detected.

A case in which extrinsic pressure on the oesophagus by lymph-nodes enlarged by sarcoidosis caused dysphagia was reported by Cook *et al.* (1970). A woman aged 29 complained of food sticking with pain at mid-thoracic level; chest radiograph showed a characteristic bilateral hilar and right paratracheal lymph-node enlargement, and a barium swallow showed extrinsic compression at this level; biopsy of a supraclavicular lymph-node showed sarcoid tubercles, and a tuberculin test with 100 IU was negative; treatment with prednisone led to relief of symptoms, subsidence of the enlarged nodes, and normal appearance on barium swallow.

Cases in which granulomatous infiltration of the cricopharyngeus muscle and upper opening of the oesophagus caused dysphagia which was relieved by myotomy have been reported by Siegel *et al.* (1961) and Panosetti and Lehmann (1979), in women aged 66 and 73 years. In neither case was there past or present clinical evidence of involvement at any other site; in the case of Siegel *et al.* biopsy of the gastrocnemius muscle showed granulomas, and in that of Panosetti and Lehmann a Kveim test was reported to be positive.

Narrowing of the oesophagus by partly granulomatous inflammatory changes has been reported in Crohn's disease (Dyer *et al.*, 1969). The diagnosis of Crohn's disease in such cases depends not only upon compatible histology of the oesophageal lesion but also upon the recognition of characteristic changes in the ileum and elsewhere in the gut, just as the diagnosis of sarcoidosis depends upon evidence of characteristic granulomatous changes in other organs known to be commonly involved.

INTESTINE

Small intestine

Very few cases in which granulomatous changes in the small intestine giving rise to symptoms in patients having other evidences of sarcoidosis have been reported. In the absence of such evidence, and especially when the ileum is involved, differential diagnosis from Crohn's disease is difficult.

In some cases reported as intestinal sarcoidosis, evidence of generalized granulomatosis was lacking. Williams and Nickerson (1935) mentioned two cases, both in women, in which intestine resected for regional ileitis was found to have the histological pattern of sarcoidosis, but gave no information about other findings. Watson *et al.* (1945) described two cases, in which long segments of small intestine resected from young women who had presented with a clinical picture of 'non-specific ileo-jejunitis' showed sarcoid histology, both in the gut and in local lymph-nodes; both were tuberculin-negative, but no other localizations of sarcoidosis were found. Cowdell (1954) mentioned a similar case in a girl, aged 15, in whom laparotomy performed because of recurrent abdominal colic showed tubercle-like structures and flat white plaques over most of the ileum, together with enlarged mesenteric lymph-nodes, biopsy showing 'appearances typical of sarcoidosis'; there was no mention of other localizations; during 13 years' subsequent observation, the symptoms subsided.

In a case reported by Clague (1972) there was acceptable evidence both of generalized sarcoidosis and of granulomatous ileitis. A woman aged 36 had bilateral parotid gland enlargement, generalized lymphadenopathy, and an abnormal chest radiograph; a clinical diagnosis of sarcoidosis was made and prednisone treatment led to rapid subsidence of the parotid swellings and gradual resolution of the lung shadows, and was continued for two and a half years. One year later, a megaloblastic anaemia with low vitamin B12 level was successfully treated with cyanocobalamin. Eight months later, she developed epigastric pain and vomiting and lost weight; there was complete achlorhydria, but no anaemia, and the chest radiograph had become normal. Because of radiographic evidence of abnormality in the prepyloric region of the stomach, laparotomy was performed. The first part of the duodenum was thickened with many pin-head pale nodules on its red peritoneal surface, and similar changes were seen in three segments of the lower ileum, each 8–10 cm in length, with 16–30 cm of normal-looking intestine between them. Biopsy of one of these abnormal segments showed sarcoid type tubercles with giant cells of both Langhans and foreign-body type throughout the intestinal wall, with few lymphocytes. No such changes were found in the stomach. There was a dramatic response to treatment with prednisone. The distribution of the intestinal changes in this case was concordant with that regarded as typical of Crohn's disease, but the predominantly granulomatous histology, the clinical features of the earlier stage, and the prompt response to corticosteroid treatment are more compatible with a diagnosis of sarcoidosis with late localization in the intestine.

Because the complex histological picture of Crohn's disease includes epithelioid and giant cells, sometimes arranged in a tuberculoid pattern (Homans and Hass, 1933; Comfort *et al.*, 1950; Crohn *et al.*, 1932), the possibility that this disease might be pathogenetically related to sarcoidosis was suggested by some pathologists, notably by Hadfield (1939). Snapper (1938) denied this possibility on the grounds that the small intestine was not affected in sarcoidosis and that patients with regional ileitis did not show any of the features commonly observed in sarcoidosis. Blackburn *et al.* (1939) studied 22 and Phear (1958) 40 cases of regional ileitis without finding any evidence of generalized sarcoidosis, though in both groups of patients the level of tuberculin sensitivity was lower than would be expected. It cannot be decided whether the very few cases, like those mentioned above, in which an apparently isolated ileitis has the histological picture of sarcoidosis should be regarded as examples of regional ileitis in which the histological pattern is unusually tuberculoid, or as cases of sarcoidosis in which other localizations were present but not discovered. In most of the cases acceptable as sarcoidosis of the alimentary tract, the stomach has been the part most evidently affected, while there are relatively few reports of Crohn's disease of the ileum with associated changes in the stomach (Martin and Carr, 1953; Richman *et al.*, 1955; Pryse-Davies, 1964).

Concurrence of sarcoidosis and Crohn's disease

Cases in which clinical and histological features of Crohn's disease have co-existed with clinical features and disseminated granulomatous changes characteristic of sarcoidosis are very rare.

Morland (1947) reported the case of a young man with miliary lung shadows and uveitis who developed abdominal pain and a mass in the right iliac fossa; the much thickened terminal ileum was removed, and showed histologically increase in lymphoid tissue, infiltration with lymphocytes and eosinophils, and only two follicular collections of mononuclear cells, while a meseteric lymph-node showed the histological patrtern of sarcoidosis. The same case appears to have been described also by Neubert (1946). A few cases have been reported in which Crohn's disease and sarcoidosis occurred in the same patient with an interval of several years between them. Dines *et al.* (1971, Case 1) and Padilla and Sparberg (1972) described cases in which typical Crohn's disease, confirmed by histology of resected bowel, was followed by sarcoidosis involving lungs and lymph-nodes histologically confirmed by biopsy of lung and of scalene lymph-node respectively after intervals of 14 and seven years. In Case 2 of Dines *et al.* (1971), sarcoidosis of lungs and hilar lymph-nodes, not confirmed histologically but radiologically following a typical course, was followed after seven years by regional ileitis, treated by resection of the involved ileum and adjacent colon.

The very small number of reports of sarcoidosis and Crohn's disease in the same patient does not seem more than might be expected by chance, especially since the concurrence of two relatively uncommon diseases, both of unknown cause is likely to be recorded. Nevertheless, Crohn's disease shares with sarcoidosis not only the granulomatous elements in its histology but also depression of delayed hypersensitivity reactions; and a proportion of patients with Crohn's disease give granulomatous reactions to some validated Kveim test suspensions (Chapter 21, p. 475).

Families in which sarcoidosis and Crohn's disease occurred in different members have been reported by Willoughby *et al.* (1971) and Grönhagen-Riska *et al.* (1983). In the first of these, two of three brothers had sarcoidosis, both with BHL and lung infiltration and one with uveitis, and the third had typical Crohn's disease, confirmed by laparotomy and histology of the resected ileum; the parents and one sister showed no evidence of either disease. All family members except the father were non-reactive to tuberculin, 100 IU; all were Kveim-tested, only one of the brothers with sarcoidosis giving a granulomatous reaction. In the family described by Grönhagen-Riska *et al.* (1983) the father had sarcoidosis affecting skin, spleen and kidneys, with hypercalcaemia. Six years later, a daughter had BHL and a son a period of ill-health with hypercalciuria and raised serum angiotensin-converting enzyme, attributed to sarcoidosis, both recovering spontaneously, and another son developed typical Crohn's disease confirmed by histology of resected bowel. The mother and the third son were unaffected; the affected members of the family had a common haplotype, including B8 and DR3.

APPENDIX

In most of the few cases reported as sarcoidosis of the appendix, it seems likely that acute appendicitis occurred in a patient with a symptomless scarcoid infiltration of the appendix. The rarity of this occurrence is indicated by the finding of only one example of sarcoidosis in a study of 50 000 surgically removed appendices by Collins (1955).

Cases in which both granulomas and acute inflammation were found when the appendix was removed for acute appendicitis in patients with known sarcoidosis were reported by MacLeod *et al.* (1965) and Munt (1974); and similar changes were found in a patient reported by Sheinfield and Rubinov (1964) who had no past or currently-evident other manifestations of sarcoidosis.

In the case reported by Byström (1968) infiltration of the appendix and gross enlargement of the lymph-nodes in the ileo-caecal region by non-caseating epithelioid and giant-cell granulomas appeared to be the cause of recurrent episodes of abdominal pain in a 20 year old man. A mobile mass was palpable in the right lower quadrant of the abdomen, and barium meal showed narrowing of the distal ileum. Removal of the appendix and of a lymph-node for biopsy was followed by relief of symptoms; no clinical or radiological evidence of other manifestations of sarcoidosis was found. Granulomatous disease apparently localized to the appendix region is a possible, though rare presentation of Crohn's disease (Allen and Biggart, 1983); differential diagnosis depends largely upon search for other localizations, and upon observation of the course.

COLON

Only a few cases which can be accepted as sarcoidosis involving the colon and causing symptoms have been reported.

Aaronson *et al.* (1957) reported the case of a black woman aged 37 in whom the diagnosis of sarcoidosis had been established by biopsy of a skin infiltration, and there was radiological evidence of changes in the lungs and the bones of the hands; investigation of increasing constipation by barium enema showed an annular constriction at the junction of the descending and sigmoid parts of the colon; the narrowed part of the colon with 4 cm on either side was removed, and showed induration with nodular foci of epithelioid cells, a few giant cells and some fibroblasts in submucosa and mucosa. This patient had had treatment for menorrhagia by radium insert into the uterus six months previously; this suggests the possibility that radiation may have determined the localization of granulomas in the colon in a patient with generalized sarcoidosis. Kohn (1980) reported the case of a 55 year old woman with bilateral parotid gland enlargement, lung infiltration and hypercalcaemia, and recent anorexia with loss of weight. Investigation showed a stenotic zone in the sigmoid colon and a mass in front of the pancreas. At laparotomy the affected part of the colon was removed, as was a large lymph-node over the pancreas, and a biopsy of the liver which showed many yellow nodules, was taken. All these specimens showed many sarcoid-type granulomas. Post-operatively, corticosteroid treatment was started; serum calcium levels returned to normal, and three months later, the patient felt well.

In other cases reported as sarcoidosis of the colon, the colon was the only detected site of granulomatosis; e.g. in those described by Raven (1949) and by Gourevitch and Cunningham (1959), in both of which the colon, removed on a provisional diagnosis of carcinoma, was found to be infiltrated with granulomas. In a case reported by McFarlane (1955) a man aged 53 with a 13 year history of peptic ulcer type symptoms was found at laparotomy to have a mass in the caecum with nodules on the adjacent peritoneum, and hypertrophy of the pyloric muscle. Right hemicolectomy and pyloroplasty were performed. In the operative specimen, a mass about 2.5 × 2.5 cm protruded into the caecum; histologically, there were non-caseating granulomas both in the gut wall and in lymph-nodes; no acid-fast bacilli were found, and a tuberculin test with 10 IU was negative.

In cases described by Debray *et al.* (1967, Case 2) and by Tobi *et al.* (1982) rectal biopsies in patients with other evidences of sarcoidosis showed unspecific inflammatory changes with some granulomas, interpreted in that of Tobi *et al.* as compatible with Crohn's disease.

A few examples of patients who had both sarcoidosis and ulcerative colitis have been reported. In that recorded by Watson *et al.* (1971) sarcoidosis preceded ulcerative colitis. A woman first noted dyspnoea at the age of 39, and two years later was found to have BHL and lung changes, scalene-node biopsy showing sarcoid-type granulomas. A year later she developed intermittent bloody diarrhoea and abdominal pain. Investigated at the age of 52, she was found to have radiographic, sigmoidoscopy and biopsy evidence of extensive ulcerative colitis. In the case reported by Theodoropoulos *et al.* (1981) a man aged 64 with ulcerative colitis, typical in clinical features, endoscopic appearances and histology, for four years was found to have BHL, enlarged peripheral lymph-nodes, histologically sarcoid on biopsy, and chorioretinitis. The two diseases appeared to be concurrent in complex cases reported with necropsy findings by Trujillo *et al.* (1967) and Jalan *et al.* (1969). In the first of these a man died at the age of 38 after an illness starting when he was aged 30 with ulcerative colitis, BHL and hepatosplenomegaly, followed two years later by jaundice, pruritus and cutaneous xanthomas; at this time laparotomy showed a finely nodular liver, biopsy of which was interpreted as showing biliary cirrhosis with only one well-formed granuloma, and large lymph-nodes showing many epithelioid-cell granulomas around the cystic duct but not obstructing it. Portal hypertension was demonstrated, and a Kveim test was positive. Later, a porto-caval shunt was performed for severe haematemesis. He died at the age of 38 after persistent rectal bleeding. At necropsy, the principal findings were chronic ulcerative colitis with extensive fibrosis, enlargement of lymph-nodes in the mediastinum and the hila of the lungs and at the porta hepatis obstructing the common bile duct, and an enlarged finely nodular liver. The lymph-nodes microscopically contained non-caseating granulomas, and the liver showed periportal fibrosis, sparsity of bile-ducts, and scanty granulomas. In the case reported by Jalan *et al.* (1969), a man developed ulcerative colitis at the age of 25; persistent symptoms and premalignant changes in a rectal polyp led to proctocolectomy at the age of 34. In addition to the changes of ulcerative colitis, the operative specimen showed an adenocarcinoma in the terminal ileum; none of the regional nodes showed tumour, but some contained non-caseating granulomas. The patient died of pulmonary embolism after a further operation to remove more ileum; at necropsy, non-caseating granulomas were found in mediastinal and mesenteric lymph-nodes lungs and spleen.

PERITONEUM

Becker and Coleman (1961) described the cases of two black women with extensive sarcoidosis and peritoneal involvement. In one, aged 24, plaques of sarcoid histology were found on the visceral surfaces of the abdominal viscera at laparotomy for removal of a large spleen; no abdominal symptoms appeared during seven years' subsequent observation. In the other, aged 39, ascites and multiple peritoneal nodules reminiscent of tuberculous peritonitis were found at laparotomy; she died four years later of pulmonary fibrosis and at necropsy the diagnosis of sarcoidosis was confirmed, but the peritoneal changes were no longer evident. Wong and Rosen (1962) reported a similar case in a man, aged 24, in whom just over two years after the appearance of bilateral parotid swellings with sarcoid histology, gross ascites developed; at laparotomy many hard white nodules were seen on the peritoneum and were shown to consist of sarcoid granulomas with some central eosinophil necrosis; the tuberculin test was negative. Papowitz and Li (1971) reported the case of a black woman aged 28 who developed abdominal distension and ankle oedema in the seventh month of pregnancy; after delivery she was found to have ascites and at laparotomy ten litres of serous fluid, with many small nodules on the serous surfaces of the much enlarged spleen, the pancreas, the greater omentum and mesentery were found. The spleen was removed, and it and biopsies of portal lymph-node, the tail of the pancreas and liver all showed sarcoid-type granulomas, all except those in the spleen looking recent. The chest radiograph showed normal lungs; the skin did not react to 250 IU of PPD; a Kveim test was later reported to be positive. During one year's further observation, ascites did not recur.

In several of the cases reported as sarcoidosis of the intestine, e.g. those of Cowdell (1954) and Clague (1972), tubercles or plaques were seen on serosal surfaces of affected gut. In a case described by Robinson and Ernst (1954), the abdomen was explored because of a lump in an old cholecystectomy scar; the mass consisted of a number of white nodules, 1–5 cm in diameter, and the peritoneum over the intestine, the liver and pelvic organs were studded with small nodules, of the same sort; and the nodules were found to be composed of non-caseating tubercles but no information about involvement of other organs was given.

INTRA-ABDOMINAL LYMPH-NODES

Intra-abdominal lymph-nodes enlarged by sarcoidosis may give rise to palpable masses, which may be tender; and occasionally appear to be the cause of pain or other symptoms.

Rakov and Taylor (1942, Case 3) described the case of a black man with generalized sarcoid lymphadenopathy and lung infiltration in whom recurrent attacks of upper abdominal pain were associated with a mass of lymph-nodes greatly enlarged by sarcoid infiltration, the liver also being infiltrated. Long-cope and Freiman (1952, Case 3) recorded the case of an Italian boy with widespread sarcoidosis of superficial lymph-nodes, confirmed by biopsy, who developed abdominal pain associated with an epigastric mass of increasing size; laparotomy showed this to consist of sarcoid-infiltrated lymph-nodes. The tuberculin test was negative to 10 mg OT. He became febrile, with further increase in the size of the abdominal mass, and died one year after the laparotomy; there was no necropsy. In the case of oesophageal sarcoidosis described by Davies (1972) and mentioned above (p. 371), abdominal pain was probably related to enlarged lymph-nodes around the coeliac axis.

One of us (JGS) has observed two patients with abdominal symptoms attributable to sarcoidosis of lymph-nodes. The first was a man who at the age of 34 was found to have widespread mottling in a routine chest radiograph. Shortly after this he developed recurrent episodes of lassitude, nausea and vomiting. The serum calcium level was normal. The symptoms responded to corticosteroid treatment, but relapsed after its withdrawal. When he was aged 41, a laparotomy was performed because in one of these episodes there was abdominal pain and tenderness in the right iliac fossa. This showed a normal appendix and enlarged lymph-nodes, in which histologically the normal structure was replaced by sarcoid tubercles. Three years later, he continued to have recurrent episodes of a similar sort, controlled by corticosteroid treatment.

The second was a man who at the age of 40 developed cough, slight dyspnoea, and later tiredness, anorexia and low fever. He was found to have bilateral hilar node enlargement with some streakiness radiating into the lung fields, a palpable spleen and somewhat enlarged liver. The fever settled with rest in hospital. The skin gave no reaction to tuberculin 100 IU. A scalene node biopsy showed typical sarcoid changes. One year from the onset, he developed pain in the left hypochondrium, nausea, abdominal distension and tenesmus. The spleen was now enlarged two fingers' breadth below the costal margin, and rounded discrete masses were felt in both iliac fossae, above the inguinal ligaments, presumably enlarged iliac lymph-nodes. Of the superficial lymph-nodes, the epitrochlear and axillary were palpably enlarged. Predniso-lone treatment led to subsidence of the enlarged lymph-nodes and of the spleen, and to relief of the symptoms. It was continued for two and a half years, and then withdrawn without relapse. He remained well without gastro-intestinal symptoms, and with slight fibrotic changes in the lungs causing no disability as the only residue of the sarcoidosis, during two years' further observation.

Miller *et al.* (1981) reported the case of a 27 year old woman who presented with dyspnoea and pleuritic pain, apparently due to pulmonary emboli conse-quent on oral contraceptive use. This was treated with heparin. Extensive superficial lymphadenopathy, hepatosplenomegaly, epigastric tenderness, nausea and vomiting were noted. Barium meal, followed by computed tomog-raphy and ultrasound, showed compression of the greater curvature of the stomach by enlarged periaortic lymph-nodes. Biopsy of a cervical node and needle biopsy of the para-aortic mass both showed sarcoid-type granulomas; treatment with prednisone led to relief of symptoms and decrease in size of the abdominal mass.

Schwarzschild and Myerson (1968) reported a case in which pressure on mesenteric veins by hyalinized sarcoid lymph-nodes led to gangrene of part of the jejunum. The patient was a black man, aged 46, who had been suffering from sarcoidosis involving lungs, eyes, liver, spleen, lymph-nodes and skin for 19 years; many manifestations had regressed spontaneously, and he had been symptom-free for nine years, when he developed post-prandial abdominal pain and nausea, and during hospital investigation became febrile. At lapar-otomy a segment of gangrenous bowel about 50 cm from the beginning of the jejunum was resected. The gangrenous part, about 40 cm in length was sharply demarcated; enlarged nodes in its mesentery appeared to be occluding veins. Microscopically, the veins were congested and some thrombosed and the bowel showed haemorrhagic infarction; the lymph-nodes showed many hyali-nized foci compatible with 'burnt-out' sarcoidosis.

Chapter 18

The Genito-urinary System, excluding Kidney; the Breast

UTERUS AND ADNEXA

In view of the widespread distribution of sarcoid granulomas in the active stages of sarcoidosis, it is surprising that few references have been made to the finding of sarcoid tubercles in the uterus, and more especially the endometrium which is so frequently subjected to curettage and biopsy in women in the age group most susceptible to sarcoidosis.

Few reports of necropsies in women with sarcoidosis have mentioned the finding of granulomas in the genital organs. In the case of uveo-parotid fever described by Garland and Thomson (1933) and mentioned on p. 310, the uterus was found to be extensively infiltrated with non-caseating tubercles, most numerous in the serosa and the endometrium. In Naumann's (1938) case of extensive sarcoidosis in an infant (p. 313), subserous tubercles were found in the uterus. Cowdell (1954) briefly mentioned that in a woman, aged 21, who died suddenly of myocardial sarcoidosis, the Fallopian tubes were among the organs infiltrated with sarcoid tubercles.

The finding of epithelioid cell granulomas in endometrial curettings must be interpreted with caution, since in endometrial tuberculosis the tubercles may be of non-caseating type, difficult or impossible to distinguish from those of sarcoidosis. Possibly the cyclic shedding of the endometrium does not allow time for the tubercles to attain a caseating stage (Haines, 1952). Tubercle bacilli may be discoverable, either by microscopy or by culture, in endometrium or menstrual fluid (Sutherland, 1960). To establish the diagnosis of sarcoidosis, not only should search for tubercle bacilli be unsuccessful, but evidence of concurrent or past manifestations of sarcoidosis elsewhere be found. In women known to be suffering from sarcoidosis, it is a reasonable assumption that granulomas found in the endometrium obtained by curettage are part of this disease, as in a case mentioned by Longcope and Freiman (1952). Other cases in which curettage for gynaecological indications in women known to have sarcoidosis showed endometrial granulomas have been reported by Winslow and Funkhauser (1968), Chalvardjian (1978) and Ho (1979). In all these cases, hysterectomy was later performed for various indications; granulomatous endometritis was confirmed, and some granulomas were found in the myometrium, noted to be sparse in Chalvardjian's case.

> Chalvardjian's patient was post-menopausal, and had been found to have pulmonary, lymph-node and skin sarcoidosis 16 years previously; both ovaries were removed with the uterus, and were found to contain groups of granulomas up to 1 mm in diameter deep in the cortex. In the case described by Winslow and Funkhauser (1968), a black woman had been found to have pulmonary sarcoidosis, confirmed by lymph-node biopsy, at the age of 28; six years later, premenstrual spotting led to the discovery of carcinoma-in-situ of the cervix and granulomas in the endometrium; at operation, the right ovary was found to be adherent to the uterus, and was removed with it; granulomas were found in myometrium, ovary, Fallopian tube, and appendix.
>
> Altchek *et al.* (1955) described the case of a black woman, aged 39, who underwent hysterectomy for fibromyomas; five years previously she had had BHL and lung shadowing; the uterus contained subserous fibromyomas, and showed small pinkish areas in the myometrium and thickening of the endometrium; and in both myometrium and endometrium, epithelioid cell granulomas with occasional giant cells, a few with asteroids, without acid-fast bacilli, were found.
>
> In some reported cases, the finding of granulomas in the endometrium has been the first evidence of sarcoidosis. Taylor (1960) described two such cases. In the first of these, that of a woman, aged 26, evidence of sarcoidosis was found elsewhere, in the form of BHL, and later iridocyclitis, with sarcoid changes in a conjunctival biopsy, and a Kveim test was positive. In the second, there was also miliary shadowing in the lungs, not responding to antituberculosis drugs; a negative Mantoux test with 1:100 OT and a positive Kveim test; a mass behind the uterus in this case was found at laparotomy to be due to an old tubal pregnancy, but in the operative specimen no histological evidence of sarcoidosis was found. This patient, who had already borne two children became pregnant again after the surgical procedures, and the pregnancy went successfully to term.

If there is neither a past history nor concurrent evidence of sarcoidosis in other organs, categorization of non-caseating granulomatous changes in tissue obtained by uterine curettage or hysterectomy as sarcoid should be provisional, with the possibility of confirmation by observation of the clinical course. Several reported cases should be regarded in this way. Englehard (1946) described two.

> One case was that of a woman, aged 64, in whom other relevant findings included a weakly positive Pirquet test, unilateral hilar lymph-node enlargement and rounded areas of rarefaction in the bones in radiographs of the

hands and feet. The other was that of a woman who had had a pleural effusion ten years earlier, but nevertheless had a negative Pirquet reaction; no other possible manifestations of sarcoidosis were found in this case. Castoldi and Giudici (1955) reported the case of a 44 year old woman submitted to hysterectomy for an intramural uterine fibroid with adnexal masses; the latter were found to have the histological structure of sarcoidosis with entirely typical features, including Schaumann bodies, but no other manifestations of sarcoidosis were recorded. Zachwiej *et al.* (1956) described a case in which the uterus was removed because of menorrhagia, and found to be irregularly enlarged and infiltrated throughout with sarcoid-type granulomas, and another in which endometrium obtained by curettage was three times found to contain granulomas; but in neither case was there evidence of granulomatous changes elsewhere.

The diagnosis of sarcoidosis was corroborated by the clinical course in patients described by Kay (1956) and by Jaumandreu *et al.* (1964). Kay's patient was a woman, aged 28, investigated for sterility and a vaginal discharge and found to have a pelvic mass; at laparotomy, there were small nodules on the peritoneum, and grossly enlarged and distorted Fallopian tubes, especially on the right side. Biopsy of a nodule from the omentum showed a giant-cell granuloma without caseation or optically active inclusions; chest radiographs showed slight enlargement of hilar nodes with increasing mottled shadows in the lower parts of the lungs; there was no response to antituberculosis chemotherapy, the Mantoux test with 1:100 OT was negative, and the spleen became palpable. The patient whose case was described by Jaumandreu *et al.* (1964) was aged 54 when she had a hysterectomy for fibroids, and granulomas were found principally in the endometrium, with a few in the myometrium; five years later, left axillary lymph-nodes became enlarged, and biopsy showed sarcoid-type granulomas.

PREGNANCY AND SARCOIDOSIS

There is no evidence that sarcoidosis affects fertility, apart of course from the apparently very rare cases of severe involvement of the uterus and Fallopian tubes. Among 136 patients whose course was followed for five years by Scadding (1961b) there were 45 married women of child-bearing age; 12 pregnancies were observed during this time in ten of these women. Subsequently, this series was extended to 28 pregnancies going to term in 24 women with sarcoidosis. Eight pregnancies occurred in seven patients after lung changes had resolved; in all instances, the chest radiograph remained clear during gestation and after delivery. Six occurred when lung changes appeared to be resolving; resolution became complete during the pregnancies and remained so afterwards. In four women, lung changes interpreted as inactive fibrotic residues of old-standing sarcoid infiltration persisted unchanged during and after pregnancy. Five women became pregnant at a time when widespread mottling suggestive of active sarcoid infiltration was evident in their chest radiographs, two of them twice and one three times; during these nine pregnancies the shadows resolved partly or completely,

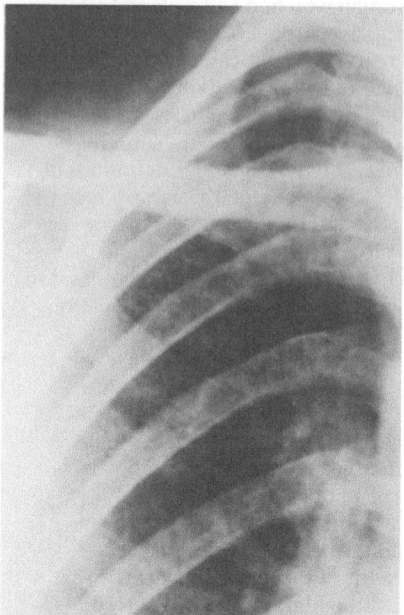

Figure 18.1   BHL and lung infiltration in a woman aged 29.

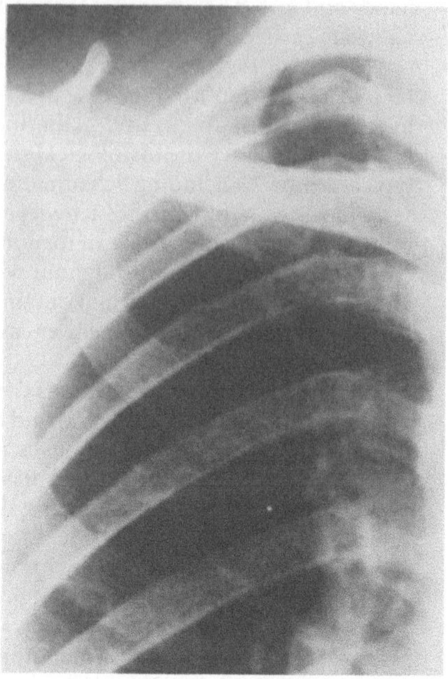

Figure 18.2   The same, eight months later, at the end of a pregnancy. Both BHL and infiltration have cleared.

reappearing 3–6 months later in eight instances (Figs 18.1 to 18.5, which show the effects of two pregnancies on a labile sarcoid infiltration of the lungs). One woman with long-standing sarcoidosis which had caused fairly severe fibrosis of the lungs was under corticosteroid treatment, not only because of the sarcoidosis but also for a concomitant extrinsic atopic asthma; her condition remained unchanged. All except one of the 28 pregnancies resulted in a healthy child; the exception was a twin pregnancy, which resulted in stillbirths, for which no cause was found. No other obstetrical complications were reported; three of the deliveries were by Caesarian section, performed twice in the patient whose case is illustrated in Figs 18.1–18.5 because of disproportion, and once in a patient who was pregnant for the first time at the age of 37.

These observations are in agreement with those of others. Mayock *et al.* (1957) observed 16 pregnancies in ten patients with sarcoidosis. There was some improvement in one or more of the manifestations of sarcoidosis during eight of the pregnancies, and four women developed new manifestations after delivery. Among the children one was stillborn, one had congenital heart disease and two minor congenital digital deformities. Reisfield

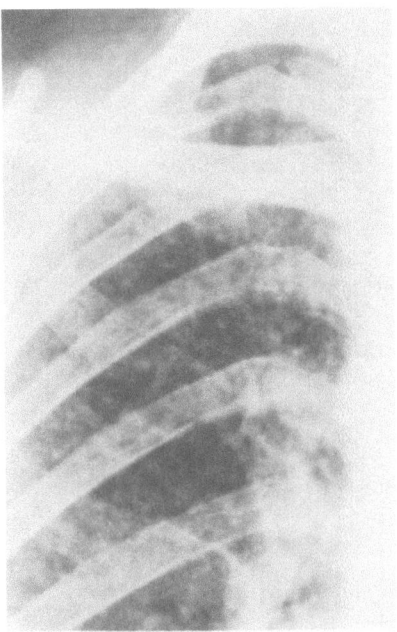

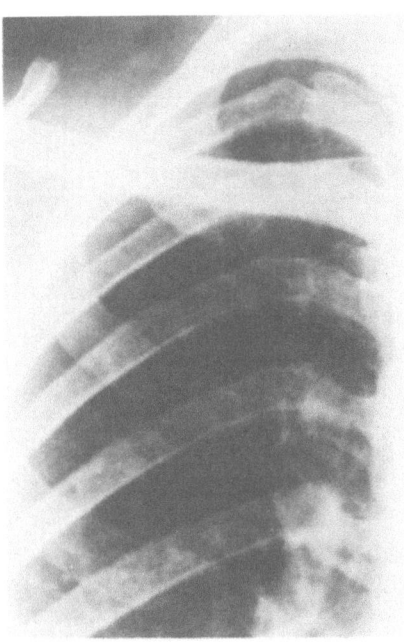

Figure 18.3   The same, six months after Fig. 18.2; the pulmonary infiltration has reappeared, and is denser.

Figure 18.4   The same, eight months after Fig. 18.3, in the fourth month of a second pregnancy; the lungs appear normal.

(1958) reported 17 pregnancies in ten patients; there were two spontaneous miscarriages, three terminations by hysterotomy, and 12 healthy infants, nine delivered normally and three by Caesarian sections near term because of disproportion. The material from the three hysterotomies and the placenta and cord from two of the normal deliveries was extensively examined, but no sarcoid lesions were found. O'Leary (1962) reported 28 pregnancies in 23 patients; there were two miscarriages, not related to sarcoidosis, two neonatal deaths, and 24 living children. No complications were observed in the mothers, of whom 11 received corticosteroid treatment; 22 of them showed no change during pregnancy, and five were thought to have improved. Franz and Wurm (1962) made similar observations on 48 pregnancies in 41 women with pulmonary sarcoidosis: the lung changes improved in about two-thirds and became worse in none during pregnancy, but relapses were observed in a few after delivery. Jörgensen (1963b) reported similar findings in the course of 39 pregnancies in 35 women with sarcoidosis. Improvement was noted during 26 of these pregnancies, but some deterioration occurred after delivery in 18. Hosoda *et al.* (1971) reported that in all but one of 40 pregnancies observed in 30 women with

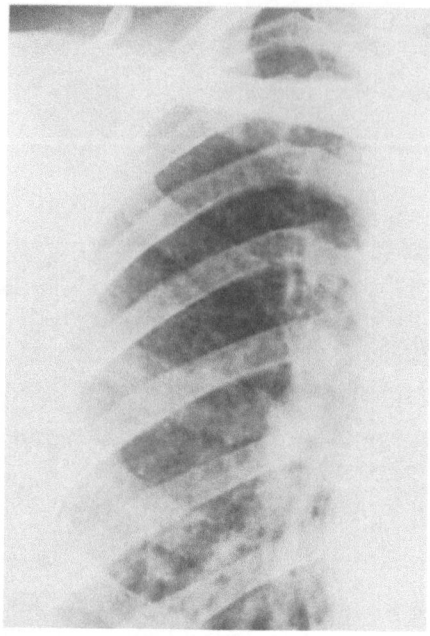

Figure 18.5   The same, seven months after delivery. The infiltration has reappeared. During a third pregnancy, one year later, the lungs cleared again, and remained clear during two years' subsequent observation.

sarcoidosis in Japan, improvement occurred during pregnancy, with relapse to the former state after delivery in 12; stationary fibrotic lung changes were unaffected.

No systematic study of the placenta in parturient women with sarcoidosis has been made. Kelemen and Mandi (1969) reported the study of the placenta from the second successful pregnancy in a 24 year old woman who had been found to have hilar lymph-node and pulmonary sarcoidosis at the age of 18. Her lung condition had improved during pregnancy. Granulomas were found in the placenta, although pregnancy and delivery had been uneventful, and the infant was healthy.

Thus the available evidence suggests that sarcoid lesions in a resolving phase continue uninterruptedly to resolve during and after pregnancy; that when sarcoidosis has already undergone clinical resolution, pregnancy does not cause recrudescence; that in some cases in the active stage of the disease, reversible elements in sarcoid lesions may be suppressed during pregnancy with symptomatic improvement; and that in such cases, there is a tendency for relapse towards the original state during the few months after delivery. There is no evidence that maternal sarcoidosis has any effect on the foetus. It may be concluded that pregnancy has no effect on the long-term prognosis in sarcoidosis; and that women with sarcoidosis, even in active stages, can bear healthy children.

It is a legitimate speculation, which has been made by several authors, that the observed tendency of sarcoid lesions to improve during pregnancy and to relapse towards their original state after delivery may be associated with the higher levels of corticosteroids in the blood during pregnancy, since it resembles so much the effect of a limited period of corticosteroid treatment; but no direct support is available for this speculation.

MALE GENITAL SYSTEM

Longcope and Freiman (1952) among 30 necropsy cases of generalized sarcoidosis found involvement of the testis in two, of the epididymis in two and of the prostate, seminal vesicles and spermatic cord each in one case. In four cases, nodules were felt during life in the epididymis, and in two of these they were confirmed at necropsy to have the histology of sarcoidosis. These were incidental findings in patients with extensive sarcoidosis. In clinical series, the proportion of cases in which abnormalities have been found in the male genital system is low, and of symptomatic changes even lower. Singer *et al.* (1959) among 45 men with sarcoidosis in a military hospital found thickening of the epididymis in two. One of these, a black man aged 31, presented with painful swelling of the left testis, accompanied by transient tender red nodules on the right leg; the swelling subsided on treatment with antibiotics, leaving nodular thickening in the epididymis; other findings included BHL, left iritis, splenomegaly, and slight enlargement of superficial lymph-nodes; and biopsy of scalene lymph-node and of the epididymis showed sarcoid-type granulomas.

Epididymis and testis

Other cases in which sarcoidosis of the epididymis or testis was clinically evident have been reported by Krauss (1958), Hines *et al.* (1961), McGowan and Smith (1967), Winnacker *et al.* (1967), Mikhail, *et al.* (1972), Rudin *et al.* (1974), Heffernan and Blenkinsop (1978), and Opal *et al.* (1979). All were in black men with extensive active sarcoidosis.

Krauss's (1958) patient was found at the age of 41 to have multiple subcutaneous sarcoids and BHL; two years later, the right testis became enlarged to four times its normal size, with thickening of the distal part of the cord, and generalized superficial lymphadenopathy and radiographic changes in the distal phalanx of a finger were found; the affected testis was removed and showed granulomas mainly in the epididymis, with atrophic changes in the body of the testis, and an ovoid swelling in the cord was also granulomatous. The patient described by Hines *et al.* was aged 21, and had subcutaneous nodules on the limbs, showing sarcoid histology involving also muscle on biopsy, generalized lymphadenopathy and bilateral epididymal thickening and nodularity. There was azoospermia. Biopsies of epididymis and cervical lymph-node showed granulomas, while the testis showed only slight atrophy. There was spontaneous improvement, the subcutaneous nodules and epididymal thickening subsiding within 18 months, and a sperm count of 15 000 000/ml was recorded. In the case described by McGowan and Smith (1967), a black man aged 38 who had been suffering from sarcoidosis for five years, being treated for fibrosing pulmonary changes with corticosteroids, and having had the left index finger amputated because of bone involvement, presented with a tender indurated scrotal mass; orchidectomy was performed, the epididymis being found to be predominantly involved in woody swelling shown on section to consist of granulomas with many giant cells containing crystalline and conchoidal inclusions within dense bands of fibrous tissue, extending from the epididymis into the body of the testis. The case described by Mikhail *et al.* (1972) was that of a black man aged 41 with sarcoidosis involving hilar lymph-nodes, lungs, parotid and lacrimal glands, subcutaneous nodules, nasal mucosa and larynx, with electrocardiographic evidence of myocardial involvement; both epididymes were enlarged, firm and irregular, biopsy showing extensive replacement by non-caseating epithelioid and giant-cell granulomas: corticosteroid treatment led to diminution in the size of the epididymal swellings and improvement in the electrocardiogram. The 29 year old man whose case was reported by Rudin *et al.* (1974) developed bilateral nodular epididymal swellings ten months after the diagnosis of sarcoidosis involving mainly lungs and lymph-nodes; the nodular mass was excised from the right epididymis and shown to be infiltrated by non-caseating granulomas; additionally, several areas of granulomatous reaction to necrotic sperm heads, and a group of fibrous structures with calcified centres thought to be calcified microfilariae were seen. Heffernan and Blenkinsop (1978) reported briefly the case of a black man aged 35 with uveo-parotid fever, nasal and skin sarcoidosis, and painful enlargement of the right epididymis, shown on biopsy to contain periductal non-caseating granulomas. The patient whose case was described by Opal *et al.* was a black man aged 20 with sarcoidosis of hilar lymph-nodes and lungs, bronchial and transbronchial lung biopsies showing granulomas, enlarged lacrimal glands, arthropathy of the right knee, and polydipsia and polyuria with evidence of hypothalamic dysfunction, and nodules in the upper poles of both testes; at surgical exploration, several small nodules were found beneath the tunica albuginea of the right testis, the epididymis and cord appearing normal; biopsy of a nodule showed non-caseating granulomas; and improvement in all symptoms, including regression of the testicular nodules, followed corticosteroid treatment.

The case described by Winnacker *et al.* (1967) was unique in presenting with recurrent episodes of epididymitis occurring every 2–4 weeks and each lasting a few days, unilaterally or bilaterally, for 11 years; the patient, a black man aged 33, had been known to have sarcoidosis of at least the same duration, with BHL, a transient lung infiltration and granulomatous changes in a scalene lymph-node removed for biopsy. Both epididymes were diffusely indurated and tender; the left was removed, with the vas, and found to contain many granulomas, coalescent in places, with some hyalinization, and dilatation of some epididymal ducts and interductal fibrosis. Bronchial, skeletal muscle and liver biopsies also showed granulomas. Under treatment with small doses of prednisone, the patient remained free from further episodes of epididymitis for 15 months, but recurrences of right-sided epididymitis then led to removal of the right epididymis, in which similar changes were found, the testis itself appearing normal.

Geller *et al.* (1977) reported a case of concurrent sarcoid BHL and malignant testicular tumour. A 35 year old white man presented with a painful swelling in the left side of the scrotum, found on biopsy to be due to a malignant teratoma. BHL was found on chest radiography. Gallium scan showed uptake in the hilar but not in the scrotal region, and mediastinal node biopsy showed sarcoid-type granulomas. Radical orchidectomy was followed by retroperitoneal lymph-node dissection, the removed nodes containing neither tumour nor granuloma.

In a case reported by Hausfeld (1961) it is doubtful whether the lesions described were local sarcoid reactions or part of a generalized sarcoidosis. A boy aged five developed a swelling in one side of the scrotum, thought to have followed an insect bite; it was excised, and found to be adherent to the tunica albuginea. Both it and slightly enlarged lymph-nodes removed at the same time contained non-caseating epithelioid and giant-cell granulomas. A tuberculin test with 10 IU was positive, and the only other possible evidence of sarcoidosis was a chest radiograph showing doubtful enlargement of hilar shadows.

Prostate

Clinically evident sarcoidosis of the prostate is excessively rare. Hardebeck (1953) reported the case of a man, aged 50, in whom irregular enlargement of the prostate was found on biopsy to be due to infiltration with sarcoid-type tubercles; the serum calcium was 12.9 mg dl^{-1} and the Mantoux test produced a reaction only with 1:10 OT. There was a localized infiltration in the lower lobe of the left lung. While it is possible, it cannot be regarded as proved that this was a case of generalized sarcoidosis.

Brock and Grieco (1972) described the case of a Haitian, aged 56, known to have sarcoidosis involving lymph-nodes, lungs, skin, liver and spleen, who presented with retention of urine after a few days of frequency and dysuria. The right lobe of the prostate was enlarged; transurethral prostatectomy was performed, and the resected tissue showed both micro-abscesses and granulomas; structures resembling cryptococci were seen both in giant cells and among inflammatory cells, and *C. neoformans* was cultured from urine and sputum. Treatment with 5-fluorocytosine for 28 days led to negative cultures, and the patient remained well during 12 months' observation. There was no other sign of cryptococcal infection; the cerebro-spinal fluid was examined in the acute stage, and found to be normal. This appears to have been a coincidental cryptococcal prostatitis during the course of unrelated sarcoidosis.

A case of coincidental adenocarcinoma of the prostate in a man, aged 78, who had been found to be suffering from cutaneous sarcoidosis, biopsy-proved, three years previously was reported by Todd and Garnick (1980). Biopsy of a prostatic nodule showed a well-differentiated adenocarcinoma and a chronic granulomatous reaction, not described in detail. A serum calcium level of 14.2 mg dl^{-1} was recorded, though a 24 hour urine collection contained only 101 mg of calcium. There was bilateral iritis with

glaucoma and dense band keratopathy in the left eye. Treatment with prednisone was followed by return of serum calcium to normal, resolution of
cutaneous lesions, and improvement in renal function. It seems likely that in
this case the prostatic granulomas were part of the generalized sarcoidosis,
probably independent of the adenocarcinoma, but the possibility that they
were a local reaction to the carcinoma cannot be excluded.

Penis

Nodular infiltrations of the skin of the penis were found by Longcope and
Fisher (1942) in a black man with very extensive sarcoidosis who died
suddenly, from cardiac involvement. Vitenson and Wilson (1972) described
the case of a black man with sarcoidosis shown to involve lymph-nodes, lung,
liver, kidney and skin, who, three years from the onset, developed slowly-
growing nodules on the glans penis alongside the meatus. Biopsy when they
had been present 18 months confirmed that they were sarcoids. Carli (1955)
reported the case of a man, aged 28, who presented with a nodule in the sulcus
between the glans penis and the prepuce, with the histological structure of
sarcoid granuloma on biopsy. The inguinal lymph-nodes were enlarged, and
other superficial nodes palpable; no information is available about chest
radiograph or tuberculin test.

Burns and Sarkany (1976) reported the case of an Indian who at the age of
65 presented with bilateral paratracheal lymphadenopathy, and a diagnosis of
sarcoidosis was made by lymph-node biopsy showing non-caseating epithelioid-cell granulomas, a positive Kveim test, and a negative tuberculin test
with 100 IU. He was treated with prednisone with improvement in cough and
dyspnoea. Two years later, while taking 10 mg prednisone daily, he developed
painful ulceration in the coronal sulcus on the dorsum of the penis; mottled
shadowing appeared in the middle zones of the lungs, the skin reacted to 10 IU
of tuberculin, acid-fast bacilli were found in the sputum, and biopsy of the
ulcer showed a caseating granuloma with a few acid-fast bacilli. Treatment
with antimycobacterial drugs led to rapid healing of the ulcer. The relationship of mycobacterial infection to the non-caseating granulomatous phase of
this patient's illness remains debatable.

URINARY BLADDER

There seems to be no recorded case of symptomatic sarcoidosis of the
bladder, or study of the incidence of symptomless granulomas in the bladder
in active sarcoidosis.

Radewill (1943, Case 2) and French and Mason (1951) reported cases in
which extensive generalized sarcoidosis of the skin, with involvement also of
liver, spleen and lungs in the case of French and Mason, was associated with
the peculiar plaque-like or nodular infiltration of the bladder described as
malakoplakia (McDonald and Sewell, 1913; Yunis *et al.*, 1967). Knoop
(1958) described the case of a woman aged 54 in whom the diagnosis of
malakoplakia was established by cystoscopy and biopsy after recurrent
attacks of cystitis for five years; she had 'healed Boeck's disease' in the lungs,
and a scalene fat pad dissection produced one hyalinized lymph-node with
small epithelioid granulomas. Brashear and Carman (1969) reported concur-

rent malakoplakia of the bladder and sarcoid BHL, followed by pulmonary infiltration, in a 47 year old black woman. The significance of the very occasional association of this granulomatous disease of the bladder with systemic sarcoidosis is unknown; it may well be fortuitous.

BREAST

Reisner (1944) mentioned two cases, and Longcope and Freiman (1952) one case, in which isolated nodules in the breast of women with active sarcoidosis were presumed to be of sarcoid origin. In Reisner's cases the nodules were described as firm, non-tender and mobile, and the supposition that they were sarcoidal was supported by their spontaneous regression. Scott (1938) described the case of a woman, aged 38, who was found to have a mobile well-defined swelling 5 cm × 4 cm in the right breast; it was removed, and both it and a lymph-node were found to show the histology of sarcoidosis. She subsequently developed a uveo-parotid syndrome, and later still was found to have become myxoedematous; her case appears also to have been reported by Stallard and Tait (1939).

A patient under the case of one of us had a histologically confirmed sarcoid nodule in the breast. At the age of 43, she was found to have widespread reticular and mottled shadows in a chest radiograph, having had progressively increasing shortness of breath on exertion for some years; the appearances suggested an already predominantly fibrotic infiltration (Fig. 6.25). Five years later a small nodule, resembling and initially thought to be a fibroadenoma, was removed from the left breast; it showed a mass of well-defined non-caseating epithelioid cell tubercles lying within the acinar tissue of the breast. The Mantoux test was negative to 250 units of PPD. No further changes were noted in the breast; she died ten years later of fibrotic pulmonary sarcoidosis.

Rigden (1978) reported the case of a woman who at the age of 22 had a symptomless radiographic abnormality in the right lung, with negative tuberculin test to 10 IU, though reacting to 100 IU, negative studies for acid-fast bacilli, no response to antimycobacterial drugs, and subsequent spontaneous clearing; at the age of 29 she was found to have a nodule in the right breast which on excision showed the histology of sarcoidosis. Neither at that time nor during four years' further observation was any other possible manifestation of sarcoidosis found.

Dalmark (1942) reported the case of a woman, aged 28, who noticed a nodule in the right axilla shortly after the end of lactation. On removal, this was found to be a lymph-node infiltrated with non-caseating epithelioid and giant-cell tubercles, and the adjacent breast tissue showed scattered similar tubercles. The tuberculin test was positive, and radiographs of the chest and of the hands and feet showed no abnormality. In the absence of evidence of possible sarcoid changes elsewhere, categorization of this case can only be provisional.

Chapter 19

The Kidneys and Calcium Metabolism

The kidneys may be affected in several ways, directly or indirectly, in sarcoidosis. They may be infiltrated by granulomas, but these rarely cause symptoms or signs. The most frequent cause of impairment of renal function in sarcoidosis is the hypercalcaemia that occurs in a minority of patients and may cause a nephropathy, at first reversible but later leading to irreversible and possibly progressive changes. In many cases with this hypercalcaemic nephropathy, granulomas are also present in the kidneys, and it is thus appropriate to consider renal changes and the disordered calcium metabolism together.

An acute transient interstitial nephritis has been reported accompanying the BHL-erythema nodosum-arthropathy syndrome; and nephritis of various sorts may occur during the course of sarcoidosis, probably no more frequently than might occur by chance, but giving rise to speculation about possible pathogenetic links.

GRANULOMATOUS INFILTRATION OF THE KIDNEYS

Granulomas are undoubtedly present in the kidneys in many patients in the active stage of sarcoidosis without causing symptoms, as they are known to be in many other organs; but the proportion of patients so affected is unknown, since renal biopsy is justifiable only if there is reason to suspect renal disease to the diagnosis of which it will contribute. Lebacq *et al.* (1970) reported the results of 25 percutaneous renal biopsies in 25 patients selected from 152 investigated for evidence of renal involvement; ten contained epithelioid-cell granulomas. MacSerraigh *et al.* (1978) investigated 90 patients with sarcoidosis and found evidence of impaired renal function in nine; epithelioid granulomas were seen in five of eight submitted to renal biopsy.

The earliest reference to renal changes at necropsy appears to have been by Schaumann (1933) in a man who died at the age of 45 after having suffered from sarcoidosis involving skin, eyes and lungs for 16 years; the capsule of the right kidney was infiltrated with granulomas and adherent to the liver, but the kidney itself was not affected. Ricker and Clark (1949) found granulomas in the kidneys in four of 22, and Longcope and Freiman (1952) in four of 23 necropsies in cases of generalized sarcoidosis. In a review of 117 published necropsy reports, Branson and Park (1954) found that granulomas in the kidneys were mentioned in eight (6.8%).

Only a few cases in which symptoms could be attributed to granulomatous changes in the kidneys, uncomplicated by hypercalcaemic or other forms of nephropathy, have been reported. Some of these occurred in patients already known to have sarcoidosis in whom renal biopsies were performed either because routine investigations had shown proteinuria or raised blood urea or creatinine, or because of symptoms related to renal failure or to hypertension. In such cases, corticosteroid treatment has generally led to improvement both clinically and biochemically, and renal biopsies when repeated after treatment have usually, but not always, shown disappearance of granulomas with variable persistence of hyalinized remnants, and sometimes with persistent non-granulomatous glomerular and interstitial changes.

Berger and Relman (1955) described the case of a black man aged 37 who had sarcoidosis involving skin, lymph-nodes, lungs and conjunctiva. Heavy proteinuria led to open renal biopsy, which showed many epithelioid and giant-cell granulomas, with some thickening of glomerular basement membranes and minor changes in proximal convoluted tubules. Treatment with cortisone led to improvement in the clinical signs of sarcoidosis and diminution in proteinuria, but a second renal biopsy showed no change.

Ogilvie *et al.* (1964) reported the case of a man, aged 27, with fever, generalized lymphadenopathy showing the histology of sarcoidosis on biopsy, and uveitis. A trace of proteinuria and some granular casts were found in the urine, and renal biopsy showed many small granulomas, without changes in glomeruli or tubules. Treatment with prednisolone was followed by improvement; in biopsies one and two years later, no granulomas were seen, but there were increasing numbers of hyalinized glomeruli.

The patient whose case was reported by Coburn *et al.* (1967) was a 19 year old black man with extensive sarcoidosis, involving hilar and peripheral lymph-nodes, lungs and nasal mucosa, biopsy of the latter and of liver showing sarcoid granulomas. Initially, a trace of protein and many granular casts were found in the urine. Treatment with prednisone was followed by disappearance of these, and return to normal of slightly diminished creatinine clearance. On withdrawal of prednisone, renal function deteriorated and proteinuria, 2.8 g/day reappeared. Intravenous pyelography showed enlarged kidneys. Renal biopsy showed extensive granulomatous changes. Reinstitution of prednisone treatment led to improvement in renal function; biopsies 14 weeks and seven months later showed patchy but in places confluent areas of hyaline fibrosis involving glomeruli and some interstitial fibrosis, but no granulomas.

In the case reported by Turner *et al.* (1977), the diagnosis of sarcoidosis was made in the investigation of hypertension. An albino black girl in her 14th year developed headaches, dizziness and scotoma, and later severe epistaxis, and was found to be severely hypertensive, with nitrogen retention, slight proteinuria, left ventricular enlargement and pericardial effusion. Needle biopsy of the enlarged liver showed non-caseating granulomas. Lowering of the blood pressure was followed by fall in blood urea and creatinine levels. Needle biopsy of the kidney showed infiltration by granulomas and more diffusely by epithelioid cells and lymphocytes with some interstitial fibrosis; glomeruli and vessels appeared normal, and no evidence of deposition of immunoglobulins or C3 was found. Treatment with prednisone was complicated by hypertension, but eventually a stable state on moderate dosage was attained, with controlled renal failure and mild hypertension. Repeat renal biopsies first showed disappearance of the granulomas; during relapse on reduction of prednisone dosage, there were extensive granulomatous interstitial changes, with involvement of small arteries and necrotizing changes in a medium-sized artery, and C3 but no immunoglobulin in some scarred glomeruli.

In a few cases, granulomatous infiltration of the kidneys has led to a clinical picture of nephrogenic diabetes insipidus, responding to corticosteroid treatment. Panitz and Shinaberger (1965) reported the case of a black man aged 25 with BHL, who had polyuria and polydipsia resistant to pitressin and with normal serum and urinary calcium levels, and was found by biopsy to have granulomas in the kidney; prednisolone treatment controlled the symptoms. Bourke and Barniville (1973) described the case of a 21 year old man with polydipsia and polyuria. He was found to have a daily urine output of 4–5 litres, but reduced by fluid deprivation, with a SG of 1007, not significantly increased by pitressin; raised blood urea and reduced creatinine clearance; normal serum calcium and phosphate levels and urinary calcium output; bilateral iridocyclitis; and bilateral hilar lymphadenopathy. Lymph-node biopsy showed non-caseating granulomas. Renal biopsy showed many granulomas throughout the cortex, with normal glomeruli and some displacement and atrophy of tubules near the granulomas. Treatment with prednisone led to normal urine volumes, and regression of the iridocyclitis and the BHL. A second renal biopsy one month after the end of nine months' treatment with prednisone showed a few areas of increased fibrous tissue or inflammatory cell infiltrations, one hyalinized glomerulus, but nine others appearing normal.

In a few cases, patients have first sought advice for symptoms attributable to renal failure, the diagnosis of sarcoidosis being first suggested by renal biopsy, with subsequent discovery of involvement of other organs.

King *et al.* (1976) recorded the case of a woman aged 51 who had been treated for three years with a diuretic for hypertension, and for four months had been losing weight, with anorexia, nausea and lethargy. She was found to be normotensive, with a hypochromic anaemia, proteinuria without cells or casts, normal calcium and raised creatinine levels in the blood. Renal biopsy showed many non-caseating granulomas, with scattered infiltration of lymphocytes, histiocytes and a few plasma cells in the interstitium, with some fibrosis and consequent tubular atrophy, but no important glomerular changes. Treatment with prednisone led to rapid clinical and biochemical improvement, with relapse on discontinuance. A second biopsy during this relapse showed similar changes with increase in fibrosis and a number of sclerosed glomeruli. Reinstitution of prednisone and continuation of a small dose was followed by maintained improvement. At the time of relapse, search for other evidences of sarcoidosis led to biopsy of liver, which was normal, and of mediastinal lymph-nodes, which contained granulomas.

Vanhille *et al.* (1977) investigated a man aged 34 who was found to have proteinuria and uraemia after a short history of general ill-health and nocturia. Chest radiography showed widespread reticulo-nodular shadows without hilar node enlargement. Renal biopsy showed non-caseating epithelioid and giant-cell granulomas. This led to biopsy of liver and of prescalene lymph-nodes, both of which showed similar granulomas. Treatment with prednisone was followed by diminution in proteinuria and in blood urea and creatinine levels and regression of the lung shadows.

Cases 1 and 2 of Wambergne *et al.* (1978), both in men, presenting similarly with renal insufficiency. In Case 1, there had been episodes of iridocyclitis and rheumatism in the past, and the liver, spleen and inguinal lymph-nodes were enlarged. Renal biopsy showed epithelioid and giant-cell granulomas on a background of interstitial nephritis; biopsies of gum and liver showed similar granulomas. Corticosteroid treatment led to disappearance of the hepatosplenomegaly, the inguinal node enlargement and the iridocyclitis and improvement in blood urea and creatinine levels and in creatinine clearance. Repeat biopsy showed persistent chronic interstitial changes but no granulomas. In Case 2, widespread reticulo-nodular shadows in the chest radiograph and granulomatous changes in liver and scalene lymph-node biopsies were found during investigation of renal insufficiency: renal biopsy showed epithelioid and giant-cell granulomas and interstitial inflammation. Corticosteroid treatment led to improvement in renal function and clearing of the lung shadows, but had to be discontinued because of necrosis of the femoral head.

The youngest patient with sarcoid infiltration of the kidney and impaired renal function appears to be a girl aged four and a half years, reported by Toomey and Bautista (1970). She also had hypercalcaemia, and is mentioned below (p. 396).

A presumptive diagnosis of renal sarcoidosis is justified in a few cases in which characteristic granulomatous changes are found in the kidney and corticosteroid treatment leads to improvement, but attempts to discover evidence of granulomatous changes elsewhere are unsuccessful. In such cases a granulomatous response to a Kveim test would be useful supporting evidence; and diagnostic categorization should be provisional, and open to revision if indicated by subsequent findings.

The case reported by Bolton *et al.* (1976) can be accepted in this way. A 46 year old woman with a six month history of anorexia, nausea and tiredness was found to have much reduced renal function. Renal biopsy showed many non-caseating granulomas and some large multinucleated cells, some moderately shrunken tufts and increase in mesangial matrix in glomeruli, and cellular infiltration and fibrosis in the interstitium. No other site of granulomatous disease was identified clinically or radiologically, or in biopsies of scalene lymph-node and bone-marrow. Dramatic improvement followed predisone treatment, creatinine clearance rising from 4–62 ml min^{-1}.

Distortion of the renal outline or of the calices by sarcoid granulomatousis may lead to pyelographic appearances suggesting renal tumours, tuberculosis or polycystic disease.

Leng-Levy *et al.* (1965) reported the case of a woman aged 56 who had a transient facial palsy and parotid gland enlargement, followed by loss of weight and anorexia. She was found to have generalized enlargement of superficial lymph-nodes, biopsy of one showing sarcoid-type granulomas; proteinuria and raised blood urea; and normal calcium levels. Intravenous pyelography showed distortion of calyceal pattern and irregular outline of the left kidney suggesting neoplasm. Open biopsy showed interstitial nephritis with many epithelioid and giant-cell granulomas. Treatment with prednisone led to improvement with lowering of blood urea towards normal.

Guédon *et al.* (1967) reported the case of a woman who after two episodes of left renal colic, the second with haematuria, had an intravenous pyelography which suggested polycystic disease. Surgical exploration showed a large kidney and enlarged para-aortic lymph-nodes. The kidney was removed. There were isolated and confluent greyish-white nodules with reddish centres thoughout its substance; histologically these were composed of epithelioid and giant-cell tubercles without caseation. Although no tubercle bacilli were found, treatment with isoniazid and para-aminosalicylic acid was given. Four years later, when the patient was aged 36, right renal colic led to further investigation. There was slight proteinuria and moderate elevation of blood urea; bilateral micronodular shadows in the chest radiograph; and evidence of old iridocyclitis. In a Mantoux test, the skin reacted to 50 IU but not to 10 IU. Calcium levels were normal. On a revised diagnosis of sarcoidosis, corticosteroid treatment was given, and led to immediate disappearance of lung shadows; no information about long-term follow-up was given.

Granulomatous changes in arterial walls, mentioned incidentally in some reports – e.g. by Turner *et al.* (1977) in a case summarized above – may be prominent, and tend to be associated with hypertension.

Rosenthal (1949) described a case in which granulomatous changes in vessel walls in the kidneys were the principal cause of renal failure and hypertension. A black man, aged 22, had been ill for two years with widespread lymphadenopathy, conjunctival and ocular changes, BHL and lung mottling, and a negative tuberculin test, and died with hypertension and renal failure. Several lymph-node biopsies had shown sarcoid granulomas, one with invasion and occlusion of a medium-sized blood vessel. At necropsy, sarcoid granulomas were found in lungs, kidneys, liver, lymph-nodes, brain and meninges; in the kidneys, granulomatous panarteritis had caused ischaemic infarcts.

Bottcher (1959) reported the necropsy findings in a woman who died at the age of 58 after an eight year illness with asthma, arthritis, abdominal pain, hypertension and terminal uraemia. There was widespread granulomatous infiltration of lungs, heart, kidneys, with involvement of large blood-vessels, including those in the mesentery; giant cells contained many Schaumann and asteroid inclusions.

In some reported cases presenting initially with reno-vascular disease and with both granulomas and non-granulomatous changes in the kidneys, it seems possible or even probable that sarcoidosis and reno-vascular disease were pathogenetically unrelated. Rutishauser and Rywlin (1950) described the necropsy findings in the case of a woman, who died at the age of 49 of a cerebral haemorrhage, having been observed to have a blood pressure of 270/150, hypertensive retinopathy and a blood urea of 125 mg dl^{-1}. The kidneys were small and scarred and showed both sarcoid granulomas in all stages of evolution and hyalinization and capsular adhesions in the glomeruli; sparse sarcoid granulomas, many hyalinized, were found in liver, spleen, lymph-nodes and tonsils. In this case it seems likely that an unrelated glomerulonephritis was concurrent with sarcoidosis; possibly the damaged kidneys were unusually liable to sarcoid infiltration, just as scars in the skin are known to be.

Falls *et al.* (1972) reported the case of a black man who was found to be hypertensive at the age of 46 at the time of an operation for duodenal ulcer. No evidence of other disease was found at that time. Three years later, he was investigated for weight loss and nocturia of six months' duration. He was found to have a blood pressure of 160/100, BHL and pulmonary mottling, chronic anterior uveitis, slight proteinuria, impaired renal clearances, normal calcium levels, negative tuberculin test, and non-caseating granulomas in bronchial and scalene node biopsies. Needle biopsy of the kidney showed interstitial mononuclear cell infiltration with considerable fibrosis and some atrophic changes in tubules; no granulomas were seen. Prednisone, initially 40 mg daily, led to rapid clearing of lung shadows and of uveitis and improvement in renal function. On reduction to 7.5 mg, there was deterioration. Open renal biopsy at this stage showed several epithelioid cell granulomas; there was hyperplasia of the media and reduplication of the internal elastica of some arterioles and small arteries; glomeruli showed only mild hypercellularity, and increase in mesangial PAS-positive material. Increase in prednisone dosage once again led to improvement.

NON-GRANULOMATOUS NEPHROPATHY

Hypercalcaemic nephropathy

The hypercalcaemia that occurs in some patients with sarcoidosis, and is discussed below, like hypercalcaemia of other causes, may lead to impaired renal function, and is probably the most frequent cause of renal failure in sarcoidosis.

Among the earliest reports of renal failure due to the hypercalcaemia of sarcoidosis are those of Schüpbach and Wernly (1943, Case 1), Klinefelter and Salley (1946), Howard *et al.* (1949), Markoff (1951), Longcope and Freiman (1952), Dent *et al.* (1953) and Citron (1954, 1955). The clinical picture is characterized by polydipsia and polyuria, the specific gravity of the urine being low and fixed. In the earlier stage, the blood pressure remains normal, and the blood urea is usually slightly to moderately raised. At this stage, the renal function will improve if the calcium levels return to normal, either spontaneously or in response to treatment. Insoluble calcium salts tend to be deposited, especially in and around collecting ducts and distal tubules, but may be seen in proximal tubules, glomeruli and blood vessels. Degenerative changes in tubules and glomeruli and fibrosis round calcium deposits may be irreversible; this damage may prove progressive even though calcium levels return to normal, leading to renal failure and hypertension. In some patients, calcium deposits become large enough to be detectable in plain radiographs as small dense flecks within the renal outlines; the appearances have been described by Davidson *et al.* (1954).

The relationship between impairment of renal function and hypercalcaemia was clearly demonstrated by Löfgren *et al.* (1957). They carried out biochemical studies and renal biopsy in 16 patients with pulmonary sarcoidosis. Among six in whom at some time a serum calcium higher than 12.0 mg dl^{-1} was recorded, there was impairment of renal clearance of p-aminohippuric acid, and to a less extent of creatinine and inulin, and in three a raised blood non-protein nitrogen, without significant symptoms or hypertension; the renal biopsies showed hyalinization of Bowman's capsule, scattered calcium deposits in tubules and in interstitial connective tissue, and in three sarcoid granulomas in the interstitial tissue. Among the ten with lower serum calcium levels, some had minor depression of the renal clearances, minor histological changes only were found in the renal biopsies, only one showing a few small sarcoid granulomas, and none calcium deposits. MacSerraigh *et al.* (1978) in their study of renal function in 90 patients with sarcoidosis found a close correlation between hypercalcaemia, nephrocalcinosis and creatinine clearance. Renal biopsies were performed in eight of nine with impaired function: granulomas were found in four and nephrocalcinosis in five, both being found in one. The remaining patient with impaired function had hypercalcaemia and died with end-stage renal disease and hypertension: at necropsy, the kidneys showed nephrocalcinosis but no granulomas. In Rømer's (1980a) series of 42 patients with sarcoidosis referred for special study, 16 were found to have both abnormal calcium levels and renal failure, three renal failure without calcium abnormality, and three calcium abnormality without renal failure.

In patients with sarcoidosis and impaired renal function, the concurrence of hypercalcaemia with the finding of granulomas in renal biopsy material is evidently not infrequent. Both may be expected to respond to corticosteroid treatment. For instance, Toomey and Bautista (1970) reported the case of a white girl aged four and a half years who presented with an extensive rash, swollen joints, band keratopathy and synechiae in both eyes, hepatomegaly, proteinuria and granular casts and hypercalcaemia. Biopsies of skin, synovial membrane and kidney all showed granulomas. Corticosteroid treatment led to relief of symptoms and signs; renal biopsy three months later showed no granulomas, but some periglomerular and interstitial fibrosis.

Similarly, the effects of hypercalcaemia and granulomas may be found together in the kidneys at necropsy; e.g. in cases reported by Horton *et al.* (1939), Longcope and Freiman (1952, Case 14) and Scholz and Keating (1956, Case 3). In the latter two cases, there was evidence also of pyelonephritic scarring. In long-standing cases, the effects of nephrocalcinosis, renal calculi, granulomatous infiltration of the kidneys and secondary reno-vascular hypertension may be inextricable. Sorger and Taylor (1961) reported the necropsy findings in a man who died at the age of 49, after an illness starting 14 years earlier with left renal pain and the finding of hydronephrosis. Over the following years, he was found to have a pulmonary infiltration, lymphadenopathy with sarcoid histology on biopsy, splenomegaly, hypercalcaemia, proteinuria and calculus in the left kidney. In spite of initial response to prednisone, he died of renal failure with severe hypertension; at necropsy there was widespread sarcoidosis, mostly hyalinized, in lymph-nodes, lungs, liver, spleen, bone-marrow and kidneys, with severe destruction of renal parenchyma. It is unlikely that there is any direct relationship between the presence of sarcoid granulomas and of calcium deposits in the kidneys; probably they are associated because hypercalcaemia is more frequent in cases of sarcoidosis with extensive multiple organ involvement. The finding of changes interpreted as chronic pyelonephritis with those of nephrocalcinosis in some necropsy reports, and also in renal biopsies in hypercalcaemic sarcoidosis (e.g. by Dent *et al.*, 1953) raises the questions whether this pattern is necessarily related to infection, and, if so, whether hypercalcaemia predisposes to ascending infection in the kidney. These questions are outside the scope of this discussion.

Renal calculi

These may develop in patients with hypercalcaemic sarcoidosis.

Van Creveld (1941) described the case of a girl, aged 12, with salivary gland enlargement, splenomegaly, hilar node and lung changes, negative tuberculin test and hyperglobulinaemia, the diagnosis of sarcoidosis being supported by an axillary lymph-node biopsy: she had slight proteinuria and cylindruria and reduced urea clearance; the serum calcium was elevated, being estimated as 15.6 and 15.0 mg on two occasions; and a calculus developed in the pelvis of the right kidney and was successfully removed. He mentioned briefly several other patients with sarcoidosis and hypercalcaemia, one of whom had bilateral renal calculi. Albright and Reifenstein (1948) in a discussion of hyperparathyroidism referred to the diagnostic difficulties in the case of a young woman with recurrent renal calculi and hypercalcaemia; exploration of the parathyroids showed only normal glands, but she had miliary shadows in the lungs and splenomegaly and evidently was suffering from sarcoidosis. Two of the seven cases of nephrocalcinosis in sarcoidosis reported by Davidson *et al.* (1954), and five of the eight of renal insufficiency in sarcoidosis reported by Scholz and Keating (1956) had evident renal calculi.

In a patient under the care of one of us (JGS), recurrent attacks of renal colic were a leading feature. A man aged 30 had sarcoidosis involving lung, hilar nodes and spleen, with bilateral uveitis and granulomas in a liver biopsy. Serum calcium levels ranged from 12.0–14.0 mg dl^{-1} and daily urinary calcium excretion from 300–500 mg. Corticosteroid treatment led to reduction in calcium levels, and cessation of the attacks of renal colic. Two years later, after sun-bathing, he developed headache, nausea, anorexia, excessive thirst and left-sided abdominal pain. Serum calcium was again raised, and calculi were found radiologically in both kidneys. In spite of corticosteroid treatment, left renal colic recurred, and required treatment by ureterolithotomy.

The reported frequency of renal calculi in large series of patients with sarcoidosis varies greatly. Among the 160 cases of sarcoidosis reviewed by Longcope and Freiman (1952), five were found to have renal calculi, the serum calcium being known to have been raised in all but one. Lebacq *et al.* (1970) found evidence of calculi in as many as 21 (14%) of 152 patients. On the other hand Murphy and Schirmer (1961) found calculi in four (1.3%) of 306 cases, a proportion no greater than they thought was to be expected in a general population.

Non-granulomatous, non-hypercalcaemic nephropathy

Non-granulomatous nephropathy of a wide variety of histological patterns and modes of presentation has been reported in patients with sarcoidosis. The inconstancy of the clinico-pathological patterns makes generalization about them difficult, and much of the available information can be presented only as individual case-reports.

In a number of reported cases, a nephrotic syndrome or symptomless proteinuria has been associated with concurrent or recent BHL, in some with erythema nodosum or febrile arthropathy (Etienne-Martin *et al.*, 1962; McCoy and Tisher, 1972, Cases 3 and 4; Salomon *et al.*, 1975; Briner and Gartmann, 1978; Lee and Michael, 1978; Mariani *et al.*, 1978; Taylor *et al.*,1982, Case 3), and renal biopsies have shown various non-granulomatous changes. In six of these cases, membranous glomerulopathy was found; in two, that of Briner and Gartmann and Case 3 of McCoy and Tisher, proliferative glomerulonephritis; and in one, that of Lee and Michael focal glomerular sclerosis. Of the nine cases, all but one were in men. Prognosis, to judge from the limited information given in the reports, appears to be that expected for the renal disease. In all those treated with corticosteroids, sarcoid changes in lungs, lymph-nodes and elsewhere showed the expected favourable response, even though in some the response of the renal changes was unsatisfactory.

In Cases 1 and 2 of Taylor *et al.* (1982), both in young men, the diagnosis of glomerulonephritis preceded that of sarcoidosis by five years and two years.

Selroos and Kuhlbäck (1972) noted transient proteinuria in patients with erythema nodosum and arthropathy in the early acute stage of sarcoidosis. They referred briefly to a young man with this syndrome in whom because renal function was slightly impaired a renal biopsy was performed and showed interstitial infiltration with mononuclear cells and a few granulocytes without changes in glomeruli, tubules or vessels. Prednisone treatment led to return of normal renal function, which was maintained when it was stopped.

Other reported cases in which non-granulomatous renal changes were found early in the course of sarcoidosis include those of Toomey and Bautista (1970, Case 1) and of Palestro (1975). In the first of these, a girl aged 14 with very extensive sarcoidosis involving lymph-nodes, lungs, eyes and bones of the

skull was found to have membranous glomerulopathy; she also had hypercalcaemia and calcification of renal tubular epithelial cells. Palestro's patient was
a man aged 18, who presented clinically with glomerulonephritis, and was
found to have an abnormal chest X-ray and sarcoid granulomas in a liver
biopsy; renal biopsy showed prominent epithelial crescents and hyalinization
of some glomeruli, and a few sarcoid granulomas. Renal function deteriorated
so that dialysis was instituted one year later.

In many of the reported cases in which renal disease developed late in the
course of sarcoidosis, factors such as hypercalcaemia, hypertension preceding the overt evidence of renal disease, and terminal cor pulmonale complicate the picture.

Teilum (1951) reported the case of a woman who died at the age of 49 of cor
pulmonale due to long-standing sarcoidosis, and at necropsy was found to
have widespread sarcoidosis with much hyalinization, and in the kidneys
hyaline deposits in glomerular tufts and in some arterioles, but no granulomas
or other vascular changes. He drew attention to the similarity of these lesions
to those seen in some cases of systemic lupus erythematosus (SLE) and
suggested that they were related to immunological hyper-activity and hyperglobulinaemia. Correa (1954) reported the case of a woman who died five
years after the onset of sarcoidosis involving skin, lungs and lymph-nodes, and
one year after the appearance of respiratory insufficiency with oedema and
proteinuria leading to renal failure. A raised serum calcium was noted, and she
had received dihydrotachysterol for a time early in her illness. At necropsy,
there was extensive hyalinizing sarcoidosis in spleen, lymph-nodes, lung and
pleura, myocardium, salivary glands, skin, liver, stomach and colon, thyroid
and meninges. In the kidneys, there were no granulomas, but widespread
glomerular changes, with adhesions between capillary loops and capsule,
crescent formation and polymorph infiltration; there was also some calcinosis
in renal tubules. In Cases 1 and 2 of McCoy and Tisher (1972) proteinuria
was found 18 and 13 years after diagnosis of sarcoidosis; both were fatal, one
from respiratory failure and the other apparently from renal failure, six and
11 years after the first sign of renal disease; in both, the kidneys showed the
histological pattern of proliferative glomerulonephritis; Case 1 was complicated by nephrolithiasis followed by hypertension early in the course, and by
the finding of focal calcium deposits in the renal medulla at necropsy. Cases 5
and 6 of McCoy and Tisher were both found to have chronic glomerulonephritis with severe vascular changes at necropsy, but the picture was
complicated by severe hypertension in both, and by diabetes mellitus and
terminal staphylococcal septicaemia in one and by hypercalcaemia in the
other.

Waldek *et al.* (1978) reported the case of a woman who at the age of 43
developed tiredness, weight loss, anorexia and pains in the joints, and was
found to be anaemic with mild proteinuria and creatinine clearance reduced to
3 ml min^{-1}. Eighteen years earlier, she had been found to have pulmonary
sarcoidosis by lung biopsy, and had been treated with costicosteroids. Renal
biopsy showed mesangioproliferative glomerulonephritis; no calcification was
seen and serum calcium was normal. Liver biopsy showed granulomas persisting 18 years after the original diagnosis. Treatment with prednisolone led to
improvement in renal function. In the case reported by Taylor *et al.* (1979) the

renal changes developed during 'maintenance' corticosteroid treatment for pulmonary sarcoidosis in a man aged 57 who developed oedema, heavy proteinuria and diminished creatinine clearance five years after the diagnosis of pulmonary sarcoidosis by lung biopsy; renal biopsy showed membranous glomerulopathy with epithelial crescents.

It is certain that during the often prolonged course of sarcoidosis, an unrelated glomerulonephritis must occur in a few cases. But the prominence of complex immunological factors both in sarcoidosis and in the several kinds of glomerulonephritis suggests that in at least some cases some common factor of this sort underlies the association. As noted above, Teilum (1951) described hyaline deposits in glomeruli and in renal vessels in sarcoidosis, and suggested an analogy with the renal changes in SLE. McCoy and Tisher (1972) found them in four of their six patients, and MacSerraigh *et al.* (1978) in six of eight renal biopsies in patients with sarcoidosis and impaired renal function; and Salomon *et al.* (1975), Lee and Michael (1978) and Taylor *et al.* (1979) also commented on the resemblance of changes in the kidneys in some cases of sarcoidosis to those of SLE, which are associated with immune-complexes. Since it is in the early stages of sarcoidosis, especially those with erythema nodosum that immune-complexes may be demonstrable (Chapter 20), it seems likely that if they are involved in renal changes in sarcoidosis it would be principally in those occurring early in its course. In a comparison of the reported histology of glomerulonephritis associated with sarcoidosis in 33 published cases with two large control groups from nephrology units, Taylor *et al.* (1982) found an excess of the membranous pattern; among those patients who presented with a nephrotic syndrome, this excess, 60% of those with sarcoidosis and 12% in a control series, was highly significant. This suggested that the pattern of renal change was affected by some factor, presumably immunological, common to the sarcoidosis patients. Until the pathogenetic factors concerned are more completely known both for sarcoidosis and for glomerulonephritis, so that they can be identified in individual cases, the question of the relationship of non-granulomatous, non-hypercalcaemic renal changes to sarcoidosis in the few cases in which they occur must usually be left open.

Renal changes: summary

Hypercalcaemic nephropathy has been found to be the most frequent cause of impaired renal function in sarcoidosis both in unselected series of cases (Löfgren *et al.*, 1957; Lebacq *et al.*, 1970; MacSerraigh *et al.*, 1978), and in cases referred for special study to nephrological clinics (Bear *et al.*, 1979), and to medical clinics (Rømer *et al.*, 1980a). The frequency of granulomatous infiltration of the kidneys is unknown, but it certainly occurs without causing symptoms or signs; very rarely it may cause impairment of function and symptoms. In such cases, it is likely that not only the profusion of the granulomas, but also their location in relation to structural elements in the kidney and their variable association with non-granulomatous changes, glomerular, tubular and interstitial, are concerned in determining the pattern of functional impairment. The occasional association of non-granulomatous renal changes with sarcoidosis raises questions which cannot in the existing state of knowledge be answered about possible pathogenetic relationships; the infrequency of this association makes it likely that any such relationship is an indirect one.

Both the frequent association of hypercalcaemic nephropathy with granulomas in the kidneys, and some reported cases of sarcoid infiltration of the kidney in which it seems likely that there was pre-existing reno-vascular disease, raise the question whether in the kidney there may be the tendency seen elsewhere for granulomas to develop in scar tissue.

In many reported series, there is an excess of males, both for hypercalcaemia and for renal impairment, and a survey of reported individual cases is concordant with this.

Favourable response to corticosteroid treatment can be expected if renal function is impaired by hypercalcaemia or by granulomatous infiltration, provided irreversible damage is not already present, but, as with other manifestations of sarcoidosis, it must be continued throughout the unpredictable duration of the active phase of the disease process. With other forms of renal involvement response is variable, and in most reported cases in which the histological pattern has been studied has been in accordance with expectation from this.

CALCIUM METABOLISM:
HYPERCALCAEMIA AND HYPERCALCIURIA

The disturbance of calcium metabolism which occurs in some patients with sarcoidosis is characterized by hypercalciuria and hypercalcaemia. The high calcium level in the blood is accompanied by normal or slightly raised inorganic phosphorus levels. The alkaline phosphatase is generally normal, but may be slightly elevated; when elevated, it may be of liver origin, and its level cannot be correlated with that of calcium. Calcium excretion in the faeces is generally low. In most cases, the disorder of calcium metabolism is of limited, but possibly prolonged, duration, often with short-term variations in severity; and apart from a general association with widespread sarcoidosis, its occurrence cannot be correlated with that of other manifestations of sarcoidosis.

Frequency

Reports of the proportions of patients so affected vary greatly. The number with symptoms evidently attributable to hypercalcaemia is agreed to be low; e.g. five (1.8%) of 275 followed for periods up to 20 years by one of us (JGS). Estimates of the proportion with abnormal biochemical values depend upon the number of estimations and the period of observation for each patient, as well as the range of values accepted as 'normal'. In serial studies of 11 patients, Harrell and Fisher (1939) found that the calcium level was above 11 mg dl^{-1} at some time in six, the highest figure recorded being 14.8 mg. Longcope and Freiman (1952) reported that of 23 patients at the Johns Hopkins Hospital, six showed values above 11 mg and of 21 at the Massachusetts General Hospital, five showed values above 12 mg dl^{-1}. Mather (1957) reported a much lower prevalence of raised serum calcium levels among 86 untreated patients with sarcoidosis in London; four of them showed levels above 11 mg dl^{-1}, and of these, one had evidence of nephropathy. In Finland, Putkonen *et al.* (1965a) found that 207 serum samples from 60 patients with sarcoidosis gave a mean calcium level of 9.95 mg dl^{-1}, compared with 9.81 mg for 100 from control subjects; only two specimens from sarcoidosis patients gave values above 11.0 mg and both of these gave lower values in subsequent tests. However, some sarcoidosis patients showed high urinary calcium excretion; three out of 39 repeatedly excreted more than 420 mg daily, the highest daily excretion found among 51 control subjects being 324 mg. One of us (JGS) found that among 62 patients newly investigated in London with a final diagnosis of sarcoidosis, none had symptoms or signs attributable to hypercalcaemia, and serum calcium estimated routinely varied from 8.6–11.6 mg dl^{-1}, exceeding 11 mg in six. Goldstein *et al.* (1971) reviewed published studies of hypercalcaemia in sarcoidosis. Among those defining hypercalcaemia as a level above 11 mg dl^{-1} and including more than 50 patients, the proportion with hypercalcaemia ranged from 3.8–35.4%. Among 243 patients in Philadelphia whose records they surveyed retrospectively, it was only 2.9%. Of 137 patients whom they studied prospectively, only two had levels above 11 mg dl^{-1} which persisted, though nine more had single measurements at this level. Lebacq *et al.* (1970) found that a rather higher proportion, 17 (11%) of 152 patients had at least one measurement of serum calcium above this level.

Most observers have found that hypercalciuria is more frequent than hypercalcaemia, but there are equally wide differences in estimates of its frequency. Since calcium excretion varies with dietary intake, there are variations between individuals on uncontrolled intakes. Goldstein *et al.* (1974a) studied 18 patients with active sarcoidosis and normal serum calcium levels on four levels of calcium intake ranging up to 5120 mg/day; the urinary calcium outputs varied with intake from 75–207 mg daily, and were not significantly different from those found in 12 control subjects. At the other end of the scale, Lebacq *et al.* (1970) found that hypercalciuria, which they defined as an excretion of more than 200 mg daily on an intake of 400 mg, occurred in 36 (62%) of 38 patients with sarcoidosis and in 7.5% of normal subjects.

Reiner *et al.* (1976) found that very few patients with sarcoidosis had hypercalcaemia, but hypercalciuria was more frequent, and abnormalities of calcium metabolism were demonstrable in balance studies in more than half those studied. Of 66 patients seen consecutively in a chest clinic during a period of ten years, only one was hypercalcaemic. Of 13 with untreated sarcoidosis, all normocalcaemic, five excreted more than 300 mg of calcium in the urine daily.

Since those patients with sarcoidosis who are liable to hypercalcaemia are very sensitive to vitamin D, small amounts of which can cause elevation of serum calcium levels (see below), local customs in relation to self-medication with vitamin preparations may have an important effect on the observed prevalence of high serum calcium levels. Similarly, it has been shown that exposure to sunlight raises calcium levels in patients with sarcoidosis. Taylor *et al.* (1963) found that among 345 such patients in North Carolina, the mean level during the winter months was 9.89 mg and during the summer months 10.26 mg dl^{-1}, whereas among 12 027 controls the levels in winter and in summer did not differ significantly. Among their sarcoid patients, levels above 11 mg dl^{-1} were observed in 28.6% in summer and 10.6% in winter. Goldstein *et al* (1971) in Philadelphia and Putkonen *et al.* (1965a) in Finland found no evidence of higher mean values among sarcoidosis patients in summer; possibly greater exposure to sun in North Carolina than in the urban environment of Philadelphia or the northerly latitude of Finland accounts for this difference. Another factor that must be expected to affect the proportion of patients with abnormal calcium levels in any series is the number receiving corticosteroid treatment, since this tends, even in small doses, to correct abnormal levels in sarcoidosis.

The cause of hypercalcaemia and hypercalciuria in sarcoidosis

Several factors that have been considered to account for the high levels of calcium in the blood and urine of some patients with sarcoidosis can be excluded. The possibility that they are due to mobilization of calcium from the bones by widespread sarcoid involvement is controverted by the complete lack of association between radiologically evident bone changes and hypercalcaemia, the combination of low faecal and high urinary calcium excretion, the normal phosphatase level, and the observation that the serum calcium falls if the dietary intake of calcium is lowered. Mather (1957) found that among 120 sarcoid patients, nine showed bone changes in routine radiographs of the hands and feet; none of these nine had disturbed calcium metabolism. Radiologically evident bone lesions do not appear to have been noted with any greater frequency among recorded cases of sarcoidosis with hypercalcaemia than would be expected by chance. Of the five patients in the series of 275 reviewed by one of us (JGS) who showed symptoms and signs of hypercalcaemia, none had radiological evidence of bone sarcoid lesions. Moreover, a similar abnormality of calcium metabolism occurs in chronic beryllium disease, of which bone changes are not a feature (Tepper *et al.* 1961).

The increased level of calcium in the blood cannot be accounted for by protein binding. When the plasma proteins are high in sarcoidosis, it is the globulins that are increased, and of that part of the serum calcium which is protein-bound, the greater proportion is bound to albumin (Gutman and Gutman, 1937); increased binding of calcium to protein could not account for hypercalciuria; and hyperglobulinaemia and hypercalcaemia cannot be correlated (Harrell and Fisher, 1939; Longcope and Freiman, 1952). Moreover, Hahnemann *et al.* (1967) found that in repeated estimates ionized calcium was elevated more frequently than total calcium in the blood of seven patients with sarcoidosis. Similarly, Goldstein *et al.* (1971) studied 137 patients, of whom only four had persistent elevations of serum calcium above 11 mg dl^{-1}, and found that the mean level of ultrafiltrable calcium was slightly higher in the 93 in whom it was measured than in control subjects.

Both indirect evidence (Transbøl and Halver, 1967; Hornum and Transbøl, 1976; Reiner *et al.*, 1976) and measurement of parathyroid hormone (PTH) in the blood (Cushard *et al.*, 1972; Labacq *et al.*, 1977; Handslip *et al.*, 1980) show that abnormal function of the parathyroid glands cannot account for high calcium levels in sarcoidosis. Cushard *et al.* (1972) found that PTH levels were unmeasurably low in 19 of 26 sarcoidosis patients, of whom six were hypercalcaemic. In two patients with high PTH levels parathyroid adenomas were found and removed surgically. Other observers have found low or normal levels of PTH in hypercalcaemic sarcoidosis patients (Bell *et al.*, 1979; Papapoulos *et al.*, 1979); when the serum calcium falls after corticosteroid treatment, PTH levels rise, showing the expected response of normally-functioning glands to the change in calcium level. The concurrence of hyperparathyroidism and sarcoidosis is discussed below.

The hypercalcaemia and hypercalciuria of sarcoidosis have generally been found to be associated with low faecal calcium excretion (Dent *et al.*, 1953; Henneman *et al.*, 1954; Anderson *et al.*, 1954; Bell *et al.*, 1964; Bell and

Bartter, 1967), implying an abnormally high absorption of ingested calcium from the gut. This, with the normal or slightly elevated serum phosphorus and generally normal phosphatase level is similar to the picture of vitamin D intoxication, and suggests that hypersensitivity to vitamin D may be the underlying abnormality (Anderson *et al.*, 1954). It is known that some patients with sarcoidosis are in fact hypersensitive to this vitamin.

In the past, calciferol was widely used in the treatment of lupus vulgaris, and was tried as a therapeutic agent in sarcoidosis. Intolerance was frequently noted (Curtis *et al.*, 1947; Scadding, 1950; Larsson *et al.*, 1952). Between 1946 and 1952, one of us (JGS) investigated the possible therapeutic effect of calciferol in 36 patients. Of these, 11 tolerated 100 000–150 000 units daily for three or four months without symptoms or evident biochemical upset; seven tolerated only smaller doses, of the order of 50 000 – 100 000 units; 18 became nauseated and developed rises of serum calcium on smaller doses, and administration of the vitamin had to be discontinued after periods ranging from five days to a fortnight. In the most strikingly intolerant, 50 000 units daily led to a rise of serum calcium to 16 mg and of blood urea to 80 mg dl^{-1} from normal levels in six days. There was thus a very wide variation in the responses of individual patients, ranging from what appeared to be normal tolerance to almost complete intolerance. Larsson *et al.* (1952) had similar experiences in treating 24 patients with doses of calciferol ranging between 30 000 and 140 000 units daily; half of them developed toxic reactions, occasionally severe, and usually accompanied by a transitory nephropathy. By contrast, the incidence of toxic reactions among patients with lupus vulgaris receiving large doses of calciferol was considerably lower. Anning *et al.* (1948) estimated that about 20% of such patients had toxic reactions, not all requiring cessation of treatment. Some sarcoid patients with hypercalcaemia have been found to be in the habit of taking vitamin D preparations without medical advice (Dent, 1970).

As noted above, serum calcium levels of patients with sarcoidosis may be increased abnormally by exposure to sunlight (Taylor *et al.*, 1963), and Dent (1970) reported that in two hypercalcaemic sarcoidosis patients, a brisk rise in serum calcium was produced by whole-body ultra-violet light irradiation. These effects are presumably due to photosynthesis of vitamin D in the skin. Hendrix (1963) put two patients with sarcoidosis, hypercalciuria and hypercalcaemia on vitamin D deficient diets and shielded them from sunlight; in six to eight weeks, the serum calcium levels fell to normal, urinary excretion diminished and faecal excretion increased. Henneman *et al.* (1954) and Henneman *et al.* (1956) suggested that there might be excessive endogenous production of vitamin D-like substances or deficient capacity to inactivate vitamin D. But blood levels of antirachitic activity were found to be normal in three sarcoid patients with hypercalcaemia by

Thomas *et al.* (1959), who found normal levels also in hyperparathyroidism and the milk-alkali syndrome, but, as would be expected, high levels in patients with hypercalcaemia due to excessive vitamin D intake. Bell *et al.* (1964) investigated four sarcoid patients with low faecal and high urinary calcium excretion. Serum antirachitic activity was low or normal. The administration of 10 000 units of vitamin D daily caused a diminution in the already low faecal excretion of calcium, without an abnormal increase in serum antirachitic activity; the same dose of vitamin D had no effect on calcium absorption in normal subjects. Prednisone diminished the absorption of calcium, whether or not additional vitamin D was given.

These observations led to the suggestion that the abnormal response to vitamin D might be due to hypersensitivity at cellular level in target organs: in the gut increasing calcium absorption (Anderson *et al.*, 1954; Taylor *et al.*, 1963; Bell *et al.*, 1964), in the bones, increasing resorption (Hendrix, 1966; Bell and Bartter, 1967), and in the kidneys, increasing excretion (Dent, 1970). On the hypothesis that the abnormal calcium metabolism of sarcoidosis is due to target-organ hypersensitivity to vitamin D metabolites, the effect of corticosteroids in lowering high calcium levels can be explained by established effects of corticosteroids on the target-organs, especially the gut (Harrison and Harrison, 1960; Kimberg, 1969; Kimberg *et al.*, 1971; Wall and Peters 1971) and on vitamin D metabolism (Avioli *et al.*, 1968).

The variable relation between hypercalcaemia and hypercalciuria has led to doubt whether target-organ hypersensitivity to vitamin D can be the sole explanation for the abnormal calcium metabolism of sarcoidosis (Henneman *et al.*, 1954; Jackson and Dancaster, 1959). Since increase in urinary calcium excretion in hypercalcaemic sarcoidosis patients is greater than increase in intestinal absorption, and hypercalciuria often occurs with normal serum calcium levels, Jackson and Dancaster suggested that there was a defect in renal tubular resorption of calcium. Lebacq *et al.* (1970, 1977, 1980) have emphasized the frequency of normocalcaemic hypercalciuria. Since they found urinary hydroxyproline levels to be normal, they concluded that bone resorption was unlikely to be a factor. In renal biopsies from 25 patients with sarcoidosis, granulomas were found in ten. They were present in 55% of 18 patients who had hypercalciuria, but in only 33% of nine who had hypercalcaemia, suggesting that the presence of granulomas might lead to increase in calcium excretion. Two patients showed histological changes interpreted as chronic pyelonephritis; both of these showed evidence of impaired tubular function. Thus it seemed likely that in addition to increased intestinal absorption of calcium due to hypersensitivity to vitamin D, a defect in tubular resorption of calcium contributes to hypercalciuria in sarcoidosis, and may be a principal factor in some without hypercalcaemia. But Dent (1970) has pointed out that the first action of vitamin D is increased urinary excretion, as well as gut absorption, of calcium, and that in normal subjects hypercalcaemia is an effect of larger doses of the vitamin and arises from the effect on bone: thus hypercalciuria alone, as well as with hypercalcaemia, could be due to hypersensitivity to vitamin D.

Reiner *et al.* (1976) studied calcium metabolism in 13 normocalcaemic sarcoidosis patients, of whom five had hypercalciuria. Calcium absorption was high in six. Bone turnover of calcium was studied in ten, and found to be high in six. Calcium absorption correlated well both with calculated bone uptake and with urinary excretion. It seemed likely that target-organ hypersensitivity to vitamin D in gut and bone could account for these findings, and was common in sarcoidosis, though only a few patients who are most severely affected develop hypercalcaemia.

Hornum and Transbøl (1976) performed calcium balance and turnover studies on four patients with sarcoidosis. One of these showed a pattern similar to that shown by a patient recovering from vitamin D intoxication. This led to the suggestion that the varying patterns seen in sarcoidosis might be explained by periods of activity in which there is hyperabsorption of calcium, hypercalcaemia and hypercalciuria and periods of remission when hyperabsorption ceases, but high calcium levels are maintained in the blood and urine by mobilization of reversible metastatic calcification. This possibility would not explain the frequency of hypercalciuria in patients who have never shown symptoms suggestive of hypercalcaemia, nor the long duration of normocalcaemic hypercalciuria in some such patients. It has important practical implications since if, indeed, normocalcaemic hypercalciuria is associated with remission from the active phase of hypercalcaemia, there is no indication for treating it unless it is complicated by stone-formation.

The possibility that abnormal metabolism of vitamin D may be a factor in the disturbance of calcium metabolism in sarcoidosis has been studied with conflicting results. The most active metabolite, 1, 25-dihydrocholecalciferol (1, 25$(OH)_2D_3$) is produced in the kidney from 25-hydroxycholecalciferol (25$(OH)D_3$), which is produced in the liver (Mawer *et al.*, 1971). Mawer *et al.* found low levels of antirachitic activity in the blood of two hypercalcaemic sarcoidosis patients, with no evidence of excessive formation of 25$(OH)D_3$ or 1, 25$(OH)_2D_3$; and Avioli and Haddad (1973) reported normal levels of these compounds and of cholecalciferol in sarcoidosis patients. Bringel *et al.* (1980) found that serum levels of 25-hydroxycholecalciferol were normal in sarcoidosis patients, whether or not they were hypercalcaemic, and were not affected in hypercalcaemic patients by dexamethasone which reduced calcium levels to normal; there was no correlation between levels of 25-hydroxycholecalciferol and of calcium. On the other hand, Bell *et al.* (1979) found in three patients with sarcoidosis and hypercalcaemia that plasma levels of 1, 25$(OH)_2D_3$ were raised when calcium levels were high and fell when prednisone was given and calcium levels returned to normal. Oral vitamin D caused a sharp increase in plasma 1, $25(OH)_2D_3$ in three sarcoidosis patients with a history of hypercalcaemia, but did not increase levels of this compound beyond the normal range in seven normal subjects or five sarcoidosis patients without a history of hypercalcaemia. Administration of 1, $25(OH)_2D_3$ raised urinary calcium excretion in all subjects, irrespective of serum levels. Papapoulos *et al.* (1979) studied a young man with sarcoidosis, known to affect lungs, liver and an infiltrated tattoo scar, who had episodes of hypercalcaemia in four successive summers, controllable by corticosteroid treatment, and exacerbated by small doses of vitamin D; serum levels of 1 $25(OH)_2D_3$ were greatly raised during hypercalcaemic episodes.

Barbour *et al.* (1981) reported the case of a man aged 32 who had been known to have sarcoidosis for four years when he developed Henoch-Schönlein purpura with a nephrotic syndrome. Hypercalcaemia led to exploration of the neck for a parathyroid adenoma, without success; a lymph-node was removed and confirmed the diagnosis of sarcoidosis. Calcium levels fell with corticosteroid treatment. Renal failure required haemodialysis; bilateral nephrectomy was performed. Hypercalcaemia persisted unless controlled by corticosteroid treatment. Both before and after nephrectomy, 1, $25(OH)_2D_3$ levels were high during hypercalcaemia and fell when it was controlled, with reciprocal changes in parathyroid hormone levels. Since these findings persisted after nephrectomy, synthesis of 1, $25(OH)_2/D_3$ must have occurred elsewhere than in the kidney; possibly in the sarcoid granuloma.

Further evidence that abnormal levels of 1, $25(OH)_2D_3$ occur in at least some cases of sarcoid hypercalcaemia is provided by a case reported by Mitchell *et al.* (1983). A woman, aged 28, who had hypoparathyroidism requiring treatment with vitamin D since the age of 19, presented with erythema nodosum, BHL and a positive Kveim test, and was found to have become hypercalcaemic; on cessation of vitamin D, calcium levels returned to normal, but the administration of hydrocortisone led to hypocalcaemia; the plasma 1, $25(OH)_2D_3$ level was measured and found to be three times the highest recorded in patients with hypoparathyroidism under treatment with vitamin D. A patient reported by Zimmerman *et al.* (1983) who had had hypoparathyroidism for 25 years was able to discontinue vitamin D treatment with maintenance of normal serum calcium levels when she developed sarcoidosis.

It is perhaps not surprising that studies of the disturbance of calcium metabolism in sarcoidosis are difficult to interpret, in view of its variability and of the complexities of the metabolism of calcium and of vitamin D. This disturbance affects only a minority of patients, who at present cannot be identified by any other characteristic, and in those affected is unpredictable in its course and duration. It is possible that different combinations of causal factors are operative in different cases, and at different times during the course of the same case; for instance, renal excretion of calcium may be affected by progressive hypercalcaemic or granulomatous nephropathy.

Clinical features

Hypercalcaemia gives rise immediately to such symptoms as anorexia, depression, nausea, vomiting, polydipsia and polyuria in varying combinations. Later, symptoms may arise from secondary changes in the kidneys and from calcinosis of soft tissues. It is a striking feature of the early stages of the hypercalcaemia of sarcoidosis that both the symptoms and the biochemical abnormalities are relieved by corticosteroids (p. 412), response to which is diagnostically helpful (p. 410). If the high calcium levels persist, irreversible renal changes occur; these are reviewed above (p. 395). They may prove progressive, leading to renal failure and/or hypertension, even though calcium levels return to normal either in the natural course of the disease or in response to corticosteroid treatment. As with other forms of hypercalcaemia, renal calculi and soft tissue calcinosis may develop.

Renal calculi may cause renal colic and/or haematuria; their reported frequency in patients with sarcoidosis varies greatly (p. 398).

Calcinosis of soft tissues may become evident clinically as hard nodules in fingers or toes, especially the pulps of the terminal phalanges (Klatskin and Gordon, 1953; Davidson, 1954) and presents a characteristic radiographic appearance (Fig. 22.3). It has also been reported in subcutaneous tissues in the axilla (Lathan *et al.*, 1968), the cartilage of the ear (Batson, 1961), and the sternomastoid muscle (Fujita *et al.*, 1974). Calcareous deposits may develop in the ear-drums, causing chalky white areas; in two patients under the care of one of us (JGS), such areas were observed to diminish in size with control of hypercalcaemia by corticosteroid treatment. Nephrocalcinosis may cause small dense flecks of opacity within the renal outlines in plain radiographs of the abdomen.

Calcinosis of the cornea and of the conjunctiva may occur (Chapter 8, p. 223).

Differential diagnosis

When hypercalcaemia appears in an individual with evident sarcoidosis, no diagnostic problems should arise, apart from the rare instances, discussed below, of co-existent sarcoidosis and hyperparathyroidism. Serum and urinary calcium estimations are often included in the initial investigations of patients with suspected sarcoidosis, but it is only rarely that the serum calcium level is found to be elevated in the absence of relevant symptoms.

In patients known to be suffering from sarcoidosis any suspicious symptom, such as unexplained anorexia, nausea or other gastric disturbance, polyuria and polydipsia, or loss of weight should lead to examinations of serum calcium and of urinary calcium excretion. But a patient with hypercalcaemia and without overt evidence of sarcoidosis may present considerable diagnostic problems. Other possibilities to be considered include vitamin D intoxication, hyperparathyroidism, the 'milk-alkali' syndrome resulting from excessive intake of antacids and milk (Burnell *et al.*, 1949; Scholz and Keating, 1955), osteolytic metastases of malignant disease in bone, multiple myeloma and Paget's disease of bone, and the hypercalcaemia occasionally associated with malignant disease without bone metastases (Plimpton and Gellhorn, 1956; Connor *et al.*, 1956; Myers, 1956; Lucas, 1960). The combination of raised calcium, normal or even slightly high phosphate and normal phosphatase levels in the blood and high urinary calcium excretion which is characteristic of the hypercalcaemia of sarcoidosis is found also in vitamin D intoxication, but this is unlikely to cause confusion.

Difficulty has arisen most frequently in the differentiation between the hypercalcaemia of sarcoidosis and hyperparathyroidism. In a number of recorded cases in which hypercalcaemia was eventually shown to be associated with sarcoidosis, the parathyroids have been explored surgically and found to be normal (Albright and Reifenstein, 1948; Howard *et al.*, 1949; Westra and Visser, 1949; Klatskin and Gordon, 1953, two cases; Anderson *et al.*, 1954, Case 3; Scholz and Keating, 1956, Case 1). Winnacker *et al.* (1968) found published reports of 21 patients with sarcoidosis who had unnecessary operations for suspected hyperparathyroidism. In hyperparathyroidism, characteristic bone changes may be evident radiologically, the serum phosphate level is low and the phosphatase high.

The response to corticosteroid administration constitutes a most striking difference between hyperparathyroidism and the hypercalcaemia of sarcoidosis. The effect of corticosteroids in reducing calcium levels to normal in hypercalcaemic sarcoidosis, with improvement in renal function, was first reported by Shulman *et al.* (1952), Dent *et al.* (1953) and Phillips (1953), and has subsequently been generally confirmed. Within a few days of starting effective doses of a corticosteroid (100–150 mg of cortisone or the equivalent dosage of an alternative compound), the urinary excretion of calcium falls, the faecal content rises, and the serum calcium starts to fall towards normal. Unless there is permanent renal damage, the blood urea, if raised, returns to normal. Corticosteroid treatment has generally been found to antagonize the effects of vitamin D on calcium metabolism in sarcoidosis (Anderson *et al.*, 1954; Mather, 1957; Bell *et al.*, 1964; Dent,

1970) just as it does in vitamin D intoxication (Connor *et al.*, 1956; Dent, 1956; Verner *et al.*, 1958). By contrast, Dent *et al.* (1953) and Dent (1956) found that cortisone had no effect on calcium levels in six patients with hyperparathyroidism. Connor *et al.* (1956) studied the effect of cortisone and corticotrophin on 23 patients with hypercalcaemia. In those with sarcoidosis, with vitamin D intoxication and with the milk-alkali syndrome the calcium fell within seven days of starting the hormone, but rose again when it was stopped. In those with hyperparathyroidism there was no response; while in those with hypercalcaemia associated with malignant disease, the response was variable. Dent and Watson (1968) have suggested that for a standard test, hydrocortisone 40 mg three times daily for ten days should be used, since this would avoid the confusing factor of defective conversion of other corticosteroids to this active compound in patients with liver involvement. Blood should be taken from the fasting patient in the morning before, and five, eight, and ten days after starting hydrocortisone. Fall of calcium levels to normal is strong evidence against hyperparathyroidism and compatible with the hypercalcaemia of sarcoidosis or vitamin D excess; it is equivocal in relation to the hypercalcaemia of malignant disease.

Dent's observation that a few patients with hypercalcaemic sarcoidosis respond better to hydrocortisone than to cortisone has not been further investigated.

Discrimination from hyperparathyroidism is complicated by the occasional concurrence of sarcoidosis with hyperparathyroidism, proved by the demonstration of adenomas or hyperplastic parathyroid glands surgically removed, followed by return to normal calcium levels (Snapper *et al.*, 1958; Burr *et al.*, 1960; Bernstein *et al.*, 1965; Dent and Watson, 1966; Pedersen, 1967; Hahnemann *et al.*, 1967; Lief *et al.*, 1967; Winnacker *et al.*, 1968; Dent, 1970; Bohnen *et al.*, 1971; Robinson *et al.*, 1980). Schweitzer *et al.* (1981) reported that among 600 cases of primary hyperparathyroidism they had observed one with concurrent sarcoidosis, as shown by granulomas in lymph-nodes and in a parathyroid adenoma removed, and one who developed BHL and a pulmonary infiltration, without hypercalcaemia, five years after successful removal of a parathyroid adenoma. Dent (1970) thought that the concurrence of hyperparathyroidism and sarcoidosis might be more frequent than would be expected by chance, and speculated whether sarcoidosis might in some way stimulate the production of adenomas in the parathyroids; but in view of the frequency of symptomless sarcoidosis, the number of reported cases is perhaps not beyond expectation. As noted above, blood levels of parathyroid hormone, estimated by radioimmune assay, have been found to be low in hypercalcaemic sarcoidosis patients, in sharp contrast to the high levels in hyperparathyroidism, and this provides a definitive discriminatory test, especially useful when sarcoidosis and hyperparathyroidism co-exist (Bohnen *et al.*, 1971; Cushard *et al.*, 1972).

Treatment of hypercalcaemia and hypercalciuria

Persistent hypercalcaemia constitutes one of the most definite indications for corticosteroid treatment in sarcoidosis; but before such treatment is started, it should be established that the hypercalcaemia is in fact persistent, and that excessive dietary intake of calcium or vitamin D, or exposure to sunlight are not factors in its causation. The dietary intake of milk and cheese, the chief sources of calcium, should be limited and care should be taken that extra vitamin D is not taken in any form. Unnecessary exposure to full sunlight should be avoided.

Although hydrocortisone may be preferred in a diagnostic test, the hypercalcaemia of sarcoidosis nearly always responds to the more generally used prednisolone or prednisone, which are to be preferred when long-term treatment is required. Treatment can be initiated with the usual dosage (Chapter 27), and continued with the smallest dose that maintains normal calcium levels. Fortunately the maintenance dose required is in most cases small or moderate, of the order of 5–12.5 mg of prednisolone daily. Like other manifestations of sarcoidosis, the disorder of calcium metabolism is of unpredictable duration, not necessarily related to that of other clinically evident features, and efficient control of treatment therefore depends upon measurement of serum calcium and urinary calcium excretion.

Chloroquine has been found to have a similar effect on the abnormal calcium metabolism of sarcoidosis to that of corticosteroids, but of slower onset and less reliable (Hunt and Yendt, 1963; Hendrix, 1964). Hunt and Yendt found that hypercalcaemia might be corrected only after four or five weeks of treatment, and hypercalciuria even more slowly. The use of chloroquine in sarcoidosis is discussed in Chapter 27. In general, it is indicated only in exceptional cases in which corticosteroid treatment is advisable, but for some reason contraindicated; and since the dose of corticosteroid required to control hypercalcaemia is usually low the need to consider an alternative to it should seldom arise.

Similarly, other measures that have been used to lower calcium levels in hypercalcaemic patients rarely need to be considered in sarcoidosis. These include sodium phytate, which acts in part by combining with calcium in the gut to form an insoluble salt which is excreted in the faeces, and in part by partial hydrolysis with adsorption of the phosphate moiety; it has been used in dosage of 9.0 g daily (Henneman *et al.*, 1954; Roelsen and Paulsen, 1964). Inorganic phosphates have been shown to lower high calcium levels in a variety of hypercalcaemic states (Goldsmith and Ingbar, 1966; Hebert *et al.*, 1966) and have been used successfully by oral administration in long-term treatment of hypercalciuric sarcoidosis (Thomas, 1969).

Opinion is divided about whether hypercalciuria unaccompanied by hypercalcaemia or renal stone formation requires treatment. Lebacq *et al.*

(1980) recommended that the urinary calcium excretion should be reduced, reinforcing dietary restriction of calcium by giving 5 g daily of cellulose phosphate by mouth, or by the administration of hydrochlorothiazide. On the other hand, Dent (1970) expressed the view that unless there is evidence of calculus formation, which is dependent on factors additional to sarcoidosis and present only in some patients, urinary calcium excretion above the accepted range of normal does not require treatment; limitation of milk and cheese in the diet and avoidance of vitamin D supplements should of course be advised.

Chapter 20

The Immunology of Sarcoidosis

The immunological responses of patients with sarcoidosis, as a group, differ from those of healthy individuals in important ways. An early finding was that a much higher proportion of them than of the populations from which they were drawn had negative tuberculin tests, and this has proved to be one aspect of generally lower ability to acquire and express delayed Type IV hypersensitivity. Their capacity to develop and express Type I hypersensitivity appears normal, and to produce antibodies normal or even enhanced. Hyperglobulinaemia and changes in immunoglobulin levels are usual in active cases. These abnormalities, their relationship to clinical aspects, and changes in immuno-competent cells underlying them have been intensively studied, and are discussed in this chapter. The Kveim reaction, which evidently detects some sort of altered reactivity, but cannot at present be interpreted in terms of recognized types of hypersensitivity, is discussed in Chapter 21.

REACTIVITY TO AGENTS CAUSING DELAYED TUBERCULIN-TYPE SKIN RESPONSES

Tuberculin*

Boeck (1916) noted that two of his original three patients showed no skin reaction to tuberculin. Subsequently it was found that groups of patients with sarcoidosis showed a lower level of tuberculin sensitivity than was

*Some earlier studies of tuberculin sensitivity were performed with old tuberculin (OT), dosage being stated in terms either of the dilution of OT used for a test with 0.1 ml or of the amount of OT contained in this volume. More recent studies used purified protein derivative (PPD). To avoid prolixity, we quote dosages in terms of international units (IU), using admittedly approximate conversion factors where necessary.

prevalent in the populations from which they were drawn. Studies by Reisner (1944) in New York, Bjornstadt (1950) in Oslo, Longcope and Freiman (1952) in Baltimore and Boston, Cowdell (1954) in Oxford, Israel and Sones (1958) in Philadelphia, and Würm (1963) in Germany found that proportions ranging from 45–70% of patients with sarcoidosis were non-reactors to tuberculin, 100 IU, at times when the large majority of the relevant populations were reactors to 10 IU or less. From London, Hoyle *et al.* (1954) reported a comparison of 90 patients with sarcoidosis with age- and sex-matched control subjects not suffering from tuberculosis or any disease likely to affect tuberculin reactivity; they found that 44% of the sarcoidosis patients and 21% of the controls were non-reactors to 100 IU. Also from London, Scadding (1956) reported that of 140 sarcoidosis patients 3% reacted to 1 IU, 13% to 10 IU, and 16% to 100 IU, while 68% were non-reactors; in a matched control group, only 20% did not react to 100 IU.

This series was later extended to 260 cases of sarcoidosis with completed serial tuberculin tests; of these, 4% reacted to 1 IU, 14% to 10 IU, 21% to 100 IU, and 61% were non-reactors. As in some other European series, the proportion of reactors was higher in patients with BHL at the early stages of the disease; only 50% of those with erythema nodosum (EN) and BHL, and 54% with symptomless BHL were non-reactors to 100 IU, proportions not far removed from the 47% found by Löfgren and Lundback (1952) for patients with BHL in Stockholm. Würm (1963) found that among German patients with acute onset, the proportion of non-reactors was even lower, only 18.6% of 129 with EN, arthropathy or fever not reacting to 100 IU; and that the proportion of cases of intrathoracic sarcoidosis failing to react to 10 IU increased with increasing chronicity from 68.2% of those with BHL to 85.9% of those with fibrosis. In the United States, this relationship between depression of tuberculin sensitivity and chronicity was not observed either in Philadelphia (Sones and Israel, 1954) or in New York (Chusid *et al.*, 1971). Sones and Israel re-tested 170 patients after an average interval of six years, and found that the proportion of non-reactors to 250 IU changed only from 74.1–77.7%, and that in individual patients changes in either direction were not correlated with the course of the disease. Similarly, Chusid *et al.* re-tested 91 patients and found no change in the proportion of reactors, although in one-third reactivity changed without evident correlation with the clinical course. Reports about changes in tuberculin sensitivity in patients regarded as having 'recovered' from sarcoidosis are difficult to interpret, since 'recovery' may refer to anything from rapid resolution of BHL to the attainment of a stable state with symptomless fibrotic residual changes after a prolonged course. From the United States, Israel and Sones (1965) and Chusid *et al.* (1971) reported that with 'recovery' the proportion reacting to tuberculin was little changed, while from

Sweden, France and Japan it has been reported that tuberculin sensitivity reappears in some (Nitter, 1953; Turiaf *et al.*, 1968; Hosoda *et al.*, 1967).

In cases in which bacteriologically confirmed tuberculosis develops in the course of sarcoidosis (reviewed in Chapter 23), changes in tuberculin sensitivity are variable. In most, tuberculin sensitivity either appears or is already present, possibly increasing; but in some the skin remains non-reactive (Scadding, 1960b, 1971; Israel and Sones, 1965; Kent *et al.*, 1970; Chusid *et al.*, 1971).

There has been little systematic study of changes in tuberculin sensitivity at the onset of sarcoidosis, although it is generally recognized that a previously positive tuberculin test may become negative at this time. Turiaf *et al.* (1968) found that among 90 patients with previous tuberculin tests, of which 61% had been positive, after the onset of sarcoidosis only 21% reacted. Hannuksela and Salo (1969) in a study of 283 patients with sarcoidosis found that the degree of depression of tuberculin sensitivity as compared with controls was the same in 91 whose history suggested that they were initially reactors, as in those who had no such history. During the long-term follow-up of over 54 000 young adults in a trial of BCG vaccination, Sutherland *et al.* (1965) observed 52 cases of intrathoracic sarcoidosis. They found that the onset of sarcoidosis was not related to previous tuberculin test or tuberculosis vaccination status. Among those who developed sarcoidosis in each skin test or vaccination group, the trend of tuberculin sensitivity before the onset of sarcoidosis was closely similar to that among those who remained healthy, though there was a tendency for tuberculin sensitivity to be depressed at or shortly after the first evidence of sarcoidosis.

There is little information about the important question whether the proportion of reactors to tuberculin among patients with sarcoidosis in a defined area changes with changes in the proportion among the general population. Scadding (1971a) reported that among patients with BHL attributed to sarcoidosis in London between 1950 and 1967, during which time there was a considerable diminution in the proportion of young adults reacting to tuberculin, the proportion of patients with BHL attributed to sarcoidosis reacting to 10 IU did not change: 30% of 74 who had BHL between 1950 to 1962, and 29% of 75 between 1962 and 1967 reacted. In Denmark, Fog and Wilbek (1974) noted that the proportions of sarcoidosis patients reacting to tuberculin, and the distribution of sizes of reaction among the reactors, were similar among those who had and those who had not been BCG-vaccinated.

Response of patients with sarcoidosis to BCG vaccination
The generally lower tuberculin sensitivity in patients with sarcoidosis as compared with the levels in the population from which they come is an index of depression of established sensitivity resulting from past mycobac-

terial infection. Ability to develop tuberculin sensitivity is also depressed, as shown by the response of patients with sarcoidosis to BCG vaccination. The usual course of events is that the local reaction proceeds, as in tuberculin-negative normal subjects, to the formation of a papule, which may show some ulceration, and may be accompanied by enlargement of regional lymph-nodes; but the skin either remains non-reactive, or develops only low reactivity to tuberculin which is transient (Lemming, 1940; Leider and Sulzberger, 1949; Israel *et al.*, 1950; Carnes and Raffel, 1949; Harris and Shore, 1952; Borrie, 1952; Forgacs *et al.*, 1957). If a tuberculin-positive sarcoidosis patient is vaccinated, the local reaction is accelerated, its early phase resembling a Type IV hypersensitivity reaction, as in other tuberculin-positive subjects (Leider and Sulzberger, 1949; Ustvedt and Aanonsen, 1949; Forgacs *et al.*, 1957). Failure to develop hypersensitivity after BCG vaccination may persist after all evidence of active sarcoidosis has disappeared (Israel and Sones, 1965). Biopsy of the local papule and of regional lymph-nodes shows tuberculoid granulomas (Lemming, 1940, 1942; Leider and Hyman, 1950; Rostenberg *et al.*, 1953) in which acid-fast bacilli may be seen, and from which BCG may be cultured (Rostenberg *et al.*, 1953; Forgacs *et al.*, 1957). Löfgren *et al.* (1954) traced the migration of BCG labelled with radio-active phosphorus from the sites of intradermal injections: the rate of removal varied with tuberculin sensitivity similarly in sarcoidosis patients and controls. Persistent or spreading local infiltrations of the skin have been reported exceptionally at the site of BCG vaccination in patients with sarcoidosis (Lemming, 1942; Leider and Hyman, 1950).

Reactions to other agents causing delayed, Type IV, hypersensitivity

Depressed sensitivity to tuberculin is one aspect of a general depression of the ability of sarcoidosis patients, as a group, to react to agents causing delayed hypersensitivity. Friou (1952) studied mumps virus, a *Candida albicans* antigen, and trichophytin, prepared from a species of the pathogenic skin fungus *Trichophyton*. All these agents cause delayed skin reactions in a high proportion of normal adults; they caused fewer and less intense reactions in patients with sarcoidosis. These observations were confirmed by Sones and Israel (1954), who added similar observations with a pertussis antigen. They found further that among those who failed to respond to pertussis antigen, immunization with pertussis vaccine led to positive reactions to skin tests in all the controls but in only 45% of the sarcoid patients; moreover in most of the sarcoid patients the skin reactivity was transient. Citron (1957) studied reactions to an antigen prepared from *Candida albicans*; it gave reactions in 90% of 60 control subjects, and in 40% of 30 patients with sarcoidosis. Among the controls 80% reacted to tuberculin, 100 IU, as compared with 18% among the sarcoid patients.

Among those who reacted, the mean size of Candida reactions was significantly less in the sarcoid patients than in the controls. Only 2% of the controls gave no reaction to both Candida antigen and tuberculin, as compared with 43% of the sarcoid patients.

Quinn *et al.* (1955) tested the responses of patients with sarcoidosis to past mumps infection by complement fixation tests (CFT) for humoral antibodies, and by skin tests with mumps virus antigen for delayed hypersensitivity. Most normal adults gave positive responses to both of these. Of seven sarcoidosis patients all had positive CFT, but only one a positive skin test. Thus six of seven showed the unusual combination of serological evidence of a past mumps virus infection, without evidence of delayed hypersensitivity.

Lordon *et al.* (1968) compared skin-test reactions to a range of tuberculins, fungal antigens and mumps virus in 50 sarcoidosis patients and 50 control subjects. Unusually, they found little difference between these groups in proportions reacting to human tuberculin, to mumps virus antigen, or to trichophytin; but there was a large difference in tests with other tuberculins, only 2.5% of tests on patients with tuberculins prepared from *M. intracellulare* and from a scotochromogenic mycobacterium being positive, while 39% and 49% of controls reacted to these. Tests with 250 IU human tuberculin, with mumps virus antigen, with trichophytin and with candida antigen were positive in a rather higher proportion of patients with inactive than with active sarcoidosis.

Contact sensitization

Epstein and Mayock (1957) found that the incidence of skin sensitivity to poison ivy allergen, a potent natural sensitizer, was similar in sarcoid patients and controls. On the other hand, they studied induced skin sensitivity to two less potent contact sensitizers, 2, 4-dinitrochlorobenzene and p-nitrosodimethyl aniline, and found a lower frequency of sensitization in sarcoid patients. Their procedure sensitized 68% of normal subjects and 35% of sarcoidosis patients to dinitrochlorobenzene. Similar findings were reported by James (1966). In a study in England, Verrier-Jones (1967) found that none of 14 patients with active sarcoidosis developed sensitivity to DNCB, whereas all of five with healed sarcoidosis were sensitized; these five patients had all had negative tuberculin tests (100 IU) during the active phase, but three became tuberculin sensitive at the time of DNCB testing. Thus, changes in reactivity to different antigens do not necessarily follow a similar course.

The abnormality of cell-mediated immune reactions in sarcoidosis is best described as depression of cell-mediated hypersensitivity. Since patients with sarcoidosis are not more susceptible than others to viral or fungal infections, in defence against which cell-mediated reactions are important, they cannot correctly be said to show depression of cell-mediated immunity.

HUMORAL ANTIBODY RESPONSES

Humoral antibody responses

Patients with sarcoidosis have been found to produce levels of circulating antibodies after vaccination with pertussis and with typhoid-paratyphoid vaccines similar to those in normal subjects (Sones and Israel, 1954; Persellin *et al.*, 1966). In response to primary vaccination with tetanus toxoid, they produced a rather lower titre than controls, but to re-vaccination a similar or rather higher titre (Greenwood *et al.*, 1958). They produced a higher titre of isoagglutinins after small intravenous injections of mismatched blood than did controls; those under treatment with corticotrophin did not show this enhanced response (Sands *et al.*, 1955).

Antibodies to commonly encountered infective agents have been found in the blood of sarcoidosis patients at levels at least similar to, and sometimes higher than, those found in normal subjects. Greenwood *et al.* (1958) found similar levels of staphylococcal haemolysin in sarcoidosis patients and in controls. Titres of antibody to herpes-like virus have been found to be higher than in controls, irrespective of the duration of the disease in most studies (Wahren *et al.*, 1971; Byrne *et al.*, 1973; Niitu *et al.*, 1974; Mitchell *et al.*, 1974), but lower in one (Hirshaut *et al.*, 1970) especially in those with long-standing sarcoidosis. Similar elevation of antibody titres to other viral antigens, herpes simplex, rubella, measles and para-influenza 1, 2 and 3 have been reported (Byrne *et al.*, 1973). Elevations of viral antibody titre have been found to be greatest in female and in black patients, but could not be correlated with clinical or radiological features or the course of the disease (Byrne *et al.*, 1973; Niitu *et al.*, 1974c; Mitchell *et al.*, 1974). A higher proportion of patients with sarcoidosis than of those with other diseases or of healthy blood-donors have been found to have detectable antibody against mycoplasma, strain 215 M (Yansson *et al.*, 1972). Johnson *et al.* (1977) found complement-fixing antibody to histoplasma yeast antigen in nine of 50 sarcoidosis sera and in only one of 50 control sera. Morison *et al.* (1975) found IgG antibodies to wart virus antigen in 18 of 20 of sarcoidosis patients, but in only 37% of 41 controls; although four of the patients had a past history of warts, none had *in vitro* evidence of cellular reactivity in leucocyte migration inhibition tests.

Antibodies to mycobacterial antigens

Using complement-fixation tests with a number of antigens from tubercle bacilli, Carnes and Raffel (1949) found positive tests with at least one antigen in 61.7% of 26 sera from tuberculosis patients, 27.3% of 22 from sarcoidosis patients, 33.3% of 30 from tuberculin-positive normal subjects, and none of 29 from tuberculin-negative normal subjects.

Müller *et al.* (1958) found antibodies to tubercle bacilli by haemagglutination and complement fixation tests more frequently in the sera of 111 patients with sarcoidosis than in normal subjects but rather less frequently than in patients with tuberculosis. There was no correlation between the presence of antibodies and the tuberculin sensitivity of the skin or the site, activity and duration of the disease or the serum protein abnormalities in the sarcoidosis patients. Chapman (1961) found precipitins against concentrated culture-medium filtrates from mycobacteria of Runyon Types I, II or III in 88 of 112 sera from patients with sarcoidosis, but against human old tuberculin in only seven. Chapman and Speight (1964) extended this study to a wider range of unclassified mycobacteria; testing against 24 strains, they found precipitins in 80% of 280 sera from sarcoidosis patients, as compared with 31% of 770 control sera. In 16 patients, reactions were negative or weakly positive in the early acute stage, and became positive later. In serial studies in 30 patients, it was found that precipitins decreased in those with a favourable course, and persisted in those with continued activity or progression of the disease (Chapman and Speight, 1967).

Pepys *et al.* (1962) found precipitating antibody to crude mouldy hay extract in 16 of 50 sera from patients with sarcoidosis, though none reacted with more specific antigens of the thermophilic actinomycetes concerned in the pathogenesis of farmer's lung (Pepys *et al.*, 1963); this seems to be best explained as the result of abnormally active antibody production to a variety of antigens in the crude extract.

Changes in plasma proteins

In 1935, Salvesen reported hyperproteinaemia and hyperglobulinaemia in three patients with florid widespread sarcoidosis, and this finding was soon confirmed (Harrell and Fisher, 1939; Ricker and Clark, 1949; Longcope and Freiman, 1952). Electrophoretic studies showed that the increase in globulin was principally in the γ fraction, and that it was often associated with low albumin levels; the α_2 fraction might be increased, but not to the same level as in active pulmonary tuberculosis (Fisher and Davis, 1942; Seibert and Nelson, 1943; Seibert *et al.*, 1947; Jencks *et al.*, 1956; Gilliland *et al.*, 1956). In the United States, these changes were especially prominent in blacks: in one study (Sunderman and Sunderman, 1957), 35 black patients with sarcoidosis showed a large increase in total protein with a mean value for γ-globulin nearly twice that found in 91 normal black subjects, while 57 white patients had a mean value for total protein similar to that of 100 normal white subjects, small increase in globulin being balanced by diminution in albumin. In 32 white patients with sarcoidosis at various stages, but most with multiple organ involvement, in London one of us (JGS) found similarly small changes in plasma proteins in this ethnic group; compared with 52 normal subjects, they showed only slightly higher α-globulin, very slightly higher $α_2$ globulin, and very slightly lower albumin levels. Norberg (1964) studied 82 patients with sarcoidosis in Stockholm, and found that albumin was low when the disease was progressive; γ globulin was high especially in those with progressive lung changes leading to fibrosis; β globulin tended to be high with BHL and progressive disease; and $α_2$ globulin was high at all stages.

Reports of levels of individual immunoglobulins present a rather confusing picture, not only because levels change during the course of the disease, but also because they vary greatly with age and between racial groups. Variations commonly found in the course of sarcoidosis tend to be less than those due to either of these factors (Buckley and Dorsey, 1970). Both in the United States (Goldstein *et al.*, 1969) and in Great Britain (Mitchell, *et al.*, 1977a), those of African descent show much greater changes than those of Caucasian descent. The most consistent are those in patients with BHL and erythema nodosum, who both in Sweden (Norberg, 1967) and in England (Mitchell *et al.*, 1977) showed a considerable rise in IgM and IgA. Those with BHL not accompanied by erythema nodosum showed similar but less marked changes in Sweden (Norberg, 1967) and the United States (Buckley and Dorsey, 1970).

In Sweden, it was found that in patients with BHL and progressive lung infiltration IgG and IgA were raised (Norberg, 1967). In groups including patients with various forms of active sarcoidosis, observers in the United States have reported high mean levels of IgG, IgA and IgM (Buckley *et al.*, 1966; Celikoglu *et al.*, 1971), in IgA and IgM in black but not in white patients (Goldstein *et al.*, 1969), in IgG and IgM especially in back females (Buckley and Dorsey, 1970); and in IgG alone (Patnode *et al.*, 1966). Niitu (1974c) found in Japan that IgG, IgM and IgA were all elevated at the early stage of sarcoidosis and fell during the course of the disease. Mustakallio *et al.* (1967) in Finland found high levels of IgM and of haptoglobin in patients with BHL and erythema nodosum, and of IgG and IgA in many patients with lung involvement. Return of elevated levels towards normal has generally been found in serial studies as the disease becomes less active, and it has been reported that IgG tends to fall first, becoming normal while IgA and IgM are still elevated (Norberg, 1967; Celikoglu *et al.*, 1971). On the other hand, in London, it was found in a study of changes in a group of patients observed for an average period of five years that during this time there was a mean rise in IgG, a fall in IgM and little change in IgA (Mitchell *et al.*, 1977). In a later study in London, Saint-Remy *et al.* (1983) found in 63 patients, of whom 11 were West Indian, that Ig levels were normal in those with BHL only; IgG and IgA tended to be raised in those with lung infiltration especially if the disease were long-standing and active, and especially in the West Indians. Administration of corticosteroids seems to lead to fall in the level especially of IgG (Celikoglu *et al.*, 1971; Mitchell *et al.*, 1977).

Levels of IgD in normal subjects are low, fall with age, and may be undetectable; and the function of this immunoglobulin is unknown. In one study (Buckley and Trayer, 1972) it was found that in sarcoidosis the mean level was lower and in tuberculosis higher than in controls; but in another (Goldstein *et al.*, 1974b), while the high level in tuberculosis was confirmed, normal levels were found in sarcoidosis, both in tuberculin-positive and in tuberculin-negative patients.

Bergmann (1973) found that serum IgE levels were rather higher in patients with sarcoidosis than in those with tuberculosis or in controls; while Yagura *et al.* (1975) found lower levels than in controls, and in a few with low levels and normal levels of other immunoglobulins, fewer responses to a standard set of skin tests for reaginic hypersensitivity than controls. Available evidence suggests that among patients with sarcoidosis the incidence of IgE-mediated atopic diseases is similar to that in the general population. Buck and McKusick (1961) in an epidemiological study found a similar incidence of asthma, hay fever, eczema and drug allergies in sarcoidosis patients and in matched controls. Among 275 patients under the care of one of us (JGS) there were seven with asthma and/or hay fever, one also with eczema; in four the symptoms of the atopic disease and of sarcoidosis were concurrent.

Rheumatoid and anti-nuclear factors

In a study of some hyperglobulinaemic states, Kunkel *et al.* (1958) found positive latex fixation tests (LFT) for rheumatoid factor (RF) in six of 61 patients with sarcoidosis, though the Rose-Waaler test was negative in all. Müller *et al.* (1961) found positive LFT for RF in 18.4% of 244 cases of sarcoidosis, the proportion increasing with the duration of the disease from 11.7% to 32% after five years. Israel *et al.* (1964) found positive LFT at titres ranging from 1:80 to 1:5120 in three of 16 and 21 of 35 women with sarcoidosis; all but two of their patients were black. The proportion with positive tests was slightly lower among those with BHL alone, but no other correlation with clinical stage was found. Oreskes and Siltzbach (1968) found that 38% of 64 patients with sarcoidosis had positive tanned red cell tests for RF, compared with 8% of a control group; 3% had positive Rose-Waaler tests; positive tests were found twice as often in women as in men and were more frequent in those with active disease and with persistent lung changes.

Anti-nuclear factor may be found in low titre in the serum in a few patients with sarcoidosis – e.g. in two of 39, with a speckled pattern of immunofluorescence by Spilberg *et al.* (1969); but no more frequently than among control subjects (Turner-Warwick, 1974).

Immune complexes

Hedfors and Norberg (1974) detected immune complexes (IC) by the platelet aggregation test in the sera of six of 20 patients with sarcoidosis. IC were associated with acute early manifestations, being found in four of seven patients with recent erythema nodosum and in five of ten with bilateral hilar lymph-node enlargement. The complexes were 19 S or larger, a size which has been shown to be pathogenic in animals (Cochrane and Hawkins, 1968). Hedfors (1975) suggested that circulating IC were associated especially with the early acute stage of sarcoidosis, while changes in lymphocytes, with diminution in number of circulating T cells and increase in atypical lymphocytes occurred with increasing chronicity. Verrier Jones *et al.* (1976) studied 22 patients with erythema nodosum, of whom 19 had bilateral hilar node enlargement. Eighteen of the 22 showed disturbances of serum complement initially. Total haemolytic complement activity (CH_{50}) was reduced in four of 18 patients; anticomplementary activity was found in eight of 16; C3 activation products were found in 14 of 18; and the platelet aggregation test was positive in six of ten. Of 13 followed with serial studies, all but two returned to normal levels within 40 days; changes paralleled those in sedimentation rate. Daniele *et al.* (1978) tested the sera of 44 patients with sarcoidosis for IC by the Raji cell method. Complexes were found in the sera of 12 of 26 patients with acute sarcoidosis of less than one year's known duration, of two of ten with longer-standing but still active disease, and in none of eight with apparently complete resolution or of 12 control subjects. Among those with recent active disease, there was no correlation with clinical features or skin reactivity to tuberculin, or to Candida or mumps antigens. These studies suggest that IC may be important in early acute stages of sarcoidosis. On the other hand, Buckley *et al.* (1966) and Sheffer *et al.* (1971), in patients most of whom had long-standing chronic sarcoidosis found that serum complement levels were high or normal, suggesting that if complement is being utilized, there must be a compensatory increase in synthesis. Gupta *et al.* (1977) examined sera from 53 patients with pulmonary sarcoidosis for IC by the Raji cell and the monoclonal rheumatoid factor methods; raised levels were detected in 27 by one or both at all stages, but in a higher proportion at Stage III. Among those who had complexes in the earlier stages, most had extrapulmonary manifestations, notably erythema nodosum. In their study of 63 patients, mentioned above, Saint-Remy *et al.* (1983) found that raised levels of IC were associated with recent acute onset, especially with EN and BHL; and raised levels of C3 with long-standing disease and independently with extrathoracic sarcoidosis.

Immunohistology

Wanstrup and Elling (1968) looked for immunoglobulins in lymph-nodes from ten patients with sarcoidosis by the fluorescent antibody technique, and found immunoglobulins of all classes in granulomas, without correlation with disease activity: $\beta 1_c$ globulin (C3) was found principally in older lesions and especially those with hyalinization. In further studies of mediastinal lymph-nodes from four patients with early active sarcoidosis they found a high immunoglobulin content in comparison with normal nodes, with IgG, IgA and IgM in and around granulomas; IgD was found especially within the granulomas and, in contrast with other immunoglobulins, was not found in hyalinized tissue (Elling and Wanstrup, 1969).

Ghose *et al.* (1974) found clumps of immunoglobulin and complement in granulomas in lung biopsies from three patients with pulmonary sarcoidosis; the immunoglobulin was predominantly IgG with some IgM. Among 36 biopsies from patients with other diseases, but including none with active tuberculosis, similar deposits were seen in only one, with extrinsic allergic alveolitis.

Quismorio *et al.* (1977) studied the immunohistology of eight sarcoid skin infiltrations. IgM was found in vessel walls in five and at the dermo-epidermal junction in two, and IgG in and around granulomas in two. Biopsy of a Kveim test site showed similar changes. They noted that IgM deposits at the dermo-epidermal junction have also been reported in lepromatous leprosy and in lupus erythematosus. The localization of deposits in vessel-walls and their elimination by acid but not by neutral buffer suggested that they might be immune complexes. Kataria *et al.* (1978) in similar studies of nine cutaneous sarcoids found fibrinogen in an arborizing pattern, but no evidence of immunoglobulins of any class within the granulomas.

INTERPRETATION OF THE IMMUNOLOGICAL ABNORMALITIES

Depressed Type IV hypersensitivity reactions

Some of the early hypotheses about the depression of ability to react with delayed skin responses are of historical interest only.

Michael *et al.* (1950) suggested that low tuberculin sensitivity might be due to selective incidence of sarcoidosis in those who have not been exposed to infection with tubercle bacilli. This is disproved by common clinical experience. In areas where tuberculosis is the common cause of calcified foci in lungs and hilar lymph-nodes, such foci are seen with the expected frequency in patients with sarcoidosis (Scadding, 1961a; Israel *et al.*, 1961); the occurrence of sarcoidosis in patients who have had proved tuberculosis in the past is well documented (Citron and Scadding, 1957; Scadding, 1960b, 1961a, 1971); and in the United States, blacks who are especially susceptible to sarcoidosis are certainly no less liable to tuberculosis than whites.

The idea that sarcoidosis was a form of tuberculosis characterized by cutaneous anergy due to the presence of substances in the blood in some way inhibiting reactions to tuberculin ('anticutins') was at one time rather widely held by dermatologists, who classified skin sarcoids among tuberculides (Jadassohn, 1913; Jadassohn, 1932). In one study (Martenstein, 1921, 1924) serum from two patients with lupus pernio was found to inhibit tuberculin reactions in sensitive subjects when mixed with tuberculin in Pirquet tests, whereas serum from three patients with sarcoids of Boeck did not; and several investigators (Horton *et al.*, 1939; Pinner *et al.*, 1943; Wells and Wyllie, 1949; Stirling, 1950) studied the effect of sarcoidosis sera mixed with tuberculin in intradermal tests, in most cases finding inhibition, but in some, enhancement. The most detailed study was by Magnusson (1956), who found that the tuberculin reaction was diminished in 11.7% of tests with sarcoidosis sera and in 14.1% of those with control sera, and that in different subjects the same serum might enhance, diminish or have no effect on the reaction. He found that the degree of inhibition was related to the extent of the early wealing reaction that occurred in some subjects with some sera. Wealing reactions of any sort are known to diminish later tuberculin reactions (Pepys, 1955). Thus the evidence which suggested the possibility that sarcoidosis sera might contain substances specifically neutralizing tuberculin is explicable on other and more general grounds.

The possibility that the skin of sarcoidosis patients might be intrinsically non-reactive is excluded by several observations. They show a normal inflammatory response to a croton-oil patch test (Tannenbaum *et al.*, 1976b). Their response to immediate wealing reactions including those produced by histamine and by passive transfer of reaginic sensitivity by the Prausnitz-Kustner method is normal (Urbach *et al.*, 1952). Intradermal tests with phytohaemagglutinin, a non-specific stimulant of lymphocyte transformation *in vitro*, produce in normal subjects reactions grossly and histologically resembling delayed hypersensitivity reactions (Blaese *et al.*, 1973). In patients with sarcoidosis (Bunforte *et al.*, 1972; Kataria *et al.*, 1975) and with tuberculosis (Barbolini *et al.*, 1977) they produce similar reactions. That these are not banal reactions to an irritant is shown not only by their histology but also by the finding of depressed responses in children with congenital defects of cellular immunity, in some adults with immunodeficiencies, and in Hodgkin's disease. Thus the skin in patients with sarcoidosis is fully capable of displaying both immediate Type I and delayed Type IV reactions.

That some residual tuberculin sensitivity persisted in some patients with sarcoidosis who failed to react to a Mantoux test was demonstrated by

Seeberg (1951) by intradermal tests with 'depot' preparations in which tuberculin is incorporated in an oily emulsion. James and Pepys (1956) reported that of 19 patients with sarcoidosis who did not react to aqueous tuberculin, 13 reacted to a depot preparation; the specificity of these reactions was supported by the finding of negative reactions in 18 tuberculin-negative normal subjects, and of positive reactions appearing in normal subjects at the site of previous intradermal injection of the depot preparation about ten days after BCG vaccination.

Observations on the effect of cortisone on skin sensitivity to tuberculin in sarcoidosis and in tuberculosis also suggest that in many cases of sarcoidosis showing no reaction to conventional tuberculin tests some residual tuberculin sensitivity persists. Pyke and Scadding (1952) observed that a few days after cortisone treatment had been started typical tuberculin reactions developed in a few patients at the site of previously negative intradermal tuberculin tests. They found that a similar phenomenon occurred if cortisone were injected locally with tuberculin in an intradermal test, and therefore studied it further by simultaneous intradermal tests with cortisone acetate suspension plus tuberculin and with the same dose of tuberculin alone. Fifty per cent of tuberculin-negative sarcoid patients reacted to tuberculin mixed with cortisone, to give a reaction similar to a normal positive tuberculin test. These findings were confirmed in a larger series of patients with sarcoidosis and compared with the findings in patients with pulmonary tuberculosis, together with control groups (Citron and Scadding, 1957). In those with tuberculosis, the degree of inhibition of tuberculin reactions by added cortisone varied directly with tuberculin sensitivity. Reactions to 1 IU in highly sensitive patients were greatly reduced or inhibited; those of similar size produced by 5 IU or 10 IU in less sensitive patients were slightly diminished; those produced by 100 IU in patients of low sensitivity showed no average reduction in size. Fourteen of 28 patients with sarcoidosis who did not react to 100 IU produced reactions when tested with cortisone plus tuberculin. Patients with sarcoidosis who were sensitive to 100 IU reacted like patients with pulmonary tuberculosis with low tuberculin sensitivity; the cortisone had little effect on the size of their tuberculin reactions. In the few who reacted to smaller doses of tuberculin, there was partial or complete inhibition of the reaction. Sixteen patients with pulmonary tuberculosis who had been desensitized to tuberculin by graded doses of tuberculin subcutaneously, under the cover of antibacterial drugs, so that the skin no longer reacted to 100 IU, were tested with cortisone plus tuberculin; 11 of them produced positive reactions. A control series of healthy tuberculin-negative subjects showed no reactions to tuberculin plus cortisone. Thus, tuberculin-negative sarcoidosis patients behaved more like desensitized tuberculosis patients than like tuberculin-negative normal subjects. Gross (1973) studied another group of patients with sarcoidosis in London 20 years after the initial observations of Pyke and Scadding and found that in spite of the reduction in the local prevalence of *M. tuberculosis* infection, the proportion of tuberculin-negative sarcoidosis patients who reacted to tuberculin-plus-cortisone remained about one-half. He suggested that the stimulation of a reaction to tuberculin by cortisone might be called a paradoxical response; his studies of the mechanism of this response are discussed below. Paradoxical responses have been reported in a high proportion of tuberculin-negative sarcoidosis patients in one study in the United States (VA-Armed Forces Study, 1963). On the other hand, in 62 patients with Hodgkin's disease in London, Fairley and Matthias (1960) found that only 8% responded in this way.

Passive transfer of tuberculin sensitivity

Urbach *et al.* (1952) showed that tuberculin sensitivity could be transferred to tuberculin-negative sarcoidosis patients by intradermal injection of leucocytes from a tuberculin-positive subject, a procedure which had been shown by Lawrence (1949) to transfer tuberculin sensitivity to normal tuberculin-negative subjects; the sensitivity was transient, lasting only a few weeks. Kohout (1976a) found that 10×10^6 lymphocytes from healthy, strongly tuberculin-positive donors transferred tuberculin-sensitivity to 19 out of 20 healthy tuberculin-negative subjects. Among 27 patients with active sarcoidosis, only a few responded to 10×10^6 cells, but 21 of 25 receiving 50×10^6 cells showed reactivity to tuberculin tests in the opposite arm; as compared with the healthy subjects, ten of whom remained sensitive one year later, they retained this reactivity for a shorter time, only two showing it at one year. Patients with inactive sarcoidosis could be sensitized more readily and retained reactivity longer. After the discovery by Lawrence (1959, 1969, 1970) of 'transfer factor', a low molecular weight, dialysable, heat labile material which can be extracted from sensitized human lymphocytes and which can cause other lymphoid cells to become specifically antigen-responsive, Lawrence and Zweiman (1968) reported that in five of seven sarcoidosis patients, transfer factor (TF) from cells of tuberculin-positive donors conveyed local hypersensitivity, though this was less intense than in healthy subjects, and was accompanied by a weak sensitization remotely in only two. Horsmanheimo and Virolainen (1976) prepared transfer factor dialysate from cells from strongly tuberculin-positive donors, and injected doses estimated to be the extract from 0.9×10^8 cells into eight tuberculin-negative sarcoidosis patients; six acquired transient sensitivity to 100 IU, the longest duration being nine months. Among three control subjects suffering from skin diseases other than sarcoidosis, two became sensitized, and in one sensitization persisted for two years.

'Skin-window' studies

The Rebuck 'skin-window' technique consists in the study of the cells adhering to a cover-slip applied to a lightly-abraded area of skin; the proportion of cells of various types, their variation with time, and responses to antigenic or other stimuli may be studied. In normal subjects, the predominant cells in the first few hours are granulocytes; mononuclear cells transforming to macrophages become more numerous over the first 24 hours (Rebuck and Crowley, 1955). Mlczoch and Kohout (1962) found in 31 patients with sarcoidosis that the number of mononuclear cells increased to 60% by 12 hours, as compared with just over 30% in normal subjects. Rechardt and Mustakallio (1965) found that, compared with controls, patients with active sarcoidosis, Kohout (1976b) confirmed the high propor-adherent macrophages at six hours, while those in whom sarcoidosis was stationary had similar numbers to controls; they found that the macrophage count correlated well with the rapidity of development of nodular reactions to Kveim tests. In skin windows at sites where alcian blue had been injected intradermally two weeks previously, many of the adherent macrophages were stained; this was taken to indicate that they were derived from tissue histiocytes rather than from cells circulating in the blood. Among 402 patients with active sarcoidosis, Kohout (1976b) confirmed the high proportion of macrophages appearing in skin windows. He found correlations between high numbers of macrophages and granulomatous Kveim-test responses, high immunoglobulin levels, and high levels of B and low levels of T lymphocytes in the peripheral blood. In 150 patients with inactive sarcoidosis, he found low counts of macrophages in skin windows; and passive transfer of tuberculin sensitivity was effected more readily in these than in those with active disease and high macrophage counts in skin windows.

Gange *et al.* (1977, 1979) studied the migration of cells from dermal abrasions into small chambers filled usually with 50% autologous serum. The predominant cells were neutrophils. Throughout the 26 hours of observation, the number emigrating in patients with sarcoidosis was about one-third of that in control subjects. Patients with two localized granulomatous skin diseases, granuloma annulare and necrobiosis lipoidica, showed a smaller reduction to about one-half of the number in controls.

Circulating lymphocytes

In patients with active sarcoidosis, the number of lymphocytes in the peripheral blood is reduced. Hoffbrand (1968) found that 20 of 61 sarcoidosis patients, but only one of 100 controls, had counts below 100 mm^{-3}, the difference in mean counts between the two groups being highly significant, while the mean counts for both neutrophils and monocytes were similar.

Among the sarcoidosis patients those who were anergic to tuberculin had lower counts than the reactors. Similar findings were reported by Böttger (1971).

Hedfors *et al.* (1974) showed that T rather than B lymphocytes are diminished. They studied blood lymphocytes from 33 patients with pulmonary sarcoidosis. The proportion recognized as T cells by the formation of rosettes with sheep red blood cells was significantly lower, and that recognized as B cells by the demonstration of surface immunoglobulin higher than in 18 healthy controls; because of an absolute lymphocytopenia, the number of B cells was normal while the T cells were greatly reduced in number. A small proportion, from 10–20% of lymphocytes were atypical, resembling those seen in acute viral diseases, infectious mononucleosis and Hodgkin's disease. No correlation was found between the numbers of cells in these subpopulations and the clinical stage of the disease, except that large atypical cells tended to be more numerous with long-standing disease. The depression of total numbers of lymphocytes and of T cells has been confirmed by others (Ramachandar *et al.*, 1975; Sørensen *et al.*, 1976; Daniele and Rowlands, 1976; Tannenbaum *et al.*, 1976a). Ramachandar *et al.* found few cells without B- or T-cell markers ('null' cells), but Daniele and Rowlands reported that in patients with active disease, both recent and long-standing, such cells constituted up to a quarter or more of the total lymphocytes, of which a proportion, up to 32%, were morphologically atypical.

Studies of lymphocytes in culture indicate that a higher than normal proportion of the small number of circulating lymphocytes in patients with active sarcoidosis is activated, with a high rate of spontaneous blast transformation, of DNA synthesis, and of production of macrophage migration inhibition factor (MIF) (Hirschorn *et al.* 1964; Siltzbach *et al.*, 1971a; Topilsky *et al.*, 1972; Kataria *et al.*, 1973; Hedfors, 1974). Biberfeld and Hedfors (1974) found that the atypical blood mononuclear cells were morphologically heterogeneous, cytochemically were not monocytes, and were probably of both B- and T-cell origin. Rossman *et al.* (1978) confirmed the low numbers of circulating lymphocytes and especially of T-cells in a comparison of seven patients with active sarcoidosis of recent onset with ten matched controls. They found that a much higher proportion of peripheral lymphocytes formed stable rosettes at 37°C in the sarcoidosis patients than in the controls, and that the rosetted lymphocytes were morphologically atypical; and concluded that though the total number of T cells was reduced, the proportion activated was increased.

Responses of cells to stimulation *in vitro*

In general, the responses of cells from sarcoidosis patients *in vitro* to antigens causing delayed hypersensitivity reactions parallel skin sensitivity to relevant antigens; while to non-specific mitogens they are less than those in controls subjects.

Citron (1958) studied the effect of tuberculin on the migration of blood leucocytes into culture-medium, and found that cells from tuberculin-negative individuals, whether normal or patients with sarcoidosis, were unaffected. Leucocytes from patients with pulmonary tuberculosis were inhibited to a degree related to the activity of the disease. Those from the few sarcoidosis patients who reacted to tuberculin showed a degree of inhibition varying with their tuberculin sensitivity. Heilman *et al.* (1970) cultured spleen and lymph-node tissue obtained surgically from patients with sarcoidosis and studied the effects of PPD and histoplasmin on macrophage migration and the outgrowth of fibroblasts; in general, they found that both were inhibited in parallel with skin sensitivity to the relevant antigens. Siltzbach *et al.* (1971a) found a close correspondence between skin sensitivity to tuberculin and lymphocyte transformation in response to tuberculin in 35 patients with sarcoidosis. Horsmanheimo (1974) found strong correlation between tuberculin-induced lymphocyte-transformation *in vitro* and skin reactivity in 87 patients with sarcoidosis and 64 controls, with similar responses *in vitro* of cells from patients and from controls with similar skin-reactivity. Among patients, the levels of skin-test sensitivity to tuberculin, of tuberculin-induced transformation and of spontaneous transformation were higher in those with erythema nodosum. On the other hand Mangi *et al.* (1974a) found that skin reactivity and *in vitro* lymphocyte response to Candida antigen correlated poorly in sarcoidosis patients, although they correlated well in controls, and there was generally lower reactivity in the patients.

Tannenbaum *et al.* (1976a) found a general correlation between negative delayed hypersensitivity skin tests and failure of lymphocytes *in vitro* to produce MIF or incorporate thymidine in response to the relevant antigen; MIF production was a better correlate than thymidine incorporation. The *in vitro* responses could not be correlated with numbers of lymphocytes, total T or B, in peripheral blood.

Buckley *et al.* (1966) studied lymphocytes from 11 patients with sarcoidosis, all anergic to tuberculin. The proportion transforming in response to phytohaemagglutin (PHA) was much lower than in controls in those with active disease, but not in those in remission. Sharma *et al.* (1971) confirmed the low level of PHA-induced lymphocyte-transformation in 21 patients with sarcoidosis, 19 showing little response as compared with one of 21 controls; they failed to induce DNCB sensitivity in 15 of the sarcoidosis patients, but in only three of the controls. Topilsky *et al.* (1972) demonstated the low response of sarcoid lymphocytes to PHA, using ^{14}C-leucine uptake as an index of stimulation. Kataria *et al.* (1973) found that lymphocytes from patients with sarcoidosis involving extra-thoracic organs, but not those with intrathoracic changes only, showed a low response to PHA, as judged by transformation, by thymidine uptake and by glucose metabolism; and that the *in vitro* responsiveness to PHA was not correlated with cutaneous anergy to antigens. Hedfors (1974) reported that though unfractionated peripheral lymphocytes showed a high level of spontaneous DNA synthesis, separated T-lymphocytes showed a reduced response to stimulation by PPD or concanavalin-A (conA). Haslam (1978) studied the response of lymphocytes to graded doses of PHA by measurement of thymidine uptake; eight patients with sarcoidosis showed an unstimulated uptake at the lower end of the normal range, and three of them showed no response to PHA up to 10 mg ml^{-1}. In a study of 75 patients, Goldstein *et al.* (1978) found that the *in vitro* response of lymphocytes to PHA and conA was decreased in those with chronic active sarcoidosis.

Responses of lymphocytes *in vitro* to sarcoid-tissue suspensions validated for use in the Kveim test are considered in Chapter 21, p. 476.

Faguet (1978) studied the responses of lymphocytes from 15 sarcoidosis patients and 15 controls to leucoagglutinin. The binding capacity and affinity of lymphocytes for the lectin were similar in patients and controls; but the induced DNA synthesis was impaired in all but four patients. In the patients as a group there was a significant reduction in circulating T-lymphocytes, but in individuals there was no correlation between the number of T-lymphocytes and the metabolic response to lectin, suggesting an intrinsic defect of effector cell function.

Circulating lymphocytes in pulmonary tuberculosis

Humber *et al.* (1980) in a comparison of 33 African patients with newly diagnosed pulmonary tuberculosis and 41 healthy contacts found changes in circulating lymphocytes similar to those reported in sarcoidosis and reviewed above; the total count, the proportion of T cells, the mitogenic response to PHA and antigen-specific transformation to tuberculin were reduced in patients, while the primary antibody response to tetanus toxoid and pneumococcal polysaccharide was enhanced. After the inception of antimycobacterial chemotherapy, cellular responses returned to normal.

Helper and suppressor cells

Human T-lymphocytes may have receptors for the Fc portion of immunoglobulins (Moretta *et al.*, 1976, 1977). Those with IgG receptors have an inhibitor or suppressor effect, and those with IgM receptors an enhancing or helper effect on the stimulation of B cells by poke-weed mitogen (PWM) to produce immunoglobulin and on some other lymphocyte functions. Katz *et al.* (1978) compared seven patients with 25 controls. The patients showed a diminished number of T cells in the peripheral blood, with an increased proportion of T_G (suppressor) and a diminished proportion of T_M (helper) cells; the proportion having neither receptor did not differ significantly from that in controls.

Monocytes

Peripheral blood monocytes of sarcoidosis patients have been shown to have suppressor effects on lymphocyte responses. Katz and Fauci (1978) used a plaque-forming cell (PFC) assay of the ability of lymphocytes to produce anti-sheep red blood cell IgM antibody after activation with poke-weed mitogen (PWM): in this system, activation of B lymphocytes to produce antibody is T-cell dependent and is regulated by a balance between 'helper' and 'suppressor' activity. Sarcoid lymphocytes showed a much lower response than controls. Removal of glass-adherent cells having characteristics of monocytes resulted in increase in response to the normal range. Goodwin *et al.* (1977) demonstrated the presence in the blood of normal subjects of glass-adherent cells which secrete prostaglandin E2 (PGE2) and suppress the response of T cells to mitogens *in vitro*. Goodwin *et al.* (1979) found that the response of peripheral blood mononuclear cells from 16 patients with active sarcoidosis to PHA, measured by ^{3}H-thymidine uptake, was less than that of 12 healthy controls; four patients receiving corticosteroids did not differ in response from those untreated. The addition of indomethacin, a prostaglandin synthetase inhibitor, to the cultures increased the response, more in patients than in controls. The removal of glass-adherent cells led to a large increase in the response to PHA in the patients and a small decrease in the controls. Johnson *et al.* (1981) in studies of circulating white cells in 26 patients with sarcoidosis confirmed lymphopenia and impaired lymphocyte transformation to conA; a lower proportion of mononuclear cells than in controls formed E rosettes, irrespective of the activity of the disease, and among those with active disease a higher proportion had IgG receptors. Twenty per cent of E-rosetting cells had the characteristics of monocytes, and removal of these by plastic adherence, or the addition of indomethacin to the medium increased transformation to conA, but not to normal levels. Thus, it appears that the suppressor effect of monocytes contributes to the depressed lymphocyte responses in sarcoidosis. Activation of circulating monocytes in three granulomatous diseases, tuberculosis, sarcoidosis and Crohn's disease, was demonstrated by Douglas *et al.* (1976) and Schmidt and Douglas (1977) in studies of monocyte receptor activity for IgG and C_3. The proportion activated in sarcoidosis was less than that in tuberculosis and greater than that in Crohn's disease.

The role of macrophages in tuberculin-induced lymphocyte transformation was investigated by Horsmanheimo and Virolainen (1974). They found that macrophages from tuberculin-negative sarcoidosis patients were as effective as autologous macrophages in enhancing the blastogenic response to tuberculin of lymphocytes from tuberculin-sensitive subjects. Thus impairment of antigen-induced lymphocyte transformation in sarcoidosis does not seem to be associated with functional deficiency of macrophages as has been reported in Wiskott-Aldrich syndrome and in Hodgkin's disease.

Humoral inhibitory factors

Factors in the sera of sarcoidosis patients inhibiting cellular processes concerned in immune responses have been described by several investigators.

Mangi *et al.* (1974b) studied the effect of plasma from patients with sarcoidosis on the response of lymphocytes to PHA, measured by ^{3}H-thymidine incorporation. They found that lymphocytes from 13 of 26 patients responded better when cultured in normal than in autologous plasma, and that plasma from 14 of 25 sarcoidosis patients reduced the response of normal lymphocytes, even in the presence of optimal concentrations of normal serum; and concluded that the plasma of sarcoidosis patients contains an inhibitor of lymphocyte stimulation.

Umbert *et al.* (1976) found evidence of an inhibitory factor for guinea-pig macrophages in the sera of nine out of ten patients with sarcoidosis, and 11 of 14 with granuloma annulare.

Daniele and Rowlands (1976) found that nine of 15 sarcoidosis sera reduced the capacity of normal T cells to form E rosettes with sheep red blood cells by an average of 25%, and that IgG and IgM antibodies to T cells were present in seven of the 15 sera. They suggested that these antibodies might have a selective effect on T_M (helper) cells.

Maderazo *et al.* (1976) tested the sera of sarcoidosis patients for chemotactic factor inactivation. Normal serum contains small amounts of inactivators of bacterial chemotaxis for leucocytes. In 19 of 20 sarcoidosis patients inactivator levels were higher than normal, but they were less elevated than in Hodgkin's disease and cirrhosis of the liver, in which four-fold increases have been reported; the inactivator differed from that in normal sera in being heat-labile. Increases in chemotactic inactivator have been found also in Crohn's disease (Segal and Loewi, 1976) and in leprosy (Ward *et al.*, 1976) and in patients with cutaneous anergy associated with acute illness (Van Epps *et al.*, 1974).

Campbell *et al.* (1977) studied the leucotactic function of monocytes in 25 untreated patients with sarcoidosis. Responses to lymphokine produced by PHA stimulation of normal human lymphocytes and to zymosan-activated human serum were depressed; the depression was greatest in Stage I patients, but otherwise was not correlated with activity, extent or duration of disease. Incubation of normal monocytes with sarcoid plasma diminished leucotaxis. The leucotactic activity was non-dialysable and heat stable; and small amounts of similar activity were found in normal serum. There was good correlation between the defect in monocyte leucotaxis and the leucotactic inhibitory factor in plasma. Campbell suggested that the apparent discrepancy between the depressed leucotaxis of blood monocytes and the early migration of monocytes in 'skin-window' studies may be explained by the demonstration by Rechardt and Mustakallio (1965) that many of the cells appearing in skin windows are of local tissue origin.

Faguet (1978) advanced evidence that though serum factors may contribute to abnormal lymphocyte response in sarcoidosis, they do not act by blocking or masking membrane receptors. The binding capacity and affinity of lymphocytes from 15 patients with sarcoidosis for leukoagglutinin were similar to those of 15 controls, but the metabolic response to bound lectin was impaired in 11. Thus there appeared to be an intrinsic defect of effector cell function distal to the membrane receptor.

Williams *et al.* (1982) found evidence of interaction between immune complexes (IC) and T-suppressor cells in sarcoidosis. Among 31 patients, they found IC in 12 of 23 by Raji cell assay and 11 of 19 by polyethylene glycol precipitation. The presence of IC was not related to the stage of the disease, but was correlated with low numbers of T-suppressor cells, identified by the demonstration of receptors for IgG. The proportion of such cells among sarcoid T-cells was increased by incubation with trypsin. The proportion among normal lymphocytes was increased by incubation with sarcoid IC, which also reduced blastogenic response to conA. Fractionation of sarcoid serum showed two inhibitory factors. One with a molecular mass of more than 300 000 daltons was thought to be the IC; the other with a mass of less than 60 000 daltons contained no identifiable immunoglobulin (Davies *et al.* 1982).

Corticosteroids and immune responses

In vitro studies of the paradoxical response to corticosteroids added to tuberculin in tuberculin-negative sarcoidosis patients described above (p. 426) have been reported by Gross (1973), Valdimarsson and Gross (1973) and Gross and Holt (1977). A lymphokine preparation was produced by stimulation of lymphocytes *in vitro* with concanavalin A, and caused a delayed skin response in 93% of normal subjects. Eight patients with sarcoidosis who were paradoxical responders failed to react to it, but six of them reacted when cortisone was added. By contrast, four patients with anergic lymphoma responded to the lymphokine preparation. The response to PPD of lymphocytes from each of ten paradoxical responders was measured by both thymidine uptake and MIF production. All responded on at least one occasion, but at a lower level than that for normal control lymphocytes. Hydrocortisone added to the lymphocyte cultures abolished thymidine uptake and MIF production, and lymphocytes obtained after oral administration of prednisone showed similarly depressed responses. Thus, in addition to the defect in lymphocyte responsiveness to antigen, there seems to be a defect in ability to express delayed hypersensitivity; while the responsiveness of the sensitized lymphocyte to antigen is further depressed by cortisone, the defect beyond this is corrected by cortisone to a degree sufficient to permit a reaction to appear in the paradoxical responders.

The complexity of the actions of cortisone on the cells involved in the immune response is illustrated by the study by Katz and Fauci (1979) of the effects of an intravenous dose of 400 mg hydrocortisone sodium succinate in four patients with sarcoidosis and four controls. There was a transient absolute T-cell lymphocytopenia with a relative increase in T_G (suppressor) and decrease in T_M (helper) cells in patients and controls. In the patients the absolute number of T_G cells showed little change, whereas there was a profound fall in T_M (helper) cells four hours after hydrocortisone. Nevertheless, at this time the depressed ability of sarcoidosis lymphocytes to produce anti-SRBC antibody after PWM activation was strikingly increased, so that PFC responses similar to those of normal subjects were obtained; normal lymphocytes showed no significant change in this response after hydrocortisone. Since Katz and Fauci (1978) had shown that the depression of PFC response in sarcoidosis lymphocytes was corrected by the removal of monocytes, it appeared that hydrocortisone acted by reducing the suppressor effect of these cells.

BRONCHO-ALVEOLAR LAVAGE

Broncho-alveolar lavage (BAL), a safe, relatively non-invasive and repeatable procedure provides a means by which cells, mainly from pulmonary acini, can be obtained for study, and has been an important source of information about immuno-competent cells in diseases diffusely affecting the lungs. This has been the subject of several reviews (Hunninghake *et al.*, 1979a; Gee and Fisk, 1980; Keogh and Crystal, 1982). The following discussion concerns those findings that are relevant to the pathogenesis of sarcoidosis by throwing light on the behaviour of immuno-competent cells at the sites of granulomatous change (Crystal *et al.*, 1981; Crystal *et al.*, 1983).

Cell types

In normal subjects, macrophages are predominant among the cells obtained by lavage, with a small proportion of lymphocytes; smoking increases the number of cells recovered and diminishes the proportion of lymphocytes

(Reynolds and Newball, 1974; Warr *et al.*, 1976). In sarcoidosis, the proportion of lymphocytes is increased. Yeager *et al.* (1977) compared lavage fluids from 14 patients with sarcoidosis with those from 20 healthy volunteers. Lymphocytes constituted 19.6% of the cells from non-smoking sarcoidosis patients, and only 8.1% from non-smoking controls. Reynolds (1978) in a study of 16 sarcoidosis patients found that the number of lymphocytes was higher in those with active disease; in them a standard lavage procedure produced an average of 13.6×10^6 cells of which 32% were lymphocytes, compared with 3.8×10^6 and 11.3% respectively in those with inactive disease. Similar findings were reported by others (Dauber *et al.*, 1979; Mahé *et al.*, 1979; Arnoux *et al.*, 1980).

Cells obtained by BAL are often called 'lung' or even 'alveolar' cells. With normal airways, this is probably a justifiable approximation. In a case reported by Rossman *et al.* (1981), exuberant changes in bronchial mucosa were found in a non-smoking patient with BHL and pulmonary infiltration of recent origin; they were accompanied by extreme changes in lymphocyte populations in BAL and in blood of the sorts generally found in pulmonary sarcoidosis, and bronchial biopsy showed extensive granulomatous changes with much mononuclear infiltration. In this case, it is likely that the bronchi were an important source of the BAL lymphocytes.

T- and B- lymphocytes

Hunninghake *et al.* (1979a), reviewing more than 400 broncho-alveolar lavages, reported that in normal non-smokers $93 \pm 5\%$ of the cells were macrophages, $7 \pm 1\%$ lymphocytes, and less than 1% polymorphonuclear cells. Of the lymphocytes, the proportions with T characteristics averaged 73%, and with B 7%. In eight non-smoking sarcoidosis patients, all with recent active disease, Hunninghake *et al.* (1979b) found that there was a great increase in lymphocytes, to an average of 58%; of the lymphocytes in BAL, the proportion with T characteristics averaged 90%, very significantly higher than in the peripheral blood, in which the proportion was 55%. The proportions identified as B cells were 5% in BAL and 20% in blood. By comparison, in normal subjects the proportions identified as T and B cells in BAL and in blood were similar, averaging 70% and 10% respectively. In six patients with idiopathic pulmonary fibrosis (cryptogenic fibrosing alveolitis) there was a very significant increase in polymorphonuclear neutrophils, to an average of 21%. Other studies of cryptogenic fibrosing alveolitis have shown similarly high numbers of polymorphonuclear cells, mainly neutrophils but possibly also eosinophils (Reynolds *et al.*, 1977; Weinberger *et al.*, 1978; Haslam *et al.*, 1980 a and b). The proportion of lymphocytes in this and other non-granulomatous lung disease did not differ from that in normal subjects.

In the relatively few studies of granulomatous lung diseases of known cause that have been reported, an increase in lymphocytes in BAL similar to or higher than that seen in sarcoidosis has been found. These diseases include pulmonary tuberculosis (Clot *et al.*, 1979; Lenzini *et al.*, 1980; Hunninghake *et al.*, 1979a); extrinsic allergic alveolitis (chronic hypersensitivity pneumonitis) due to fungal contamination of ventilation systems (Reynolds *et al.*, 1977) and in bird-fanciers (Tonnel *et al.*, 1979; Arnoux *et al.*, 1980; Valenti *et al.*, 1982); and talc granulomatosis caused by intravenous injection of crushed pentazocine tablets (Farber *et al*; 1982). In the latter study, four men in whom the diagnosis of talc granulomatosis was established by the history of intravenous drug abuse and by transbronchial lung biopsy were found to have 18%–32% of lymphocytes in BAL fluid, in which talc crystals were present; they also had high serum ACE levels and positive gallium lung scans.

'Activation' of lymphocytes

The lymphocytes obtained by BAL from the lungs of patients with active sarcoidosis show evidences of activation, such as a high rate of spontaneous incorporation of tritiated thymidine, high proportions forming rosettes with sheep erythrocytes at 37°C and having receptors for the Fc fragment of IgG, and spontaneous release of lymphokines of various sorts (Hunninghake *et al.*, 1979b; Hunninghake *et al.*, 1980a; Arnoux *et al.*, 1980, Crystal *et al.*, 1981; Pacheco *et al.*, 1981).

Hunninghake *et al.* (1980b) found a chemotactic factor for monocytes in supernatants of cultures of lung lymphocytes from all of six patients with sarcoidosis; their blood lymphocytes produced a much lower level of similar activity. The molecular mass of the monocyte chemotactic factor was estimated to be the range 10 000–16 000 daltons. Supernatants from lymphocytes from lung and blood of control subjects and of patients with 'idiopathic pulmonary fibrosis' showed no monocyte chemotactic activity. T-cell-enriched fractions of BAL cells from sarcoidosis patients had enhanced, and T-cell-depleted fractions diminished chemotactic activity, implying T-cell origin. Sarcoid lung T-lymphocytes were found to secrete spontaneously an average of 25 times the amount of this factor as blood T-lymphocytes. Monocyte chemotactic factor attracts not only monocytes but also polymorphs, which are insignificant in sarcoid granulomas and in BAL from sarcoid lung; the selective attraction of monocytes in sarcoidosis may be explained by the finding that T-lymphocytes from sarcoid lung also secrete a factor with a molecular mass of 68 000 daltons which inhibits the migration of polymorphonuclear leucocytes but has no effect on monocytes (Hunninghake *et al.*, 1979b).

Pinkston *et al.* (1983) studied the release of interleukin-2, a factor stimulating proliferation of T-lymphocytes, from BAL cells from 27 sarcoidosis patients, three with interstitial pulmonary fibrosis, and ten normal subjects. Ten of the sarcoidosis patients were judged to have 'high-intensity alveolitis' (see Chapter 27, p. 588). In nine of these, but in no other patients or controls, release of interleukin-2 was detected, at a rate varying with the proportion of T-cells in BAL.

'Suppressor' and 'helper' T-cells

As noted above (p. 431), the proportion of the usually reduced number of lymphocytes in the blood in patients with sarcoidosis having suppressor function, as indicated by Ig receptors, is higher, and having helper function lower than normal. Ginns *et al.* (1982) used the OKT series of monoclonal antibodies to study T-lymphocyte subsets in blood and BAL. These mouse monoclonal antibodies reacting with cell surface antigens of human T-lymphocytes were prepared by the hybridoma technique (Kung *et al.*, 1979; Reinherz *et al.*, 1979; see also reviews by Reinherz and Schlossman, 1980; Kung and Goldstein, 1980). The series of antibodies prepared was numbered, and the subsets of lymphocytes reacting with some of them have been shown to be functionally distinct. Those reacting with OKT_3 (designated $OKT3^+$) appear to be mature circulating T-lymphocytes (Chang *et al.*, 1981). $OKT4^+$ cells constitute a helper-inducer subset, and are not cytotoxic (Reinherz *et al.*, 1979, 1981), while $OKT8^+$ cells have cytotoxic and suppressor functions (Friedman *et al.*, 1981), although these subsets do not correspond exactly with subsets defined by other tests of these functions. Ginns *et al.* (1982) found, in accordance with expectation, that peripheral lymphocyte counts were low in 11 patients with sarcoidosis, and slightly but not significantly low in eight with idiopathic pulmonary fibrosis (IPF), as compared with 45 normal subjects; the proportions of $OKT3^+$ (mature T-lymphocytes) and of $OKT4^+$ (helper-inducer) cells were reduced in both sarcoidosis and IPF patients. BAL was performed in six sarcoidosis and four IPF patients. Lymphocytes constituted 67% of the cells from the lung in the sarcoidosis patients, and 36% in the IPF patients. In sarcoidosis $OKT4^+$ cells averaged 66%, and $OKT8^+$ 10%, while in IPF the proportions were 27% and 34% respectively. The ratio of $OKT4^+$ to $OKT8^+$ cells, the helper/suppressor ratio, in BAL averaged 6.5 for sarcoidosis and 0.9 for IPF; in the peripheral blood it was 2.2 for sarcoidosis and 1.7 for IPF, not significantly different from 1.9, found in the normal subjects. The relatively small discrepancy between the findings of Katz *et al.* (1978) for T_M and T_G receptor-bearing cells and the $OKT4^+/OKT8^+$ ratio in peripheral blood is presumably explained by differences in the constitution of the subsets of cells defined by these two methods. The striking finding by the monoclonal antibody procedure is the great preponderance of $OKT4^+$, helper-inducer, cells in the lung lymphocytes in sarcoidosis. Findings by this technique in granulomatous lung disease of known cause will evidently be of great interest.

Immunoglobulins

A high level of IgG, as shown by a high Ig/albumin ratio was reported in BAL fluid in patients with sarcoidosis by Reynolds (1978), as compared with controls. Weinberger *et al.* (1978) reported similar findings in sarcoidosis; rather higher levels were found in patients with interstitial pulmonary fibrosis, and considerably higher in those with hypersensitivity pneumonitis (extrinsic allergic alveolitis), who were the only group in whom IgM was found. IgA content was variable within groups. In normal subjects the absence of IgM is not surprising, in view of its high molecular mass; both IgG and IgA might appear by transudation from the serum, while IgA might come in part from local production in the respiratory mucosa. In extrinsic allergic alveolitis, it seems likely that the IgM and at least some of the IgG comes from the local reaction to the causal antigen that is going on in the lung. In sarcoidosis, Hunninghake and Crystal (1981a) found that a high proportion of lymphocytes obtained by BAL was secreting IgG or IgM, but not IgA. The proportion of cells secreting Ig was directly related to the number of cells in BAL. Co-culture of T-cells from sarcoid patients with high proportions of T-cells in BAL with normal blood mononuclear cells caused these cells to differentiate into Ig-secreting cells, an effect that was not observed with blood lymphocytes from the sarcoidosis patients, or with BAL lymphocytes from patients with low proportions of T-cells in BAL. These findings suggest that in active pulmonary sarcoidosis the lung is an important site of Ig production, activated T-lymphocytes modulating local antibody production and leading to polyclonal hyperglobulinaemia. Rankin *et al.* (1983) confirmed and extended these findings. In 11 normal subjects, they found, as expected, that there was rather more IgA than IgG in BAL, presumably because of local synthesis of IgA, and very small amounts of IgM, presumably because its high molecular mass limits its movement to the alveolar surface; there was a weak correlation between the number of cells in BAL secreting IgA and the level of this Ig, but none between the numbers secreting IgG or IgM and levels in BAL or blood of these immunoglobulins. In 17 patients with sarcoidosis, there were highly significant correlations between the number of Ig-secreting cells and both the IgG/albumin ratio in BAL, and the serum IgG level. The IgG/albumin ratio was higher in BAL than in serum in the patients, but equal at these two sites in the normal subjects. The proportion of IgG-secreting, but not of IgA- or IgM-secreting cells in BAL was higher in the patients than in normal subjects, and was higher in BAL than in blood in the patients.

'Activation' of macrophages

Macrophages obtained by BAL from patients with sarcoidosis show several signs of 'activation'.

Yeager et al. (1977) found that among sarcoidosis patients about 10% (slightly higher in non-smokers and lower in smokers) of macrophages obtained by BAL showed spontaneous attachment of one or more lymphocytes, compared with about 2% in controls. Neither the number of lymphocytes bound, nor the proportion of macrophages with adherent lymphocytes could be correlated with clinical features. Reynolds (1978) observed macrophages with two or more adherent lymphocytes in BAL in four of 16 patients with sarcoidosis. Lussier et al. (1978) studied in vitro binding of peripheral blood lymphocytes by alveolar macrophages from normal subjects; with optimal conditions, 7% of macrophages acquired adherent lymphocytes. Yeager et al. (1979, 1980) using these optimal conditions, studied alveolar macrophage-blood lymphocyte (AM-L) binding in smoking and non-smoking sarcoidosis patients and controls. They found that smokers showed a lower level of AM-L binding than non-smokers. Non-smoking sarcoidosis patients showed a higher level than non-smoking controls. In three patients with positive skin tests to recall antigens, AM-L binding was increased in the presence of the antigen. Kveim-test suspensions partially inhibited it in sarcoidosis patients, but slightly increased it in controls; a normal spleen suspension caused a slight but not significant increase in patients and controls.

Gee et al. (1978) and Hinman et al. (1979) found that BAL macrophages from patients with sarcoidosis contained about five times and from normal smokers about three times, as much angiotensin convertase activity as those from normal non-smokers. They found no evidence that alveolar macrophages in culture secrete ACE. Hinman et al. (1978) also found a high level of lysozyme in sarcoid alveolar macrophages (AM), 2.5 times that found in normals. The high level of ACE may be correlated with their evolution towards an epithelioid cell structure, since ACE is present in the epithelioid cells of sarcoid granulomas, especially those at the periphery (Chapter 2, p. 31). Gupta et al. (1982) could not confirm the high level of ACE in sarcoid AM; they found that the content of ACE in these cells from patients with active and inactive sarcoidosis and from normal subjects did not differ significantly, although serum ACE levels were higher in those with active sarcoidosis, and the proportion of lymphocytes higher in those with sarcoidosis, as expected. Perrin-Fayolle et al. (1981) found higher levels of ACE in BAL fluid from 16 patients with sarcoidosis than in controls. Serum ACE levels were raised in nine of the patients. ACE levels were correlated with the BAL lymphocyte counts and with clinical activity, but not with radiographic 'staging'. Rossman et al. (1982) found similarly that in 22 sarcoidosis patients there were strong correlations between serum ACE levels and proportions of lymphocytes and of T-lymphocytes in BAL; but ACE was increased in only seven of the patients, and was normal in ten with high proportions of lymphocytes in BAL. Since there is evidence that cells of the macrophage series are the source of the elevated ACE levels in sarcoidosis, the role of the lymphocytes can only be indirect, through activation of macrophages.

Other possible evidences of macrophage activation are the release of interleukin-1 (Hunninghake *et al.*, 1981) and enhanced presentation of antigen to T-cells (Venet *et al.*, 1982). Production of fibronectin (Rennard *et al.*, 1981) and of a factor causing fibroblast replication (Bitterman and Crystal, 1981) are common to sarcoidosis and idiopathic and other forms of pulmonary fibrosis; while a neutrophil chemotactic factor that has been shown to be produced by macrophages from these fibrosing lung diseases has not been found in sarcoid AM (Hunninghake *et al.*, 1981).

Some other tests of macrophage 'activation' studied by Dubois *et al.* (1981) gave negative results in AM obtained by BAL from 18 patients with sarcoidosis, but suggested some activation in 29 with cryptogenic fibrosing alveolitis (CFA). In both sarcoidosis and CFA, receptor sites for C36 were reduced; in sarcoidosis, intracellular and extracellular levels of β-D-glucosamidase, a lysosomal enzyme, were similar to those in controls, while in CFA the extracellular level was higher in some cases; and AM from sarcoidosis showed similar degrees of spreading on glass to controls, while those from CFA showed significantly more. Evidently, various tests of 'activity' test different aspects of cell function; Ridley *et al.* (1979) found that ingestion of BCG causes macrophages to lose C3 receptors temporarily.

Hunninghake *et al.* (1981) showed that after intravenous injection of gallium-67 preparatory to scanning, 95% of the isotope in lung effector cells is contained in macrophages, and that AM from patients with active sarcoidosis take up ^{67}Ga more rapidly than those from normal subjects or patients with inactive sarcoidosis. This finding suggests that ^{67}Ga uptake is a measure of the activity of cells of the mononuclear phagocyte series.

In a study of the ultrastructure of BAL cells from eight sarcoidosis patients and 11 healthy subjects, Hawley *et al.* (1979) found interaction between macrophages and lymphocytes more frequently in the sarcoidosis patients, irrespective of smoking habits; sarcoid AM had a more irregular cell surface, more membrane-bound inclusions and fewer lysosomes and phagolysosomes, though the number of these was greatly affected by smoking. Danel *et al.* (1983) studied the ultrastructure of BAL cells from 28 sarcoidosis patients and 17 control subjects and of lung tissue granulomas in five patients. They found that both macrophages and lymphocytes in BAL from sarcoidosis patients showed a general increase in size compared with the controls. A proportion varying between 10 and 70% of macrophages showed morphological changes suggesting 'activation'. In sarcoidosis, 6.4% of macrophages were in close contact with lymphocytes, compared with 1.6% in the control subjects. At the points of contact between macrophages in sarcoidosis patients, but not in controls, paired subplasmalemmal linear densities, similar to those more commonly seen between epithelioid cells, giant cells and macrophages in granulomas, were sometimes seen. Cells having the appearance of epithelioid cells were not seen in BAL, but AM in sarcoidosis showed larger pseudopodia, more polarization of cytoplasmic membranes, larger and more numerous lysosomes and less nuclear heterochromatin.

IMPLICATIONS FOR THE PATHOGENESIS OF SARCOIDOSIS

The relevance of the findings obtained by BAL to the pathogenesis of sarcoidosis is dependent upon whether the cells in BAL can be accepted as representative of immunocompetent and inflammatory cells at sites of disease, not only in the lung but also at other localizations of sarcoidosis.

Haslam *et al.* (1980) found in 21 cases of cryptogenic fibrosing alveolitis that there was a correlation between the percentages found in BAL and in extracts from lung biopsy samples which attained statistical significance for neutrophils, the most prominent cell in this disease, and fell just short of it for eosinophils and lymphocytes; no correlation was found between scores for numbers of cells seen in histological sections and percentages in BAL. Hunninghake *et al.* (1981) found that the proportions of macrophages, of lymphocytes and their sub-sets, and of polymorphonuclear cells in BAL fluid were similar to those in suspensions prepared from lung biopsies in patients with sarcoidosis and with idiopathic pulmonary fibrosis and from normal lung obtained from patients undergoing thoracotomy for removal of localized lesions, and could thus be regarded as representative of the populations of such cells in the periphery of the broncho-alveolar tree. It has generally been found that BAL performed in different parts of diffusely affected lungs shows similar proportions of cell-types (Weinberger *et al.*, 1978). In three cases of pulmonary sarcoidosis with patchy radiographic changes, Cantin *et al.* (1983) found great differences in lymphocyte percentages, from less than six to high figures ranging from 21–49 in BAL performed in different lobes, indicating that cellular changes in the lungs are localized to involved parts.

Corroborative evidence of T-cell changes similar to those found by BAL in the lung at other localizations of sarcoidosis is difficult to obtain. Alario *et al.* (1977) obtained biopsy samples from cutaneous sarcoids in a 68 year old woman. Lymphocytes were separated from the minced granulomatous tissue; 84% were found to be T-cells, compared with 34% in the blood, in which the total lymphocyte count was low, 540 mm^{-3}.

Acceptance that the cell content of BAL is generally representative of events at sites of granuloma formation in pulmonary sarcoidosis has led to the formulation of the view that activated lymphocytes play a central role in the inception and maintenance of the granulomatous changes (Hunninghake *et al.*, 1980b; Hunninghake and Crystal, 1981b; Crystal *et al.*, 1981; Crystal *et al.*, 1983). T-lymphocytes accumulate in the lung (and presumably at other sites of sarcoidosis) in response to some as yet unidentified stimulus or agent(s), and become activated. They produce monocyte chemotactic factor, in response to which monocytes accumulate at affected sites and become transformed into epithelioid cells which aggregate into epithelioid and giant-cell granulomas. The low level of T-lymphocytes found in the peripheral blood is accounted for by the segregation of large numbers at the sites of active sarcoidosis; and this sequestration of immune effector cells contributes to the depression of peripheral expression of tuberculin-type hypersensitivity which is commonly found in sarcoidosis. Activation of B-cells in the lung and other affected tissues containing lymphoid tissue may lead to polyclonal secretion of immunoglobulins and accounts for the hyperglobulinaemia seen in some cases.

Some of the phenomena described in this picture of events in the evolution of pulmonary sarcoidosis have been observed in the few studies of granulomatous lung disease of known cause that have been reported, notably the prominence of activated T-lymphocytes. This raises the question how far the changes are to be regarded as peculiar to sarcoidosis, rather than to a general class of granulomatous reactions to known and as yet unidentified agents. Current immunological findings, including those obtained by BAL, seem compatible with the possibility that sarcoidosis is a response to a replicating agent of some kind. Hypotheses about the inciting stimulus to granuloma formation in sarcoidosis are considered in Chapter 25.

Chapter 21

The Kveim Reaction

In 1941, Kveim, working in Danbolt's department of dermatology is Oslo, reported that the intradermal injection of a heated suspension of tissue particles prepared from a sarcoid lymph-node caused a nodule to develop within nine days to four weeks in 12 out of 13 patients with sarcoidosis; that these nodules might increase in size for several weeks and persist for several months, and on biopsy showed histological changes resembling those of sarcoidosis; and that no reactions occurred in control subjects, including some with lupus vulgaris. Williams and Nickerson in 1935 briefly reported that they had prepared a suspension from a sarcoid skin lesion, and used it in the hope of obtaining a reaction in patients with sarcoidosis analogous to the Frei test in lymphogranuloma inguinale; and that in four patients thought to be suffering from sarcoidosis, a papule appeared in 24–36 hours and persisted for about a week, while in four control subjects there was no reaction. The clinical account of their four patients is very brief, but it seems arguable that two of them may have been suffering from regional ileitis. Harrell (1940) prepared suspensions from three sarcoid lymph-nodes; one gave 'questionably positive' reactions (presumably papules of the sort described by Williams and Nickerson) in three sarcoidosis patients, and the other two gave no reaction in four. Appel (1941) stated that Nickerson had used a sarcoid spleen suspension, and had found granulomatous changes on biopsy of the induced nodule. There is no question, however, that Kveim's account, published in 1941, was the first description of a reaction to intradermal injection of a sarcoid tissue suspension resulting in a slowly developing nodule with sarcoid histology, and was remarkably complete; and that his name has been justly associated with this reaction.

This reaction has been investigated intensively. As a result, it is now known that sarcoid tissue suspensions vary greatly in their ability to cause granulomatous reactions selectively in patients with sarcoidosis; that the probability that a patient with sarcoidosis will give such a reaction varies with the evolution of the disease; that some sarcoid tissue suspensions cause reactions unselectively; and that some suspensions selectively causing granulomatous reactions in sarcoidosis patients cause similar reactions in a proportion of patients with some other diseases, notably Crohn's disease. There is general agreement about the proportions of sarcoidosis at various stages giving granulomatous reactions, but reports about the frequency of such reactions in patients with other diseases vary widely; and the reasons for the selectivity of a 'good' suspension and the significance of the Kveim reaction in relation to the aetiology of sarcoidosis remain undetermined.

KVEIM REACTANT TISSUE SUSPENSIONS

Suspensions from a variety of tissues have been prepared and tested for ability to cause granulomatous reactions in sarcoid patients. It has generally been found that spleen and lymph-node are most likely to provide satisfactory suspensions. The original method of preparation described by Kveim (1941), Putkonen (1943), Danbolt (1948) and Nelson (1948) consisted in grinding the tissue in a mortar with sterile physiological saline solution to make a suspension of known strength, usually one part by weight of wet tissue to ten of the final suspension; allowing the larger particles to separate by sedimentation and discarding them; and using the supernatant particulate suspension as the test-material after sterilization by heating to 56°C – 60°C for one hour on two successive days and the addition of a preservative, usually 0.25% phenol. Subsequent workers have adopted more refined methods, but it has been found that only particulate suspensions are active, and conventional Kveim reagent remains a relatively crude suspension of human sarcoid tissues.

The active component is particulate and not water-soluble. It does not pass a Berkefeld or Seitz filter (Putkonen, 1943; Danbolt, 1948, 1951a). Rogers and Haserick (1954) found that the opalescent supernatant after centrifugation at 2500 rpm retained activity, but the clear supernatant after ultracentrifugation at 30 000 rpm was inactive. Chase and Siltzbach (1961) reported that particles sedimenting from their spleen suspension in 15 minutes on centrifugation at 5500 G had the highest activity, 450 μg of this fraction constituting an effective dose, and 30 μg producing a reaction in some patients. Particles sedimenting on further centrifugation at 10 000 G showed only one-ninth of the activity, weight for weight, of the larger particles. As described below (p. 446), Chase (1961) prepared a suspension, designated Type I, in which the active component was concentrated by washing and differential centrifugation by a factor of two or more.

Removal of lipids by extraction in the cold with ether (Rogers and

Haserick, 1954) or with chloroform-methanol (Chase and Siltzbach, 1961) does not reduce activity; Rogers and Haserick found that ether extraction increased activity somewhat. Nelson (1957) reported that repeated extractions with a series of hot organic solvents destroyed activity, and thought that this was probably due to the disruption of lipoprotein linkages. Boiling in aqueous suspension may reduce but does not destroy potency (Putkonen, 1943, 1945; Danbolt, 1948, 1951a; Rogers and Haserick, 1954). Chase and Siltzbach removed nucleoprotein by 2M sodium chloride, apparently without reducing potency; the separated nucleoprotein fraction was not active. Exposure to alkali destroys potency (Danbolt, 1948). Siltzbach and Ruttemberg (1971) reported that exposure to NaOH at a concentration as low as 0.05 mol l^{-1} for only 90 sec. at 0°C greatly reduced activity; by contrast, exposure to H Cl, 1.0 mol l^{-1}, for four days at 37°C only slightly reduced it. Proteolytic enzymes, nucleases, hyaluronidase and neuraminidase had little effect.

Chase and Siltzbach (1967) sought to concentrate the active component of their Type I suspension by physico-chemical methods. A validated suspension was extracted with alcohol, ether and water, dispersed by sonication, and digested with pepsin, the remaining undigested particles, amounting to about 90% of the initial dry weight, being suspended in phenolized buffer. This new suspension, designated Type III, was found to produce granulomatous reactions in parallel tests with the original Type I suspension in reactive sarcoidosis patients; doses of 20–50 μg were effective, the active component having been concentrated ninefold. A normal spleen similarly processed produced a suspension that was inactive but of similar dry weight, indicating that the active component constituted only a very small proportion of the sarcoid spleen suspension.

Cohn *et al.* (1967) investigated the distribution of Kveim-test activity in subcellular fractions from sarcoid lymph-nodes. Homogenates prepared from lymph-nodes of patients with sarcoidosis were fractionated by differential or sucrose gradient centrifugation. After adjustment to similar protein concentrations, fractions were examined by phase contrast and electron microscopy, and tested for Kveim activity by tests in parallel with a validated suspension in both reactors and non-reactors. The active principle sedimented almost completely at 15 000 G, and equilibrated between 50% and 70% glucose. Electron microscopy and acid phosphatase assays suggested that activity was located in membrane – bound dense bodies, probably lysosomal.

Early investigators found that many suspensions retained activity after prolonged storage, though some appeared to lose potency or selectivity. Putkonen (1943) found that a suspension stored for three years in a refrigerator remained active. Siltzbach and Ehrlich (1954) reported that a suspension stored at room temperature remained active after three years, but thought that storage might increase the incidence of 'non-specific' reactions. Nelson and Schwimmer (1957) found that one splenic suspension retained potency for seven years, but another lost it after 22 months; three lymph-node suspensions retained potency until they had been expended after six to nine months, and another lost selectivity after nine months. More recent experiences with some widely-used splenic suspensions are discussed below (p. 467).

HISTOLOGY OF THE KVEIM REACTION

Early descriptions of the histology include those of Putkonen (1945), Rogers and Haserick (1954), Siltzbach and Ehrlich (1954), James and Thomson (1955), Nelson (1957), and Steigleder *et al.* (1961). It is generally agreed that the typical reaction, consisting in well-formed tuberculoid collections of epithelioid cells with or without giant cells, and with limited or negligible lymphocytic infiltration, begins to develop within two weeks but does not attain a fully characteristic appearance until later.

Rogers and Haserick (1954) described the evolution of the reaction to Kveim test suspension in serial biopsies of two reacting and two non-reacting subjects. In the non-reactors, the tests sites showed only slight perivascular infiltration with lymphocytes in the early stage, a small collection of lymphocytes with a few small multinucleated cells at 13 days in one, and virtually normal skin in both at 42 days. In the reactors, one of whom eventually developed an intense reaction with some central necrosis, the changes at three days were similar to those in the non-reactors. At six days, there was a dense perivascular infiltration containing large pale-staining histiocytes, small deeply-staining mononuclear cells, and some atypical pleomorphic cells. At ten days, some central collagen degeneration with a few foci of necrosis was seen, the affected area being infiltrated with polymorphonuclear leucocytes, and surrounded by mononuclear leucocytes and histiocytes and pleomorphic cells. At 13 days, the atypical cells had diminished and lymphocytes increased in number, and small collections of epithelioid cells, surrounded by lymphocytes, were recognizable near vessels, together with a few giant cells of Langhans type. At 16 days, epithelioid cell tubercles were more evident, and lymphocytes less numerous. These changes had progressed at 25 days to large aggregations of epithelioid cells with scanty peripheral lymphocytes, and at 42 days to almost confluent epithelioid cell tubercles. By this time, the central necrotic area was well-defined and acellular. Siltzbach (1964a) studied the histology of developing Kveim reactions by serial injections at intervals of 1–4 weeks. At one week, the reaction consisted of mononuclear cells with small numbers of neutrophils, eosinophils and plasma cells. During subsequent weeks, the neutrophils, eosinophils and plasma cells diminished in numbers, and

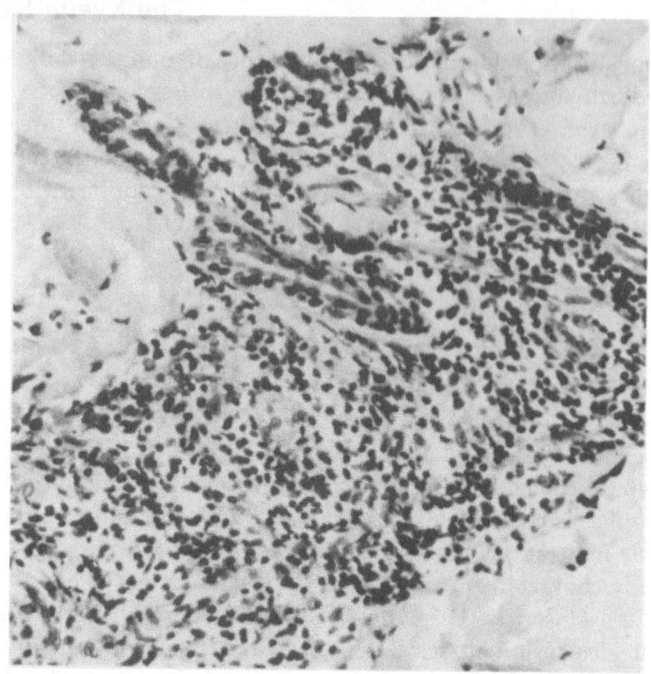

Figure 21.1 Evolution of Kveim reaction; aggregations of mononuclear cells with dark-staining nuclei at ten days. H & E. × 240.

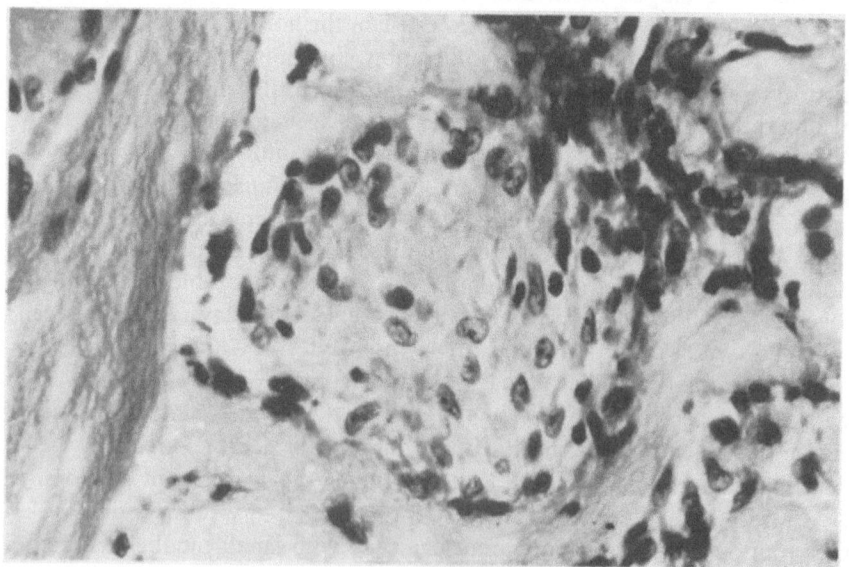

Figure 21.2 Developing epithelioid cell follicle at 18 days. H & E. × 350.

epithelioid cells appeared: whether these arose from the mononuclear cells which had been observed earlier, or from cells that replaced them was not clear. At three weeks, epithelioid cell follicles appeared and later matured. Over the following months, these follicles became surrounded and eventually replaced by hyalinized connective tissue, as in the healing of spontaneous sarcoid granulomas.

Our own findings are in keeping with those of Siltzbach. In the evolution of a granulomatous response to a Kveim test in a patient with sarcoidosis, the salient features are the presence of large aggregations of mononuclear cells with dark-staining nuclei at about ten days (Fig. 21.1), and the gradual development of epithelioid cell follicles, starting about 18–21 days after the injection (Figs. 21.2 and 21.3).

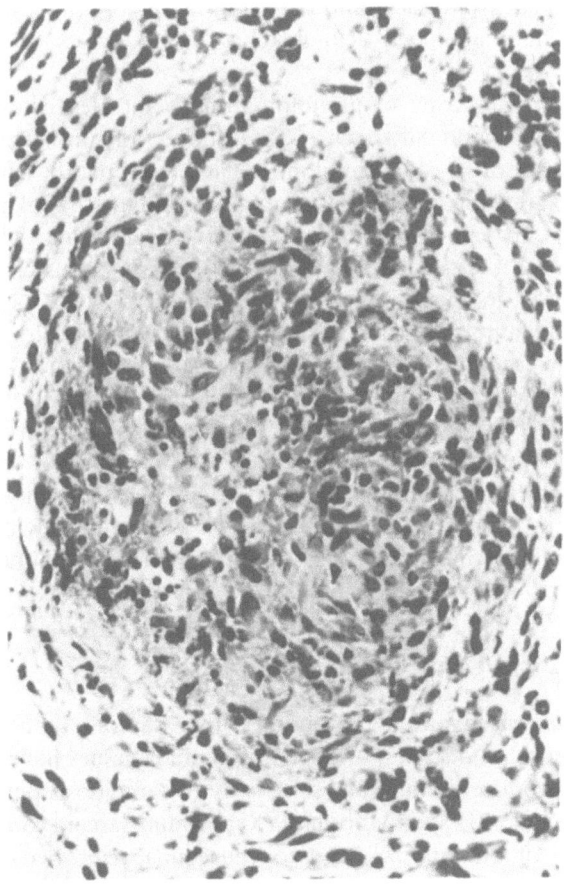

Figure 21.3   Kveim reaction: epithelioid cell granuloma at 28 days. H & E. × 210.

Asteroids may rarely be seen in multinucleated cells in a Kveim reaction, but Schaumann bodies do not occur (Siltzbach and Ehrlich, 1954).

Reactions resembling foreign-body granulomas may occur. It may be possible to attribute them unequivocally to extraneous material, such as fibres from cotton swabs used in sterilizing skin, fragments of plastic from disposable syringes, mineral particles incorporated in the suspension during its preparation, or fragments of keratin from the epidermis. Procedures for the use of the reaction as a diagnostic test (see below) should minimize these possibilities, and the presence and nature of discrete particles in giant cells and elsewhere in the reaction may be determined by microscopy, including the use of polarized light. Kenney and Stone (1963) observed that reactions with many giant cells, some containing doubly-refractile particles, might occur in patients with sarcoidosis in response to test-suspensions shown to contain no such particles; and our experience confirms this. Thus, doubly refractile material in a Kveim reaction is not necessarily of extraneous origin.

Electron microscopy of granulomatous Kveim test sites (Hirsch *et al.*, 1967; Douglas and Siltzbach, 1974) shows an ultra-structure generally similar to that of sarcoid granulomas (Chapter 2, p. 30), with the exception that there are more cytoplasmic organelles suggestive of phagocytosis or pinocytosis. In one case, Hirsch *et al.* mixed carbon particles with the test suspension; in the granuloma at six weeks, carbon particles were found in large vacuoles in epithelioid cells.

Salo and Hannuksela (1972) studied the immunohistology of granulomatous Kveim reactions in 20 patients. In vessel walls inside, but not outside, granulomas IgM was found in 19, IgG in one, and IgA in none; and C3 in nine of 12. Fibrin was present in a fine fibrillar network in the ground substance of granulomas. In an earlier study, Paronetto, reported by Siltzbach (1964a) found fibrinogen around granulomas in eight of ten Kveim test sites, and in two sarcoid lymph-nodes; it was present within granulomas only in areas of fibrinoid necrosis. No abnormal amounts of IgG or of complement were found.

SOURCES OF KVEIM-REACTANT MATERIAL

As well as spleen and lymph-node, other sarcoid tissues, lymph-nodes affected by other diseases, and normal human tissues have been tested for ability to produce granulomas selectively in sarcoidosis patients.

Putkonen (1943) and Danbolt (1951a) found sarcoid tonsil to be weakly productive of granulomas, and to cause unspecific reactions in control subjects; skin sarcoids were difficult to process into suspensions, might or might not be active, and provided only small amounts of material. A suspension prepared by Danbolt (1951a) from a sarcoid bone lesion was active. Siltzbach and Ehrlich prepared suspensions from 15 tissues from sarcoidosis patients; three from lymph-nodes and two from skin were inactive, and eight from lymph-nodes and two from spleens of variable activity.

Danbolt (1948) found that a suspension prepared from granulomatous papule at a previous test-site produced a similar, though smaller, reaction.

It is evident that the granuloma-producing potency of sarcoid tissues varies greatly, and cannot be predicted from their histology; an exuberantly granulomatous tissue may produce a suspension of low potency, while a tissue showing much hyaline scarring and poorly-formed granulomas may be potent. A study by Putkonen (1967) suggests an explanation for this apparent discrepancy. He prepared suspensions from enlarged lymph-nodes excised from patients with sarcoidosis before, immediately after, and three weeks after three weeks' intensive treatment with prednisone. The nodes diminished greatly in size during, and enlarged again after, the treatment-period; and histologically epithelioid cells gave place to hyalinization. Tests in patients with sarcoidosis showed that the concentration of the active material increased as the nodes diminished in size, and returned towards the original level when they enlarged again, roughly in inverse proportion to their size. Thus the granuloma-inducing material, presumable located in the cells of the fresh granuloma, was not removed when these cells disappeared, but persisted in the residual hyalinized tissue. Further evidence on this point, derived from the study of spleens used to produce diagnostic suspensions, is discussed below (p. 466). Similarly, the granuloma-producing potency of a sarcoid tissue correlates poorly with the clinical features of the patient who provides it. Putkonen (1943) prepared a suspension from a lymph-node from the neck of a patient in whom, although the node had the histology of sarcoidosis, there was no other evidence of sarcoidosis, a Mantoux test was strongly positive, and there was no reaction to a potent Kveim antigen; nevertheless this suspension gave granulomatous reactions in sarcoidosis patients. Moreover, the potency of a suspension is not dependent upon the Kveim-reactivity of the patient from whose tissue it is prepared. Putkonen (1964) tested suspensions from lymph-nodes of 16 sarcoidosis patients and found that the most potent were obtained from patients who responded weakly to a Kveim test. This finding is in line with our experiences in the validation of test-suspensions from spleens, though it conflicts some-what with the earlier observations of Siltzbach and Ehrlich (1954). They found that eight patients whose tissues had produced active suspensions, all themselves reacted, four to autologous suspensions, while of four whose tissues had produced inert suspensions, two failed to react.

Ripe *et al.* (1980) compared reactions to simultaneous tests with suspensions prepared from sarcoid spleen and from mediastinal lymph-nodes obtained by mediastinoscopy. All 15 patients tested gave granulomas reactions to the lymph-node suspension, but four gave negative reactions to the spleen suspension, and reactions to the spleen suspension were weaker than those to the lymph-node suspension. Histologically, the spleen showed necrotizing granulomas, suggestive of acute changes. These findings are consistent with those of Putkonen (1964, 1967) suggesting that the active component may be present in greater quantity in chronic than in recent active lesions.

A suspension which contains the component causing granulomatous reaction in patients with sarcoidosis may contain also components producing granulomatous or simple inflammatory reactions of various sorts unselectively. Chase (1961) described one such suspension. It was derived from lymph-nodes from a tuberculin-negative sarcoidosis patient, and gave responses interpreted as positive in sarcoidosis patients, but with prominent early inflammation. In tuberculin-positive human subjects and guinea-pigs, it produced a tuberculin-type delayed skin reaction.

Suspensions made in a similar manner from normal tissues, or tissues affected by other diseases have been tested by a number of observers. While most of them have reported negative results, a minority have found that these suspensions caused nodules, sometimes granulomatous, in the sarcoid patients used as test subjects. Putkonen (1943) and Lomholt (1943) stated that a suspension prepared from a lymph-node from a patient with lymphatic leukaemia produced characteristic reactions. Danbolt (1951a) found that a suspension prepared from lymph-nodes affected by Hodgkin's disease was inactive. Nelson (1948, 1949) prepared suspensions from 12 normal human spleens, and found that two produced reactions in sarcoidosis patients who were reactive to a sarcoid spleen suspension, and ten were inert; suspensions of normal human lymph-node and of defatted human muscle were inert. Siltzbach and Ehrlich (1954) tested suspensions of normal human spleen and lymph-node and found them inactive, as did Rogers and Haserick (1954) in suspensions of human lymph-node. Kenney and Stone (1963) studied the reactions produced by suspensions prepared from sarcoid lymph-node and skin, and from normal lymph-node and skin, the histology being interpreted by four pathologists unaware whether the biopsies of the reactions came from patients with sarcoidosis or not. Of the 43 patients with active sarcoidosis, 41, and of 18 with inactive sarcoidosis, six gave reactions to the sarcoid lymph-node suspension, interpreted by at least three of the pathologists as positive; of ten controls, none gave such reactions. Of those reacting in this way, ten were tested with the sarcoid skin suspension, and nine gave 'positive' reactions; 14 were tested with the normal lymph-node suspension and five gave 'positive' reactions. Among those reacting to the normal tissues, most showed relatively feeble reactions; nevertheless they were interpreted as positive by a majority of the pathologists. These varied findings indicate that some apparently normal human spleens, lymph-nodes and skin may contain in small amounts components capable of eliciting selectively granulomatous responses in reactive sarcoidosis patients.

Attempts to mimic the effects of Kveim-test suspensions by intradermal injection of material derived from sources other than human tissues have been unsuccessful. Nelson (1949) found that sarcoidosis patients gave no unusual reactions to chick embryo lymphogranuloma venereum antigen, to *Pityrosporon ovale*, to soy-bean phosphatides, to calcium sulphate, or to collodion particles. Exceptionally, Gilroy (1971) stated that standard typhoid-paratyphoid vaccine administered intradermally in six young men with BHL and early sarcoid lung changes produced nodules at 4–6 weeks read as positive Kveim reactions by several pathologists, but this observation does not appear to have been repeated or further investigated.

The possibility that tubercle bacilli or products derived from them might produce unusual reactions in patients with sarcoidosis has been extensively investigated, with generally negative results. Sarcoid-like granulomas were reported to have developed in patients with sarcoidosis at the site of BCG vaccination in one case by Lemming (1942) and at the sites of intradermal injection of killed human tubercle bacilli by Warfvinge (1945); but in a critical study of intradermal tests with killed tubercle bacilli of human, bovine and BCG strains in patients with sarcoidosis and with cutaneous tuberculosis and in tuberculin-negative and tuberculin-positive normal subjects, Bjornstad (1948) found that the histological pattern of the reaction depended upon tuberculin sensitivity. Some of the tuberculin-negative subjects showed a sarcoid-like pattern, but there was no systematic difference between the histology of the reactions in the sarcoidosis patients and in the rest. Others also have concluded that the character of reactions produced by acid-fast bacilli varies similarly with the level of tuberculin sensitivity in normal subjects, in patients with tuberculosis and in those with sarcoidosis (Israel *et al.*, 1950; Bernstein and Spoor, 1952; Rostenburg *et al.*, 1953; Forgacs *et al.*, 1957).

Billings and Shapiro (1954) reported the appearance of a spreading reaction composed of many small papules around a positive tuberculin test and reaching a diameter of 2 cm after one month in a woman with multiple sarcoids of the skin; on biopsy the induced lesion had a sarcoid histology, and a second tuberculin test caused a similar response. This was evidently in a peculiarly reactive patient. Schaumann and Seeberg (1948) performed biopsies of the injected sites four to eight weeks after Mantoux tests with 0.1 mg OT, which had produced no evident reaction, in four patients with sarcoidosis. Small epithelioid cell foci were found, in three without necrosis, and in one with some foci of necrosis.

Visible late reactions at the sites of tuberculin tests must be excessively rare, in view of the routine use of such tests in sarcoid patients. Sandor

(1958) reported a remarkable case in a man, aged 54, the upper lobe of whose right lung was removed for a carcinoma of very limited extent. In the removed lobe there were 'nodular masses' which showed the histological picture of healed sarcoid, and in the lymph-nodes at its hilum typical discrete sarcoid tubercles. He remained well under observation after the operation; the spleen became palpable. Mantoux tests soon after, 17 and 23 months after the operation, were at first positive weakly only with 1:100 OT, and later became strongly positive with 1:1000; at the sites of these tests, indolent infiltrations appeared, having the histological structure of sarcoids when excised for biopsy at four weeks, seven weeks and in one instance after six months. Hurley and Shelley (1960) found that in five of 50 healthy black men, painless papules persisted four weeks after tuberculin tests, and on biopsy showed epithelioid cell granulomas. Biopsies were performed at four weeks in 15 of those without a papule and no granuloma was observed. Repeat tests were done on four of those who produced papules, up to nine months after the first, and showed similar histological changes.

THE KVEIM REACTION AS A DIAGNOSTIC TEST

The Kveim reaction is in wide, but not universal, use as a diagnostic test for sarcoidosis. The following section deals with the preparation of validation and of test suspensions, the technique of the test, and the factual basis for its diagnostic use. Its role and significance in the diagnosis of sarcoidosis are discussed in Chapter 26.

Preparation of test-suspensions

Though there is some evidence that sarcoid lymph-node may produce a more potent suspension than spleen (Jones-Williams *et al.*, 1976; Ripe *et al.*, 1980), spleen offers the advantage of providing a large volume of tissue, desirable in view of the time and effort required for validation. For this reason, spleens removed surgically for such indications as hypersplenism, thombocytopenia or abdominal discomfort (Chapter 12) or, less often, at necropsy have been found to be the best starting point for the preparation of Kveim test suspensions. The donor patient should have no history of transmissible disease, especially hepatitis. Bacteriological cultures and microscopy should show no pathogens. The spleen should be cut into narrow slices and rinsed free of blood with cold sterile normal saline. Supensions of Type I of Chase and Siltzbach (1961) are generally prepared by the technique described by Chase (1961). It is convenient to process 30–35 g of spleen at a time. On the first day, the tissue is thawed, teased, scissored and disintegrated in buffered saline at 0–4°C. On the second day, it is washed twice by centrifugation at 5500 G for 20 minutes on each occasion, after which it is suspended, dispersed and strained through 40-mesh, 80-mesh and 100-mesh sieves. It is then suspended and, after adjustment of pH to 7.2–7.4, heated in a water-bath to 58°C for 75 minutes. It is held overnight at 4°C, its sterility is checked, and an aliquot precipitated with alcohol and vacuum-dried to determine its dry weight. On the third day, second and third heatings to 58°C for 75 minutes are carried out, sterility and pH are finally checked, the concentration is adjusted as required (see below), and phenol is added to 0.25% concentration; the suspension is finally dispensed in sealed ampoules of 1.5 ml. Mitchell *et al.* (1974a) showed that ^{60}Co irradiation of a Type I suspension with 2.5 megarad, the customary steriliz-ing dose, did not change levels of reactivity and selectivity for sarcoidosis, as shown by simultaneous tests with non-irradiated suspension. All ampoules of Kveim test suspension issued from the Standards Laboratory for Serolo-gical Reagents in London are now irradiated in this way as an extra safeguard against the hazards of injection of material derived from human tissues.

The concentration of particles in an undiluted suspension prepared in this way ranges up to 8 mg or more per ml, as measured by alcohol precipitable dry weight; but the reactant potency as well as the selectivity of a suspension can be assessed only by biological assay in man. It is advisable to adjust the concentration of a suspension which is to be validated for diagnostic use after preliminary tests of its potency. The standard to be expected of a 'good' suspension is the induction of granulomatous reactions in 60% or more of patients with active sarcoidosis, and no more than 2–3% of other subjects (Siltzbach, 1976); the special problem of reactivity of some suspen-sions in patients with inflammatory bowel disease is considered below (p. 475). Suspensions from the New York spleen J attain this at a concentration of 3.0 mg ml^{-1}, giving 450 μg in a test dose of 0.15 ml. Mitchell *et al.* (1976) compared lot 10 of spleen J with suspensions from two spleens, designated K12 and K13, in a statistically designed study in 18 patients with active and 18 with inactive sarcoidosis, similar numbers with active and quiescent pulmonary tuberculosis, and 18 healthy subjects, all groups matched for age and sex. The K12 and K13 suspensions had concentrations of 8.3 mg and 5.9 mg ml^{-1}. K12 undiluted, giving 1250 μg in a test dose, K12 in half-dilution, test dose 625 μg, K13 giving 880 μg in a test dose, and the reference spleen J suspension, test dose 450 μg, gave reactions in similar proportions of patients with sarcoidosis; over all, reactions interpreted as positive were found in 67% with active, and 22% with inactive sarcoidosis. Among 36 patients with pulmonary tuberculosis, two tests with spleen J and one with undiluted K12 were interpreted as equivocal, and none as positive. Among nine normal subjects, one reaction to undiluted K12 was interpreted as positive, all others being negative. It thus appeared that half-dilution of K12 increased the selectivity of this suspension for sarcoidosis. In the routine validation of a suspension for diagnostic use, the elaborate design of this study is, of course, unnecessary; a few tests in parallel with a validated suspension in sarcoidosis patients will suffice to indicate the optimal concentration of a potent source tissue for further tests in patients with sarcoidosis at various stages, and with other diseases, both granulomatous and non-granulomatous. In these tests, histology must be assessed by an experienced observer unaware whether the reaction was produced by a validated or the unvalidated suspension, and of the clinical features of the subjects.

Performance of the Kveim Test

Sterile 1 ml disposable syringes and short shank needles of gauge adequate to allow passage of the particulate suspension, usually 26 gauge, are convenient. We have found that the use of disposable, rather than glass, syringes is convenient, and does not lead to an unacceptable incidence of refractile material or foreign-body granulomas at the test site. Occasionally a sliver of foreign-body material showing 'rainbow' birefringence may be seen in sections from the test site when examined by polarized light. The frequency of this occurrence is diminished by routinely sluicing the assembled syringes and needles with sterile normal saline before drawing up the test suspension. Chase (1961) advocated the use of needles with Huber point and closed bevel to minimize the incidence of keratin implants, but we have found disposable short-shank 26 gauge needles with a short bevel to be satisfactory. We have observed keratin implants in only 16 (0.3%) of over 5000 tests; nine of these were in papules 5–8 mm in diameter. The injection is most conveniently made on the ulnar side of the upper part of the forearm, so that any residual scar will be inconspicuous. The skin at the test site should be cleaned with an alcohol dab; the use of cotton-wool or gauze should be avoided to minimize the risk of introduction of cotton-fibres into the skin. The vial containing the test suspension is thoroughly shaken, and the test dose of 0.15 ml drawn into the sluiced syringe, and injected intracutaneously and as superficially as possible, to raise a papule with a 'peau d'orange' appearance. The epidermis at the test site is then marked by a tattoo mark made by a sterile needle dipped into autoclaved Gunter-Wagner Pelikan ink; the mark should be made at a point about one-third of the radius of the papule from its centre. This marker will be within the edge of a visible reaction, and will ensure that tiny areas of induration are not missed, or permit routine biopsy in 4–6 weeks even in the absence of visible or palpable reaction.

Evolution of the macroscopic reaction

An area of induration about 3–4 mm in diameter with some surrounding erythema usually develops in the day or two after the injection; it is attributable to inflammatory response to trauma and to a particulate suspension, and is unrelated to Kveim reactivity. In Kveim reactive subjects, it is slowly replaced, usually during the second week, by an area of palpable induration which may develop into a dusky red papule and attain a diameter of up to 5 mm by 14 days. Thereafter it persists and may increase in size for a variable time, up to eight weeks. It is usually excised for biopsy at 4–6 weeks. If it is not completely excised, the residue in most cases gradually subsides over the next few months, leaving only a little pigmentation and a small scar at the test site. Occasionally, a visible and palpable reaction persists as long as the sarcoidosis remains active. Danbolt (1951b) reported the case of a young man with sarcoidosis of the skin, eye, lungs and bones, in whom a Kveim reaction increased over the course of two years to an infiltration 17 × 15 mm, which on excision was found to have a structure similar to that of the skin sarcoids. Møller (1952) recorded the persistence of a Kveim reaction for nine years, and Rogers and Haserick (1954) for four years.

Rarely, the appearance of a papule at the test site is delayed. Putkonen (1952) recorded the development of reaction papules at the site of injection five years after a Kveim test; his patient was regarded as a case of skin tuberculosis. Rogers and Haserick (1954) stated that they had observed reactions to develop as late as one and a half years after the injection of the test suspension, these late reactions usually developing during a recrudescence of activity of sarcoidosis.

The scar at the site of a previous Kveim test biopsy may become indurated with resurgence of activity of sarcoidosis. This is sometimes observed after pregnancy, since the activity of sarcoidosis tends to be suppressed during pregnancy (Chapter 18, p. 381). Re-biopsy of a scar showing new induration may show typical granulomas.

Most observers have found that ulceration is very rare, though papules may show some crusting, and few undergo central softening (Siltzbach and Ehrlich, 1954). Some early workers observed ulceration in vigorous reactions. The illustrations in Putkonen's (1943) monograph show many ulcerated reactions. It is possible that he may have been dealing with highly reactive patients, and that the method of preparing the suspension which he then used may have led to the inclusion of silica particles, increasing the intensity of the reaction. Later, the incidence of ulcerated reactions among his patients appears to have diminished, for in 1952 he noted only that ulceration, healing only with remission of the sarcoidosis or under corticosteroid treatment, might occur in some large Kveim papules. In over 5000 tests, one of us (DNM) has observed ulceration on only four occasions. In general, the severity of the reaction depends not only upon the reactivity of the subject, but also upon the qualities of the test-suspension; and a suspension causing more than very few necrotic reactions would not now be thought suitable for diagnostic use.

Siltzbach (1964a) found that the average size of developing Kveim papules was greater in black than white patients. Among those with less than two years' known duration of sarcoidosis the reaction papule at six weeks was 5 mm or more in diameter in 30% of white males and 17% of white females as compared with 70% of black males and 60% of black females.

Karlish (1967) related the size of reaction papules to histology and to duration of sarcoidosis in 180 patients. Reactions interpreted as positive were found in two (6%) of 32 with no papule; in 11 (29%) of 38 with 1–2 mm papules; in 44 (71%) of 62 with 3–4 mm papules; and in 73 (91%) of 80 with 5 mm or larger papules. Papules 5 mm or more in diameter were found in 55% of patients with sarcoidosis of less than two years' duration, and in 19% of those of longer duration.

Effect of corticosteroids

Rogers and Haserick (1954) found that the injection of hydrocortisone, 5 mg, either with the test-suspension or into an ten day old test site, inhibited the Kveim reaction; they noted, however, that patients with active sarcoidosis under treatment with corticosteroids but showing a poor response might develop granulomatous responses to Kveim tests. In general, it has been found that the administration of corticosteroids, either locally with the test-suspension or systemically, diminishes and in sufficient dosage abolishes Kveim reactivity (Nelson, 1957; Siltzbach, 1961, 1964a). Siltzbach *et al.* (1971b) studied the effects of 20 mg prednisone or 2.4 mg betamethasone daily by mouth on Kveim papules in 30 reactive sarcoidosis patients, using each as his own control. The mean diameter of control papules was 6.6 mm. In 11 patients, corticosteroid administration was started on the day of a repeat test; the mean diameter of the papule at six weeks was 2.1 mm, and only six were interpreted histologically as 'positive'. In 16, the corticosteroid was started 14 days after the second test; the resulting papules averaged 3.1 mm in diameter, and seven were histologically 'positive'. When corticosteroid administration was delayed until four weeks after the test 11 of the 14 produced responses interpreted as positive. Karlish (1971) found in studies on 18 patients at various stages of sarcoidosis that prednisolone 10–15 mg daily by mouth had an inhibitory effect on both the size and the histology of Kveim reactions; in patients presenting with erythema nodosum, Kveim nodules were generally larger, and were less inhibited by prednisolone in the given dosage. Our experience is in keeping with these findings. Although a strongly reactive subject may show a granulomatous response in spite of corticosteroid administration at conventional dosage, a patient with active sarcoidosis receiving corticosteroids in dosage sufficient to maintain optimal suppression usually fails to show a granulomatous response to a Kveim test. The implications of this for the diagnostic use of the Kveim test are discussed in Chapter 26.

Biopsy of the test site

Some of the earlier investigators accepted the appearance of a reaction papule in the appropriate time as indicating a positive test; e.g. Danbolt (1951a) accepted a papule distinctly visible at one month and persisting for several months. But later observers have concluded that because of the frequency of unspecific reactions and of the possibility that a granulomatous reaction demonstrable by biopsy may be impalpable, biopsy is essential (Siltzbach and Ehrlich, 1954; James and Thomson, 1955; Nelson, 1957; Anderson *et al.*, 1963b). In our experience, many Kveim test papules are small, measuring no more than 2–3 mm in diameter; and without the evidence obtained by microscopy including the use of polarized light, it would be impossible to determine whether such small lesions were banal inflammatory or foreign body responses or sarcoid-type granulomas. Small granulomatous reactions may cause so little induration that they can be overlooked on inspection and palpation even at marked test sites. During the eight years 1973–1981, one of us (DNM) performed 5244 tests by the technique described below. Of these, 319 showed no macroscopic reaction at the time of biopsy; nevertheless, biopsy showed histological changes interpreted as granulomatous in 17 (5%) and as equivocal in ten (3%).

Biopsy is performed 4–6 weeks after the injection. The skin is swabbed with 70% alcohol. About 0.15 ml of 1% procaine with adrenaline to minimize capillary oozing is injected into the skin at the marked site; this does not appear to distort the histological pattern. With a no-touch technique, a 3 mm or 4 mm diameter skin biopsy punch of Hays-Martin type is applied to encircle the centre of any reaction or the test site marker and gently rotated to cut through the full thickness of the skin. If it is necessary to cut through a large papule, the residual rim of granulomatous tissue will heal satisfactorily. A very large papule, which may contain extensive central collagen necrosis, may be cut through obliquely to avoid the possibility that insufficient of the surrounding granulomatous tissue is included. The pedicle of the biopsy fragment is then stretched gently with fine non-toothed forceps, and dissected clear with scissors; the fragment is placed in neutral

10% formalin for fixation. Haemostasis is maintained by a 'band-aid' or similar approximating adhesive dressing, and a simple gauze dressing secured by adhesive strapping; both can be removed by the patient after five days.

The fixed 4 mm core of tissue is embedded in paraffin wax, and serial sections, 5–7 μ thick, cut at right angles to the epidermis. Depending on the amount of tissue, every 8th to 20th section is mounted in ribbon formation and stained with haematoxylin and eosin (H and E).

Interpretation of the test

Interpretation of the test necessitates microscopy of representative serial sections by an experienced observer who is unaware of clinical features. He can be informed of the presence and characteristics of a visible or palpable reaction; he can usually deduce its size from the extent of histological changes.

Microscopically, the essential feature of a response supporting a diagnosis of sarcoidosis is the presence of one or more granulomas composed principally of epithelioid cells. Granulomas may be discrete or confluent; there may be epithelioid cells infiltrating diffusely between collagen bundles, with one or more satellite granulomas. In a florid reaction, granulomas may show central fibrinoid necrosis, or may surround an area of fibrinoid necrosis

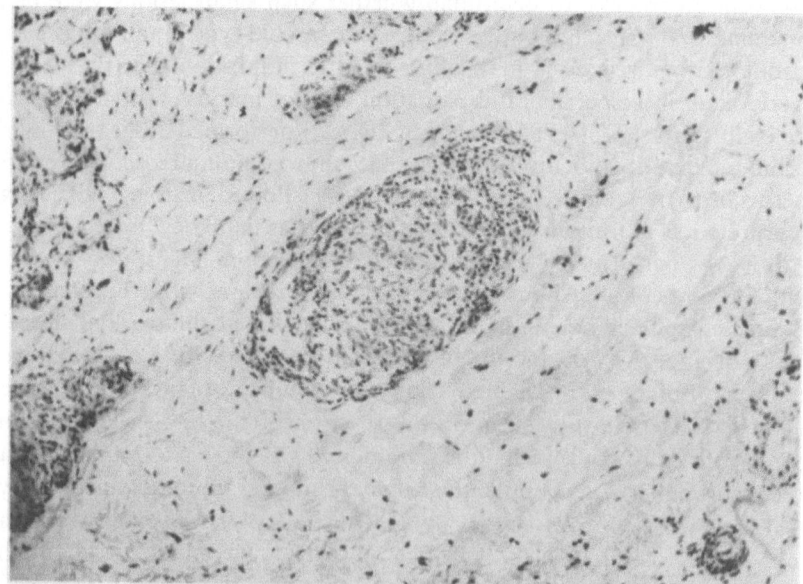

Figure 21.4 A single well-formed epithelioid cell granuloma in response to a Kveim test; minimal requirement for a granulomatous response. H & E. × 112.

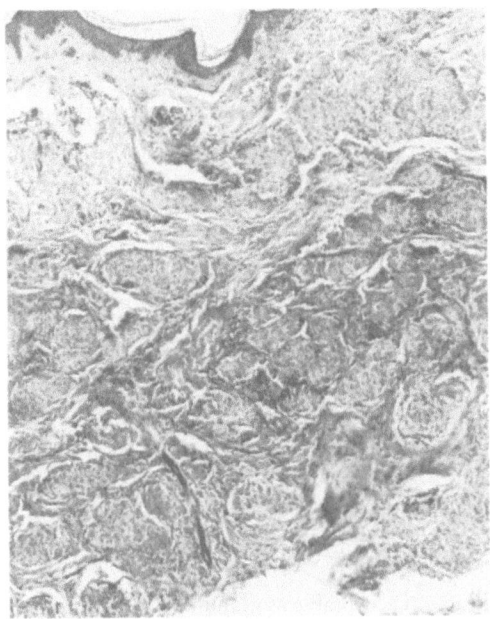

Figure 21.5   An exuberantly granulomatous response to a Kveim test.
H & E. × 39.

devoid of cells and staining pink in sections stained with H and E; it is
especially important to examine by polarized light for birefringent foreign-
body material in such reactions. Surrounding granulomas, there is cellular
infiltration of variable extent, in which lymphocytes predominate, with
some histiocytes, neutrophils and occasional eosinophils or plasma cells.
Kveim granulomas are usually sited in the middle and deeper dermis,
whereas spontaneous sarcoid granulomas usually extend into superficial as
well as deeper layers. Some Kveim reactions contain brown granules or
fibres, or doubly refractile particles, not apparently of foreign body origin;
these are not seen in skin sarcoids. Though the finding of doubly refractile
material should lead to consideration of the possibility that granulomas may
be a foreign body reaction, it does not exclude the possibility that they are
specifically related to sarcoidosis (Figs. 21.4 and 21.5). In some reactions,
epithelioid cells are seen infiltrating diffusely between collagen bundles,
without satellite granulomas; and in others the infiltrating cells are predominantly histiocytes, with less abundant cytoplasm and smaller round nuclei,
in focal collations with few or no epithelioid cells. Reactions of these types
must be regarded as doubtfully granulomatous and equivocal. A localized
reaction to evident foreign particles, an infiltration of mixed inflammatory
cells, which may be lymphocytes, mononuclear cells, neutrophils, plasma
cells or eosinophils, or a scar with fibroblasts and fibrocytes, constitute a

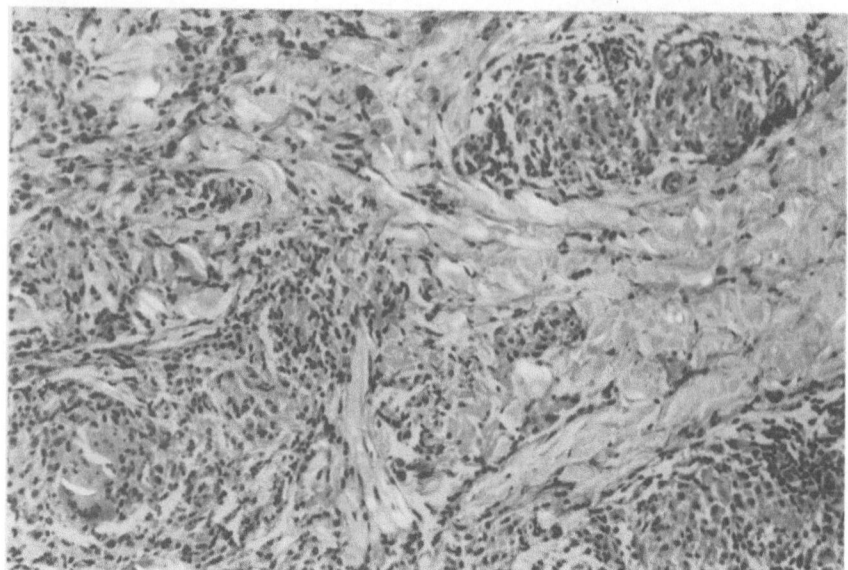

Figure 21.6   A reaction acceptable as granulomatous, in spite of the presence of some bifringent material H & E. × 126. Note well-formed granulomas, and a birefringent body in a giant cell; also collagen birefringence.

non-granulomatous, 'negative' Kveim test response (Figs. 21.6 and 21.7).

It is evident that a fairly wide range of histological patterns may be acceptable as 'specific' reactions in the interpretation of the Kveim test, which consequently is subject to a certain amount of observer variation. Steigleder *et al.* (1961) reported that of 83 reactions which they accepted as specific, rather over one-third showed granulomas of typically sarcoid appearance; among the rest about one-half showed similar granulomas but with some necrosis and banal inflammatory reaction, and one half a less well-formed tuberculoid granuloma. Reactions with many giant cells, some containing doubly refractile particles, are especially liable to varied interpretation. Steigleder *et al.* observed such reactions in eight of 99 patients with proved or probable sarcoidosis, and Kenney and Stone (1963) observed that they might occur in patients with active sarcoidosis in response to suspensions shown to contain no doubly-refractile particles, and thought that they were related to specially active disease. Kenney and Stone submitted each biopsy to four pathologists for independent study. Decision whether the test was to be regarded as positive or negative depended upon agreement by at least three of the four pathologists; it was noted that 'in no reading was there an equal division of interpretation between the four pathologists'. When 15 of the biopsies, accepted in this way as positive but showing some deviation from the strict criteria, were resubmitted later as 'skin biopsy', 11 were called 'granuloma of unknown origin' and four 'foreign-body giant-cell granuloma'. Not surprisingly, better agreement is possible if pathologists adopt agreed criteria, but discordant readings still occur. Jones Williams *et al.* (1976) reported that two pathologists working in the same centre and reading Kveim biopsies in three categories, positive, equivocal and negative, agreed completely in the categorization of 229 (75%) of 306 tests; 70 read as either positive or negative by one were read as equivocal by the other; while seven were read as positive by one and negative by the other. Mitchell *et al.* (1976) reported a similar level of disagreement between two observers working in the same centre and to agreed criteria; of 180 paired readings, 156 were concordant, 20 were graded unequivocally by one reader and as equivocal by the other, and four as positive by one and negative by the other.

The assessment of the histology of Kveim reactions in groups of participants in the Medical Research Council BCG trials (D'Arcy Hart *et al.*, 1964) provided a striking example of disagreement between observers. In this study, other aspects of which are discussed below (p. 469), 64 biopsies were assessed by a very experienced observer who classified 16 as positive, five as equivocal, and 43 as negative; and by one of us (JGS) who placed eight, five and 51 respectively in these categories. Since no clinical evidence of sarcoidosis was found or subsequently appeared in any of the subjects studied, there was no means of determining which observer's assessments were more 'correct'. Such experiences suggest to us that in reports of the histology of Kveim test reactions, it is advisable to avoid a 'positive–negative' terminology, and to use descriptive terms. A scale ranging from granulomatous, though partially granulomatous and simple inflammatory, to no reaction is appropriate; and reports should describe mixed reactions, and refer to such

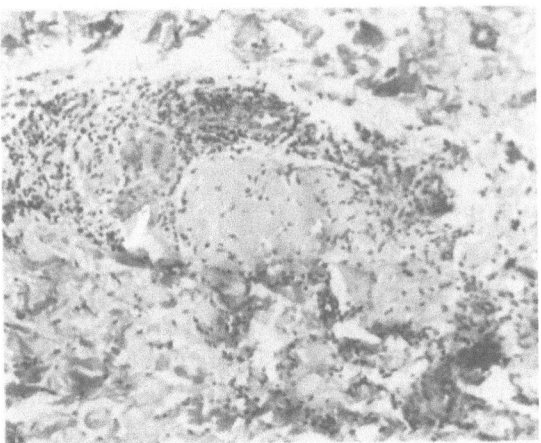

Figure 21.7   A foreign-body reaction at a Kveim test site. H & E. × 112.

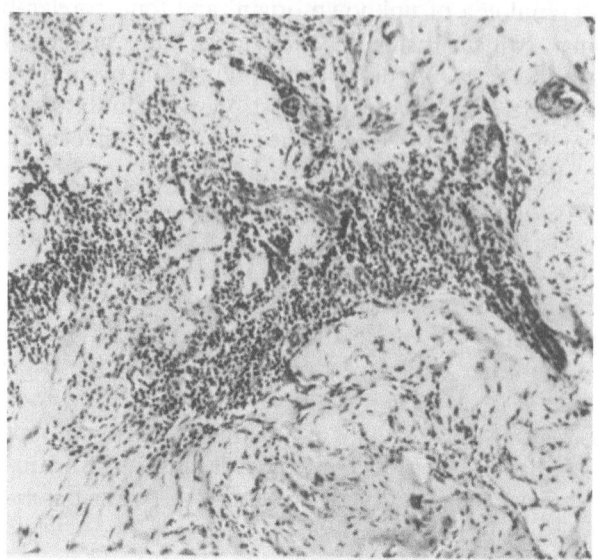

Figure 21.8   A mixed cellular reaction at a Kveim test site. H & E. × 98.

special features as the presence of foreign material, especially birefringent, of large numbers of giant cells and their character, and of necrosis. The diagnostic significance of the test depends upon the correlation of these findings with clinical features (Chapter 26). The size of reaction papules may have some diagnostic implications, although this has not been specially investigated. In the study of Mitchell *et al.* (1976) mentioned above (p. 455), the mean size of papules read microscopically as 'negative' was greater in patients with sarcoidosis, active or inactive, than in those with tuberculosis; and of 72 tests in patients with pulmonary tuberculosis, 41 produced papules, none interpreted as positive and three as equivocal, while in 36 in normal subjects, only one produced a papule, which was interpreted as positive.

Validation of test-suspensions

A spleen or other tissue which is a potential source of Kveim test suspension must be assessed for potency and selectivity by tests in parallel with a validated suspension in patients with sarcoidosis at various stages and individuals not suffering from sarcoidosis, preferably including some with mycobacterial tuberculosis, inflammatory bowel disease, and lymphodenopathy of various sorts.

Siltzbach (1964a) found that less than half the new suspensions tested were satisfacory. Of 38 suspensions prepared for possible diagnostic use,

Table 21.1 Percentages of 'positive' reactions to some widely-used validated Kveim test suspension in patients with sarcoidosis. The figures in brackets refer to the total numbers on which the percentages are based.

	Patients diagnosed as sarcoidosis			Duration		Chest radiograph[1]				Controls[2]
	All	With biopsy	Probable	< 2 yr	> 2 yr	I	II	III	0	
Hirsch et al. (1961) New York	70% (122)	79% (47)	57% (85)	75% (71)	61% (51)					9% (85)
Siltzbach (1961) New York	64% (447)	84% (165)	52% (282)			90% (144)	89% (115)	41% (80)	21% (109)	1% (303)
Anderson et al. (1963) London		62% (148)	38% (216)	70% (63)	56% (85)					2% (245)
Turiaf et al. (1980) Paris	58% (471)	74% (255)								0.2%[3] (530)
Kataria et al. (1980) 4 cities in USA	67% (228)			73% (143)	56% (84)	73% (97)	91% (43)	44% (54)	53% (34)	0 (94)
Bradstreet et al (1980) London	56% (3071)	72% (309)	54% (2762)	57% (2755)	42% (316)	76% (1351)	71% (304)	34% (207)	26% (684)	1.3% (219)
International studies										
Siltzbach (1967)	52% (1716)	61% (1124)	35% (592)	62% (453)	38% (310)	62% (311)[4]	48% (225)[4]	38% (154)[4]	50% (51)[4]	0.7% (668)
Hurley and Sullivan (1974)[5]	59% (639)			66% (395)	51% (294)					6% (287)
Middleton and Douglas (1980a)	70% (913)						75% (677)		55% (236)	1% (698)

[1] I = hilar lymph-node enlargement only
II = hilar nodes + lung infiltration
III = lung infiltration only
0 = normal chest radiograph

[2] Controls = patients with other diagnoses and normal subjects
[3] 19 histologically 'doubtful'
[4] Biopsy-confirmed cases only
[5] Early lots of CSL suspension

only 18 were acceptable; 11 were not sufficiently potent, and nine were non-selective. The unpublished experience of one of us (DNM) is similar. Of 17 spleen suspensions, nine have been found to be acceptable; four were rejected because they produced reactions non-selectively, one because it was only weakly selective, two because they were both poorly selective and of low potency, and one because of low potency. Siltzbach (1964a) stated that he preferred spleens showing relatively fresh granulomas and no more than minor degrees of hyalinization; but we have found no consistent relationship between the potency and selectivity of a suspension and the profusion of granulomas or the prominence of fibrosis in the spleen from which it was derived. Of the nine spleens which provided acceptable suspensions, four showed extensive haline fibrosis. One of these (K12), which was validated alongside lot 10 of Siltzbach's spleen J and provided our reference suspension, was grossly fibrotic with almost complete obliteration of splenic architecture; while another (K41) which showed similar potency and selectivity showed a large number of follicular granulomas with central necrosis. Like Putkonen (1964), we have found no correlation between the Kveim reactivity of the donor of a sarcoid tissue and the potency and selectivity of a suspension derived from it. Of the nine patients providing spleens from which acceptable suspensions were prepared, four were Kveim-reactive and four non-reactive; the remaining donor had not been tested.

The initial validation of a spleen as a source of Kveim test suspension may be undertaken with a lot prepared from one of the portions into which the spleen has been divided for storage (Mitchell, *et al.*, 1976), or from an aliquot of a suspension prepared from the whole spleen (Douglas *et al.*, 1976). The former procedure would be justified if it were found that sequential lots prepared from other parts of a spleen behave similarly to that initially validated, as has been found to be the case with sequential lots of several sarcoid spleens in London. On the other hand, it may be that discrepant results with later lots of the Australian CSL suspension, discussed below, may be at least partly due to differences in activity of different parts of this spleen. If the whole spleen is processed at once and stored as a suspension, and there are variations between parts of it, the bulk suspension would be expected to be less potent or selective than suspensions from the 'best' parts of it.

The proportions of patients with sarcoidosis reported to have given reactions interpreted as positive in studies with some validated suspensions which have been widely used are summarized in Table 21.1. In general, two-thirds to three-quarters of patients within two years of the onset of sarcoidosis reacted, the proportion falling with increasing duration of disease. Correspondingly, up to 90% of those found radiographically to have hilar lymph-node enlargement reacted, while of those with pulmonary infiltration only, less than half reacted. Siltzbach (1961b) reported the results of tests repeated after varying intervals in 97 patients who gave 'positive' reactions initially. Of those re-tested after periods up to one year, 84% still reacted; after 1–3 years, 68%; after 3–5 years, 50%; and after longer periods up to 15 years, 38%.

Several test suspensions prepared in the manner outlined above have been reported to have been stored for prolonged periods without loss of potency or selectivity. Siltzbach (1976) found that vials of suspensions prepared from spleen J kept at 4°C for eight years and at room temperature for five years had retained these qualities. One of us (DNM) has performed tests after storage at room temperature, at 4°C and at −20°C for periods up to seven years with lot 1, and up to ten years with lot 5, of spleen K12; all, including those stored at room temperature, continued to produce granulomatous reactions in the expected proportions of patients with sarcoidosis.

Kennedy (1967) found that a test-suspension could be freeze-dried and reconstituted without loss of potency; but in view of the keeping qualities of suspensions, freeze-drying does not appear to offer sufficient advantage to justify the extra steps involved.

The behaviour of later lots of the Australian CSL suspension differed from that of earlier lots, results of an international study with which were in line with those with other widely-used suspensions, and are included in Table 21.1. This suspension was prepared from a spleen weighing 1.2 kg and containing many epithelioid and giant-cell granulomas, removed from a woman with a six year history of sarcoidosis because of haemolytic anaemia (Hurley and Bartholomeusz, 1968). Lots 004 and 005 from this spleen produced granulomatous reactions not only in higher proportions of patients with sarcoidosis at various stages than earlier lots, but also in considerable proportions both of patients with a wide range of other diseases, and of normal subjects (Hurley and Sullivan, 1974; Izumi *et al.*, 1974; Hurley *et al.*, 1975). Four possible explanations of these findings have been suggested:

(1) In the original validation of this spleen, a test site at which there was no visible or palpable reaction was not submitted to biopsy, the test being recorded as negative. In view of the selectivity of early lots of CSL, with very low proportions of 'positive' reactions in non-sarcoid subjects reported in the international study, failure to biopsy unremarkable sites in the validation study could not account for the different behaviour of some later lots.

(2) In the preparation of lots 004 and 005, which were more potent and much less selective in induction of granulomatous reactions, the additional step of filtration through muslin was introduced. This might

conceivably have given rise to foreign-body reactions, though the published reports contain no reference to the finding of fibres in the microscopy of the reactions. But Hurley *et al.* (1975) prepared a further lot 006, without this filtration, and this lot, while slightly less potent than lot 005, showed almost as poor selectivity.

(3) Different parts of the spleen, which had been stored deep-frozen in approximately 100 g portions from which successive lots were prepared, might differ in content of various granuloma-producing components. No further lots were prepared after lot 006, and there is thus no evidence relevant to this possibility for this spleen. Kooij *et al.* (1976) studied six suspensions prepared from portions of one spleen, and found wide differences in potency with patients with sarcoidosis.

(4) Changes might have occurred in the spleen during storage.

The available evidence suggests that the probable explanation is either (3), (4), or a combination of these. This indicates the need for close monitoring of suspensions from successive portions of a spleen when they first come into use, in addition to the initial full validation.

GRANULOMATOUS RESPONSES NOT ASSOCIATED WITH SARCOIDOSIS

Test-suspensions that have been validated satisfactorily may produce granulomatous reactions in a few individuals with no evidence of sarcoidosis. Such reactions are often called 'false positives', implying that the Kveim reaction is 'specific' for sarcoidosis. This usage is undesirable, for two reasons. Until pathogenesis, both of sarcoidosis and of the Kveim reaction is elucidated, the sense in which this reaction can be said to be specific remains unclear, and its occurrence with special frequency in patients with sarcoidosis is best described as selectivity for sarcoidosis. And among individuals not suffering from sarcoidosis, granulomatous reactions do not occur randomly, but with special frequency in certain specifiable groups. They have been reported more frequently with some well-validated suspensions than with others.

Mycobacterial infections

Although those sarcoid tissue suspensions that have been validated for their selectivity for sarcoidosis cause few reactions in patients with mycobacterial tuberculosis, some suspensions have been reported to cause granulomatous reactions in a higher proportion of tuberculosis patients than of other subjects. Israel and co-workers reported a remarkable difference in this respect between two suspensions prepared at different times from the cervical lymph-nodes of the same patient with sarcoidosis. That first prepared produced granulomatous nodules in 12 of 57 tests in 28 patients with sarcoidosis, in 14 of 27 in 33 patients with tuberculosis, and in two of 24 other subjects (Israel and Sones, 1955). Two years later, a second suspension prepared from much-enlarged nodes from the neck of the same patient gave well-defined granulomatous reactions in 13 of 46 patients with sarcoidosis, and none of 29 with tuberculosis (Israel *et al.*, 1958). Daniel and Schneider (1962) tested ten patients with active tuberculosis, two with histoplasmosis and one with coccidioidomycosis with a Kveim suspension which had been found to give reactions in more than 90% of a large series of patients with sarcoidosis and in about 2% of a larger control series. Eight of the 13 patients, in all of whom the diagnosis of the specific infection was undoubted, gave reactions containing well-formed epithelioid cell granulomas and interpreted as positive by two independent observers, one of whom regarded an additional reaction as positive.

Patients with sarcoid-like clinical features from whose tissues or secretions *M. tuberculosis* is isolated (Chapter 23) may give granulomatous responses to a Kveim test, which thus in these circumstances is not decisive in diagnostic categorization. Kent *et al.* (1970) reported 30 patients with sarcoid-like clinical, radiographic and histological features who were intensively investigated for identifiable aetiological agents. *M. tuberculosis* was isolated by culture from tissues or from secretions in 17; in five of these, Kveim tests were performed, and produced granulomatous responses in four. Granulomatous responses in patients with tuberculous lymphadenitis have been reported by Israel and Goldstein (1971) and Mikhail and Mitchell (1971). The three patients reported by Mikhail and Mitchell all showed some sarcoid-like clinical features, though they reacted to tuberculin; the diagnosis of tuberculosis was made by mediastinoscopy, lymphnodes removed showing in two histological changes interpreted as caseating tuberculosis with subsequent culture of tubercle bacilli, and in the third sarcoid-like granulomas with central necrosis and acid-fast bacilli, though cultures were negative.

BCG vaccination

Granulomatous reactions to Kveim tests were found in a high proportion of a small group of healthy individuals who had failed to become tuberculin-positive ('convert') after two vaccinations with BCG (D'Arcy Hart *et al.*, 1964). Of 13 598 who had been vaccinated with BCG at the beginning of a multi-centre study of its protective effect, only 58 remained persistently tuberculin-negative during 8–10 years' observation. Of these, 19 were available for further study, and were revaccinated; seven converted and 12 failed to convert. Both those who converted after this second vaccination and those who did not, and representative small groups, both of subjects who had converted after one vaccination and of those who had originally been reactors and non-reactors to tuberculin and had not been vaccinated, were tested with a well-validated suspension, lot 8 of spleen J. Among 12 subjects who had failed to convert after two BCG vaccinations, ten produced nodules ranging from 5–8 mm in diameter four weeks after the intradermal injection of the Kveim suspension. Of these ten nodules, seven were read histologically as positive, one equivocal and two negative by one assessor, and four as positive, three as equivocal and three as negative by the other. Among seven subjects who had failed to convert after one BCG vaccination, but had converted after a second, three produced small nodules, 1–4 mm in diameter; three were read histologically as positive, one as equivocal and three as negative by one assessor, and two as positive and five as negative by the other. Among 25 subjects vaccinated once, either in the past or recently, and converting, 18 showed nodules ranging from 1–6 mm in diameter; five reactions were read histologically as positive, two as equivocal and 18 as negative by one assessor, and two positive, two equivocal and 21 as negative by the other. Among 15 subjects who had not been vaccinated with BCG, but were naturally reactors to tuberculin, 12 produced nodules 1–4 mm in diameter: one of these was read histologically as positive and one as equivocal by one assessor only, and these were both in weak reactors to tuberculin. Among eight tuberculin-negative and unvaccinated subjects, no nodules appeared, and no biopsies were assessed as positive. Thus there was a systematic difference in the levels of the reading of the two assessors; but both read a high proportion of reactions as positive in subjects who had failed to convert after two BCG vaccinations, and a small proportion in those who had converted after vaccination, while among the unvaccinated, no tuberculin-negative subject reacted and one initially tuberculin-positive subject had a reaction interpreted as positive by one observer.

The proportion of the subjects who had failed to convert after two BCG vaccinations reported by one of the assessors to show a positive Kveim reaction was of the same order as that reported with the same suspension in patients with sarcoidosis. Detailed study of all these subjects was not possible, since they were quite healthy; but complete physical examination and chest radiographs at the time of this study and at irregular intervals during the period of about ten years which had elapsed since the beginning of the BCG trial in all of them, and biochemical studies and slit-lamp examination of the eyes in some who were available for such studies showed no abnormalities. Moreover, none of them had had any evident illness or symptoms in the past, such as erythema nodosum or an unexplained inflammatory disease of the eye, which might have been a manifestation of sarcoidosis. It thus seems improbable that their peculiar reactivity could be explained on the ground that they were suffering from some inapparent form of sarcoidosis. Two other possible explanations must be considered.

Some healthy individuals might for reasons at present unknown be normally, or become temporarily, non-converters to BCG and Kveim reactors and thus the process of BCG vaccination in the trial selected natural Kveim reactors; or BCG vaccination may increase Kveim reactivity. These are not mutually exclusive. The hypothesis that BCG vaccination was a cause of the Kveim reactivity received support from the finding that among those vaccinated once, and converting normally, a small proportion produced granulomatous nodules. But this alone cannot explain all the observations. If BCG vaccination were the sole factor, those vaccinated twice would be expected to show a similar incidence of positive reactions whether or not they converted after the second vaccination; but in fact those vaccinated twice and converting showed an incidence of positive reactions similar to those vaccinated once and converting, while those failing to convert after two vaccinations showed more and larger reactions than either of these groups. Moreover, the latter group differed from all others in showing a generally diminished reactivity to an intradermal test with a *Candida* antigen. These observations could be explained on the hypothesis that non-conversion after BCG vaccination is due to an underlying abnormality of reactivity, of which another manifestation is an increase in a normally slight tendency to become Kveim reactive after BCG vaccination. Those in whom the underlying abnormality persisted would be expected both to fail to convert after the second BCG vaccination and to have developed a strong tendency to give a granulomatous response to Kveim test suspension, while those who had reverted to normal reactivity by the time the second BCG vaccination was performed would convert as a result of it and show only the slight effect of the vaccination alone on liability to react to Kveim suspension.

The seven subjects who did not convert after two BCG vaccinations and had large granulomatous reactions to Kveim suspension remained healthy and were retested three years later with the same suspension. Six again showed large papules, but histologically these were now assessed as positive in only one, equivocal in two, and negative in four. This is comparable to the waning of Kveim reactivity in regressing sarcoidosis; but all seven of these subjects further observed for a total of 15 years showed no evidence of overt sarcoidosis.

Attempts to repeat these observations have been unsuccessful. This may well be because it has not been, and may never be, possible to reproduce the circumstances of this study, in which a few unusual reactors were discovered during prolonged supervision of participants in a large-scale BCG trial. Mitchell *et al.* (1967) studied responses to Kveim tests in 37 subjects who had not converted to tuberculin sensitivity after BCG vaccination. At the first test, 19 showed small nodules, 1–3 mm in diameter, and 18 no visible reaction. Five months after a second BCG vaccination, a second Kveim test was given; 18 subjects now showed nodules 4 mm or more in diameter, 14 nodules 1–3 mm in diameter, and five no nodule. Histologically, all the sites after the first Kveim test were read as negative; of the tests after the second vaccination, eight showed an equivocal response, with epithelioid cells but no formed granulomas. But all 37 subjects became tuberculinpositive after the second vaccination, and thus differed from those who showed granulomatous reactions in the earlier study. The effect of repeated Kveim tests was studied in 11 subjects who had not been BCG vaccinated; two consecutive Kveim tests at five months' interval caused no nodules, and histologically all test sites were negative. It thus appeared that the 'equivocal' responses observed after two BCG vaccinations were likely to be related to these, rather than to repeated Kveim tests.

Meyer *et al.* (1967) in Paris investigated 41 subjects, aged between seven and 26 years who were found to be tuberculin-negative despite two or more BCG vaccinations, of which the first appears to have been between one and three years before the study. The total number at all ages vaccinated during this time was 2282, of which one-third, i.e. about 750, were stated to be in the relevant age-group. Thus the proportion said to be unconverted by two vaccinations was about one in 18, compared with one in 234 in the British MRC study. Moreover, the French study was performed on subjects identified retrospectively 1–3 years after the initial vaccination, while the British subjects were identified after 8–10 years' surveillance during which a very small group remained persistently tuberculin-negative. Meyer *et al.* performed 45 Kveim tests in their 41 subjects with lots 8 and 10 of spleen J, lot 7 of which had been used by D'Arcy Hart *et al.* In 29 of these tests, there was no visible or palpable reaction at 4–6 weeks, and in 12 small reactions, ranging up to a 3 mm papule, were observed. Thirty biopsies, including all the grossly evident reactions were performed; 24 were 'strictly negative', and six showed 'a follicular and giant-cell reaction' with foreign bodies in the form of birefringent filaments interpreted as dubious. Pasteur Institute BCG was used in this study. Six subjects were therefore vaccinated with the Danish vaccine used in the British study; this gave rise to brisker vaccination reactions, but the effect on Kveim reactivity was similar, one subject showing a dubious and the rest negative responses.

The probable explanation of the differences between the results reported by Mitchell *et al.* (1967) and Meyer *et al.* (1967) and those of D'Arcy Hart *et al.* (1964) is that the very stringent procedure by which the few subjects with unusual reactivity were brought to light in the latter investigation could not be reproduced in the other two.

Israel and Sones (1966) performed Kveim tests before and after BCG vaccination in patients with inactive and active sarcoidosis. Nine who appeared to have recovered from sarcoidosis gave no reaction to the Kveim test either before or after vaccination. Among five with active sarcoidosis, one reacted positively, two positively after some delay, and two negatively before vaccination, and the only change after vaccination was that one who had given a delayed positive gave a negative reaction. Thus BCG vaccination had no effect on Kveim reactivity in patients who had or had had sarcoidosis. Neither these observations, nor those of Mitchell *et al.* (1967) and Meyer *et al.* (1967), conflict with the interpretation, suggested above, of the results of the study of D'Arcy Hart *et al.* (1964).

Although there has been much discussion about sarcoidosis in BCG vaccinated individuals, considered in Chapter 23 (p. 498), BCG vaccination probably does not affect the incidence of sarcoidosis.

Leprosy

The responses of patients with leprosy to Kveim tests might be of special interest, because in leprosy a range of clinical patterns between the lepromatous and the tuberculoid correlates well with the results of the Mitsuda lepromin test, which has some analogies with the Kveim test. Both tests are performed by intradermal injection of a suspension of diseased human tissue; and both cause in reactive individuals a slowly-developing granulomatous nodule (Kooij, 1958; Kooij and Gerritsen, 1958). Although the Mitsuda test is performed with a suspension of lepromatous tissue ('lepromin') which contains many of the causal acid-fast bacilli, Kooij and Gerritsen (1958) found that a crude tissue suspension produced a larger late granulomatous reaction than a more bacillary suspension prepared by the Dharmendra method; and that a 'purified lepromin protein' prepared from the Dharmendra suspension produced only an early reaction of tuberculin type. The Kveim and Mitsuda tests, however, have different sorts of clinical inplication. The Mitsuda test does not distinguish between normal subjects and leprosy patients, for many healthy subjects react to it; among leprosy patients, it distinguishes between those with the tuberculoid pattern, in which bacilli are scanty, who react, and those with the lepromatous pattern, with very large numbers of bacilli, who do not react.

Wade (1951) stated that no macroscopically evident reaction had been observed to Kveim tests in ten patients with lepromatous leprosy in the Philippines, or in 20, some with lepromatous and some with tuberculoid leprosy, in Mexico. Kooij (1964) tested black patients with leprosy in South Africa with three sarcoid tissue suspensions; the mean size of nodules at four weeks was considerably greater in 15 with a tuberculoid pattern than in 12 with a lepromatous pattern, and, depending upon the criteria adopted, between one-third and one-half of the tuberculoid were read macroscopically as positive; three of the nodules were biopsied and showed 'a tuberculoid structure'. The absence of routine biopsy of test sites makes these early studies difficult to interpret.

In an international study of the Kveim test with the New York suspension (spleen J), tests were done on 32 leprosy patients (Siltzbach, 1967); a further 38 leprosy patients in Turkey were studied by Celikoglu and Siltzbach

(1969), using the same spleen suspension. In these studies, the only reactors to the Kveim test were found among the 15 patients in Japan; of these, two were read as positive and five equivocal among ten with lepromatous leprosy, and one as equivocal among three with tuberculoid leprosy. No reactions were observed among five patients in Finland, 11 in Israel, three in Italy, and 38 in Turkey; of these 28 were classified as lepromatous, 13 as tuberculoid, and 16 as indeterminate.

Pearson *et al.* (1969) performed Kveim tests with lots 8 and 10 of spleen J on leprosy patients, predominantly Chinese, in Malaysia. The mean diameter of nodules, both maximal and at time of biopsy was greater in nine with tuberculoid than in 21 with lepromatous leprosy. Among the tuberculoid, four were read histologically as equivocal, and among the lepromatous one as weak positive and two as equivocal. The two largest nodules, both over 5 mm in diameter, were both read as negative. Nine additional patients, eight lepromatous and one tuberculoid, who were tuberculin-negative and failed to convert after BCG vaccination, were tested; two tests were read as positive, and thus BCG vaccination did not appear to increase Kveim reactivity in this group. A special difficulty in histological interpretation was apparent in the lepromatous, but not in the tuberculoid group; among 18 read as negative, acid fast bacilli were seen at the test-sites in eight, and small foamy cell infiltrations interpreted as manifestations of leprosy in 12.

Mendes *et al.* (1976), using a Type I suspension prepared locally from a sarcoid spleen, Kveim-tested 13 leprosy patients in Brazil; no nodules were present 4–5 weeks after the test-injections, and all sites were histologically negative.

Thus it appears that, with the exception of the Chinese and the Japanese, patients with leprosy are not specially liable to give granulomatous reactions to Kveim test suspensions. In these two groups, small proportions with either tuberculoid or lepromatous leprosy have been found to give reactions interpreted as weakly positive or equivocal. The reason for the special liability of these two ethnically related groups remains unclear.

There is little information about the reactivity of patients with sarcoidosis to lepromin. Weeks and Smith (1945) found that three of ten sarcoidosis patients gave positive lepromin tests; two of the three positive reactors also reacted to tuberculin, and six of the seven negative reactors were also negative to tuberculin. This is in accordance with the general finding that in persons not suffering from leprosy there is a correlation between tuberculin and Mitsuda reactions. Harrell and Horne (1945) found that three out of five sarcoidosis patients gave weak lepromin reactions, while six out of seven with active tuberculosis gave moderate or strong reactions, as did more than half of a control group.

Lymphadenopathy

Israel and Goldstein (1971) studied the relationship of lymphadenopathy of various sorts to Kveim reactivity, testing patients with sarcoidosis with and without lymphadenopathy, and with other forms of lymphadenopathy with CSL test suspension. Fourteen with chronic sarcoid hilar lymphadenopathy, known to have been present for 3–26 years, all gave granulomatous responses; only three of 12 with subacute pulmonary sarcoidosis and little or no lymphadenopathy, and one of 11 with extrapulmonary sarcoidosis and a normal chest radiograph responded in this way. Granulomatous reactions occurred in two patients with tuberculous lymphadenitis, in two with chronic lymphatic leukaemia, and one with 'non specific' cervical lymphadenitis. Two with Hodgkin's disease and two with histoplasmosis did not react.It was concluded that Kveim reactivity was related to the degree and duration of lymphadenopathy. As noted above, others have found that patients with tuberculous lymphadenitis may react. On the other hand, Turiaf *et al.* (1974) tested 12 patients with tuberculous lymphadenitis, and 13 with other lymphadenopathies, with negative results in all but two, one with lymphosarcoma and one with 'lymphoepithelioma' who gave reactions interpreted as equivocal.

Inflammatory bowel disease

Mitchell *et al.* (1969, 1970) performed Kveim tests with a suspension, lot 5, from spleen K12 in 74 patients with Crohn's disease. This suspension, as noted above (p. 455) had been validated against lot S10 of the New York spleen J. Reactions interpreted histologically as positive were found in 38 (51%). A similar proportion of granulomatous reactions was found in patients with Crohn's disease tested with lot 14 of spleen K12 and with lot 0025 of the Australian CSL suspension, which had also been validated against spleen J. Karlish *et al.* (1970), also using CSL suspension, found 'positive' reactions in 13 of 20 patients with Crohn's disease.

Mitchell *et al.* (1974b) extended their observations to include some other chronic bowel diseases. Of a total of 117 patients with Crohn's disease tested with lot 5 of spleen K12, 52 (44%) reacted. Sixteen who had reacted were subsequently tested with CSL suspension, lot 0025, simultaneously with a second test with lot 5 of K12. Eight gave granulomatous reactions to both suspensions. Tests with lot 5 of K12 were performed in 26 patients with ulcerative colitis, two (7%) giving granulomatous reactions, and in ten with coeliac disease, of whom five reacted.

Lot 5 of K12 and the early lots of CSL used in these studies were not unselective; they had both been shown to produce acceptably low numbers of reactions in subjects not suffering from sarcoidosis or inflammatory bowel disease. It seems likely, however, that the production of reactions selectively not only in sarcoidosis but also in inflammatory bowel disease is a property of some suspensions only. Siltzbach *et al.* (1971c) found no histologically positive reactions to tests with lot 10 of spleen J and lot 1 of K12 in 16 patients with Crohn's disease.

Leucocytes from patients with Crohn's disease have been reported to react to some Kveim test suspensions *in vitro* similarly to those from patients with sarcoidosis (see below).

Brucellosis

In chronic brucellosis, granulomas may be found, especially in the liver (Chapter 11, p. 265). Williams (1974) performed Kveim tests with K12 suspension, lots 16 to 18, in patients with confirmed or suspected brucellosis. In 32 attending a brucellosis follow-up clinic, with positive brucella antibody tests, Kveim reactions were interpreted as positive in seven and as equivocal in two. In 11 who had had serological evidence of brucellosis, receding at the time of the Kveim test, reactions were interpreted as positive in one and equivocal in four; the patient in this group with a positive response was a farmer whose herd was heavily infected, whose wife was under treatment for brucellosis, and who himself had had compatible symptoms for more than two years, with an enlarged spleen although serological tests were inconclusive. None of the patients with positive or equivocal Kveim tests had clinical (including opthalmological) or radiological evidence of sarcoidosis.

IMMUNOLOGICAL STUDIES OF THE KVEIM REACTION

Although both cellular and humoral reactions to sarcoid tissue suspensions which have been validated for use in the Kveim test have been studied, results have not been entirely consistent.

Hirschhorn *et al.* (1964) and Cowling *et al.* (1964) found that the rate of morphological blast formation in cultures of lymphocytes from patients with sarcoidosis, already high in the unstimulated state (Chapter 20, p. 429) was increased by the addition of unheated unphenolized sarcoid spleen suspension. Despite this increase in blast formation, Siltzbach *et al.* (1971) found that the addition of Kveim test suspension did not increase the rate of deoxyribonucleic acid (DNA) and ribonucleic acid (RNA) synthesis in cultures of lymphocytes from patients with sarcoidosis. Zweiman and Israel (1976) studied the effect of four Kveim test suspensions on lymphocyte DNA synthesis. Responses of cells from sarcoidosis patients and from normal subjects differed significantly for the CSL and Edinburgh suspensions, but not for spleen J and Ohio suspensions. Synthesis was increased by at least one of the suspensions in cells from 14 of 45 patients with sarcoidosis, and from three of 20 normal subjects. Correlation with Kveim tests was poor; 12 of the 14 whose cells responded, and 23 of the 31 whose cells did not respond, gave granulomatous reactions to Kveim tests.

In direct *in vitro* tests, Bendixen and Søberg (1969), Hardt and Wanstrup (1969), Becker *et al.* (1972) and Kalden *et al.* (1974) found that Kveim test suspensions inhibited migration of leucocytes from patients with sarcoidosis. On the other hand, Topilsky *et al.* (1972) reported that a suspension of spleen J did not inhibit migration of cells from patients who had given granulomatous reactions to Kveim tests with a suspension from the same spleen; Horsmanheimo *et al.* (1980) had similarly negative results in direct migration inhibition tests with a suspension from another well-validated spleen, B; and Zweiman and Israel (1976) found only slight differences in direct migration inhibition tests with four Kveim test suspensions between leucocytes from sarcoidosis patients and from normal subjects. Using a test of migration inhibition in an agarose medium, Hardt *et al.* (1976) observed no inhibition of leucocytes from sarcoidosis patients by a Kveim test suspension which, however, caused reactions interpreted as positive in only seven of the 50 patients tested; on the other hand, Schubotz *et al.* (1980) using a similar technique and a sarcoid spleen suspension, whose validation was not described, found that migration of leucocytes from 25 patients with sarcoidosis was inhibited, more in the acute than in the chronic stages.

Tests for production of leucocyte migration inhibition factor (LMIF) by cells stimulated with Kveim test suspensions have given similarly variable results. Jones-Williams *et al.* (1972, 1974) found that LMIF was produced in response to lot 14 of K12 by cells from 20 of 26 patients with sarcoidosis, four of 11 with tuberculosis, four of 16 with Crohn's disease, and only one of 20 normal subjects. LMIF correlated well with response to Kveim test, with the exception that it was found more frequently in patients with long-standing sarcoidosis; it was reduced, like Kveim test reactivity, in those receiving corticosteroid treatment. Jones-Williams *et al.* pointed out that the concentration of the test suspension they used (250 μg ml^{-1}) was much higher than the 8 μg ml^{-1} used by Topilsky *et al.* (1972) in their direct migration inhibition tests which gave negative results. Horsmanheimo *et al.* (1980) studied the responses of lymphocytes from patients with sarcoidosis to three spleen suspensions; one from a sarcoid spleen that had been validated as a Kveim test suspension, one from a Hodgkin's disease spleen, and one from a normal spleen. In the two-step MIF agarose assay of Clausen (1973), no significant production of LMIF was found in response to any of these at the concentration of 100 μg ml^{-1}.

Kveim test suspensions have been shown to inhibit leucocyte migration in a proportion of patients with Crohn's disease. Brostoff and Walker (1971) found that lot 14 of spleen K12 had this effect in 14 of 30 patients with this disease; no such effect was observed in patients with ulcerative colitis. Willoughby and Mitchell (1971) reported similar findings with a suspension from spleen K19 in 12 of 18 patients with Crohn's disease, and no effect on cells from patients with ulcerative colitis. Pagaltsos *et al.* (1971), also using a K19 suspension, observed inhibition of leucocyte migration in four of ten patients with coeliac disease and 16 of 17 with dermatitis herpetiformis. As mentioned above, Jones-Williams *et al.* (1972) found that LMIF was produced in response to lot 14 of K12 by cells from four of 16 patients with Crohn's disease.

Using the complex electrophoretic method of Field *et al.* (1970), Caspary and Field (1971) found evidence that lymphocytes from patients with sarcoidosis who had negative or weak tuberculin reactions were sensitized to tuberculin and to Kveim test suspension. Lymphocytes from patients with Crohn's disease, and with systemic lupus erythematosus, and from two healthy subjects who had failed to become tuberculin-positive after repeated BCG vaccination were similarly sensitized. The addition of 1:60 sarcoid serum, but not normal serum, to the system blocked the reactions indicating sensitization, suggesting that *in vivo* sensitivity might be masked by inhibitory factors in the serum.

Attempts to demonstrate antibodies against component(s) of Kveim test suspensions have been reported by Favez and Leuenberger (1971) and Bergmann *et al.* (1979). Favez and Leuenberger (1971) sought antibodies in the sera of 75 patients with biopsy-confirmed sarcoidosis and of 90 control subjects by the passive haemagglutination method. The sarcoidosis patients showed a higher range of titres, from 1:640–1:10 240, than the controls, who ranged from no haemagglutination to 1:2560, but there was considerable overlap between 1:640 and 1:2560, 50 of the sarcoidosis patients and 22 of the controls having titres in this range. The two controls with the highest titres were both suffering from pulmonary tuberculosis, with no evidence of sarcoidosis, and non-reactive to Kveim tests. In a further study of 54 sarcoid and 30 normal sera, reactions to sarcoid and to normal spleen suspensions were compared. Antibodies to normal and to sarcoid spleen were found in both sarcoid and normal sera in similar ranges to those observed in the first study. Thus circulating antibodies were found by this sensitive technique to a component present in both normal and sarcoid spleens in many non-sarcoid sera, and at a generally higher level in patients with active sarcoids. Bergmann *et al.* (1979) sought evidence of antigenicity in Kveim test suspensions by attempting to induce antibodies in rabbits. They prepared suspensions from sarcoid lymph-nodes and spleens, and injected them intravenously five times at weekly intervals, with Freund's complete adjuvant on all but the first occasions. Sera of the injected animals showed up to three precipitation lines against Kveim test suspensions in

Ouchterlony tests; after absorption with normal lymph-node and spleen suspensions, a single band persisted. Similar results were obtained with counter-immunoelectrophoresis.

In view of the particulate nature of the granuloma-inducing component of Kveim test suspensions, these serological findings are difficult to interpret.

PATHOGENESIS OF THE KVEIM REACTION

It is well established that there exists in particulate suspensions from sarcoid tissues, both freshly granulomatous and hyalinized, though in varying amount, a component capable of causing after intradermal injection the slow development of an epithelioid cell granuloma of sarcoid character in a high proportion of patients with active sarcoidosis; that the proportion of patients giving granulomatous responses diminishes with increasing chronicity of sarcoidosis; that such reactions have not been produced consistently by any material not derived from human tissue; that other components that may be present in human tissues may cause banal inflammatory reactions, possibly with a granulomatous component, in a non-selective manner; that some suspensions shown to produce granulomatous reactions selectively in the expected proportions of patients with sarcoidosis produce similar reactions in appreciable proportions of patients with inflammatory bowel disease, especially of the Crohn's type; and that of a few normal subjects who remain persistently tuberculin-negative after two technically satisfactory BCG vaccinations, a high proportion show granulomatous responses to well-validated suspensions. The reasons for these findings and their significance in relation to the pathogenesis and aetiology of sarcoidosis remain unknown. The component responsible for selective granulomatous reactions is known to be insoluble in water or in fat solvents, to resist heat, proteolytic and some other enzymes, and moderate acidity, but to be rapidly inactivated by weak alkalinity; it is particulate and probably derived from lysosomal membranes. Its chemical constitution is unknown, but available evidence is compatible with its being a lipoprotein.

Kveim (1941) thought that the reaction he described was an allergic one, presumably caused because some component of a hypothetical causal agent of sarcoidosis was present in the affected tissue from which the suspensions was prepared; and Siltzbach (1961a) claimed that the fact that a test suspension prepared from the spleen of a single patient in New York had produced 'specific' reactions in patients with sarcoidosis in several other parts of the world 'suggests that a common primary inciting agent may be at work'. But the reaction, delayed for several weeks and consisting of an epithelioid cell granuloma, is quite different from that produced by any reagent that detects past infection by demonstrating allergy to some component of the specific infective agent. Kveim reactivity diminishes and may

disappear as the activity of sarcoidosis wanes, whereas allergic sensitivity –
e.g. to tuberculin, coccidioidin or histoplasmin – generally persists. Reid
and Gebbie (1958) tested 21 family contacts of seven patients with sarcoidosis , with uniformly negative results; if the Kveim reaction were a test
for a specific infection which might be latent, some positive results among
contacts would have been expected. Nevertheless, Reid (1964) suggested
that the Kveim reaction might be related to a specific agent if the response
was to antigenic derivatives modified by phagocytosis or by binding to
tissue elements late in the course of an infection.

The only other skin test performed by intradermal injection of a suspension of diseased tissue and producing slowly developing granulomatous
reactions is the Mitsuda lepromin test. This is not specific for infection with
M. leprae, but distinguishes among those infected and showing evidence of
disease between two reaction-patterns, the tuberculoid and the lepromatous
(see above, p. 473). Though the analogy between the Kveim and the Mitsuda
reactions is imperfect, and like all analogies must be regarded critically, it
suggests the possibility that the Kveim reaction detects a special sort of
reactivity, and not a specific infective agent. This hypothesis is entirely
compatible with all the observed facts, including the reactivity of sarcoidosis
patients all over the world to a suspension from a single source.

Attempts to demonstrate an immunological basis for the Kveim reaction
have given negative or equivocal results. Rogers and Haserick (1954) reported that the injection of Kveim suspension together with (γ) -globulin from
a patient with sarcoidosis into the skin of a normal subject caused the
delayed development of a histologically typical Kveim nodule. This observation has not been confirmed (Siltzbach, 1961b), and Webb and Mitchell
(unpublished observations) found that stored sera drawn from Kveim-
reactive patients with recent sarcoid BHL failed to elicit responses when
mixed with the same test suspension in tests of the original donors after
reactivity had wanted 18 months to two years later. Fordtran (1956) was
unable to induce Kveim reactivity in guinea-pigs or rabbits by repeated
subcutaneous and intravenous injections of an active suspension. He also
found that the electrophoretic pattern of the sera of sarcoidosis patients was
not changed by adsorption with Kveim suspension. Lebacq (1964) sought to
transfer Kveim reactivity to individuals not suffering from sarcoidosis by
intradermal injection of leucocytes from patients with active sarcoidosis
around the site at which a test-suspension derived from sarcoid lymph-
nodes was injected at the same time. The conventional suspension produced
discrete granulomatous reactions in three of four subjects; 'purification' of
the suspension by ultrasonication and ether extraction resulted in reduction
of the number of granulomatous reactions to one of four subjects tested.
This suggestive result has not been confirmed with any of the widely used
validated spleen suspensions.

The lack of a satisfactory explanation of the Kveim reaction does not detract from its value in some diagnostic contexts, discussed in Chapter 26. The elucidation of the origin and chemical nature of the component or components of an active Kveim suspension which can incite granuloma-formation selectively, and of the characteristics, possibly immunological, which distinguish individuals susceptible to induction of granulomas in this way would be an outstanding contribution to the solution of the problems of the pathogenesis and aetiology of sarcoidosis.

Chapter 22

Beryllium Disease

Exposure to beryllium and to some of its compounds is known to be associated with two sorts of disease: an acute form involving the respiratory tract in an inflammatory reaction which seems capable of complete resolution, and a chronic form, appearing at a variable and often long interval after exposure, characterized by systemic as well as lung changes having a histological structure resembling that of sarcoidosis, and generally leading to irreversible fibrotic changes in the lungs. Since these diseases have been well described in a number of publications (Vorwald *et al.*, 1950; Archives of Industrial Health, February 1959; Tepper *et al.*, 1961; Stoeckle *et al.*, 1969; Freiman and Hardy, 1970) only a brief summary of the established facts about them will be given here, as an introduction to a discussion of the resemblances and differences between chronic beryllium disease and 'idiopathic' sarcoidosis.

Sources and uses of beryllium

Beryllium is derived from the ore beryl, an aluminium beryllium silicate. Beryl itself has not been associated with disease, but metallic beryllium, beryllium oxide, beryllium sulphate and fluoride which are encountered in extraction processes, and complex silicates of beryllium and zinc at one time used as a phosphor in fluorescent electric lamps, have all been incriminated as causes of acute or chronic disease.

Beryllium has wide applications in industry. The addition of beryllium to copper in proportions up to 3% gives alloys which are strong and hard, resistant to corrosion, non-magnetic, non-sparking and with good elastic properties, while retaining high electrical conductivity. Such alloys can also be tempered and made into springs. Alloys with some other metals – e.g.

aluminium, magnesium and nickel – also have useful properties. Because of its low atomic weight, it is transparent to X-rays, and has been used in X-ray tube windows. The oxide is very stable and has good thermal conductivity, and for this reason finds applications as a refractory for special purposes. Beryllium and its oxide are good sources of neutrons under nuclear bombardment, and have uses in the atomic energy field. The use of beryllium-containing phosphors in fluorescent lamps has now been stopped, because of the high hazard not only to workers engaged in their manufacture but also to persons exposed by accidental breakage.

ACUTE BERYLLIUM DISEASE

The acute disease associated with beryllium exposure has no resemblance to sarcoidosis. Soluble salts may cause an acute rhinopharyngitis and tracheobronchitis, resolving in a few weeks. The most serious of the acute syndromes is a chemical pneumonitis. This may be caused by beryllium metal, the oxide and beryllium phosphors as well as the soluble salts. The atmospheric concentration required to produce it should now arise in industry only as an accidental occurrence; much lower concentrations may produce the delayed chronic disease. The acuteness of the disease depends upon the type of exposure. A brief exposure to a high concentration may cause a fulminating illness, starting within 72 hours and with a high mortality. Prolonged exposure to smaller concentrations causes an insidiously developing illness with cough, retrosternal pain, and progressive dyspnoea, often with low fever. Physical signs include cyanosis, rapid pulse and respiration rates, and widespread râles over the lungs. Depending upon the severity of the case, radiographic changes of variable extent and character appear one to three weeks after the first symptoms. Although the majority of patients with the acute but not fulminating disease recover, the radiographic shadows may take several months to resolve. Some persons who have recovered from the acute disease have been observed to have further attacks on subsequent exposure, but it is not known whether sensitization to beryllium necessarily follows the acute disease.

Pathologically, the lungs in fatal cases (Vorwald, 1950; Freiman and Hardy, 1970), show widespread acute inflammation, with oedema and lymphocytic and plasma cell infiltration of alveolar walls, swelling, vacuolation and desquamation of alveolar lining cells, which may become multinucleate, mixed cellular exudate and proteinaceous fluid in alveolar spaces, in some cases hyaline membrane formation and desquamation of bronchiolar epithelium; and usually less severe inflammatory changes in bronchi. In most cases, fibroblasts are present in the alveolar exudate and in alveolar walls, with focal organization of the exudate and fibrosis in alveolar walls. Giant cells may be seen, but formed granulomas are rarely if ever seen in the acute disease. The appearances are similar to those seen in response to other acute pulmonary irritants and the diagnosis is dependent upon the association with recent heavy exposure to beryllium, and the identification of beryllium in the lung tissue. In some cases, focal necrosis has been found in the liver, but no specific changes have been reported in other organs.

Recovery from the acute stage is usually complete, only a minority of patients later developing chronic beryllium disease. Tepper *et al.* (1961) stated that only 11% of those with acute beryllium pneumonitis had been reported to have developed the chronic disease.

Other acute manifestations induced by beryllium include a contact dermatitis, an acute conjunctivitis, and small localized ulcers due to implantation of crystals of a soluble beryllium compound in the skin.

CHRONIC BERYLLIUM DISEASE

Chronic beryllium disease mimics sarcoidosis, closely in some cases, and some of the early cases were at first regarded as sarcoidosis. After the first publications (Hardy and Tabershaw, 1946; de Nardi *et al.*, 1949; Slavin, 1949), the number of cases recorded in the United States rapidly increased, and in 1952 a Beryllium Case Registry was started. By 1970 this included 756 patients with beryllium disease of all sorts. Of these, 215 had the acute disease only, 47 the acute followed by the chronic, and 494 the chronic disease only (Freiman and Hardy, 1970). Early reports from Great Britain include those by Agate (1948), Sneddon (1955, 1958), Rogers (1957) and Jordan and Darke (1958); by 1971, 16 had been reported (Jones Williams, 1971). Many of the early cases occurred before the hazards of beryllium exposure were recognized, and at a time when the industrial uses of beryllium were expanding. With the introduction of control measures, and of the cessation of the use of beryllium in the fluorescent lamp industry, which had been a major source of cases, acute beryllium disease should no longer occur, except as the result of accidents. But new cases of chronic beryllium disease continue to occur, both from recent exposure in other industries and from delayed response to earlier exposure (Hasan and Kazemi, 1974).

Clinical features

Changes in the lungs are the most prominent feature, and cause the presenting symptoms and signs in nearly all cases, although evidence of involvement of other organs can be found in some. There is in many cases an interval, which may be of long duration, between last known exposure to beryllium and onset of symtoms. Tepper *et al.* (1961) found that among 334 patients, 46% developed symptoms while still exposed or within a month of the last known exposure; about half had a latent period between one and five years, while in 12 (4%) more than ten years elapsed between the last exposure and the first symptom.

The severity and rapidity of onset of symptoms is variable. Dyspnoea on exertion is the principal symptom; it may appear insidiously over many months, or may be noticed first after an intercurrent respiratory infection. Cough, usually unproductive, is the next most frequent symptom. It may be precipitated by exertion, and thus accompany the dyspnoea. In rare cases, changes in the chest radiograph have been the first evidence of disease; e.g. in three of 60 reviewed by Stoeckle *et al.* (1969). The course is variable. Most commonly, the development of fibrosis leads to gradual deterioration; in some patients the condition remains unchanged for prolonged periods; and in a very few, spontaneous improvement, short of complete radiographic clearing, has been reported.

In those with progressive fibrosis, the clinical picture is similar to that of patients with other sorts of pulmonary fibrosis, with increasing respiratory insufficiency and the development of cor pulmonale. Of the 60 patients reviewed by Stoeckle *et al.* (1969), 18 died during the observation period, nearly all of cardiorespiratory causes. Spontaneous pneumothorax occurred in ten; this is certainly more frequent than in sarcoidosis or in cryptogenic fibrosing alveolitis. Clubbing of the fingers, rare in sarcoidosis, was observed in 12 patients, but none developed hypertrophic pulmonary osteo-arthropathy.

Extra pulmonary changes include granulomatous infiltrations of the skin, of the liver, and of muscle, and hypercalcaemia and hypercalciuria. Skin infiltrations similar in appearance to small nodular sarcoids may appear without evident local cause and may disappear spontanously, unlike those due to local implantation of beryllium compounds; their histology is indistinguishable from that of sarcoidosis. Nodules of this sort appeared in the skin of four of the 60 patients reviewed by Stoeckle *et al.* (1969). The liver was palpably enlarged in 13 of these patients; biopsy or necropsy in ten of these showed granulomatous changes in only three. The spleen was palpable in four, all with severe disease; in all it later became impalpable. Peripheral lymph-nodes were palpable in the neck in three and in the axilla in one; biopsies of two palpable cervical lymph-nodes and of two out of three impalpable scalene lymph-nodes showed granulomas. The disturbance of calcium metabolism observed in a minority of cases resembles that seen in sarcoidosis. Stoeckle *et al.* (1969) found hypercalcaemia in two, and a 24-hour urinary excretion of more than 200 mg of calcium in these and nine others of their 60 patients. Renal calculi were found in four; only one of these had hypercalcaemia, and the relationship of the others to beryllium was unclear. Among 535 patients with chronic beryllium disease recorded in the Beryllium Case Registry, 6% had renal calculi.

Radiology

The radiographic changes in the lungs consist of widespread small opacities, some rounded and varying in size up to 5 mm in diameter, and some linear (Weber *et al.*, 1965; Stoeckle *et al.*, 1969). Among the 60 cases reviewed by Stoeckle *et al.* the initial findings were a mixture of rounded opacities of various sizes and linear opacities in 35, 'nodular' opacities between 1 and 5 mm in diameter in 19, and a 'granular' pattern of opacities up to 1 mm in diameter in six. Hilar lymph-nodes were enlarged in 27, but the enlargement was described as mild, less than is observed in sarcoidosis, and always accompanied by changes in the lungs. The initially-observed appearances remained unchanged during five to 15 years' observation in six cases. In the others, linear densities appeared or became more prominent, with diminution in granular or nodular shadows, evidence of contraction of densely involved parts and increased transradiancy of other parts, suggesting the development of fibrosis and emphysema. Fibrosis was evident in upper lobes in 20 and in lower lobes in seven; these changes tended to be symmetrical. Cyst-like appearances were noted in the upper lobes in ten and throughout the lungs in one; of ten patients who developed spontaneous pneumothorax, seven showed these cyst-like appearances. Calcifications were observed in hilar nodes in eight, and in lungs in eight; all those with calcification were tuberculin-negative.

In general, the range of radiographic changes cannot be distinguished from those that may be observed in the course of sarcoidosis, or of the other diseases that give rise to widespread reticulo-nodular patterns (p. 166).

Pathology

Histologically, the changes are widely distributed through the lungs, and consist of varying combinations of diffuse inflammation and non-caseating epithelioid and giant-cell granuloma-formation. The giant cells of the focal granuloma often contain inclusion-bodies; conchoidal bodies of the Schaumann type and birefringent crystals are the most frequent; asteroids may occur but are infrequent. Granulomas are seen mainly in the septa, especially at the margins of secondary lobules, beneath the pleura and in the peribronchial and perivascular spaces. The focal granuloma is indistinguishable from that of sarcoidosis (Jones Williams, 1958); it tends to undergo hyaline fibrosis just as sarcoid granulomas do in some cases. As fibrosis occurs, some peripheral air spaces become dilated forming cyst-like spaces.

The relative prominence of focal granuloma and diffuse inflammation varies. A study by Freiman and Hardy (1970) of 124 cases of chronic beryllium disease from the US Beryllium Case Registry with satisfactory histological material from the lung at necropsy or on biopsy suggested that prominent granuloma formalation may be favourable prognostically. Of a group of 25 patients, in which granuloma formation was the principal finding, with little interstitial cellular infiltration, only one died during observation for periods averaging 11 years. In 55 cases, granulomas were not found or were indistinct, the most prominent change being widespread cellular infiltration and in 44, focal granulomas accompanied diffuse inflammation. In these two groups, 85% of those without and 60% of those with focal granulomas were dead at the time of the study.

Calcific inclusion bodies of the Schaumann conchoidal type occur in about the same proportion of cases as in sarcoidosis. Jones Williams (1958, 1960a) found conchoidal or crystalline inclusions in 62% of 52 cases of chronic beryllium disease and in 88% of 17 cases of sarcoidosis. Freiman and Hardy (1970) found them in 64% of their 124 cases of chronic beryllium disease of the lungs; they were more frequent in those cases with prominent diffuse inflammatory changes than in those cases with focal granulomas as the principal finding. Whether this is due to the persistence of Schaumann bodies after granulomas have become unrecognizable in undergoing fibrosis, as in sarcoidosis (p. 140), remains uncertain.

Pathogenesis: quantitative aspects

Although there is evidence that the risk of development of acute beryllium disease is related to the concentration of beryllium in the atmosphere, and it has been suggested that concentrations of less than $100~\mu g\,m^{-3}$ cannot produce this disease, no such limiting concentration can be defined for the chronic disease. The development of this disease evidently depends upon individual liability, whether this is of the nature of acquired hypersensitivity or due to individual idiosyncrasy, or to a combination of these factors is not known. The amount of beryllium found in the tissues of patients with chronic beryllium disease varies greatly. In the lungs, quantities varying from undetectable up to as much as $4.4~\mu g\,g^{-1}$ have been reported. In one fatal case, samples from different parts of the lungs gave levels ranging from $0.001–0.282~\mu g\,g^{-1}$. In hilar nodes, the levels were generally higher, and in other organs considerably lower, than in the lungs (Tepper *et al.*, 1961). In the tissues of persons with no known beryllium exposure, the largest quantity found was $0.0008~\mu g\,g^{-1}$. In 84 cases of chronic beryllium disease without a history of the acute disease, Freiman and Hardy (1970) found that 85% had less than $0.05~\mu g\,g^{-1}$ of beryllium in the lung-tissue, 11% having between 0.05 and $0.19~\mu g$ and 4% more than $0.2~\mu g\,g^{-1}$. By contrast, three of five with acute beryllium disease had more than $0.2~\mu g$; those with chronic disease and a history of acute episodes showed an intermediate range of levels. Hasan and Kazemi (1974) gave figures ranging from undetectable to $3.1~\mu g\,g^{-1}$ dried weight of lung in six cases of chronic beryllium disease; peripheral lymph-nodes from four of these contained lower, and mediastinal lymph-nodes from two higher levels. Chamberlin *et al.* (1957) found that many lung samples from routine necropsies in the neighbourhood of a beryllium plant showed beryllium in amounts similar to those in the lungs of patients with beryllium disease.

Typical chronic beryllium disease may occur in persons who live in the vicinity of a beryllium processing plant, presumably from the minute amounts of beryllium present in the air, and among the home contacts of workers presumably from the dust carried home on their clothes. Tepper *et al.* (1961) reported that of 395 chronic cases on the Beryllium Case Registry, 47 were 'neighbourhood' cases. Of these, eight lived near a beryllium plant and were home contacts of workers, 13 lived in the neighbourhood without such contact, and 24 were contacts but lived at a distance. In two, in whom the diagnosis was suggested by the detection of beryllium in lung tissue, neither of these factors could be established. The large majority of the neighbourhood cases were in women, and the mortality among known cases was high; presumably many mild cases went undiagnosed.

In view of these facts, definition of maximum permissible concentrations is difficult and partly arbitrary. The United States Atomic Energy Commission proposed that the maximum concentrations in working places should not exceed an average of 2 μg m^{-3}, and in their neighbourhood 0.01 μg m^{-3}.N

The amount of beryllium excreted in the urine is very variable. In a large proportion, perhaps half, of the cases of chronic beryllium disease, no detectable amount is found. On the other hand, workers exposed to beryllium may excrete detectable amounts without showing evidence of disease, and hence estimation of urinary beryllium is of no value as a diagnostic aid.

Immunology

Curtis (1951) found that workers with beryllium derematitis were hypersensitive to beryllium, giving reactions to patch tests with various beryllium salts, though not to the oxide or the metal, or to inorganic salts of various other metals as controls. The test was performed by the application of a 2% solution of beryllium sulphate or nitrate to the skin for forty-eight hours, a positive reaction being evident within seventy-two hours of the application as an acute inflammatory reaction and remaining evident for at least a week. Sneddon (1955, 1958) reported that biopsy of the reaction site after several weeks showed a tuberculoid reaction with giant cells. This is an important observation, distinguishing this reaction from that observed in contact dermatitis. In half his control subjects, Curtis (1951) found that hypersensitivity was induced, a spontaneous flare appearing at the site of the test patch six to sixteen days later. He later (1959) reported that 32 patients with chronic beryllium disease had all given positive reactions while a number with idiopathic sarcoidosis and chronic interstitial fibrosis of the lungs gave negative reactions. However, in some doubtful cases the test gave results discordant with clinical possibilities, and Waksman (1959) and Stoeckle *et al.* (1969) found that in some patients with probable chronic beryllium disease it was negative. Because a positive test indicates only hypersensitivity to beryllium and does not prove that lung changes are associated with it, and a negative test does not exclude chronic berylliosis, and because of the risk of causing hypersensitivity by the application of the test, its use as a diagnostic procedure cannot be recommended.

Reports about the level of sensitivity to tuberculin in patients with chronic beryllium disease vary. Tepper *et al.* (1961) stated that 25% of their large series reacted to tuberculin, and considered that this was similar to the proportion then expected in their part of the United States. In 1967, one of us (JGS) reviewed seven published British cases with reports of tuberculin tests together with two personally observed cases, among which only two reacted, one to 10 IU, later becoming non-reactive, and one only to 100 IU; this was certainlay a lower proportion of reactors than was currently prevalent in Great Britain. Of the 60 patients reviewed by Stoeckle *et al.* (1969), 57 were tested with tuberculin; only four reacted, the reactions being weak in all.

Elevated levels of one or more serum immunoglobulin fractions have been reported in some patients with chronic beryllium disease, but with no consistent pattern or relation to clinical features. Resnick *et al.* (1970) found that IgG was raised more frequently than IgA, IgM being raised only rarely, in similar proportions of patients with chronic beryllium disease, with beryllium dermatitis, and having recovered from acute beryllium disease, and of subjects with prolonged beryllium exposure but no overt disease. Deodhar *et al.* (1973) found that IgA was raised in the majority of 23 patients with chronic beryllium disease, IgG being raised with IgA in two, and IgM with IgA in two and alone in three.

Lymphocytes from patients with dermal sensitivity to beryllium were found by Hanafin *et al.* (1970) to undergo blast transformation *in vitro* in response to concentrations of beryllium oxide or sulphate which had no effect on control lymphocytes. Van Ganse *et al.* (1971) studied lymphocyte responses in a patient with longstanding chronic beryllium disease whom they had previously (1970) shown to react strongly to a patch test. Phytohaemagglutinin response was normal, unlike that of lymphocytes from patients with sarcoidosis, which is depressed; a small proportion of lymphocytes transformed in response to beryllium in concentrations having no effect on control lymphocytes. Deodhar *et al* (1973) found that lymphocytes from 25 of 35 patients with chronic beryllium disease transformed in response to beryllium sulphate, 18 very strongly, with good correlation between severity of clinical disease and grading of blast transformation, but no correlation with immunoglobulin levels. Control groups of normal individuals, unaffected beryllium industry workers, and patients with other lung diseases showed only a very few equivocal responses. Preuss *et al.* (1980) reported tests of lymphocyte transformation in response to beryllium in 571 beryllium workers, among whom 36 showed weak reactions, none persistent on repeat tests; in 47 patients with chronic beryllium disease, of whom 27 gave persistent strongly positive responses and ten weaker positive responses; and in 25 patients with other lung diseases and 51 healthy subjects among whom only one healthy subject gave a strongly positive response, seven healthy subjects and one with lung disease giving weak positive responses.

Lung changes resembling human chronic beryllium disease can be induced in guinea-pigs by inhalation exposure to beryllium, and skin reactivity to patch testing and lymphocyte reactivity to beryllium is also induced, although the level of hypersensitivity does not correlate well with severity of lung changes (Reeves, 1980). There is thus good evidence from both human and animal observations that immunological factors are important in the pathogenesis of chronic beryllium disease, but these factors have yet to be fully elucidated.

SIMILARITIES AND DIFFERENCES BETWEEN CHRONIC BERYLLIUM DISEASE AND SARCOIDOSIS

The differential diagnosis between chronic beryllium disease and sarcoidosis has been discussed by Hardy (1956), by Israel and Sones (1959) and by Sprince *et al.* (1976).

Similarities

The histological pattern of chronic beryllium disease includes non-caseating granulomas indistinguishable from those of sarcoidosis, and like them liable to undergo hyaline fibrosis. Inclusion-bodes of crystalline and conchoidal types occur with similar frequency in both diseases.

Symptoms and signs of chronic beryllium disease of the lungs and of chronic pulmonary sarcoidosis are indistinguishable in individual cases, consisting in varying combinations of dyspnoea, dry or slightly productive cough, and loss of weight, and in symptomatic cases, similar patterns of lung function disturbance occur. In both, progressive fibrosis and disorganization of lung structure may lead to respiratory failure and right ventricular hypertrophy and eventually failure.

The liver and the spleen are enlarged, usually no more than moderately, in a minority of cases of both diseases.

Skin lesions resembling the sarcoids of Boeck, and capable of spontaneous regression may occur in chronic beryllium disease.

An identical disturbance of calcium metabolism with hypercalcaemia, hypercalciuria, nephrocalcinosis and nephrolithiasis occurs in some cases of both diseases.

Differences

The histological pattern in many cases of chronic beryllium disease includes more non-granulomatous inflammation than is usual in sarcoidosis, and in some, changes of this sort especially in alveolar walls are the most prominent feature throughout the disease.

Certain features found in some cases of sarcoidosis have not been reported in unequivocally acceptable cases of chronic beryllium disease. These include uveitis, involvement of salivary and lacrimal glands, generalized superficial lymphadenopathy, gross splenomegaly or hepatomegaly, and changes in the bones of the hands and feet. Erythema nodosum was not mentioned in connection with the large series of cases of beryllium disease reported by Tepper *et al.* (1961); the frequency of its occurrence in sarcoidosis is variable from locality to locality (Chapter 5). Case 2, described below (p. 494), appears to be exceptional in the occurrence of erythema nodosum, although in other respects characteristic of chronic beryllium disease. The proportion of patients developing disabling symptoms and the mortality rate are higher in beryllium disease; and although minor variations in severity of symptoms and in density of radiographic shadows may be observed, the course is generally slowly progressive, possibly with some prolonged periods of unchanging disability. This contrasts with the course of sarcoidosis, much more variable from one case to another, and tending in a high proportion of cases to complete or virtually complete resolution.

The radiographic appearance of the lungs in individual cases of chronic beryllium disease can be matched by those of selected cases of sarcoidosis. But as a group, chronic beryllium disease shows less hilar node enlargement occurring only in association with lung shadowing, a higher proportion with progressive fibrosis, and few, if any, with radiographic lung changes and little or no disability. Spontaneous pneumothorax is more frequent in chronic beryllium disease.

The criteria for the diagnosis of beryllium disease for the US Beryllium Case Registry (Hasan and Kazemi, 1974; Sprince *et al.*, 1976), applied indiscriminately, would result in most patients with chronic sarcoidosis affecting the lungs and with a history of significant beryllium exposure being classified as suffering from chronic beryllium disease. For this reason, isolated cases suggesting that granulomatous changes in the central nervous system or the heart, similar to those recognized as possible manifestations of sarcoidosis, may be due to beryllium (Sprince *et al.* 1976) should be viewed with reserve.

The combination of a history of exposure with a clinical and radiological picture compatible with chronic beryllium disease is an acceptable basis for the diagnosis of this disease, provided that there are no features not characteristic of this disease. Israel and Sones (1959) studied the magnitude of the problem of differential diagnosis between sarcoidosis and chronic beryllium disease. They reviewed 209 patients with an accepted diagnosis of sarcoidosis to assess the proportion in which the clinical and radiological findings were such that, if there had been a history of beryllium exposure, the question of chronic beryllium disease would have arisen. They concluded that 41 would have fallen into this category initially; subsequently the lung changes cleared completely in 20, leaving 21 in whom even after a period of observation, the diagnosis of beryllium disease would have been impossible to exclude.

The amount of help available from special investigations is limited. As noted above, the ranges of levels of beryllium in urine and in tissues in patients with chronic beryllium disease and in various control groups overlap to such an extent that the finding of beryllium in urine or in lung tissue, either at necropsy or in biopsy specimens supports but does not prove the diagnosis, and failure to detect beryllium does not disprove it. The drawbacks and limitations of the beryllium patch test have been discussed above. The Kveim reaction has been reported to be negative in all patients with chronic beryllium disease tested (Hardy, 1956; Dattoli *et al.*, 1964; Stoeckle *et al.*, 1969), but a negative response, especially in a patient with chronic lung changes is entirely compatible with a diagnosis of sarcoidosis (Chapter 21). The studies of beryllium-induced lymphocyte transformation by Deodhar *et al.* (1973) and by Preuss *et al.*, (1980), noted above, suggest that it may discriminate usefully between chronic beryllium disease and sarcoidosis.

We quote three cases to illustrate the differential diagnostic problem. All three patients had been exposed to beryllium. In the first both the initial presentation and the subsequent course were characteristic of chronic beryllium disease. In the second, the initial clinical picture was suggestive of sarcoidosis, apart from the absence of hilar lymph-node enlargement at any time with an unusually dense fine mottling in the lung radiograph, and the subsequent course was more suggestive of chronic beryllium disease. In the third, we remain uncertain whether beryllium was a causal factor.

Case 1   A woman worked for 14 months starting at the age of 19 in a factory making fluorescent lighting tubes, and was exposed to beryllium-containing phosphor. Eighteen months after leaving this occupation, she noticed breathlessness on running or brisk walking. Three months later, she developed morning cough with some mucoid phlegm, and a chest radiograph showed

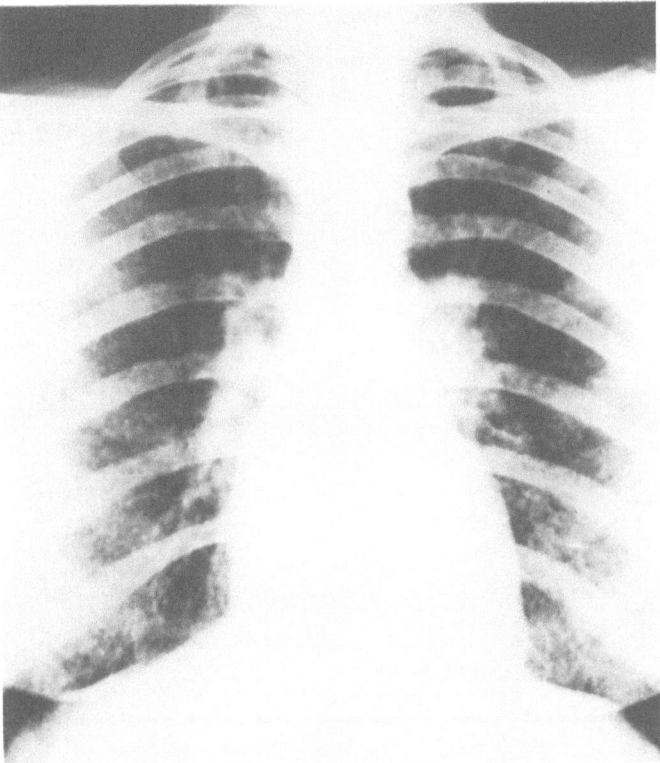

Figure 22.1   Chronic beryllium disease after exposure to beryllium-containing phosphor in fluorescent lamp manufacture, in a woman aged 21.

widespread fine mottling in the lung fields (Fig. 22.1). Eight months after her first symptom and just over two years after the end of exposure, her general condition was good, there were fine crackles over both lungs, but no other abnormal physical sign. Tomography showed evidence of slight enlargement of hilar lymph-nodes. The skin gave a moderate reaction in a Mantoux test with 1:100 OT. A liver biopsy showed no abnormality. Two 24-hour collections of urine showed no beryllium by a method capable of detecting 1.5 μg. In view of the clear history of exposure, a diagnosis of chronic beryllium disease was made. Cortisone 100 mg daily produced slight diminution in the density of the mottling in the chest radiograph and some diminution in dyspnoea on exertion. It was withdrawn gradually after six weeks, and the symptoms and radiographic appearances returned to their former state. Over the next few years, her condition remained unchanged, and she had three pregnancies, all resulting in healthy infants. Towards the end of the last pregnancy, when she was aged 32, she developed first a right-sided then a left-sided pneumothorax, and finally a recurrence of the right-sided pneumothorax, which expanded only after the induction of a chemical pleuritis. At the age of 33 she had a bacterial pneumonia which responded satisfactorily to antibiotic treatment. Thereafter, effort tolerance gradually dimin-

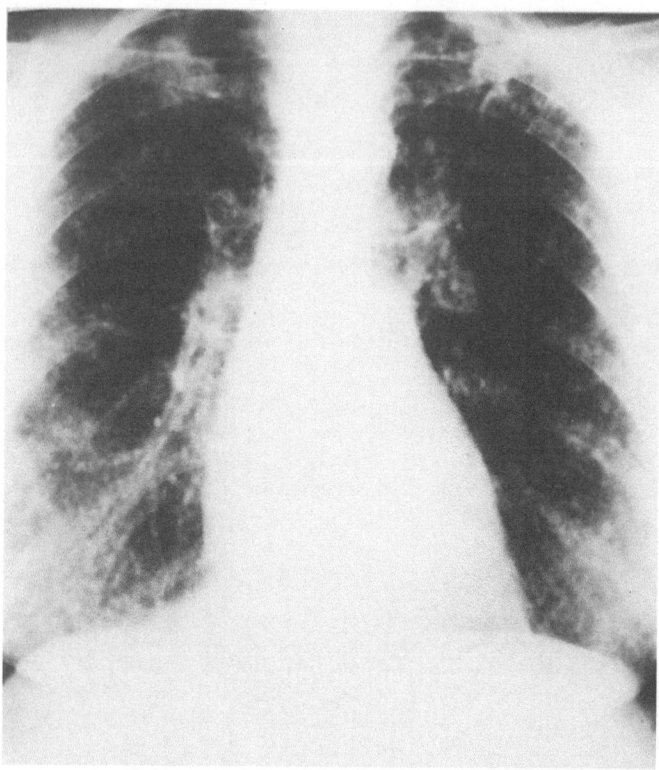

Figure 22.2   The same patient, 32 years later.

ished, but she remained able to run her home. At the age of 53, she could walk two miles at her own pace; function tests showed moderately severe impairments of ventilatory function, principally obstructive, and of gas exchange; and radiologically the only change was that the mottling had coalesced in places to form a coarser pattern, (Fig. 22.2).

Case 2   The earlier part of this case was reported by Citron (1954, 1955). At the age of 18, a woman worked for one year in a fluorescent lamp factory where a beryllium phosphor was used. Towards the end of this time, in April 1949, a chest radiograph was normal. In November 1949, she developed unproductive cough and dyspnoea on exertion, gradually increasing over two years and then diminishing. In March 1950, a chest radiograph showed widespread, fine but dense mottling throughout both lungs. In May 1950, she developed erythema nodosum on the shins, and shortly afterwards, several old scars on the fingers and hands became raised and infiltrated; biopsy of one of these showed the histological appearance of sarcoidosis. The infiltration of the scars subsided spontaneously. In January 1952, the fourth toe of the right foot became red and swollen. Radiography showed extensive soft tissue calcinosis (Fig. 22.3) confirmed by histological study of the amputated toe. Radiographs of the hands at this time showed less extensive calcinosis in the tips of the left little and right ring fingers. In 1953, she noticed frequency of micturition and nocturia, and later discomfort in the eyes. She was investigated at Brompton Hospital in October 1953, at the age of 23. She was thin but not ill, and afebrile. The positive findings on physical examination included many small white nodules in the exposed parts of the conjunctivae especially near the limbus, and chalky white areas on both tympanic membranes, though audiometry showed normal results. The chest radiograph (Fig. 22.4) showed no appreciable change compared with that of March 1950. The Mantoux test was negative up to 1000 IU. The urine contained a trace of protein, a few leucocytes and occasional hyaline, cellular and granular casts, and in a concentration and dilution test showed a range of specific gravity from 1002–1010. A radiograph of the abdomen showed two small flecks of calcification in the left kidney. The serum calcium content was 19.0 and 18.7 mg, the inorganic phosphorus 5.6 mg, the alkaline phosphatase 6.5 King-Armstrong units, the total proteins 8.5, albumin 4.3 and globulin 4.2 g dl^{-1}. There was hypercalciuria, the daily excretion ranging around 800 mg. During one month's observation in hospital, these figures showed little change, the serum calcium at the end of this time being 17.5 mg, and inorganic phosphorus 4.6 mg dl^{-1}. The blood urea remained around 50 mg dl^{-1}. On treatment with cortisone, 150 mg daily, there was a rapid fall in serum calcium and

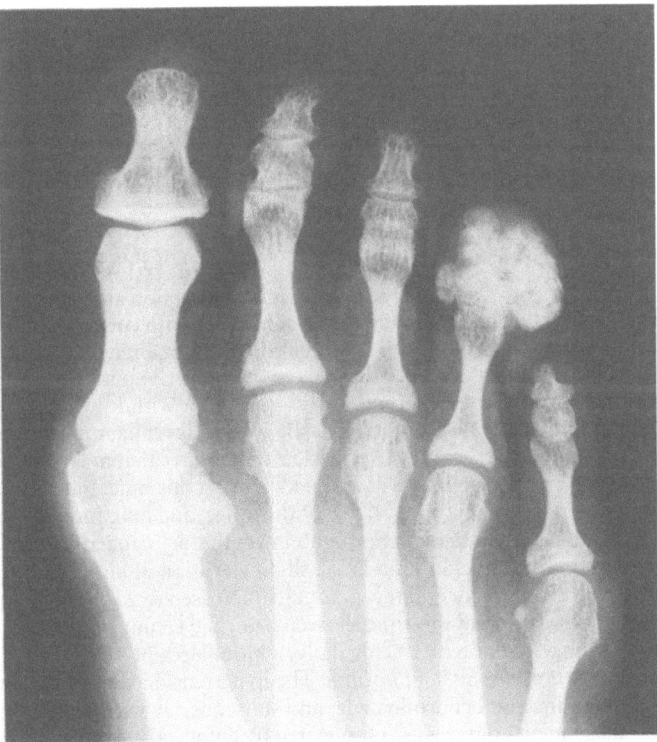

Figure 22.3   Calcinosis of soft tissues of fourth toe in a woman aged 20 with chronic beryllium disease and hypercalcaemia.

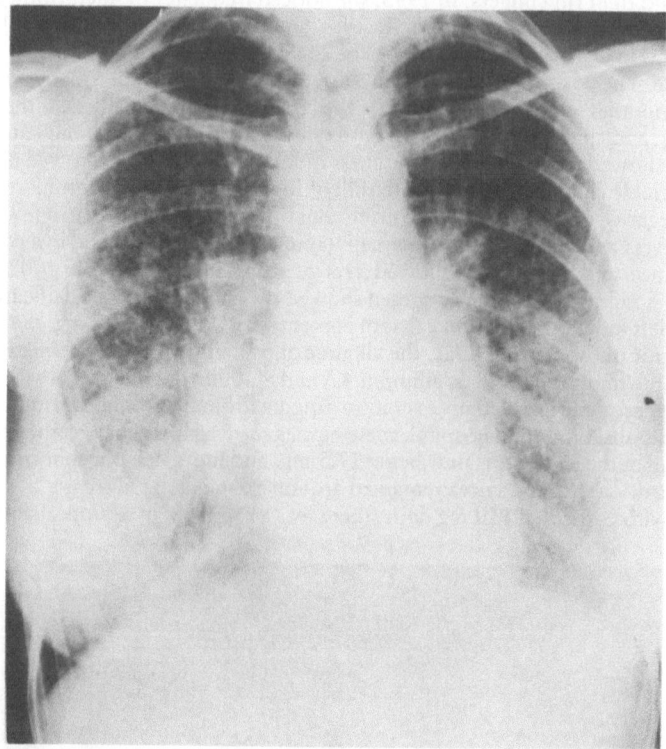

Figure 22.4   Chest radiograph in the same case, showing widespread dense stippling.

phosphorus, and a slower fall in urinary calcium excretion and in blood urea to normal levels. Over the next few years, treatment with cortisone and later prednisolone was continued with the intention of maintaining her serum calcium below 11.0 mg dl^{-1}. The dosage required varied up to 50 mg of cortisone or 10 mg of prednisolone daily. Until 1959, withdrawal of corticosteroid treatment resulted in return of the hypercalcaemia, though the blood urea remained normal; but after April 1959 the serum calcium levels remained below 11.0 mg, and treatment was stopped. During this time, there was little change in the radiographic appearance of the lungs, and lung function studies showed variable moderate reduction both in ventilatory capacity and in carbon monoxide uptake. In June 1957, slight elevation of blood pressure to 150/90 was first observed, and this gradually increased to 210/150 in September 1960. Investigation at this time showed a normal serum calcium level, a urinary calcium excretion of 300 mg daily, a blood urea of 45 mg dl^{-1}, and a urea clearance of 60% of normal. The hypertension was treated initially with guanethidine and bendrofluazide, and subsequently was easily controlled. The subsequent course was complicated by colonization of the damaged lungs by *Aspergillus fumigatus*, first evident in 1968. This was treated by natamycin inhalations. There was gradual deterioration in respiratory function, with the first episode of failure in 1976, and death in respiratory failure precipitated by infection in 1981, 32 years after the exposure to beryllium.

Case 3   A man who had been employed for ten years, between the ages of 19 and 29, as a maintenance engineer in a plant manufacturing beryllium compounds at which a number of cases of chronic beryllium disease had occurred, and whose later employment did not involve beryllium exposure, remained well until the age of 50, when he noticed increasing dyspnoea on exertion. Chest radiography showed small lungs with widespread mottling and bilateral hilar lymph-node enlargement. Function tests showed a small total lung capacity with restrictive ventilatory defect and low CO transfer factor. Mediastinoscopy showed large matted lymph-nodes; biopsy showed epithelioid-cell granulomas with giant cells many of which contained conchoidal bodies. Assay for beryllium showed less than 0.02 μg, the lower limit of the method used, in the whole sample. An itchy papular rash appeared on the back of the trunk about the same time as the dyspnoea; on biopsy it proved to be lichen planus. A Kveim test gave a granulomatous response. A test of lymphocyte transformation in response to beryllium was negative. In this case, the diagnosis of sarcoidosis appears probable, in view of the typical clinical, radiological, histological and Kveim test findings, and the 20 years interval between the end of beryllium exposure and the first symptom.

A note on nomenclature

In this chapter, the recommendations of Tepper *et al.* (1961) about nomenclature of the diseases associated with beryllium have been adopted. Several names have been used for these diseases. The term 'berylliosis' has the disadvantage of suggesting an analogy with pneumoconioses, such as silicosis and asbestosis, in which the disease is localized to the lungs and due to the specific effect of definable quantities of noxious dust in the lungs; chronic beryllium disease has features so different from this that the possible confusion is undesirable. 'Delayed chemical pneumonitis' and 'delayed pulmonary granulomatosis' similarly suggest a disease limited to the lungs.

In some of the early descriptions of chronic beryllium disease the term 'beryllium sarcoidosis' was used. The definition of sarcoidosis suggested in Chapter 3 certainly admits those forms of chronic beryllium disease with a predominantly granulomatous histological pattern in the lungs and with similar changes in lymph-nodes and possibly in liver and other organs into the category 'sarcoidosis'. But the now generally accepted term 'chronic beryllium disease' is to be preferred on several grounds. It conforms to the general rule that aetiology takes precedence over other criteria of diagnostic categorization; it covers those cases in which focal granulomas are not prominent in the histological pattern and those in which changes are detected in one organ only; and it removes the need to specify sarcoidosis as 'idiopathic' or 'cryptogenic' in discussion of differential diagnosis.

Chapter 23

Concomitant or Associated Diseases

I Infections with agents causing granulomatous inflammation

In this chapter, observed and recorded facts about the concurrence of sarcoidosis and those aetiologically defined diseases which are characterized by granulomatous inflammation will be summarized. The chief of these, of course, is tuberculosis. In the next chapter associations with diseases of other types will be considered, and the implications of any association will be discussed in Chapter 25, which concerns aetiology.

MYCOBACTERIAL INFECTIONS

Under the general heading mycobacterial infections may be considered both asymptomatic infection, past or present, with M. *tuberculosis*, or with other mycobacteria, and the disease tuberculosis, which implies specific morbid anatomical changes caused by this organism, with clinically evident manifestations.

BCG vaccination preceding sarcoidosis

Since BCG vaccination is an artificial infection with an attentuated bovine strain of M. *tuberculosis*, it is appropriate to consider here the available evidence about the incidence of sarcoidosis after this prophylactic procedure. The reaction of patients with established sarcoidosis to BCG vaccination and the effects of BCG vaccination on Kveim reactivity have been considered above (p. 416 and p. 469).

Early reports from countries where BCG vaccination was in use suggested that the expected proportion of patients presenting with sarcoidosis had been vaccinated. Among the 212 patients with BHL reported by Löfgren and Lundback (1952) in Stockholm, 25 had had BCG; of these, 17 had become negative reactors and eight remained positive reactors to tuberculin. A number of other reports of sarcoidosis, usually characterized by BHL, appearing after BCG vaccination indicated that the course of the disease in such cases was not unusual (Larsen, 1950; Pfisterer *et al.*, 1954; Birkhäuser, 1957; Fried and Genz, 1958; Jönsen, 1964a). In suspected cases of sarcoidosis appearing shortly after BCG vaccination, histological evidence from lymph-nodes related, even remotely, to the site of vaccination, or from liver must be interpreted with caution; in detailed necropsies of BCG-vaccinated persons who had died of unrelated causes, Gormsen (1956) found epithelioid cell granulomas in related lymph-nodes up to twenty months after vaccination, and in the liver in ten and in the lung in six of 20 cases studied six to forty months after vaccination. Acid-fast bacilli were found only in granulomas in the related axillary nodes and not in those in more distant sites.

Some large-scale studies of the incidence of sarcoidosis among groups vaccinated and not vaccinated with BCG have confirmed that BCG does not significantly affect the incidence of sarcoidosis. Hertzberg (1948), among 18 496 vaccinated in Oslo recognized six cases in which BCG vaccination 'coincided with Boeck's sarcoid verified by Kveim and other tests'. Oudet and Roegek (1962) examined 7500 students yearly at the University of Strasbourg, of whom 40% were BCG-vaccinated; in five years they observed nine cases of BHL, of which three were in BCG-vaccinated students. Press and Wacker (1962) vaccinated 9561 adolescents in seven years; during this time they detected only three who developed hilar or pulmonary shadows suggesting sarcoidosis, 14 months, 20 months and over two years after BCG. Sutherland *et al.* (1965) studied the incidence of pulmonary sarcoidosis in participants in the Medical Research Council Tuberculosis Vaccines Trial, to which reference has already been made in connection with the Kveim test (p. 469). The mean annual incidence of detected pulmonary sarcoidosis was rather smaller among the vaccinated than among the unvaccinated, but the differences were not significant; vaccination, either with BCG or with vole bacillus vaccine, appeared neither to protect against nor to predispose to sarcoidosis.

INFECTIONS WITH *M. TUBERCULOSIS*

Several possible associations between sarcoidosis and *M. tuberculosis* infections may be considered:

(a)   *M. tuberculosis* infection preceding the development of sarcoidosis.
(b)   Clinically evident tuberculosis preceding sarcoidosis.

(c)   Evidence of concurrent *M. tuberculosis* infection in patients showing
the clinical picture of sarcoidosis, with or without clinical features of
caseating tuberculosis.

(d)   Caseating tuberculosis developing during the course of sarcoidosis.

The true proportion of patients with sarcoidosis who have been infected
with, or have diseases evidently caused by, mycobacteria is difficult to
determine. The tuberculin test gives a probably considerable underestimate
of the proportion of them infected in the past; and it is impossible to make
unequivocal decisions about the categorization of some patients with disseminated granulomatous disease having mixed features. These include
some in group (b), in whom an illness initially typical of caseating tuberculosis, confirmed bacteriologically, imperceptibly assumes the characteristics
of, and follows the expected course of, sarcoidosis; and some in group (c) in
whom in spite of the demonstration of mycobacteria, the picture remains
that of sarcoidosis. Observers who include 'unknown aetiology' as a defining characteristic of sarcoidosis may deal with cases of these sorts in one of
three ways: (i) They may withdraw the diagnosis of sarcoidosis. This was
the procedure adopted by Kent *et al.* (1970) in the study described below, in
which they isolated mycobacteria in patients who otherwise conformed to
all normal criteria for the diagnosis of sarcoidosis. (ii) They may dismiss a
single isolation of mycobacteria as an error. (iii) They may conclude that the
patient is suffering from two diseases, tuberculosis, caused by *M. tuberculosis*, and sarcoidosis, about whose cause they profess ignorance, apart from a
conviction that it cannot be related to any already identified mycobacterial
or fungal pathogen.

Those who adopt the first procedure will exclude the case from any study
of sarcoidosis, while those who adopt the second will exclude the evidence
of mycobacterial infection. Those who adopt the third are excluding from
consideration the possibility that mycobacteria or some component or
derivative of them may be concerned directly or indirectly in the pathogenesis of sarcoidosis, if not generallly, at least in some cases.

We suspect that because evidence of mycobacterial infection in patients
with a clinical picture of sarcoidosis is often dealt with in one of these ways,
especially (i) and (ii), the published reports underestimate the frequency of
this association.

(a) *M. tuberculosis* infection preceding sarcoidosis

It is a matter of common clinical experience that in some cases sarcoidosis
occurs in the presence of evidence of old tuberculous infection either in the
form of a past or present positive tuberculin test, or of calcified residues of a
primary tuberculous infection. The proportion of cases of active sarcoidosis

showing old calcified foci in lungs and hilar lymph-nodes has been discussed in chapter 6 (p. 151). In Europe and other areas where coccidioidomycosis and histoplasmosis are not endemic, such calcification can be assumed to be associated with primary *M. tuberculosis* infection. In view of the depression of all delayed skin reactions in sarcoidosis, a negative tuberculin test in the presence of active sarcoidosis does not exclude past infection with *M. tuberculosis*.

(b) Clinical tuberculosis preceding sarcoidosis

The prevalence of tuberculosis in the past has been, and in some parts of the world at the present time still is, so high that a proportion of cases of any chronic disease affecting individuals of a wide range of ages would be expected to give a history of having suffered from tuberculosis.

Among cases of sarcoidosis with a history of tuberculosis, those in which the evidently mycobacterial disease gradually assumes the characteristics of sarcoidosis are most suggestive of a possible pathogenetic factor common to the caseating and the non-caseating granulomatous phases. Among 425 patients with sarcoidosis seen by one of us between 1945 and 1969 (Scadding, 1971a), 24 (5.6%) had a history of various forms of tuberculosis in the past; in seven of these, there was no clear interval between the phases of caseating tuberculosis and of sarcoidosis. The proportions of patients showing these features were similar among the 150 patients first seen after 1962 to those observed in the 275 in the earlier part of the series, in spite of a large reduction in the prevalence of tuberculosis in the general population during this time.

The following are three examples of cases in which features of sarcoidosis appeared gradually during the course of an illness initially showing diagnostic features of mycobacterial tuberculosis, leading to a pattern characteristic of sarcoidosis. In the first two, the initial picture was of pulmonary tuberculosis with no unusual feature:

Case 1   A woman, then aged 17 (Case 2 of Scadding, 1960b), was first examined as a contact of her husband when he was found to be suffering from pulmonary tuberculosis. Her chest radiograph was then normal. Their child, born in the following year, was tuberculin-positive at the age of one year. Seven years after the first examination, a small area of mottling was found in the upper zone of the right lung; the Mantoux test was positive to 10 IU, and tubercle bacilli were cultured once from the sputum and once from gastric contents. Despite treatment with isoniazid and para-amino-salicyclic acid, the lung shadows steadily spread eventually to involve all zones of both lungs. Two years later, the skin was found to be insensitive to 1000 IU, and a liver biopsy showed non-caseating tubercules; the addition of prednisolone to the treatment led to rapid clearing of the abnormal shadows and the subsequent course was characteristic of sarcoidosis, with relapse on withdrawal of prednisolone at first, but eventual quiescence with limited non-progressive fibrosis and no reactivation on withdrawal of prednisolone.

Case 2   A man, aged 39 (Case 1 of Scadding, 1971a), was found to have pulmonary tuberculosis, affecting the upper part of the left lung. Tomography showed a 5 cm cavity, the tuberculin test was positive with 1:1000 OT, and tubercle bacilli were found in the sputum, both on microscopy and by culture. He was treated with streptomycin, isoniazid and PAS for six months, and with the latter two drugs for a further 18 months. Tubercle bacilli disappeared from the sputum after two months of treatment, and the radiographic shadows cleared strikingly within six months. Fifteen months from the beginning of treatment, however, mottled shadowing reappeared at the site of the original disease in the middle zone of the left lung, and there was faint mottling also in the middle zone of the right lung. Over the next 18 months these shadows became denser. At this time, the tuberculin test was found to be negative to 1:100 OT, and there was an unequivocally granulomatous response to a Kveim test.

In the third case, the initial mycobacterial disease presented unusual features:

Case 3   A man, aged 52, presented with a cold abscess of the chest wall, tubercle bacilli being seen microscopically in and cultured from the pus. The chest radiograph showed mottling in the middle zones of both lungs. After nine months of treatment with antituberculosis drugs, the abscess healed. Serial chest radiographs showed progressive increase in the mottling in the lower two-thirds of both lungs. Four years later, a bronchoscopy showed some granulations in the right main bronchus; biopsy showed irregular collections of epithelioid cells, some round cells and fibroblasts, but no giant cells. An old scar on the knee was seen to be infiltrated, and on biopsy showed sarcoid changes. The eyes showed a mild iritis. The Mantoux test with 100 IU was negative. Treatment with prednisolone led to temporary suppression of the pulmonary infiltration, with recurrence on withdrawal of treatment.

The other 17 cases in which there was a clear interval between apparent recovery from caseating tuberculosis and the clinical onset of sarcoidosis are more readily explicable as chance associations. In most of them, the first evidence of sarcoidosis was the appearance of BHL, usually symptomless but in a few with symptoms. Nevertheless, where the interval between active tuberculosis and the first evidence of sarcoidosis is brief, the possibility of some pathogenetic relationship should not be excluded from consideration *a priori*, as in the following two cases:

Case 1   A woman, aged 29 (Case 2 of Scadding, 1950), was treated at a sanatorium for pulmonary tuberculosis of limited extent at the apex of the right lung, discovered after a haemoptysis. Eighteen months later, she developed symmetrical hilar lymph-node enlargement, and supraclavicular nodes became palpable. Biopsy of one of these showed non-caseating tubercles, and the Mantoux test with 250 IU was negative. Later, as the hilar nodes subsided, a faint bilateral pulmonary infiltration appeared, and this too eventually cleared completely, leaving only calcified residues at the site of the old apical tuberculosis. Six years from the first enlargement of hilar nodes, the Mantoux test was still negative to 100 IU. The following year, shortly after a successful pregnancy, there was a strong reaction to 10 IU.

Case 2   A man, aged 22, was found to have pulmonary tuberculosis. After two years of various forms of treatment, including several periods of chemotherapy, a left lower lobectomy was performed. The removed lobe showed a large caseous mass with central softening and many small caseous nodules. Four years later, he was found at routine review to have BHL, without symptoms. The Mantoux test was negative to 100 IU, and a liver biopsy showed typical non-caseating tubercles. The hilar nodes returned to normal size within a year.

In one case, the initial tuberculosis affected cervical lymph-nodes and, after the sarcoid manifestations had subsided, the cervical lymphadenopathy resumed the characteristics of caseating tuberculosis:

Case 3   A man, aged 22 (Case 1 of Scadding 1960b), had tuberculous lymphadenitis of the neck, tubercle bacilli being cultured from the pus. Four years later he developed a generalized superficial lymphadenopathy, BHL, fine mottling in the middle zones of the lungs, splenomegaly and uveitis. The skin gave a moderate reaction to 100 IU. Biopsy of a lymph-node showed non-caseating tubercles. All the sarcoid manifestations subsided within six months. Five years later, a lymph-node in the neck enlarged and softened, sterile pus being aspirated from it, and the skin now gave a very brisk reaction to 10 IU.

The appearance of sarcoidosis after clinically evident tuberculosis is likely to be thought worth recording only if the interval is brief, or the tuberculosis has unusual features. Among reported cases may be mentioned those of Hiatt (1948) in which hilar node and pulmonary sarcoidosis followed two and a half years after primary tuberculosis; of Nestman (1949, Case 7) and of Lindig (1954), in which bilateral hilar node enlargement and skin sarcoids appeared during treatment of proved pulmonary tuberculosis; of Emerson and Young (1956) in which pulmonary tuberculosis with rather unusual features but proved bacteriologically and by response to specific chemotherapy was followed shortly by BHL, splenomegaly, and sarcoid changes in a palpable cervical lymph-node; of Kerbrat and Cellerier (1954) in which miliary tuberculosis merged into sarcoidosis; of Ståhle (1958) in which skin sarcoids appeared three years after successful chemotherapy of pulmonary tuberculosis; of Seshul and Grubb (1960) in which after a very long history of tuberculosis of various organs, including the prostate and the spine, but not the lungs, typical sarcoid BHL appeared; of James (1961) in which BHL and pulmonary infiltration, with sarcoid histology in a scalene node biopsy, developed during chemotherapy of pulmonary tuberculosis; the two cases of Werner (1962) and one of Malecki (1965) in which BHL closely followed successful chemotherapy of pulmonary tuberculosis; and Cases 1 and 3 of Fischer *et al.* (1979) in which pulmonary infiltration having the characteristics of sarcoidosis, with 'positive' Kveim tests appeared in patients under treatment for bacteriologically confirmed pulmonary tuberculosis. The case reported by Lim (1961) in which four episodes of BHL and transient pulmonary infiltration were observed after successful treatment of pulmonary tuberculosis has been noted in Chapter 5, p. 96. Haroutunian *et al.* (1964) described 14 black patients in whom various combinations of features of caseating tuberculosis and of sarcoidosis were observed; five presented with features of caseating tuberculosis, merging into a sarcoid phase. Aberg (1964) observed five cases in which 'post-primary' tuberculosis was followed by sarcoidosis. In Case 2 of Turiaf *et al.* (1965), a young woman was treated for pulmonary tuberculosis with a cavity in the upper lobe of the left lung, and three years later developed BHL followed by widespread infiltration leading to fibrosis complicated by pyogenic infection; at necropsy, there was evidence of sarcoidosis in lymph-nodes with hyalinization of mediastinal nodes, in the spleen, and in the sclerotic stage in the lungs, with cavities containing aspergillus mycelium. Oldershaw and Edmondson (1978) reported the case of a 17 year old man in whom renal tuberculosis, proved by biopsy and demonstration of acid-fast bacilli presented with hypertension; one year after initiation of antimycobacterial chemotherapy, uveitis, generalized lymphadenopathy and lung changes appeared, and axillary lymph-node biopsy showing non-caseating granulomas and negative tuberculin test led to the diagnosis of sarcoidosis.

(c) Evidence of *M. tuberculosis* infection concurrently with sarcoidosis

Two groups of cases may be considered under this heading; those in which at a time when the evident manifestations remained those of sarcoidosis, tubercle bacilli were isolated from secretions or tissues, and those which showed a mixture of features, some associated with caseating tuberculosis and others with sarcoidosis. Both these types of case present difficulties of interpretation. In the first, the possibilities to be considered are that an isolated positive report of an examination for tubercle bacilli is an error in or on the way to the laboratory; that sarcoidosis of unknown cause co-exists with clinically and radiologically inapparent tuberculosis which nevertheless 'leaks' a few detectable tubercle bacilli; or that sarcoidosis is related to a mycobacterial infection in which the bacilli are few and difficult to demonstrate. In the second, unless the non-caseating features affect several organs and are entirely characteristic of sarcoidosis, argument is likely to develop about the validity of the diagnosis of sarcoidosis; and if they constitute a syndrome unmistakably that of sarcoidosis, the point of dissension is likely to be whether all the manifestations are related to the mycobacterial infection, or the caseating ones to this and the non-caseating to some unknown and independent agent or agents. Among the 425 cases of sarcoidosis reviewed by Scadding (1971a), 22 were found to have either tubercle bacilli on culture or acid-fast bacilli on microscopy of sputum, bronchial aspirate, gastric contents or tissues at least once, at a time when all features were characteristic of sarcoidosis. In 14 of these, cultures of sputum or gastric contents produced tubercle bacilli, in one on two occasions; in five, acid-fast bacilli were seen microscopically in sputum but cultures were negative; in one, microscopy of the sputum during life showed acid-fast bacilli, and at necropsy guinea-pig inoculation from lung showing only the non-caseating histology of sarcoidosis, with much hyaline fibrosis, produced human-type *M. tuberculosis*; and in three, acid-fast bacilli were seen in lymph-nodes with the histology of sarcoidosis. In the five instances in which tubercle bacilli isolated by culture were typed, they were of human type and normal virulence for the guinea-pig. In all cases, the clinical course remained characteristic of sarcoidosis as the following brief summaries show:

Case 1   A young man, aged 18, was found at a routine examination to have grossly enlarged hilar and right paratracheal lymph-nodes. A
cervical node removed for biopsy having shown only reactive hyperplasia, an anterior mediastinal node was removed through a small thoracotomy; histologically this showed typical non-caseating tubercles of sarcoid type, but one small clump of acid-fast bacilli was seen in it. Unfortunately, no cultures had been done before the material was fixed. The Mantoux test was negative with 100 IU. Without treatment, the nodes subsided completely within six months. He was known to be well, with a normal chest radiograph and leading an extremely active life three years later.

Case 2   A woman, aged 23, had erythema nodosum with BHL followed by widespread pulmonary infiltration. A cervical lymph-node removed for biopsy showed a sarcoid histology. The Mantoux test was negative with 100 IU. At the time of these investigations, seven months after the erythema nodosum, tubercle bacilli, shown to be of human type and of normal virulence for the guinea-pig, were isolated by culture from one of several specimens of sputum. The subsequent course of this patient's case was typical of sarcoidosis: temporary resolution occurred during a short period of cortisone treatment and later the extrathoracic manifestations regressed spontaneously. About two years from the onset, a group of papules of sarcoid histology appeared on the lower legs. These faded within a year. Last seen six years from the onset, she remained well and free from evidence of disease.

Case 3   A man, aged 26, was examined because his wife had been found to have pulmonary tuberculosis. He had no symptoms, but the chest radiograph showed a localized shadow in the upper zone of the right lung. Although tubercle bacilli were not found at this time, the appearance was so characteristic of a small tuberculous infiltration that in view of the known recent contact he was treated with antimycobacterial drugs for six months. During this time, mottled shadowing extended over the lung fields, although he remained symptom-free. Towards the end of the six months, one out of four cultures of gastric lavage produced tubercle bacilli, fully sensitive. The skin did not react to tuberculin, 250 IU. Liver biopsy showed sarcoid-type tubercules. Without further treatment the lung shadowing gradually cleared, and six years from first observation, he remained well and the chest radiograph was normal.

Case 4 (Case 3 of Citron and Scadding, 1957). A woman, aged 48, who had noticed cough for three years and dyspnoea on exertion for one year was found to have enlargement of the right paratracheal lymph-nodes. One of these removed at thoracotomy showed a central mass of fibrous tissue with peripheral epithelioid and giant-cell tubercles. In one of 23 sputum specimens acid-fast bacilli were seen; 22 cultures were negative. At bronchoscopy, the upper lobe bronchus was distorted and narrowed; acid fast bacilli were seen on microscopy of aspirated bronchial secretions, but not isolated on culture. Antimycobacterial treatment was given. Two years after the thoracotomy, the Mantoux test was found to be negative to 100 IU; an enlarged lymph-node was removed from the neck for biopsy and showed non-caseating tubercles. The scar left at the site of insertion of a towel-clip on the back had become swollen and red, and on biopsy was seen to be infiltrated with similar tubercles. At this time, one out of 14 sputum cultures produced human-type tubercle bacilli of normal virulence for the guinea-pig. Bronchography showed stenoses of the proximal parts of several segmental bronchi of the sort described in Chapter 6, p. 143. Some symptomatic relief of the dyspnoea and wheezing caused by these bronchial changes was produced by corticosteroid treatment, but the patient felt that this did not outweigh the side-effects of the treatment, and eventually it was withdrawn. Nine years after the thoraco- tomy, a gastrectomy was performed for a large gastric ulcer histolo- gically to be malignant; a lymph-node removed at this operation showed sarcoid changes. She died two years later with hepatic metastases from the gastric carcinoma; no necropsy was performed.

Case 5 A woman, then aged 34, was first seen with a history of cough for three years, increasing dyspnoea for one and a half years, gradually increasing tiredness and weakness, and loss of 28 lb in weight. She was found to have low fever, generalized slight enlargement of superficial lymph-nodes, a very large spleen and a palpable liver. Biopsies of an inguinal lymph-node and of the liver both showed sarcoid changes. The Mantoux test was positive to 10 IU. The chest radiograph showed slight enlargement of hilar shadows with widespread mottling in the lungs. During a brief period of treatment with cortisone 100 mg daily, there was temporary improvement. Three months later, one sputum specimen produced tubercle bacilli on culture. When she was aged 36, she was investigated again. The spleen remained very large, and the chest radiograph still showed widespread mottling. The serum protein level was raised to 9.1 g dl^{-1}, of which 5.85 g was globulin. A few small areas of pinkish-brown infiltration had appeared on the skin of the thighs, and biopsy of one of these showed sarcoid. Once again, one of a number of sputum cultures produced tubercle bacilli. Treatment with corticotrophin, streptomycin and isoniazid resulted in defervescence, reduction in fever, in sedimentation rate and in the size of the spleen; but all these manifestations returned when the corticotrophin was withdrawn. Several similar remissions were induced by corticotrophin or cortisone treatment during the next two years, after which it became clear that prolonged corticosteroid treatment was required. The lung changes progressed to fibrosis associated with episodes of bacterial infection causing considerable disability; the spleen became impalp- able; no new skin lesions appeared. She was last seen at the age of 47, 13 years from first observation.

Case 6 A full account of this case has been published (Clinico-pathological Conference, 1950). A woman, aged 40, was found to have extensive mottling in the lungs with evidence of fibrosis, especially in the middle thirds, and with extensive irregular cavitation. Two of many examinations of sputum showed acid-fast bacilli, but these were not grown on culture. The Mantoux test was negative to 1:10 OT. A palpable supraclavicular lymph-node removed for biopsy showed a central mass of hyalinized fibrosis with a peripheral zone of non-caseating tubercles. She died with respiratory insufficiency probably exacerbated by secondary bacterial infection. At necropsy, old-standing sarcoid changes with much hyalinization in most organs was found in lungs, spleen, liver, lymph-nodes and tonsils. Cultures for tubercle bacilli from several organs were all negative; but a guinea-pig inoculation from the lung produced after more than three months tuberculosis shown to be due to human-type bacilli.

In those instances in which mycobacteria were found at a single examination only, the possibility of laboratory or other error must of course be considered. If this explanation is correct, the proportion of such errors in this series must have been exceptionally high; and doubt would be thrown on the validity of the acceptance of a single isolation after many negative examinations as confirmatory evidence of mycobacterial infection in patients with clinical pictures considered to be compatible with caseating tuberculosis. And it is generally recognized that in those cases of indolent chronic tuberculosis that most nearly resemble sarcoidosis, such as those quoted in Chapter 6, p. 166 and p. 168, bacilli are usually very scanty and difficult to demonstrate.

Many cases have been recorded in which tubercle bacilli were found on a single occasion, or in a few of many examinations though clinical and other features were typical of sarcoidosis. The first seems to have been Case 5 of Boeck (1905), that of a young woman, aged 18, with sarcoids of the skin of the nose and cheek, involving also the nasal mucosa, together with enlargement of upper cervical lymph-nodes. In a biopsy of the nasal mucosa, acid-fast bacilli were seen, and inoculation of a guinea-pig gave a delayed positive result. Other early reports of the isolation of tubercle bacilli from tissues of patients with sarcoidosis include those of Von Gebsattel (1920), Mylius and Schürmann (1929), van Hasselt (1935), Berblinger (1939), Bernstein and Oppenheimer (1942, Case 6), Ricker and Clark (1949, Case 9) and Granström *et al.* (1946) in which bacilli were found by culture or guinea-pig inoculation from mediastinal lymph-nodes or spleen at necropsy. Berblinger (1939) found tubercle bacilli only by serial inoculation of guinea-pigs, and Granström *et al.* (1946) were unable to culture bacilli from the tuberculous lesions of an inoculated guinea-pig. Mylius and Schürmann (1929) and Berblinger (1939) stated that the bacilli fround were of human type. Isolation of tubercle bacilli from biopsy specimens has been recorded by Cavara (1928) in a case of uveo-parotid syndrome with lung changes; by Ramel (1934) from a skin sarcoid and also from urine in a young man with generalized sarcoidosis; and by Reid and Lorriman (1960) from a lung biopsy. The latter case is of great interest; at the age of 21 a woman developed a pleural effusion. This absorbed without specific treatment, but increasing patchy mottling appeared in the lungs. Fourteen months after the effusion, the Mantoux test was negative with 100 IU, but culture of gastric contents produced tubercle bacilli. The lung biopsy showed typical sarcoid lesions, but both culture and guinea-pig inoculation produced tubercle bacilli. The lung shadows showed no response to streptomycin, but later resolved spontaneously. Šimeček (1970) reported that mycobacteria were found by guinea-pig inoculation in tissue obtained from mediastinal lymph-nodes by perbronchial biopsy in three of 196 patients showing histological and clinical features of sarcoidosis; they were identified as *M. tuberculosis* in two. Kent *et al.* (1970) reported the results of 'aggressive' aetiological investigation in 30 patients with clinical and radiological features of sar-coidosis, supported by histological evidence from biopsies. Open lung biop-sies were performed in most cases, and repeated in one. All biopsy material was intensively cultured for mycobacteria; this resulted in the isolation of *M. tuberculosis* in 12 cases and of mycobacteria other than *M. tuberculosis* in two. *M. tuberculosis* was cultured at some stage from sputum in a further four cases, and from drainage from a joint in one. Five of the patients from whom tubercle bacilli were isolated received a Kveim test; of these four were positive. These findings led Kent *et al.* to reject the diagnosis of sarcoidosis; but in all other respects than the discovery of mycobacteria on one occasion, most of their cases conformed to all normal criteria for this diagnosis. Addrizzo *et al.* (1971) in a series of 40 patients with intrathoracic sarcoido-sis submitted to scalene node biopsy, mediastinoscopy with biopsy of mediastinal nodes, and open biopsy of the lingula found acid-fast bacilli in mediastinal nodes in two and in the lingula in four; *M. tuberculosis* was cultured from the lingula in one.

Tubercle bacilli were isolated by culture or guinea-pig inoculation from sputum in cases of sarcoidosis reported by Schaumann (1924, two cases, later described again as Cases 4 and 5 in a paper published in 1934), Warfvinge (1943), Lees (1956), Taylor (1958, Case 2) and Reid and Lorri-man (1960, Case 3). In all these cases, the clinical picture remained that of sarcoidosis, and tuberculin tests were negative, though in Lees' case, it became positive six months later. The isolated bacilli were stated to be of bovine type in one of Schaumann's cases and of human type in Warfvinge's. Other cases in which *M. tuberculosis* was cultured from the sputum, although other features and the course of the disease were compatible with the diagnosis of sarcoidosis include those reported by Di Benedetto and Lefrak (1970), Baum *et al.* (1973, Case 5), and Fischer *et al.* (1979, Cases 5 and 7).

Acid-fast bacilli (AFB) were seen in tissues, without confirmation by guinea-pig inoculation or culture, by Kyrle (1921), Ruete (1922), Hudelo *et al.* (1925) and Dittrich (1931, two cases) from skin sarcoids, by Tanner and McCurry (1934, Case 2) in parotid tissue from a case of uveo-parotid syndrome, and by Souter (1929) with difficulty in the myocardium in a case of uveo-parotid syndrome with myocardial infiltration. The observations of Kyrle (1921) have been quoted frequently.

> A man, aged 22, had a recurrent eruption of multiple lesions having the histology of sarcoids on limbs, trunk and face, each recurrence being heralded by a few days' fever. Cervical, epitrochlear and hilar nodes were slightly enlarged, but the lungs were radiographically normal. Serial biopsies showed non-specific inflammatory changes with many acid-fast bacilli on the fourth and tenth days of the eruption; aggregations of epithelioid cells without giant cells and only a few AFB on the 21st day; and a typical sarcoid histological picture without AFB on the 36th day. By the 94th day, only atrophic residua of unspecific appearance were seen. Guinea-pigs inoculated with tissue in which AFB had been seen did not develop tuberculosis, but one of two inoculated with blood taken during the initial fever died of tuberculosis.

The absence of convincing evidence of sarcoidosis elsewhere, and the brief duration of the skin lesions in spite of their showing at one stage of their development a sarcoid histology make the interpretation of this much-quoted observation conjectural.

Koch and Cote (1965), in a comparison of fluorescence microscopy with Ziehl-Neelsen staining, found AFB in the lungs, but not in liver, spleen or heart, in all of six patients with 'an unchallenged autopsy diagnosis of generalized sarcoidosis' by the fluorescence method, but in only two by Ziehl-Neelsen. By prolonged search, Vaněk (1968) found AFB in all of 70 lymph-nodes showing non-caseating epithelioid cell granulomas, without evidence of fibrosis; 23 came from patients with clinical and other findings compatible with sarcoidosis affecting at least two sites. Similar findings were reported by Vaněk and Schwarz (1970) in a further 30 cases; in this series of 29 lymph-nodes and one lung biopsy, 13 came from patients with a clinical picture and course suggesting sarcoidosis involving at least two sites. Rosen *et al.* (1977b) in a series of 128 open lung biopsies from patients with a final diagnosis of sarcoidosis found AFB in three; in all three, tuberculin tests were negative, and no mycobacteria were isolated on culture.

Greenberg *et al.* (1970) in electron-microscopic studies of lung biopsies from five patients with sarcoidosis found inclusions in epithelioid cells which they thought might be atypical or mutant forms of mycobacteria. Leake and Myrvik (1971) commented that similar structures could be found in alveolar macrophages from rabbits injected intravenously with BCG in oil, and suggested that they were cell-derived organelles.

In a few cases, clinical or pathological features of caseating tuberculosis, as well as the demonstration of a few acid-fast bacilli or of scanty myco-bacteria in culture or guinea-pig inoculation co-exist with clinical and histological features of sarcoidosis. In some recorded necropsies in patients whose course during life had been characteristic of sarcoidosis, both caseating and non-caseating lesions were found; e.g. in the case of sarcoidosis involving the skin, optic nerves and orbital tissues reported by Reis and Rothfeld (1931) and by Lenartowicz and Rothfeld (1930) and summarized in Chapter 8, p. 224. Other cases with a clinical picture of sarcoidosis but some caseating lesions as well as sarcoid-type tubercles at necropsy were recorded by Wahlgren (1936) in a patient with lupus pernio and diabetes insipidus, also reported by Tillgren (1935) and Schaumann (1936, Case 3); by Hollister and Harrell (1941); by Erickson *et al.* (1942) in a patient with sarcoid arachnoiditis mentioned in Chapter 14, p. 320; by Ustvedt (1948, Case 3); and by Longcope and Freiman (1952, Case 14) and Davidson *et al.* (1954, Case 6) in a black man with florid generalized sarcoidosis with hypercalcaemia, who had a tuberculous sinus in the axilla. In a patient under the care of one of us (JGS) with persistent cutaneous and pulmonary sarcoidosis who died of malignant lymphoma, a well-encapsulated focus of caseation was found at necropsy in an adrenal gland (Chapter 24, p. 535).

Coincidence of clinical features of sarcoidosis and of caseating tuberculosis has probably occurred much more frequently than it has been recorded. Cases with such mixed features include Salvesen's (1935) Case 4 in which a small cavity developed in the lung in a woman with old-standing skin sarcoids, AFB were found in the sputum, and Bjornstad (1948) later reported that an inoculated guinea-pig developed tuberculosis, and that the patient developed tuberculosis of the spine although the skin sarcoids persisted; Stuart's (1944) Case 3; Larsson's (1951) case in which a man with lupus pernio, nasal granulomas, BHL and lung infiltration died of generalized tuberculosis; case 16 of Rösgen and Heigl (1952); Taylor's (1958) Case 1; three cases of Favez (1963); Cases 12, 13 and 14 of Haroutunian *et al.* (1964); Case 7 of Baum *et al.* (1973); and Cases 5, 6 and 7 of Fischer *et al.* (1979).

Jacobsen (1937) reported the cases of two black sisters who died after illnesses undoubtedly of tuberculous aetiology, but presenting bizarre features, some resembling those of sarcoidosis. They had both been in prolonged contact with their father who died of open pulmonary tuberculosis. Both showed generalized lymphadenopathy of non-caseating tuberculous histology, from which guinea-pig inoculation was negative. One developed cyst-like rarefactions in metacarpals and phalanges and in several long bones, and at this time had a negative tuberculin test, though both earlier and later it was positive, and eventually died of tuberculous peritonitis, tubercle bacilli of human type being isolated. The other repeatedly had negative tuberculin tests, but eventually died of tuberculous meningitis.

In Taylor's (1958) Case 1, a clinical picture characteristic of sarcoidosis occurred during the long course of an illness undoubtedly mycobacterial tuberculosis:

A woman, aged 42, had tuberculous peritonitis confirmed at laparotomy and treated with streptomycin; four years later she developed BHL, irregular infiltration and a small cavity in the lungs, and a small pleural effusion, and tubercle bacilli were cultured from the sputum although the skin gave no reaction to 1:100 OT. Antituberculosis drugs were given; the tubercle bacilli disappeared for a time from the sputum, but reappeared later, although the skin remained insensitive to tuberculin, and histologically typical sarcoids appeared on the arms. Later, the cavity in the lung became larger, skin sensitivity to tuberculin appeared, and shortly afterwards, the skin sarcoids disappeared. After further anti-tuberculosis treatment, the lung changes became fibrotic, and tuberculin sensitivity diminished again.

In a case observed by one of us (JGS), symptomless BHL characteristic of sarcoidosis was accompanied by a partly calcified primary complex of tuberculosis with positive tuberculin test and demonstrable tubercle bacilli.

Blair (1967) reported the case of a girl aged three with indolent ulcerating skin lesions on the limbs and multicystic changes in phalanges of a finger and both great toes. Biopsy of the skin showed, beneath superficial unspecific inflammation, multiple non-caseating epithelioid and giant-cell granulomas, in which on special search AFB were found and from which human-type tubercle bacilli were cultured. A tuberculin test 11 months from the onset of symptoms was negative to 100 IU, but another, six weeks later, was strongly positive. Two small opacities appeared in the chest radiograph in the upper part of the left lung. Treatment with isoniazid and PAS was followed by improvement, with eventual calcification of the lung foci.

Patients showing mixed features of caseating tuberculosis and of sarcoidosis are by no means infrequent, and we suspect that doubt about categorization leads to many of them going unrecorded. Most of those reported from North America are black (Haroutunian *et al.*, 1964), and in our experience many of those seen in London are of West Indian, Asian, or African origin. Most of them present with varying combinations of hilar and superficial lymphadenopathy, patchy infiltration of the lungs, low fever, and constitutional symptoms. They may have non-caseating granulomatous infiltrations of the skin or uveitis. The intermediate or mixed features include a histologic pattern in which there is some central necrosis, of a degree that gives rise to argument about whether it should be called 'granular necrosis' and accepted as consistent with sarcoidosis, or must be regarded as so extensive that it must be called caseation and entail a diagnosis of caseating tuberculosis. In most of these cases, tuberculin sensitivity is of low degree or even absent. Acid-fast bacilli may be demonstrated on microscopy, and mycobacteria may be isolated on culture. In the presence of both these findings a diagnosis of tuberculosis (defined in terms of aetiology) is, of course, made, and the 'sarcoid-like' features are attributed to an unusual reaction to a mycobacterial infection. But in some instances, the only direct evidence of mycobacterial infection is the finding of a very few acid-fast rods on microscopy with negative culture or possibly a single culture producing a few colonies of mycobacteria after prolonged incubation. In such cases, differences of opinion about diagnostic categorization are likely, partly because some observers will accept and others reject the equivocal bacteriological evidence. In other cases, no acid-fast bacilli or mycobacteria are demonstrated; in the presence of low tuberculin sensitivity, a diagnosis of sarcoidosis may be accepted in spite of the rather prominent central necrosis. We have found that the Kveim test produces granulomatous responses in some cases of all these subcategories, especially if lymphadenopathy is prominent, and thus does not help in distinguishing between them.

(d) Caseating tuberculosis developing during the course of sarcoidosis

Just as among the cases of tuberculosis preceding sarcoidosis (p. 500) every gradation can be found betweeen those in which the two phases of the history were distinct and separated by years and those in which the sarcoid phase followed immediately and without any sudden change in clinical features, so the case in which the caseating phase became evident after the sarcoid phase present every gradation between those described in the last section, in which tubercle bacilli were discovered in patients whose illnesses had all the characteristics of sarcoidosis, through those in whom in the late fibrotic stage of pulmonary sarcoidosis, tubercle bacilli appeared in sputum and the disease gradually assumed the characters of chronic fibrotic pulmonary tuberculosis, to an interesting group in whom during the course of sarcoidosis, characteristically sarcoid features disappeared as features of caseating tuberculosis appeared. Additionally, in some cases the manifestations of tuberculosis have been localized and of unusual character.

Among the 425 patients reviewed by Scadding (1971a), eight developed overt mycobacterial tuberculosis, two to 12 years from the first evidence of sarcoidosis. All had lung changes. The evidence of mycobacterial infection consisted in the finding of tubercle bacilli in sputum in seven; one of these also had a cold abscess overlying a focus of osteitis in the tibia from which tubercle bacilli were cultured, and another had radiographic and clinical evidence of tuberculosis of a lumbar vertebra. The eighth developed a cold abscess over the pubic bone from which tubercle bacilli were cultured and a chronic synovitis of the knee responding to antimycobacterial chemotherapy. In all, the skin was non-reactive to 100 IU in the sarcoid phase, and reacted to 10 IU or less in the caseating phase. One died with progressive fibrotic lung changes and right ventricular failure, with tubercle bacilli still present in the sputum, before antimycobacterial chemotherapy was available; the others attained apparent cure of tuberculosis with various amounts of fibrosis after chemotherapy.

The following are examples of these cases:

(1) (Case 3 of Scadding, 1960). A man aged 33, complained of dyspnoea on exertion and cough, and was found to have widespread mottling in the lungs.

Two years later, lymph-nodes on both sides of the neck enlarged, and on biopsy showed sarcoid-type tubercles. The following year he was investigated at Brompton Hospital. The shadowing in the lungs had become denser, especially in the middle zones of the lungs; there was widespread enlargement of superficial lymph-nodes, and biopsy once again showed sarcoid tubercles; and the skin gave no reaction to 1000 IU. Three months later, several striking events had occurred. A cold abscess the pus from which produced tubercle bacilli on culture had appeared over an area of rarefaction in the left tibia; the skin reacted briskly to 10 IU; tubercle bacilli had been cultured from a sputum specimen obtained at a time when his skin had failed to react to tuberculin, and were now evident on direct examination of the sputum; and the scattered mottled shadows in the lungs had largely cleared, leaving localized shadows mostly in the middle zones suggestive of fibrosis. Antituberculosis chemotherapy for six months resulted in subsidence of the cold abscess and disappearance of the tubercle bacilli from the sputum. Seven years later he suffered a relapse of tuberculosis, controlled by two years of chemotherapy. He was left with severe disability from pulmonary fibrosis complicated by chronic bronchitis and by hypertension. He died with a purulent exacerbation of chronic bronchitis 21 years after the first evidence of sarcoidosis and 17 years after the discovery of tubercle bacilli. At necropsy, no remnant of tubercles, either caseating or non-caseating, was found in the lungs.

(2) (Case 2 of Scadding, 1971). A man aged 35 was found to have BHL with faint mottled shadows in the middle zones of both lungs, confluent locally at the periphery of the right side. The only symptom was cough, productive of only scanty mucoid sputum. Enlarged lymph-nodes were palpable in both axillae. No tubercle bacilli were found in repeated sputum cultures. Bronchoscopy showed no abnormality. The Mantoux test was negative with 1:100 OT. Biopsy of the right scalene node showed non-caseating epithelioid cell tubercles, no acid-fast bacilli being demonstrable. A diagnosis of sarcoidosis was made, and no treatment was thought necessary. During the next three years, he remained well, though the cough continued, and the mottling in the middle zones of both lungs increased. He then started to become breathless on exertion with morning wheezing, and was found to have low fever in the evenings, a positive tuberculin test (Heaf grade II, equivalent to a moderate reaction to 1:1000 OT in a Mantoux test), and increased density of the parahilar shadow on the right side in the chest radiograph shown in the lateral view to be due to consolidation in the right upper lobe. The sputum now contained many acid-fast bacilli, shown on culture to be *M. tuberculosis*, sensitive to the commonly used antituberculosis drugs. Bronchoscopy showed narrowing of the right upper lobe orifice, and biopsy of the mucosa showed caseating tubercles with acid-fast bacilli. Antimycobacterial chemotherapy led to the disappearance of tubercle bacilli from the sputum within seven weeks, but only very slow improvement in radiographic appearances. Interestingly, there was more clearing on the right side, the site of the original localized shadow, than on the left.

(3) A student nurse, aged 19, developed fever, iridocyclitis, and BHL. The Mantoux test was negative with 1000 IU although one year previously she had been reported to be tuberculin-positive. She was treated with prednisolone 35 mg daily, together with streptomycin and isoniazid for two months before being referred to JGS. At this time, she was moon-faced, the eyes were quiet, the hilar nodes remained large but the lungs were clear, the skin gave no reaction to 100 IU, and a scalene node biopsy showed sarcoid changes. The antituberculosis drugs were stopped and the predisolone gradually with-

drawn. Eighteen months later, the eyes remained quiet, the hilar nodes had subsided, and mottling had appeared in the middle zones of both lungs. Two months later, she coughed up a little blood and complained of pain in the back. Although there was little change in the chest radiograph, many tubercle bacilli were seen in the sputum; the Mantoux test with 100 IU was positive, and there was an area of rarefaction in the fourth lumbar vertebra. She was treated with streptomycin, PAS and isoniazid for a year, and for the first three months was immobilized on a plaster bed. At the end of this time she returned to her nursing career. Seen three years later, she was well, the spine was painless and mobile, and the chest radiograph showed only faint residual streakiness in the middle zones of the lungs.

We have observed a number of other cases in which overt mycobacterial tuberculosis, in some with unusual features, appeared during the course of sarcoidosis.

(1)   In the case summarized in Chapter 7, p. 193, tubercle bacilli appeared simultaneously in sputum and in newly ulcerated skin sarcoids at the same time as the skin became sensitive to tuberculin.

(2)   In the case summarized in Chapter 12, p. 279, evidence of mycobacterial infection in the unusual form of an apparently solitary subcutaneous cold abscess appeared during the long course of an illness otherwise characteristic of chronic sarcoidosis, with lung infiltration, hepato-splenomegaly and hyper-calcaemia.

(3)   A woman, aged 42, noticed dyspnoea on exertion after a brief febrile illness with cough; a chest radiograph showed multiple opacities in the upper two-thirds of both lungs coalescent in the upper zone of the left lung. Although four sputum cultures for tubercle bacilli were negative she was treated for one year with isoniazid and PAS. At the end of this time, there had been some radiographic deterioration in spite of the chemotherapy, and the diagnosis was reviewed. The Mantoux test with 100 IU was found to be negative; three gastric lavage specimens and three laryngeal swabs were negative on culture for tubercle bacilli and a scalene node biopsy showed sarcoid tubercles. Eight months later, she complained of pain in the left buttock and fever. This was found to be due to a tuberculous osteitis of the ileum, a large subgluteal abscess communicating with a cavity in the ileum containing a sequestrum being found at operation; a biopsy showed tuberculous granulation tissue with many AFB. The sputum now contained tubercle bacilli, and the Mantoux test with 10 IU was strongly positive. Prolonged chemotherapy led to healing of the bone lesion and the associated abscess, but the pulmonary lesions continued to be active, the right upper lobe becoming atelectatic and cavitated behind an apparent bronchial stenosis.

(4)   A woman, aged 41, was found to have BHL, a scalene node biopsy showed sarcoid changes, a Kveim test was reported to be positive and a Heaf tuberculin test gave a weakly positive reaction. She also had congestive heart failure, the cause of which was obscure. Over the next few years she had several further episodes of congestive heart failure, and developed atrial fibrillation. Seven years from the onset, treatment with betamethasone was tried, on the hypothesis that the unexplained heart failure might be due to myocardial sarcoidosis. Four months later she developed fever and pain in the right buttock and leg. An abscess developed over the lower end of the right fibula; pus aspirated from it produced on culture one colony of tubercle bacilli,

sensitive to streptomycin, PAS and isoniazid; and biopsy of the wall of the abscess showed caseating tuberculosis though no AFB were seen. The skin was now extremely sensitive to tuberculin, a Mantoux test with 1:100 000 OT being positive. On treatment with isoniazid and PAS, the cold abscess subsided and she improved generally, though one and a half years later she again developed congestive heart failure. Whether the latter might have been due to myocardial sarcoidosis remained undecided.

(5) A man, aged 24, who was said to have had tuberculous cervical adenitis at the age of two, complained of thirst, polyuria, and bloodshot eyes. He was found to have BHL and fine stippling in the lung fields in a chest radiograph, a scalene node biopsy showed sarcoid changes, the Mantoux test with 100 IU was negative, the serum calcium was 11.7 mg and urea 90 mg dl^{-1}, and urinary calcium excretion 430 mg in one day. A diagnosis of sarcoidosis with hypercalcaemia was made, and treatment with prednisolone 15 mg daily was begun. A year before the beginning of this illness, he had had a lower molar tooth, and four months later a lower wisdom tooth extracted. Discharge from both sockets was continuing, and accordingly a portion of the granulation tissue was removed for biopsy; it showed giant-cell systems, in which AFB were seen. Three weeks after the beginning of prednisolone treatment, he developed tuberculous meningitis, proved by typical chemical and cellular changes in CSF, the finding of AFB in it although tubercle bacilli were not cultured, a positive Mantoux test with 1 TU, and response to antituberculosis chemotherapy.

(6) In this case, the earlier part of which has been reported by Hopkins (1974), tuberculous meningitis developed, with AFB in the cerebrospinal fluid (CSF) and the discovery of *M. tuberculosis* in the sputum by culture, during the course of an illness generally characteristic of sarcoidosis involving lymph-nodes, lungs, spleen, eyes and skin, with hypercalcaemia, with the exception that the skin infiltrations showed some ulceration and histologically some necrosis interpreted as caseation.

A woman, aged 23, who had been BCG-vaccinated at the age of 15, was found to have BHL with a negative tuberculin test. At first symptomless, nine months later she felt unwell, with left upper abdominal pain; the spleen was now palpable, and the hilar nodes had increased in size; biopsies of scalene node at that time and of a Kveim test site later both showed sarcoid-type granulomas. During the next two years, red nodular infiltrations appeared on the shins, the arms and the neck, and the scar of the node biopsy became infiltrated; mottled shadowing appeared in the lungs, splenomegaly increased; and there were bouts of low fever. Some of the skin infiltrations showed superficial ulceration, healing with slight scarring. There was little response to predisolone at a dose of 20 mg daily, but some improvement with 40 mg. Rather less than three years from the discovery of BHL, the very large spleen was removed because of abdominal pain; it weighed 3.5 kg, and contained many sarcoid-type granulomas without AFB. Multiple sputum-cultures for mycobacteria were negative. Thee weeks after splenectomy, she developed bilateral anterior uveitis, and generalized enlargement of superficial lymph-nodes was noted; chloroquine and indomethacin were added to the prednisolone she was receiving without notable improvement. Six months later she had an episode of paraesthesia in the face and left arm with mental confusion. Three months later she became febrile with consolidation in the middle zone of the right lung and purulent sputum containing *Staph. aureus*. This apparently staphylococcal pneumonia was treated with appropriate antibiotics, but she became confused with left hemiparesis and lapsed into coma. Staphylococcal cerebral abscess was excluded by normal isotope scan, carotid arteriogram and ventriculogram. Serial lumbar puncture showed increasing numbers of lymphocytes, rising protein and falling glucose, and finally many acid-fast bacilli; and *M. tuberculosis* was cultured from an earlier sputum specimen. Antimycobacterial chemotherapy with continuation of prednisolone, 40 mg daily, led to rapid improvement; but three months later the CSF still showed pleocytosis. Intrathecal streptomycin and isoniazid were added to the treatment, and the CSF gradually became normal. When prednisolone was withdrawn, uveitis recurred, and later the skin infiltrations reactivated, and new ones appeared. Biopsy of one of these showed epitheliod-cell granulomas with some caseation, but no AFB, and no mycobacteria on culture. Later events in this case included hypercalcaemia with rise in blood urea after sunbathing, responding to prednisolone; and exacerbation of uveitis and of skin infiltrations, when prednisolone was withdrawn because it was thought to be causing paranoid delusions. Investigation seven years from the detection of BHL showed multiple skin infiltrations on face, trunk and limbs; persistently active uveitis with cataract in the left eye and kerato-conjunctivitis sicca; persistent slight enlargement of hilar lymph-nodes with mottled shadowing in both lungs; hypercalciuria; and non-reactivity of the skin to tuberculin, 100 IU. Reinstitution of long-term treatment with moderate doses of prednisolone led to gradual improvement in all symptoms and normocalciuria, and five years later she was leading a normal life.

The reported frequency of the development of mycobacterial tuberculosis during the course of sarcoidosis varied greatly, even when the general incidence of tuberculosis was high. Such factors as duration of observation and diagnostic fashion were probably responsible for some of the variation. Before antimycobacterial chemotherapy was available, tuberculosis was not infrequently the reported cause of death in fatal cases. Riley (1950) reported that 13 of 52 black patients with sarcoidosis in New York ultimately developed tuberculosis; Lovelock and Stone (1953) found that among 25 cases observed over a period of three and a half years without corticosteroid treatment, tuberculosis developed in five; among 11 cortisone-treated patients, three had positive cultures for tubercle bacilli while under treatment; and Ustvedt (1948), reviewing 59 reported necropsies in cases of sarcoidosis, found that the cause of death was tuberculosis in 11. On the other hand, a few authors have considered that the incidence of overt tuberculosis was no higher among their patients with sarcoidosis than would be expected by chance. Thus Carr and Gage (1954) stated that only one of 194 cases seen at the Mayo Clinic was known to have died of tuberculosis.

In some reported cases, there has been little change in clinical features with the appearance of evidence of mycobacterial tuberculosis, especially in those with chronic lung changes as the principal localization, in which the discovery of tubercle bacilli in the sputum, usually with increase in tuberculin sensitivity may be the only new findings. In others, there are obvious changes in clinical features; specifically 'sarcoid' changes may regress, or tuberculosis may become evident at sites unaffected by sarcoidosis.

In one of the eight reported by Scadding (1971a), skin sarcoids which had been present for more than 12 years regressed shortly before tubercle bacilli appeared in the sputum; and in another (Case 1, p. 512) extensive mottled shadowing in the lungs diminished with the transition to tuberculin sensitivity and the appearance of tubercle bacilli in sputum and in pus from a cold abscess.

Schaumann (1917, Cases 1 and 3; 1924, Cases 1 and 2; and 1934, Cases 1 and 2) reported the cases of two women, aged 41 and 46, with lupus pernio, in whom the skin changes cleared when frank tuberculosis developed; in the first, pulmonary tuberculosis from which tubercle bacilli of bovine type were isolated at necropsy, and in the second, tuberculosis of two lumbar vertebrae, with strongly positive Mantoux test.

Goldschmidt (1925, Case 1) reported the case of a man, aged 27, who had had histologically typical sarcoid lesions on nose, forehead, and legs, with negative tuberculin test, enlarged hilar shadows and some pulmonary infiltration, and changes in the bones of the hands, for eight years; he then developed a painful hip with radiographic evidence of rarefaction in the great trochanter, the Mantoux test was found to be positive with 1:100 000 OT, and the skin lesions assumed the characterisitics of lupus vulgaris, both grossly and histologically. This case presents similarities to that reported by Lewis (1961) and mentioned on p. 193.

Other cases in which skin sarcoids disappeared when evidence of caseating tuberculosis appeared have been reported by Bonnevie and With (1937), Pruvost *et al.* (1941), Ronchese(1942), Kalkoff and Ehring (1948), and Winkler (1948). Leitner (1946, Case 1) described a case of uveo-parotid syndrome with lung infiltration and hypercalcaemia in which concurrently with a change in skin reactivity from negativity to extreme sensitivity, these clinical manifestations regressed; and four months later, a cold abscess appeared on the chest wall and was shown to contain tubercle bacilli, probably of human type.

Tuberculosis of bones has appeared during the course of sarcoidosis in five cases observed by one of us (JGS), including those summarized on p. 512 (Case 1) and p. 514 (Cases 3 and 4). Others include those reported by Schaumann (1924, Case 2), Goldschmidt (1925), Bonnevieo and With (1937), Lomholt (1937), Pruvost *et al.* (1941) and Castellanos and Galan (1946).

In Boelen's (1941) Case 1 a woman aged 22, who had lupus pernio with involvement of bones of the hands and BHL developed a cold abscess, associated with a rarefaction in the lower end of the humerus, from which human-type tubercle bacilli were isolated. In the case described by Müller and Pedrazzini (1948) death resulted from miliary tuberculosis ten years after the detection of BHL with negative tuberculin test; at necropsy there was recent tuberculosis of the second thoracic vertebra, miliary tuberculosis in the lungs, liver, kidneys, and spleen, and hyalinized sarcoid-type tubercles with many giant cells in thoracic and abdominal lymph-nodes. Small's (1951) Case 2 was that of a 24 year old black man who had BHL, a negative Mantoux test, sarcoid tubercles in a liver biopsy, and a positive Kveim test; shortly after forty-five days of treatment with cortisone, he complained of low backache and fever, the skin was sensitive to 1 IU, and the hilar nodes had become smaller; a month later, destructive changes were found in the second lumbar vertebra, and several urine cultures grew tubercle bacilli.

Patients in whom tuberculous meningitis has occurred during the course of sarcoidosis have been reported by With and Helweg-Larsen (1938), Schoonhoven van Beurden (1942, Case 1), Warfvinge (1945), Hopkins (1974, two cases including that summarized on p. 514), Forgan-Smith and Newton (1974) and Fischer *et al.* (1979, Case 4). The case described by Forgan-Smith and Newton was that of a man who presented at the age of 28 with fever, uveitis, parotid gland enlargement and lung shadowing, with negative tuberculin test; four years later, he developed tuberculous meningitis with AFB in the CSF and *M. tuberculosis* was cultured from gastric aspirate.

Cases in which patients with extensive sarcoidosis have eventually developed evidence of caseating tuberculosis insidiously are perhaps less striking, especially if they were observed at a time when or a place where the prevalence of tuberculosis was high. Cases of this sort have been recorded by, among others, Martenstein (1924); Funk (1933, Case 3); Jordon and Osborne (1937), in whose case the Mantoux test remained negative in spite of the development of extensive cavitating pulmonary tuberculosis; Horton *et al.* (1939); Bour (1942); Hagn-Meincke (1944), whose Case 10 developed multiple tuberculous subcutaneous abscesses; Stuart (1944, Case 3); Castellanos and Galan (1946), in a child whose case is mentioned in connection with joint changes on p. 245; Ehrner, 1946; Leitner (1946, Case 2; 1949, Case 11); Nestman (1947, Case 6); Rey *et al.* (1947); Robinson and Hahn (1947), in a black man whose brother also had sarcoidosis and developed pulmonary tuberculosis with bacilli in the sputum; van Rijssel (1947, Case 2); Frey (1948); Moldover (1938), reporting further on a case of extensive sarcoidosis with involvement of the spinal cord previously described by Reisner (1944) and mentioned in Chapter 14, p. 322; Müller and Pedrazzini (1948); Ricker and Clark (1949, Cases 9, 14 and 22); Hautschmann (1959); Longcope and Freiman (1952, Cases 10 and 15); and Lühe (1958).

The case reported by Rubin and Pinner (1944) is of interest because it showed transitions from a caseating to a sarcoid and back to a caseating phase, like Case 3, p. 503.

A black woman whose mother had died of pulmonary tuberculosis had been found at the age of 13 to have enlargement of hilar and paratracheal lymphnodes with calcification in the right paratracheal nodes and a positive Pirquet test. She remained in good health until the age of 22 when she developed a typical uveo-parotid syndrome with general enlargement of lymph-nodes, including those at both hila; biopsy of a cervical lymph-node showed sarcoid changes and the tuberculin test was negative. Two years later she developed hepato-splenomegaly; biopsy of the spleen showed tubercles, some with central caseation. An eruption resembling a papulo-necrotic tuberculide appeared. A cold abscess developed on the chest wall and pus from it showed many AFB. At necropsy both caseating and non-caseating tubercles were found; AFB were seen only in the caseating tubercles. Case 5 of Höök (1954) showed a similar sequence; a woman who had had pulmonary tuberculosis in the past developed sarcoidosis involving the central nervous system, the spleen and the liver, and two years later the pulmonary tuberculosis became active again with AFB in the sputum.

Benda *et al.* (1955) described a case in which they had observed what they called 'aller et retour entre une maladie de Besnier-Boeck-Schaumann et une tuberculose pulmonaire'.

A man, aged 27, was found to have increasing bilateral lung shadows, with negative tuberculin test and no tubercle bacilli discoverable in gastric lavage material, and sarcoid changes in an inguinal lymph-node biopsy. Two years later, the tuberculin test remained negative. Five years from the onset, tubercle bacilli were found for the first time, and the Pirquet test was positive. He was then treated with various antituberculosis drugs, but tubercle bacilli resistant to streptomycin, isoniazid and PAS were persistently present in sputum. Ten years from the onset, AFB were still seen but did not grow on culture or infect guinea-pigs, and tuberculin tests were negative.

The 14 cases of associated tuberculosis and sarcoidosis reviewed by Haroutunian *et al.* (1964) included six (Nos. 6–11) in which tuberculosis followed sarcoidosis, the clinical picture resuming some of the features of sarcoidosis after treatment of the tuberculosis. 'Sarcoid' features, especially sarcoids of skin which were present in all but one of these six patients, did not disappear during the 'caseating' phase.

The usual finding at necropsy in patients in whom overt mycobacterial tuberculosis has appeared during the course of sarcoidosis, whatever the interval between these two phases, has been a mixture of sarcoid-type non-caseating tubercles, usually with some hyalinization, and caseating foci, and generally the organ-distribution of these two types of lesion has been different.

A very sharp contrast between non-caseating and overtly mycobacterial elements was reported by Uehlinger (1945) in a man who at the age of 24 had BHL with some lung mottling which persisted with little change until six years later he developed an acute febrile illness and died; at necropsy, sarcoid changes in a fibrotic stage were found in lungs and hilar nodes, but elsewhere there were widely distributed necrotic foci with many tubercle bacilli and little tissue reaction, interpreted as 'sepsis tuberculosa acutissima'.

A few cases, in other respects characteristic of sarcoidosis, in which at necropsy, as in that summarized on p. 535, caseation was found in the adrenal glands have been described. In that described by Bergmann (1958), sclerosing sarcoidosis was found in lymph-nodes, skin and lungs, but there was ulcerating tuberculosis of the small intestine and caseating tuberculosis of the adrenals; and cultures from hilar nodes and lung grew bovine tubercle bacilli. The case described by Tangen (1954) was that of a woman who died, aged 40, after an illness characterized by increasing pulmonary fibrosis with negative tuberculin tests. At necropsy, there were non-caseating sarcoid-type tubercles in lungs and elsewhere, including pectoral muscle; only in the enlarged right suprarenal was there a caseous area both grossly and histologically, in which 'enormous numbers of acid-fast rods' were seen. In Cases 10 and 11 of Ricker and Clark (1949), caseous changes regarded by them as tuberculous were found only in the adrenal glands. In neither case were AFB seen in the caseous areas, though in Case 11 it was stated that two AFB were seen in a section from the apex of the right lung. Subsequent re-examination of material from these cases suggested that the caseous changes in the adrenals might be attributable to *Histoplasma capsulatum* (see p. 522).

INFECTION WITH MYCOBACTERIA
OTHER THAN *M. TUBERCULOSIS*

Only a few cases have been reported in which infections with mycobacteria other than *M. tuberculosis* have been found in patients with sarcoidosis. It must be remembered, however, that in the cases reviewed above in which AFB were seen on microscopy of secretions or tissues, but not cultured or isolated by guinea-pig inoculation, the identity of the presumed mycobacterium was not established.

Israel *et al.* (1961) reported the case of a black man who at the age of 30 was found to have enlarged hilar shadows and a pulmonary infiltration; the tuberculin test was negative, but the histoplasmin positive; two years later, a lymph-node biopsy showed some caseous necrosis with AFB visible, but tubercle bacilli were not cultured; when he was aged 37, biopsy of a skin lesion and of a lymph-node showed non-caseating tubercles; the skin now reacted to 10 IU; the serum calcium was 15 mg dl^{-1}; the following year, chromogenic mycobacteria were cultured from the sputum; in this case, calcification of 'egg-shell' type developed in hilar and mediastinal lymph-nodes.

Brun *et al.* (1964) found an acid-fast bacillus in the sputum of a man who had had pulmonary sarcoidosis for seven years, following a characteristic course from BHL and pulmonary infiltration towards fibrosis. The AFB were found a few months after treatment with corticotrophin had been started; they were identified as *M. kansasii*. Brun *et al.* quoted a case described by Chanial (1937) in which culture from the lung at necropsy in a case of pulmonary and skin sarcoidosis produced a mycobacterium non-pathogenic for the guinea-pig.

Wood (1964) gave a brief report of the case of a man, aged 35, in whom sarcoidosis had been diagnosed on the strength of granulomas found in lymph-node, liver and bone marrow biopsies; the skin reacted only to 250 IU. Bilateral pulmonary infiltrations were treated with prednisone and isoniazid. Air-containing spaces appeared in the upper lobes of the lungs. AFB were repeatedly found on microscopy of sputum, but only one of a number of cultures produced a growth of a Battey strain of mycobacteria.

Berger *et al.* (1968) reported the case of a black man aged 17 with sarcoidosis affecting parotid and lacrimal glands, lymph-nodes and lungs, confirmed by lymph-node biopsy and a Kveim test and a negative tuberculin test, 250 IU. From the biopsy, two colonies of scotochromogenic mycobacteria, niacin-negative, catalase-positive and resistant to streptomycin, isoniazid and PAS, were grown. At the time of the report, he had improved on treatment with prednisone.

In Case 8 of Baum *et al.* (1973), a black man with pulmonary infiltration, skin sarcoids and a cervical lymph-node biopsy showing sarcoid-type granulo-as and a negative tuberculin test, was found seven years from the onset to have *M. kansasii* in the sputum, and the tuberculin test became positive. In this case, heavy silica exposure and conglomerate shadows in the chest radiograph indicated complicating silicosis.

Bretza and Mayfield (1978) reported the complex case of a North American Indian woman aged 54, whose illness started with BHL, discovered after three attacks of pneumonia; skin tests with tuberculin and fungal antigens were negative, and non-caseating granulomas were found in biopsies of bronchial mucosa and mediastinal lymph-node. She was treated with prednisone, in part for asthma. Five years later, she presented with increasing dyspnoea and haemoptysis, and was found to have lung infiltration with a cavity in the upper part of the right lung and persisting mediastinal enlargement, and *M. intracellulare* of avian variety was cultured from the sputum.

LEPROSY

In the tuberculoid variety of leprosy lesions having the histological structure of sarcoids may appear. Pautrier (1934) reported a case of leprosy in an African from the Congo with thickening of ulnar nerves and anaesthesia, in whom a large nodular lesion on the forearm was histologically a sarcoid. Rabello (1936), working in Rio de Janeiro, stated that in 105 cases of tuberculoid leprosy examined histologically, more than half showed a pure sarcoid structure. Reenstierna (1937, 1940) concluded that leprosy might show itself as skin affections histologically identical with Besnier's lupus pernio, Boeck's cutaneous sarcoids and Schaumann's erythrodermia, and could cause radiological changes in bones like those associated with these skin affections, but that changes of sarcoid-type in other organs had not been demonstrated.

Ramasoota *et al.* (1967) studied the histology of skin infiltrations in 47 patients with cutaneous sarcoidosis (CS) and 45 with tuberculoid leprosy (TL). Granulomas tended to be scattered throughout the corium in CS, and to be confluent around nerves and vessels in TL; giant cells occurred with similar frequency, but inclusion-bodies were seen in more than a quarter of the CS cases, and only in one TL; fibrosis and fibrinoid degeneration were more frequent in CS; invasion and destruction of nerves and of arrectores pilae were much more frequent in TL; and acid-fast bacilli were seen in 24 of the 45 TL cases. Thus, while in some cases histology might permit confident categorization, in some it was equivocal. Ramanujam (1982) reported a case which illustrates the difficulty of histological discrimination; a young man in South India had widespread infiltrated patches on the skin, which gradually spread; repeated biopsies, one showing two acid-fast bacilli, were interpreted as tuberculoid or borderline tuberculoid leprosy; after 18 years, reassessment of the histology and a granulomatous response to a Kveim test led to revision of the diagnosis to sarcoidosis.

It is striking that the abundant records of *M. tuberculosis* infections and generalized sarcoidosis standing in every possible temporal relation to each other, outlined above, are not paralleled in relation to leprosy; how far the lack of sufficiently intensive medical supervision of appropriate populations contibutes to this difference must remain conjectural.

INFECTIONS WITH PATHOGENIC FUNGI

Histoplasma capsulatum

Reimann and Price (1949a; 1949b, Case 2) described a case in which the course for seven years was typical of sarcoidosis, but shortly before death, evidence of histoplasma infection appeared.

> A black woman aged 28 developed on the skin of the limbs papules and nodules up to 3 cm in diameter having the histological structure of sarcoids, enlargement of hilar shadows and nodular shadowing in the lungs. During the following seven years, shadowing in the lungs increased, and generalized lymphadenopathy, splenomegaly, and localized rarefactions in several metarsals and phalanges and in the head of the radius appeared. She then developed laryngeal ulceration, from which a biopsy was taken and showed granulations containing *H. capsulatum*, identified by culture. The old skin biopsy was re-examined and structures resembling histoplasma were seen. She died of cor pulmonale; at necropsy there was fibrosis and granulomatous involvement of the lungs, and granulomas in the liver, the mediastinal and abdominal lymphnodes and in the adrenals, but histoplasma was seen in the adrenals only.

In Cases 10 and 11 of Ricker and Clark (1949) similarly, structures resembling histoplasma were seen in the adrenals at necropsy.

> Two white men died, aged 30 and 54, after febrile illnesses lasting eight and seven months. Both showed sarcoid granulomas in caseous areas, but in one, two AFB were seen in a section from the lung. Material from these cases was subsequently re-examined by Pinkerton and Iverson (1952, Cases 1 and 3) and

by Engle (1953, Cases 19 and 20); in the caseous adrenals, some macrophages containing globular bodies, 2–4 μ in diameter, resembling *Histoplasma capsulatum* were found, and PAS staining showed that the caseous mass was packed with similar bodies. The original identification of these caseous changes as due to *M. tuberculosis* was thus not tenable, and it seems likely that they were due to *H. capsulatum*. The similarity to the case of Reimann and Price (1949b) quoted above, and to the cases of Addison's disease due to *H. capsulatum* reported by Crispell *et al.* (1956) lends support to this view.

Israel *et al.* (1952) described the case of a man who at the age of 30 was found to have a bilateral pulmonary infiltration causing no symptoms. Five years later, a cervical lymph-node removed for biopsy showed sarcoid changes. The Mantoux test was negative, and serum globulin was elevated. The following year, his throat became sore and his voice hoarse; this was found to be due to laryngeal ulceration and oedema, and biopsy showed a granuloma in which *H. capsulatum* was detected microscopically and by culture. A second cervical lymph-node biopsy again showed sarcoid granulomas, in which *Histoplasma* could not be found. Various forms of treatment were tried over the next few years. Laryngeal obstruction necessitated tracheostomy, which was followed by clinical improvement. Further biopsies of a cervical lymph-node and of a nasal ulcer showed epithelioid cell tubercles typical of sarcoidosis; at this stage, although *Histoplasma* was occasionally seen in biopsies of the laryngeal granuloma, it could not be cultured.

Crispell *et al.* (1956), discussing Addison's disease associated with histoplasmosis, described a case (no. 4) in which histoplasma infection was diagnosed on the basis of 'miliary' calcified foci typical of healed histoplasmosis in the chest radiograph; biopsies of an inguinal lymph-node, and of liver and abdominal lymph-nodes at laparotomy showed non-caseating granulomatous lesions with giant cells but without demonstrable bacilli or fungi; postoperatively acute adrenal insufficiency led to the diagnosis of Addison's disease.

Symmers (1956) reported the case of a man who at the age of 50 noticed lividity and induration of an old scar on the forehead; on biopsy this showed infiltration with sarcoid tubercles around birefringent particles. The following year he developed generalized lymphadenopathy and was found to have BHL and mottling in the middle zones of the lungs; an epitrochlear node removed for biopsy showed sarcoid changes; the lymphadenopathy and the lung shadows resolved spontaneously within a year. When he was aged 56, he noticed enlarged lymph-nodes above the left clavicle; removed for biopsy, they showed epithelioid cell collections with many large giant cells, many structures resembling *H. capsulatum* being present principally in the giant cells, and the organism was isolated on culture. No other signs of disease could be found in the patient at this time; the chest radiograph was normal; a histoplasmin skin test was strongly positive. The patient had never been outside the British Isles.

Several other cases have been reported in which a syndrome typical of sarcoid BHL was associated with evidence of *Histoplasma* infection. Bullock and Ray (1961) reported the case of a man aged 20 who presented with fever, BHL and a scalene lymph-node biopsy showing epithelioid cell tubercles with a few giant cells and some hyalinization. He improved without specific treatment, the course thus resembling that of sarcoid BHL. Although no inclusions were seen in the biopsy sections, culture from the lymph-node produced *H.*

capsulatum, and a histoplasmin skin test was strongly positive, other fungal antigens and tuberculin giving negative tests. Baum *et al.* (1973, Case 10) reported the case of a white woman, aged 29, who presented with BHL; a scalene node biopsy showed non-caseating granulomas, in which yeast cells were seen, and culture of the node produced *H. capsulatum*; the enlarged nodes subsided without treatment. Their Case 11, that of a black man aged 27, presented in a manner less characteristic of sarcoidosis, with a right hilar mass, a lymph-node removed by mediastinoscopy showing granulomas with some central necrosis, with no AFB or fungi on routine reporting; complement fixation tests for *Histoplasma* showed a rise and fall in titres, and re-examination of the biopsy showed structures resembling histoplasma; the condition resolved spontaneously.

Coccidioides immitis

Ellis (1955) reported the case of a black man in whom a characteristic syndrome of sarcoidosis appeared after the healing of disseminated cocci-diodomycosis. In the first illness, enlarged cervical lymph-nodes suppurated and an abscess appeared over an area of rarefaction in the right tibia; other bone rarefactions were seen in the skull. There was enlargement of hilar lymph-nodes and shadowing in the upper zone of the left lung. Pus from a sub-occipital abscess grew *C. immitis*, and skin and complement fixation tests with coccidioidal antigens were positive. These manifestations gradually cleared. Three years later, he presented with a generalized lymphadenopathy and multiple skin infiltrations. Biopsies of cervical lymph-nodes, nasal mucosa and skin all gave the histological picture of sarcoidosis. Guinea-pig inoculations from the biopsies were negative. The coccidiodin skin test was now negative, as were the tuberculin and histoplasmin.

Bacharach and Zalis (1963) described the case of a black man who six months after travelling through the San Joachim valley developed epididymitis; the right epididymis was removed and showed many non-caseating epithelioid cell tubercles with central giant cells, no bacilli or fungi being seen after special staining. Three months from the onset, he developed anterior uveitis. The right paratracheal and hilar lymph-nodes were enlarged. Biopsy of a submandibular lymph-node showed similar changes to those found in the epididymis. Although only one out of a series of coccidioidin skin tests gave a positive result, the titre of coccidioidal complement-fixation rose steeply over a period of four months to 1:128, and this was taken to indicate coccidioidal infection. Treatment with amphotericin B was followed by improvement.

Cryptococcus neoformans

Cryptococcosis (torulosis) is frequently an opportunistic infection, complicating Hodgkin's disease, malignant disease and other conditions in which host resistance is depressed either by specific effects on immunological reactivity or by general debility. Its reported associations with sarcoidosis have been of various sorts. In some, sarcoid-like clinical manifestations and evidences of cryptococcal infection have been concurrent; in some, overtly cryptococcal lesions, especially in bone, lymph-nodes or skin, have appeared during the course of sarcoidosis; and have seemed to evolve independently; and in others, acute cryptococcosis, usually in the form of meningitis, has been a late, and in many instances terminal, event.

One of three cases of cryptococcosis described by Fisher (1950) occurred in a patient with extensive sarcoidosis. The patient was a black woman aged 20 who had had clinical evidence of hypopituitarism with amenorrhoea and loss of body hair, BHL and lung infiltration, fever, hepato-splenomegaly and a general lymphadenopathy, a lymph-node biopsy having shown sarcoid changes with Schaumann bodies; later she developed subcutaneous abscesses and rarefactions in bones, *C. neoformans* being seen in granulation tissue and pus and cultured from pus, and ultimately evidence of meningitis. The necropsy diagnosis was sarcoidosis of lungs, heart, lymph-nodes, lever, spleen and hypophysis, and crytococcosis of meninges, brain, kidneys, adrenal, lung, bone and skin, together with a primary tuberculosis complex in the lung. In another case, the principal manifestation of cryptococcosis was bone abscesses which responded well to treatment with potassium iodide; eight months before the first abscess appeared, an enlarged lymph-node had been removed for biopsy and showed sarcoid changes; re-examination of this later showed no evidence of cryptococci.

Littman and Zimmerman (1956) in their monograph on cryptococcosis mention the case of a man, aged 41, who died of cryptococcal meningitis; *C. neoformans* was found in brain and kidney, but not in non-caseating sarcoid-type granulomas that were present in the lung and mediastinal lymph-nodes.

Cases in which cryptococcal osteitis was concurrent with a clinical and histological picture of generalized sarcoidosis were reported by Heller *et al.* (1957) and Shields (1959). That described by Heller *et al.* occurred in a 22 year old black man who presentred with generalized lymphadenopathy, including the hilar nodes, pulmonary mottling, and an osteolytic lesion in the iliac crest. Cervical and epitrochlear lymph-node biopsies showed sarcoid changes, no AFB or fungi being seen. He improved on cortisone treatment. Later, a swelling in the hip region was explored; an abscess was evacuated, and biopsy of its wall showed granulation tissue with *C. neoformans*, confirmed by culture. The Kveim test was reported to be positive. Treatment with several antifungal agents was given. McCullough *et al.* (1958) appear to have referred to the same case, and added that the parotids were enlarged. The case described by Shields (1959) was that of a black woman, aged 42, who presented with acute polyarthritis, fever, ulcers on the arms, rarefactions in bones, and enlarged hilar lymph-nodes. An axillary lymph-node biopsy showed a sarcoid pattern. *C. neoformans* was isolated from an abscess over an affected clavicle and external malleolus and from the cerebro-spinal fluid. Treated with amphotericin B, she improved. Six months later, headaches recurred, cryptococci were again found in CSF and further treatment was given. Later, because of low fever and anaemia, a spleen weighing 930 g and two accessory spleens were removed. The spleen and intra-abdominal lymph-nodes and a portion of liver removed for biopsy showed replacement by a sarcoid-type granuloma; though a few cryptococci were detected by microscopy in spleen and lymph-node, none was cultured.

In other cases, the principal manifestation of cryptococcosis has been in bone, and has developed in patients with long-standing sarcoidosis.

Leithold *et al.* (1957) reported the case of a black man, aged 27, in whom sarcoidosis, manifested by mottling in the chest radiograph and superficial lymphadenopathy with typical biopsy changes, was complicated two years from the onset by an abscess below the right scapula, proved by culture to be cryptococcal, and treated successfully by 2-hydroxystilbamidine. Later, an enlarged spleen was removed, and showed sarcoid changes, cryptococcus not being demonstrable.

Bernard and Owens (1960) reported the case of a black woman who at the age of 41 had a partial thyroidectomy for colloid adenoma; sections showed some foci of a sarcoid-type granuloma, and biopsy of an axillary lymph-node showed similar changes. Three years later, she presented with pain in the back and fever, found to be due to erosion of the fourth thoracic vertebra which was shown by surgical exploration to be due to a cryptococcal granuloma and abscess, the organism being isolated on culture. Treatment with amphotericin B led to recovery, the patient remaining well eleven months after the end of treatment.

Case 4 of Baum *et al.* (1973) was that of a black woman, aged 48, with a five year history of sarcoidosis involving skin, confirmed by biopsy, lungs and hilar lymph-nodes. She presented with a painful lytic lesion of the right femur, which on biopsy showed granulomatous osteitis with cryptococci demonstrable by special staining, and cryptococcal antibodies in the serum; no cryptococci were found in concurrent biopsy of a skin infiltration, or reviews of the previous biopsy. Both bone and skin lesions improved on treatment with amphotericin B.

Nottebart *et al.* (1973) reported the case of a black man who presented at the age of 26 with BHL and lung infiltration, a lymph-node biopsy showing sarcoid-type granulomas. Later a generalized lymphadenopathy appeared, and he was treated with prednisone. Nearly three years from the onset, he developed a painful fluctuant swelling at the lower border of the left scapula, and a lytic lesion was found radiographically in the eighth rib. Pus aspirated from this swelling showed many budding yeasts, and grew *C. neoformans* on culture. Nasal mucosal biopsy showed sarcoid-type granulomas, and no cryptococci. Treatment with 5-fluorocytosine was followed by healing of the bone lesions, but the lymphadenopathy, nasal obstruction and lung shadows increased, and skin infiltrations of sarcoid histology, without micro-organisms appeared on the elbows. Reinstitution of treatment with prednisone led to regression of the manifestations of sarcoidosis.

Belcher *et al.* (1975) reported two cases of sarcoidosis in which cryptococcal osteitis appeared, the second also with a cryptococcal granulomatous mass in the lung. Their Case 1 was that of a woman aged 49 who presented with histologically confirmed skin sarcoids on the face, scalp and legs, and was found to have BHL and pulmonary infiltration. Five years later, she developed a painful swelling below the right knee, and an osteolytic lesion was found in the fibula underlying it; biopsy of this showed bone necrosis, with granulomatous inflammation containing yeast-like organisms, and *C. neoformans* was cultured from this tissue. Treatment with amphotericin B led to healing of the bone lesion, but had no effect on skin, lung or lymph-nodes; subsequent treatment with hydroxychloroquine was followed by improvement in the skin infiltrations. In the second case, a woman aged 48 with BHL and lung infiltration later developed uveitis and skin sarcoids, the diagnosis being confirmed by biopsies of lymph-node and skin. Seven years from the onset, a localized nodule appeared in the lung, and soon afterwards a soft tissue swelling overlying an osteolytic area in the left frontal bone, and another osteolytic area was found in a rib. The lung nodule was resected. It consisted of non-caseating granulomas with many yeast-like structures; culture from it grew *C. neoformans*, and material aspirated from the forehead swelling showed encapsulated yeasts. Treatment with amphotericin B and fluorocytosine resulted in resolution of the bone lesions.

Cryptococcal lesions may appear in the skin, and in a few cases have been the only overt manifestation.

Gandy (1950) reported the case of a woman who at the age of 24 presented with a generalized lymphadenopathy, an inguinal node biopsy showing sarcoid changes, condylomata vulvae treated by vulvectomy, and nephrolithiasis treated by nephrolithomy. Four years later, blisters appeared on the face, and *C. neoformans* was isolated on culture from them. The superficial lymph-nodes were still enlarged, and biopsy of a cervical node again showed sarcoid changes. A year later, the skin lesions were healed; she had early uraemia associated with nephrocalcinosis. The evidence available does not indicate whether there was a disturbance of calcium metabolism of the sort associated with sarcoidosis.

Harris *et al.* (1965) reported the case of a black man who at the age of 25 was found to have a large mediastinal shadow, shown at thoracotomy to be due to a mass of lymph-nodes of sarcoid histology. At the age of 29 he presented with fever, scattered skin lesions and patchy mottling in the chest radiograph. Tender subcutaneous nodules appeared on the thighs. Biopsies of a lymph-node, of the liver, and of one of the skin lesions showed sarcoid tubercles; and of a subcutaneous nodule showed central necrosis with many intracellular and extracellular *C. neoformans*, confirmed by culture. The same organism was subsequently cultured from the sputum, though a lung biopsy showed the histology of sarcoidosis, and no organisms were seen in it.

In a case reported by Spivack *et al.* (1957), the only overt localization of cryptococcosis was in the kidney. A black man was found at the age of 23 to have a pulmonary infiltration, a negative tuberculin test and a sarcoid pattern in a lymph-node biopsy. He had also had uveitis. At the age of 26, he developed symptoms suggestive of right-sided pyelonephritis, and an abnormal pyelogram led to nephrectomy. The kidney contained an adherent mass in its upper part, composed of collections of macrophages and plasma cells, separated by dense collagen; structures resembling *C. neoformans* were found both in and separate from macrophages, and this organism was subsequently cultured from the discharge from the wound. A lung biopsy showed confluent sarcoid tubercles, and *C. neoformans* was not demonstrable in it.

Inguinal lymph-nodes were the only detected site of cryptococcal infection in a 53 year old man whose case was described by Baum *et al.* (1973). He had been found to have symptomless pulmonary infiltration with a positive Kveim test three years before a lymph-node abscess in the groin was incised, and yielded *C. neoformans* on culture. Treatment with amphotericin B was followed by healing of the groin lesion, without change in the chest radiographic appearance.

In two cases observed by one of us, cryptococcal meningitis was the terminal event in patients with long-standing sarcoidosis. The first has been reported in detail (Clinicopathological Conference, 1969). An army officer was found at the age of 28 to have symptomless pulmonary infiltration; investigations were inconclusive, but a provisional diagnosis of sarcoidosis was made. During the following year, he had an episode of fever, headache and vomiting, from which he recovered spontaneously; during the investigation of this the cerebrospinal fluid (CSF) was found to be normal. Just over two years from the first abnormal radiograph, after two weeks of intensive sunbathing, he felt tired, weak and thirsty, with complete anorexia, and the serum calcium, previously normal, was found to be very high. This hypercalcaemia and the symptoms associated with it responded rapidly to treatment with prednisolone; but soon afterwards, he developed fever and headache, and the CSF showed increasing lymphocytosis, and rising protein and falling glucose levels, and eventually *C. neoformans* was both seen in and grown from it. Treatment with amphotericin B led initially to improvement, but had to be interrupted because of pancytopenia; this was complicated by *Staph. aureus* infection with septic endocarditis, leading to death from cardiac arrest. At necropsy, sarcoidosis in a fibrotic stage was found in lung, lymph-nodes, liver and spleen; the renal tubules showed calcinosis; there was cryptococcal meningitis and cryptococci were seen also in the kidney; and large vegetations in which both staphylococci and cryptococci were seen grossly distorted the aortic valve.

The second presented two diagnostic problems; that of appropriate categorization when mycobacteria are found on a single occasion in a patient whose clinical picture is that of sarcoidosis, and that presented by lymphocytic meningitis in a patient with sarcoidosis. A West Indian woman presented at the age of 20 with enlarged cervical lymph-nodes which on biopsy showed granulomatous changes; she also had BHL. The following year she came to England, and at the age of 22 she was found to have enlarged cervical and axillary lymph-nodes and the hilar nodes had subsided. Biopsy of a cervical node showed non-caseating granulomas; a tuberculin test with 1:10 000 OT was positive. The following year she developed uveitis, which was treated for two years with topical corticosteroids. When she was aged 27, the uveitis recurred and required systemic corticosteroid treatment, in spite of which secondary glaucoma in the right eye required surgical treatment. At the age of 30, after a urinary tract infection she was found to have renal and ureteric calculi. At laparotomy for removal of a ureteric calculus, an enlarged pelvic lymph-node was removed and was found to contain epithelioid and giant-cell granulomas with some necrosis; acid-fast bacilli were seen, and *M. tuberculosis*, sensitive to the usual antimycobacterial agents, was cultured from it. Treatment with streptomycin, isoniazid and PAS was begun. Two months later, she complained of giddiness and headache; CSF showed increased protein, lymphocytosis, and normal glucose, and the diagnosis being thought to rest between mycobacterial tuberculous and sarcoid meningitis, antituberculosis treatment was continued. There was little change over the next five months, when severe headache, mental confusion and fever was accompanied by increase in CSF pressure and protein content, with a predominantly polymorphonuclear pleocytosis. Cryptococcus was identified in the CSF, but before treatment could be started, she died of a massive pulmonary embolism. At necropsy, the meninges were infiltrated with lymphocytes, macrophages, many Langhans giant cells and some polymorphs, with many cryptococci, both within macrophages and extracellular. There was granulomatous infiltration of both kidneys. No acid-fast bacilli were seen.

Plummer *et al.* (1957) reported the occurrence of sarcoidosis in monozygotic twins, complicated in one by cryptococcosis involving bone and later the meninges, leading to death. At the age of 31 this man had been examined as a contact of his wife who had been found to have pulmonary tuberculosis. He had then been found to have mottling in both lungs, but was not investigated until two years later, when supraclavicular lymph-nodes had enlarged and in biopsy showed sarcoid changes. The Mantoux test was negative with 1:10 OT. Treatment with cortisone was started; shortly afterwards, he became febrile, a nodule previously noted on the chest wall enlarged and later softened, and a fluctuant swelling appeared over the left acromion, associated with rarefaction in the underlying bone. These swellings were aspirated, and later *C. neoformans* was found in the aspirate, both by microscopy and by culture. Further biopsies of lymph-nodes and tonsil showed sarcoid changes. Treatment with 2-hydroxystilbamidine led to regression of the abscesses. Two years later, loss of weight, fever and splenomegaly were followed shortly by evidence of meningitis which was fatal in spite of further treatment. At necropsy, sarcoidosis in a sclerotic stage in lymph-nodes, lungs and spleen, calcified caseous lymph-nodes in mediastinum and mesentery, and cryptococcal meningitis were found. The twin, examined at the time his brother first developed symptoms, showed lymphadenopathy, with biopsy evidence of sarcoid structure, lung mottling, and negative Mantoux test, and later splenomegaly.

Lepow *et al.* (1957) reported the case of a black girl, aged ten, who presented with sarcoidosis characterized by generalized lymphadenopathy, lung infiltration, hypercalcaemia, cyst-like changes in phalanges, a number of lymph-nodes removed for biopsy all showing sarcoid changes, with no bacilli or fungi demonstrable by microscopy or culture, and a positive Kveim test. Shortly after treatment with cortisone was instituted she developed meningitis, and *C. neoformans* was cultured from the CSF. In spite of treatment with polymixin B and nystatin she died. At necropsy, sarcoid changes were were found in lungs, lymph-nodes, liver, spleen, kidneys, salivary glands and bones, calcareous deposits in the kidneys, and meningoencephalitis due to *C. neoformans*. No cryptococci were found by staining or culture in any site except the central nervous system.

Brandt and Stürup (1959) described the case of a woman aged 58 who developed cryptococcal meningitis; she had been known to have sarcoidosis for five years, confirmed by lymph-node biopsy and characterized by a lung infiltration which persisted. The meningitis responded to treatment with amphotericin B.

Sokolowski *et al.* (1969) reported a case of sarcoidosis in which early in the course there was suggestive evidence of infection by a scotochromogenic mycobacterium, and later *C. neoformans* was found in affected lung and lymph-node, in new skin lesions and in CSF. A black woman aged 32 presented with enlarged cervical lymph-nodes, splenomegaly and BHL; biopsy of a lymph-node and of a Kveim test site confirmed the diagnosis of sarcoidosis. In a second node biopsy, the histology was similar but AFB were seen; culture was negative. Serology suggested a scotochromogenic mycobacterial infection. A year later, she developed bilateral chest pain and fever, and increasing lung infiltration was found; treatment with prednisone was started. Shortly after-wards, fever recurred and a small left pleural effusion was found, and later an acneiform rash apeared on the face. Biopsies of skin and of lung, pleura and hilar nodes obtained at biopsy showed non-caseating granulomas with many budding organisms, and cultures from the tissues produced *C. neoformans.* Later this organism was found in CSF, and also in urine. Treatment with amphotericin B led to resolution of skin lesions, which had ulcerated, and normalisation of CSF, but had no effect on the chest radiographic appearances.

Case 12 of Baum *et al.* (1973) was that of a black man, aged 45, who had extensive long-standing cutaneous sarcoidosis, with lung involvement, con-firmed by biopsies of skin and lung. Nineteen years from the onset, he became febrile, with increased lung shadows, and *C. neoformans* was found both in sputum and CSF. He was treated with amphotericin, but the response was not reported.

Sporotrichum schenkii

McFarland and Goodman (1963) reported the case of a black woman, aged 33, who presented with cough, dyspnoea, multiple small raised skin lesions, generalized lymphadenopathy, and scattered opacities in the chest radio-graph. A diagnosis of sarcoidosis was made on the basis of biopsies of a skin lesion and of a lymph-node and negative tuberculin and other skin tests. Treatment with prednisolone was started, with improvement. Shortly after-wards, the skin lesions started to suppurate and ulcerate, and later areas of rarefaction appeared in bones of the foot. Biopsy of a skin lesion showed non-specific inflammatory changes with necrosis; no organisms were seen, but cultures from ulcers and from a bone lesion grew *Sporotrichum schenkii.* Treatment with potassium iodide was followed by healing of skin and bone lesions. Two years later, she was known to be well, with a normal chest radiograph. Shortly afterwards she died suddenly. Necropsy showed no cause for the sudden death; there were healed granulomas in lungs and mediastinal lymph-nodes, without demonstrable organisms, the nodes being almost entirely fibrotic.

In Case 6 of Baum *et al.* (1973), a black man was found to have sarcoidosis with uveitis and lung infiltration, confirmed by liver and lymph-node biopsies, at the age of 26; corticosteroid treatment was given for control of ocular and pulmonary symptoms. Thirteen years later, ulcers appeared on both legs after needling of a swelling near the ankle; culture from a skin lesion and from the lung (presumably from sputum) led to the diagnosis of sporotrichosis. Treatment with amphotericin B led to healing of the skin, but little effect on the lung changes.

Blastomyces dermatitidis

Baum *et al.* (1973, Cases 1 and 2) reported two cases in a black woman aged

23 and a black man aged 31, presenting with mediastinal lymph-node enlargement and lung infiltration suggestive of sarcoidosis, but without histological evidence, which were later shown to be due to blastomycosis. Hiatt and Lide (1949) described a complex case in a black man, aged 27, with BHL, lung infiltration and non-caseating granulomas in a lymph-node removed for biopsy, later showing evidence of infection by both *M. tuberculosis* and *Blastomyces*, confirmed at necropsy. In all these cases, it seems likely that the whole process was a response to the observed infecting agent or agents, and it was unnecessary to invoke a diagnosis of sarcoidosis.

Chapter 24

Concomitant or Associated Diseases

II Miscellaneous

The clinical course of sarcoidosis is in many cases prolonged, and may be preceded by a period of varying duration during which granulomatous changes are present in various organs without causing symptoms; and it is certain that some individuals go through the entire course of sarcoidosis to spontaneous resolution without, or with only trivial symptoms, although granulomas if sought would be found in involved organs. Thus it is to be expected that a proportion of patients will show evidence of some other disease during the course of known sarcoidosis; and also that during the investigation of patients found to be suffering from some other disease, evidence of previously unsuspected sarcoidosis will be found occasionally. The associations of greatest interest are those that may cause diagnostic difficulty because one disease masks the other; and those in which there is some possibility of a pathogenetic relationship through a common immunological, genetic or other factor between sarcoidosis and the other disease, or through some feature of sarcoidosis that predisposes to the other disease. If such a relationship seems possible, it is important to determine whether the association occurs more frequently than would be expected by chance. Because of uncertainty about the total incidence of sarcoidosis, including undiagnosed and asymptomatic cases, estimates of the expected frequency of associations with other diseases are subject to considerable error. Another source of uncertainty arises from the occurrence of local granulomatous reactions in adjacent tissues and lymph-nodes to malignant disease, lymphomas and some infections (Chapter 2, p. 33); because of such reactions, convincing evidence of generalized granulomatosis is required before the additional diagnosis of sarcoidosis should be accepted in patients with diseases of these sorts.

MALIGNANT TUMOURS

There is no evidence that the frequency of malignant tumours in general, or of any particular tumour with the possible exception of lymphomas, differs from expectation in patients with sarcoidosis. The idea that the immunological peculiarities of sarcoidosis might predispose to tumours, which has been suggested, was based upon a misconception; for, as discussed in Chapter 20, although the abnormality of T-cell function in sarcoidosis results in diminished ability to express delayed hypersensitivity, it does not impair immune defences.

In Denmark, where from 1962 to 1971 a central registry of cases of sarcoidosis known to chest clinics was maintained, Brincker and Wilbek (1974) correlated this with the Danish Cancer Registry. Among 2561 registered patients with sarcoidosis, 65 were also recorded in the Cancer Registry. In 17 of these, the diagnosis of malignant disease preceded that of sarcoidosis. Thus among 2544 patients with sarcoidosis and no previous history of malignant disease, 48 were subsequently registered with malignant disease. This number significantly exceeded the number expected, 33.8. The excess was attributable principally to malignant lymphoma, of which six cases, 11 times the expected number, were reported, and partly to lung cancer, of which nine cases, three times the expected number, were reported. But Rømer (1980b) reviewed these 48 cases by tracing individual case-records, and found that the diagnosis of sarcoidosis had not been established in ten, and of cancer in three. Removal of these cases reduced the numbers of cases of malignant disease of all sorts combined and of lung cancer to almost exactly the expected levels; the incidence of malignant lymphomas remained six times that expected, but the number of cases was only three. As would be expected if sarcoidosis and cancer occurred together by chance, ages at onset of sarcoidosis in those later found to develop cancer showed a distribution peaking past middle age, 94% being over 40 years old when sarcoidosis was diagnosed, as compared with the peak in young adult life seen in unselected series of patients with sarcoidosis.

It is probably because the occasional concurrence of a common cancer with sarcoidosis is not unexpected that few reports of the concurrence of lung cancer and sarcoidosis have been published, mainly to draw attention to diagnostic difficulties (Jefferson *et al.*, 1954; Goodbody and Taylor, 1957; Ellman and Hanson, 1958; Jörgensen, 1963a; Sakula, 1963; Sarkar,

1970; Schoenfield *et al.*, 1978). The following two cases illustrate the diagnostic problems that may arise. In the first, changes in radiographic appearances in the lung of a man with pulmonary sarcoidosis at first suggested coalescence of sarcoid infiltration, but were found to be due to bronchial carcinoma:

> A man aged 42 noticed cough and some breathlessness on exertion and two years later was found to have a widespread irregular mottling in the lungs; the diagnosis of sarcoidosis was confirmed by biopsy of a cervical lymph-node and a Mantoux test negative to 100 IU. Six years after the first abnormal chest radiograph, when he was aged 50, he had become so breathless that treatment with cortisone was begun. This was followed by clearing of the shadows in the left lung, but those in the right appeared to coalesce into large 'cannon-ball'-like masses. Needle biopsy of one of these showed undifferentiated carcinoma. He died with cerebral metastases; at necropsy the carcinoma appeared to have arisen in the middle lobe bronchus, and old sarcoid changes were evident in lungs, intrathoracic lymph-nodes and spleen.

In the second, symptomless sarcoid infiltration in the lungs of a man who had been treated for carcinoma of the rectum, raised suspicion of pulmonary metastasis, but proceeded towards resolution, while the carcinoma later metastasized in the lung and elsewhere:

> A man aged 66 underwent abdomino-perineal resection for carcinoma of the rectum. A year later, a chest radiograph showed widespread fine nodular shadows. A Kveim test gave a granulomatous response. Under observation the nodular shadows diminished, but six months later, a solitary rounded shadow appeared in the upper part of the left lung. At thoracotomy, a firm nodule was found in the left upper lobe which was removed, together with a large subaortic lymph-node. Histologically, the nodule proved to be an adenocarcinoma, presumably metastatic from the rectum; sarcoid-type granulomas were present in the lung, and the lymph-node showed sarcoid granulomas, but no evidence of carcinoma. Subsequently, there was no further clinical or radiological manifestation of sarcoidosis, but hepatic metastases of the carcinoma led to death one year later.
>
> Sybert and Butler (1978) reported the case of an 18 year old man who was treated for osteosarcoma of the femur by amputation, followed by one year of treatment with methotrexate and doxorubicin. At the end of this time, the chest radiograph was normal, but later there was progressive enlargement of hilar and right paratracheal shadows. Mediastinoscopic biopsy showed non-caseating granulomatous lymphadenitis, and later ill-defined nodules appeared in the lung and on biopsy were found to be due to sarcoid granulomas. In this case, sarcoidosis appeared to develop and pursue its course independently of the osteosarcoma, though the possibility that immunosuppressive treatment may have been a factor in determining its onset cannot be dismissed.

MALIGNANT LYMPHOMA

Sarcoid reactions in or adjacent to tissues affected by Hodgkin's disease and other lymphomas are discussed in Chapter 2, p. 33; and a case illustrating the diagnostic difficulty that they may cause if they are prominent in the early stages of these diseases is described in Chapter 10, p. 256.

Brincker (1972) in a survey of 1500 cases of various sorts of maligant lymphoma found five in whom the diagnosis of sarcoidosis was made on acceptable grounds, in three before and in two after the lymphoma was diagnosed. Those in which the sarcoidosis appeared first do not seem especially remarkable; in two chronic lymphatic leukaemia was diagnosed 14 and 27 years after erythema nodosum and lymphadenopathy attributable to sarcoidosis, and in the other, Hodgkin's disease developed in a patient with chronic pulmonary sarcoidosis which had been diagnosed eight years earlier. Of the two in which lymphoma appeared first, both had Hodgkin's disease, successfully treated; in one, cutaneous sarcoidosis with radiographic evidence of sarcoid changes in a metatarsal bone appeared five years later, and in the other erythema nodosum and BHL 17 years later. In both, sarcoid-type granulomas had been seen in the lymph-nodes which had provided the initial histological diagnosis of Hodgkin's disease; it is a matter for speculation whether these were a local reaction to the Hodgkin's disease, or part of a widespread sarcoid granulomatosis that later became clinically apparent.

As noted above, Brincker and Wilbek (1974) reported a high incidence of malignant lymphoma in their survey of 2544 patients with sarcoidosis, which even after review by Rømer (1980) had removed dubious diagnoses, was six times that expected for the general population; the number of cases, however, was only three. Among about 500 patients with sarcoidosis followed for varying periods by one of us (JGS), three developed malignant lymphomas nine, one and 11 years from the diagnosis of sarcoidosis which was following a chronic course.

The first was a woman who had had multiple small nodular sarcoids of the skin of the trunk and extensive sarcoid infiltration of the scalp and forehead (Fig 7.8 and Plate 11), with fibrosing pulmonary infiltration for nine years before she developed a mediastinal tumour causing dysphagia and stridor. She died at the age of 59, less than two months after the appearance of these symptoms. At necropsy, lymphosarcoma was found to have spread widely in the mediastinum, where it had apparently originated, and involved also the right iliac lymph-nodes; there were old sarcoid changes in the lungs; and the right suprarenal gland showed an area of caseation, 2.5 cm in diameter, enclosed in a firm partly calcified capsule, showing no histologically specific features, and yielding no mycobacteria on culture.

The second was a woman who at the age of 41, investigated because of cough and loss of weight, was found to have widespread fine mottling in the chest radiograph. A year later, she developed nausea, vomiting and diarrhoea which continued for six weeks, but recurred shortly afterwards. At this stage, the only abnormality on physical examination was some vague abdominal tenderness, with indefinite masses palpable in the iliac fossae, especially the right, thought to be enlarged lymph-nodes. Radiography of the chest showed the mottling to have diminished considerably. A barium meal showed no abnormality in the alimentary tract. The Mantoux test gave a positive reaction to 1:100 OT. Although a liver biopsy showed no specific changes, a diagnosis of sarcoidosis seemed likely. Two years later, when she was aged 45, the gastric symptoms, which had persisted, became more severe, and a barium meal showed a filling defect in the stomach. At laparotomy the wall of the stomach was thickened and indurated, and the spleen was considerably enlarged. Two-thirds of the stomach and the spleen were removed. The spleen, a portion of liver and a lymph-node removed for biopsy were found to be infiltrated with sarcoid tubercles. In the greater curvature of the stomach there was a large plaque of infiltration, which histologically was found to be a malignant lymphoma. After the operation, she improved, and ten years later remained in good health, without evidence either of sarcoidosis or of recurrence of the lymphoma. The latter appears to have been of the type of primary malignant lymphoma of the alimentary tract described by Allen *et al.* (1954), Azzopardi and Menzies (1960) and Jacobs (1963), in which prolonged survival after surgical treatment is possible.

The third was a patient who at the age of 38 developed lupus pernio and later other skin lesions, illustrated in Fig 7.9. She was found to have lung changes, illustrated in Figs 6.28 and 6.29. On prednisolone treatment, both these manifestations were controlled. At the age of 49, she developed acute abdominal symptoms, and laparotomy showed a perforation of the ileum, which on biopsy was found to be infiltrated by a reticulum cell sarcoma. This illness proved fatal, and at necropsy, multiple deposits of reticulum cell sarcoma were found in the lungs, apparently densest round collections of typical Schaumann conchoidal bodies, and the liver, spleen and stomach were infiltrated by a similar tumour.

A few other cases in which malignant lymphoma and sarcoidosis were associated have been reported.

Buckle (1960) reported the case of a woman, aged 28, who was found at routine radiography to have widespread mottling in the lungs, the Mantoux test being negative with 100 IU; seven months later she developed rapidly increasing enlargement of lymph-nodes in the neck, shown by biopsy to be due to an undifferentiated reticulosarcoma; in spite of radiotherapy, the disease spread rapidly; at necropsy there was extensive reticulosarcomatous infiltration of lymph-nodes, chest wall and pericardium, together with non-caseating epithelioid and giant-cell tubercles with much fibrosis in the lungs. Raben *et al.* (1961) reported the case of a woman, aged 45, with sarcoidosis of the skin, histologically proved, associated with enlargement of cervical lymph-nodes, the right parotid gland, the liver and spleen; one and a half years from the onset, she became ill with increase in the size of the lymph-nodes and the spleen, and now a cervical lymph-node biopsy showed evidence of reticulosarcoma; she died two years later, and at necropsy the diagnosis of reticulosarcoma was confirmed, the report not stating whether or not sarcoid changes persisted. Goldfarb and Cohen (1970) reported two cases in which epithelioid cell granulomas of sarcoid type were found in several organs not affected by Hodgkin's disease in patients with Hodgkin's disease. One of these patients died, and there was no necropsy, and the report gave no information about the later course of the other; interpretation of these cases must remain in doubt.

Cases in which extensive skin infiltrations initially showing the histological pattern of sarcoidosis later changed character and showed the histological pattern and course of malignant lymphoma were reported by Atwood *et al.* (1966, Case 1) and Kahn *et al.* (1974). In the first of these, the change in histological pattern occurred gradually, starting six years after the original biopsy, which had been accompanied by two 'positive' Kveim tests; lymphnodes became involved later, and a Kveim test was negative; there was persistent BHL. In spite of treatment the patient, a black man aged 49, died five years after the diagnosis of lymphoma; at necropsy, there was extensive malignant lymphoma, but no active sarcoidosis, the only residual evidence of which was fibrosis in hilar lymph-nodes. In the case reported by Kahn *et al.* (1974), there was no evidence of systemic sarcoidosis during life, and no necropsy; and the initial sarcoid histology was interpreted as an unusually florid local sarcoid reaction.

Hairy-cell leukaemia

Myers *et al.* (1979) reported the case of a woman, aged 45, who presented with erythema nodosum, fever, anterior uveitis and arthropathy, hepatosplenomegaly and BHL with lung infiltration. The blood leucocytes numbered 3300 mm^{-3}, and 34% of them were hairy cells. The spleen, weighing 415 g, was removed; it and a wedge biopsy of liver showed both infiltration with hairy cells and granulomas of sarcoid type. There was a 20 mm reaction to a tuberculin test with 5 IU; because of this treatment with isoniazid was given. After the splenectomy, the symptoms improved and six months later the chest radiograph was normal. In this case, it seems likely that sarcoidosis occurred incidentally in a patient with hairy-cell leukaemia, and resolved spontaneously, while there was the favourable symptomatic response to splenectomy often seen in hairy-cell leukaemia. The question whether the granulomatosis was a reaction to the mycobacterial infection indicated by the strongly positive tuberculin test and responded to isoniazid treatment remains open; it is relevant that infections, including those with mycobacteria, are frequent in hairy cell leukaemia (Bouza *et al.*, 1978; Golomb *et al.*, 1978).

Myeloma

Selroos *et al.* (1974) described a case in which myeloma of lambda-type IgG appeared during the course of sarcoidosis.

At the age of 48 a woman whose mother had died of a lung disease, probably tuberculosis, was found to have symptomless BHL; the diagnosis of sarcoidosis was supported by scalene node biopsy, though there was a positive reaction to a tuberculin test with 1 IU. Four years later, she developed bilateral uveitis. Investigated at the age of 54, she was found to have persistent BHL, posterior synechiae due to old uveitis, a histologically confirmed sarcoid papule on the cheek, a granulomatous response to a Kveim test, and fibrotic granulomatous changes in a mediastinal lymph-node. Over the next few months, the erythrocyte sedimentation rate rose to 95 mm, and the serum protein to 9.2 g dl^{-1}, with paraprotein amounting to 2.03 g dl^{-1}, shown to be a lambatype IgG. The finding of plasma cells amounting to 15% of nucleated bone-marrow cells, and 2% of peripheral blood leucocytes indicated a pre-symptomatic multiple myeloma.

Macrocryoglobulinaemia

Turkington and Buckley (1966) reported the case of a black man, aged 55, who presented with macrocryoglobulinaemia causing episodes of bleeding, anaemia, neurological symptoms, including a seizure, retinal changes, and Raynaud's phenomenon, in whom the finding of enlarged hilar lymph-nodes followed by a pulmonary infiltration and of granulomas in liver and lymph-node biopsies led to the diagnosis of sarcoidosis. The relation between the two aspects of this case remains speculative.

Gammaglobulin deficiency

Several cases of sarcoidosis in patients with IgA deficiency have been reported.

Goldstein *et al.* (1969), in a review of immunoglobin levels in 84 patients with sarcoidosis, mentioned two, both black women, who had no IgA; one, aged 38, had chronic pulmonary sarcoidosis, and the other, aged 39, had BHL with erythema nodosum; in neither was there evidence of undue susceptibility to infections. Davis *et al.* (1970) reported the case of a man, aged 36, who had had recurrent episodes of otitis media and two of pneumonia, and was found to have IgA deficiency; intermittent diarrhoea was assocated with nodular hyperplasia of the lymphoid tissue of the small intestine; chest radiography showed enlargement of hilar and right paratracheal lymph-nodes and rounded shadows in both lower lobes; biopsy of a scalene lymph-node showed sarcoid-type granulomas; and the hilar lymph-node enlargement and lung shadows subsided spontaneously. Sharma and Chandor (1972) described the case of a 31 year old woman with selective serum and salivary IgA deficiency in whom enlargement of peripheral lymph-nodes and lung infiltration was attributed to sarcoidosis, supported by biopsy of a scalene lymph-node. Siegler (1978) reported two patients with selective IgA deficiency who developed sarcoidosis. In the first, a man aged 47 presented with BHL and lung infiltration and arthropathy of the ankles, which subsided in a manner characteristic of sarcoidosis; he was later found to have no detectable IgA. In the second, a 21 year old woman with serum and salivary IgA deficiency who had had many severe bacterial infections of the respiratory and urinary tracts and of the skin, presented with evidence of a widespread granulomatous disease with mixed features of sarcoidosis and mycobacerial tuberculosis. In the man with sarcoidosis and auto-immune haemolytic anaemia reported by Thomas *et al.* (1982), there was a selective IgA deficiency.

Bronsky *et al.* (1965) reported the case of a black woman aged 37 who had had several episodes of pneumonia, otitis media and paronychia. BHL was noted after a pneumonia, and later she developed sarcoids of the skin, the diagnosis being supported by biopsies of scalene lymph-node and skin. She was found to have no detectable IgA or IgM, and the level of IgG was low.

In all these cases, the diagnosis of sarcoidosis was supported by a compatible course. Since the frequency of IgA deficiency of the sort reported in most of them is estimated at between one in 500 and one in 700 of the general population (Amman and Hong, 1971), the number of recorded cases is probably within that to be expected if the association occurred only by chance. Granulomas in spleen, liver and lymph-nodes may be a feature of some immunoglobulin deficiencies (Rosen and Janeway, 1966); thus not only histological evidence of granulomas, but also clinical features and course compatible with sarcoidosis are required to establish this diagnosis in patients with such deficiencies. For instance, judgement must be reserved about the case reported by Zinneman *et al.* (1954), that of a woman, aged 30, who was known to have had 44 attacks of pneumonia and two of pneumococcal meningitis, and was found to have hypogammaglobulinaemia and no isohaemagglutinins; biopsies of an axillary lymph-node and of liver, and of the spleen weighing 1130 g and removed surgically, all showed sarcoid-type granulomas.

SYSTEMIC LUPUS ERYTHEMATOSUS

Cases in which during the course of systemic lupus erythematosus (SLE) BHL and lung infiltration attributable to sarcoidosis appeared have been reported by Harrison *et al.* (1979), Hunter *et al.* (1980) and Needleman *et al.* (1982). These occurred in women aged 54, 62 and 47 after the diagnosis of SLE had been established for 16 months, eight years and four months; in all cases the diagnosis of sarcoidosis was supported by histology, of a skin papule and liver, of lung and hilar lymph-nodes, and of lung and bone-marrow respectively.

De Paola (1958) recorded the case of a woman who died at the age of 43 with SLE; at necropsy, in addition to the changes of this disease, hyalinizing sarcoid tubercles were found in hilar lymph-nodes and lungs, although sarcoidosis had not been clinically manifest.

A patient observed by one of us (JGS) presented a confusing mixture of features, criteria for the diagnosis first of sarcoidosis and later of SLE being met:

A man, aged 28, developed pain in the right side of the chest and fever. He was found to have a generalized lymphadenopathy and a palpable spleen and a chest radiograph showed enlargement of hilar nodes, especially on the right. A Heaf tuberculin test gave a strongly positive reaction. Biopsy of a lymph-node showed no specific changes. The fever did not respond to antibiotics. Three weeks from the onset, he became acutely ill, with a leukaemoid reaction and a severe haemolytic anaemia; the total leucocyte count rose to 44 000 mm^{-3}, of which a high proportion were immature cells of the granulocyte series, and the haemoglobin fell to 28%. He was treated with blood transfusions and prednisolone; because of the strongly positive tuberculin test, streptomycin and isoniazid were given also. Improvement started from the fourth day after the beginning of prednisolone treatment, and the blood count returned to and remained normal. Antituberculosis chemotherapy was continued for six months, but prednisolone was gradually withdrawn after two months. The hilar node enlargement subsided during prednisolone treatment, but within two months of its cessation, had recurred and was accompanied by widespread mottling in the lungs. Nine months from the beginning of the illness, the only symptom was slight dyspnoea on exertion. The only abnormal finding in physical examination was slight enlargement of lymph-nodes in neck, axillae and groins. The chest radiograph showed bilateral enlargement of hilar lymph-nodes with some foci of calcification on the left side and fine mottling throughout the lungs. Further lymph-node, bone-marrow and liver biopsies showed no specific change. Open lung biopsy showed a soft lung, not deflating as easily as usual, and with no gross nodularity; lymph-nodes up to 1 cm in diameter were palpable at the root of the lung; a wedge of the apical segment of the lower lobe was removed and showed aggregations of tubercles of sarcoid type along the interlobular septa and around the vessels, undergoing circumferential fibrosis; culture produced no tubercle bacilli. As the pulmonary function was little affected and he had no disability, no treatment was advised. Six months later, he became ill with fever, left pleuritic pain, cough and expectoration. The fever persisted; he developed pain and stiffness in the knee joints; the heart enlarged; and LE cells were found repeatedly in the blood. Treatment with prednisone led to prompt defervescence and relief of symptoms. Maintained on prednisone treatment, he remained symptom-free, though LE cells continued to be demonstrable in the peripheral blood.

In all these cases, the features attributable to sarcoidosis and to SLE seemed to have run expected courses independently of each other, and the number of recorded cases seems to be no greater than would be expected from the frequency of the two diseases.

CHRONIC ARTHROPATHIES

Rheumatoid arthritis

There is no reason to believe that sarcoidosis and rheumatoid arthritis (RA) occur together more frequently than would be expected by chance. As noted in Chapter 9, p. 241, Putkonen *et al.* (1965b) in a review of 94 patients with sarcoidosis found evidence of RA in two, 'definite' in one and 'probable' in one.

In the patient with chronic pulmonary sarcoidosis leading to the formation of thick-walled cavities, whose case is summarized in Chapter 6, p. 132, there were mild joint symptoms and rheumatoid nodules on the elbows, and at necropsy evidence of inactive RA in an interphalangeal joint.

Hillerdal *et al.* (1965) recorded the case of a woman with sarcoidosis, starting with erythema nodosum and BHL, and proceeding to pulmonary infiltration and fibrosis; syphilis causing pharyngeal ulcerations and later aortic valve disease; and severe rheumatoid arthritis with nodules.

Ankylosing Spondylitis

A patient observed by one of us (JGS), and mentioned in Chapter 8, p. 213, had ankylosing spondylitis and sarcoidosis, manifested by hilar lymph-node enlargement followed by lung infiltration. There was also a uveitis which might have been associated with either disease; the first symptoms of the two diseases appeared about the same time, and both diseases followed a similar course to spontaneous cessation of activity.

Verstraeten and Bekaert (1951) reported the case of a man, aged 36, who presented with ankylosing spondylitis involving the lumbar and thoracic spine, and was found to have BHL, diffuse pulmonary infiltration, a Mantoux test negative to 1:100 OT, and sarcoids of the skin of the forearm, confirmed by biopsy both of skin and of an enlarged epitrochlear lymph-node. Lovelock and Stone (1953, Case 7) mentioned briefly a black man, aged 32, with BHL, lung infiltration, an epididymal nodule, negative tuberculin and positive Kveim tests, who also suffered from Marie-Strumpell arthritis. Deshayes *et al.* (1965) reported the case of a man aged 40 with sarcoidosis, manifested by pulmonary infiltration, negative tuberculin test and typical histological changes in a bronchial biopsy, who also had ankylosing spondylitis.

Gout and psoriasis

Kaplan and Klatskin (1960) observed two patients in whom sarcoidosis, psoriasis and gout were associated.

The first had had psoriasis since the age of 20, and his first attack of gout at the age of 33; at the age of 37, he presented with widespread lung infiltration, with sarcoid-type granulomas in a liver biopsy. The second was a man who at the age of 42 had erythema nodosum, uveitis and BHL, with sarcoid granulomas in a liver biopsy, followed by a pulmonary infiltration; six years later he had his first attack of gout, and two years later still, psoriasis appeared. In a third patient with gout and psoriasis, the diagnosis of sarcoidosis was less well established.

Interested in this association, Kaplan and Klatskin reviewed 73 patients with sarcoidosis and found none with psoriasis or gout, though six of 25 in whom the blood uric acid was estimated showed a raised figure; in 100 with psoriasis they found no gout and no unequivocal evidence of sarcoidosis, though 11 had unexplained shadows in the chest radiograph, or an enlarged liver or spleen, and one had a number of odd features and a small unspecific granuloma in a liver biopsy; and in 100 cases of gout they found no psoriasis or sarcoidosis, though two had some pulmonary fibrosis.

Bunim *et al.* (1962) considered possible relationships between psoriasis, gout and sarcoidosis in discussion of a case of psoriasis with hyperuricaemia and infiltration of the liver with granulomas. There is evidence that psoriasis and gout occur together more frequently than would be expected by chance. For instance, Kuzell *et al.* (1955) stated that psoriasis occurs in a proportion estimated to be between 0.27 and 1.4% of the general population, and that among 520 patients with gout they had found 4.0% to have psoriasis; they thought that this might be due to hyperuricaemia in psoriasis caused by the rapid turnover of epidermal cells. But the bizarre assocation of these two diseases with sarcoidosis seems to have been recorded only by Kaplan and Klatskin. Zimmer and Demis (1966) examined the hospital records of 233 patients with gout, 335 with psoriasis and 79 with sarcoidosis. Although gout and psoriasis occurred together in 11 cases, no patient with sarcoidosis had either of the other two diseases.

Polyarteritis nodosa

Symmers and Gillett (1951) described the necropsy findings in a man who had suffered from pulmonary tuberculosis and died at the age of 50 after a haematemesis. This was found to have arisen from a ruptured polyarteritic aneurysm in the duodenum; similar polyarteritic lesions were found elsewhere, especially in the liver, the spleen and the kidneys. Other arteritic lesions resembling those of systemic lupus erythematosus were found elsewhere, especially in the kidneys. There was a widespread lymphadenopathy involving cervical, mediastinal and abdominal nodes, with the histological picture of hyalinized sarcoidosis, Schaumann bodies and asteroids being present. No sarcoid-like lesions were found elsewhere. In the lungs there was evidence of an old silicosis, together with banal tuberculous changes. In this case it seems probable that the sarcoid changes antedated the arteritis and were unrelated to it.

AMYLOIDOSIS

Very few cases in which sarcoidosis and amyloidosis have occurred together have been reported. In reviews of amyloidosis, Azar (1968) commented on the lack of association with sarcoidosis, and Glenner and Page (1976) found only one published case. This was reported by Swanton (1971).

> It occurred in a 30 year old man, known to have bilateral basal bronchiectasis for seven years. He presented with heavy proteinuria and hepatosplenomegaly; the diagnosis of amyloidosis was based on amyloid deposits in biopsies of liver and kidney, and in the spleen, which was removed; the diagnosis of sarcoidosis on granulomas in liver and spleen, but not in kidney, and at a Kveim test site, and on hypercalcaemia responsive to corticosteroid. This patient later died in renal failure, and there was no necropsy.
>   Subsequently other cases have been reported by Bar-Meir *et al.* (1977) and Fresko and Lazarus (1982). The patient described by Bar-Meir *et al.* was a 58 year old woman, who presented with a very large spleen, enlarged lymph-

nodes in axillae and groins, slight BHL and lung infiltration; the diagnosis of sarcoidosis was supported by biopsy of an axillary lymph-node and of liver, and a positive Kveim test; and the diagnosis of amyloidosis by histology of the axillary node, and in a rectal biopsy, but not in the liver. Treatment with prednisone led to reduction in the size of the spleen, which had caused pain, and after 18 months the chest radiograph was normal. The case reported by Fresko and Lazarus (1982) was that of a 40 year old black man, known to have had pulmonary sarcoidosis for 16 years, leading to fibrosis and episodes of pneumonia; he died in respiratory and right ventricular failure, with proteinuria; at necropsy, there was gross fibrosis of the lungs with honeycombing, showing both granulomas and inflammatory exudate microscopically, and both interalveolar septa and vessel-walls were infiltrated with amyloid; hilar lymph-nodes showed granulomas with extensive hyalinization; and amyloid was found around vessels in many organs, including heart, liver, spleen and kidneys.

In this case, it seems likely that the amyloidosis was related to chronic infection in the fibrotic lung, and in that reported by Swanton (1971) to the unrelated bronchiectasis, rather than to sarcoidosis itself.

INFECTIONS

Aspergillosis

The sort of aspergillosis which consists in the growth of a mat of mycelium in an air-containing space in the lung, causing it eventually to become filled with a rounded mass of mycelium, the so-called 'fungus ball' or aspergilloma (Hinson *et al.*, 1952) is a well-recognized complication of any chronic pulmonary disease leading to the development of such spaces. It may thus complicate the late stage of pulmonary sarcoidosis, and is discussed in Chapter 6, p. 135. There is no evidence that the liability of lungs damaged by chronic sarcoidosis to be colonized by aspergilus is different from that of lungs with similar anatomical changes due to other diseases.

Nocardiasis

Steinberg (1958, Case 1) reported the case of a black woman who at the age of 38 was found to have pulmonary and skin sarcoidosis, confirmed by skin biopsy. Fibrosis gradually developed in the lungs, and because of this cortisone was administered, with temporary improvement. Seven years from the onset, she became ill with cough, haemoptysis and dyspnoea and shortly afterwards developed meningeal signs and coma and died. At necropsy there were cavities in both lungs and bilateral cerebral abscesses, in which *Nocardia asteroides* was found both microscopically and by culture.

A similar case was reported by O'Neill and Penman (1969) in a man aged 52 with chronic pulmonary sarcoidosis, treated with varying doses of prednisone; he died of an acute meningo-encephalitis, *Nocardia asteroides* being grown from CSF shortly before death. At necropsy, the central nervous system showed the changes of nocardial disease only, while the lungs and hilar nodes showed granulomas without demonstrable micro-organisms.

In both these cases, it seems likely that Nocardia infection was an unrelated late complication of the fibrotic stage of pulmonary sarcoidosis.

Toxoplasma gondii

In a case described by Konstantin-Hansen and Arentsen (1981), a man aged 29 presented with a clinical picture of encephalitis, with high protein level in the CSF. A diagnosis of sarcoidosis was made on the chest radiograph and the finding of granulomas in a liver biopsy. Treatment with prednisone was started, but shortly afterwards serological findings indicating recent toxoplasma infection were reported, and treatment with pyrimethamine and spiramycin was added. There was symptomatic improvement, but relapse after cessation of treatment. Subsequent response to prednisone alone suggested that the nervous system changes may well have been due to sarcoidosis, the toxoplasma infection being incidental.

Herpes simplex encephalitis

Sweeney and McDonnell (1979) reported the case of a woman, aged 33, who died of herpes simplex encephalitis: at necropsy, there were severe changes attributable to this disease in the brain, and non-caseating granulomas of sarcoid-type in lungs, hilar lymph-nodes, liver and spleen.

A case in which fatal generalized herpes virus infection developed soon after the initiation of methotrexate treatment for intractable sarcoidosis of the central nervous system is mentioned in Chapter 27, p. 596.

Yersinea enterocolitica

Infections with *Yersinia enterocolitica* causing illnesses of varying severity with such features as gastro-enteritis, mesenteric lymphadenopathy, arthropathy, septicaemia, and, as mentioned in Chapter 5, p. 73, erythema nodosum (EN), have been reported mainly from northern Europe (Mollaret, 1971; Ahvonen, 1972; Hällström *et al.*, 1972). In some cases, EN has been associated with hilar lymph-node enlargement, but Hallstrom *et al.* found no granulomas in lymph-nodes removed by scalene biopsy or mediastinoscopy in three such cases. On the other hand, Agner and Larsen (1979) in a study of 55 patients with biopsy-confirmed sarcoidosis in Copenhagen found seven with serological evidence of recent infection with *Y. enterocolitica*, of Type 3 which is prevalent in Denmark. Of these seven patients, five had erythema nodosum, six joint pains, one uveitis and five fever; in all, the course over periods of 14–41 months was compatible with a diagnosis of sarcoidosis. The relation of the Yersinia infection indicated by the serological evidence to generalized granulomatosis is uncertain. It may have been a precipitating factor, or have brought to light a previously asymptomatic condition; it seems unlikely to have been directly causal.

Inflammatory bowel disease

The few recorded associations of sarcoidosis and inflammatory bowel disease (Crohn's disease and ulcerative colitis) are discussed in Chapter 17, p. 373.

Chapter 25

Aetiology

Hypotheses that have been advanced about the aetiology of sarcoidosis are of widely different sorts. Some are now of historic interest only, and some have been implied rather than explicitly stated.

Among those that are of historic interest are those implied by the names proposed by Boeck and by Schaumann. As noted in Chapter 1, Boeck at first thought that the 'multiple benign sarcoid' of the skin which he described in 1899 was a benign new growth of connective tissue, and although he later recognized that the histology was that of a tuberculoid granuloma, the name he suggested gradually crept into general use to designate the systemic disease of which the skin eruption is a possible manifestation. In 1914, Schaumann advanced the name 'lymphogranulomatosis benigna' for the generalized disease underlying sarcoids of the skin and lupus pernio, suggesting that it might be regarded as a proliferative disease of lymphatic tissue, analogous in some respects to Hodgkin's disease (Schaumann, 1934). Like Boeck, he came later to the conclusion that it was probably related to tuberculosis; this is discussed below.

DISCARDED HYPOTHESES

The sarcoid diathesis hypothesis

This postulated an inherent tendency in certain individuals to react to a variety of stimuli with non-caseating epithelioid-cell granulomas. This, the sarcoid diathesis or 'terrain sarcoidique' hypothesis can be controverted on several grounds. Apart from the tendency of old scars to become infiltrated in the active stage of sarcoidosis, and of the few reports of Kveim-like reactions to intradermal injections of certain materials not derived from sarcoid tissues (Chapter 21, p. 453), there is no evidence that patients with sarcoidosis react with a sarcoid granuloma to non-specific stimuli.

Refvem (1954) investigated granulomatous reactions to a number of agents including silica and phospholipids from hen's eggs and from human serum, and showed that patients with sarcoidosis showed no evidence of abnormal reactivity to these substances. Hurley and Shelley (1959) performed intradermal tests with sodium stearate, a large number of metallic elements and homologous blood in normal subjects and in patients with sarcoidosis and with zirconium granulomas. They found no difference in quality or intensity of reaction between the various groups, apart from the specific granulomatous response to zirconium in the patients with zirconium granulomas (Shelley and Hurley, 1958a and b), suggesting that the sarcoid granuloma is a specific response to an inciting agent or possibly one of a number of possible agents.

Non-infective causal agents

A number of non-infective factors have been considered as possible causes or contributory causes of sarcoidosis. The high incidence of sarcoidosis in the south-eastern area of the United States coincides with a high content of beryllium in the soils of this region (Gentry *et al.*, 1955); but the clinical differences between chronic beryllium disease and 'idiopathic' sarcoidosis (Chapter 22), the clear relationship between known exposure to beryllium, and the development of beryllium disease, and the absence of skin reactivity to beryllium in sarcoidosis rule out the possibility of a relationship between 'idiopathic' sarcoidosis and beryllium exposure.

A general correspondence of areas within the United States with the distribution of pine forests (Cummings *et al.*, 1956) led to much investigation of the possibility that inhalation of pine pollen might be a causal factor in sarcoidosis. Cummings and Hudgins (1958) demonstrated that pine pollen had acid-fast staining characteristics, contained an acid-fast lipid and an amino-acid resembling diaminopimelic acid, and was capable of inducing epithelioid cell granulomas in tuberculin-sensitive guinea-pigs, both at the site of intradermal injection and in the related lymph-nodes. Laboratory and epidemiological studies relevant to this hypothesis were reviewed by Cummings (1964), who concluded that they did not support it. While pine pollens had components with granuloma-producing and immunogenic potentiality in the experimental animal, no evidence was obtained that any component caused or contributed to a progressive generalized granulomatosis; and epidemiological studies in other areas showed no relation between the distribution of pine forests and the incidence of sarcoidosis.

Relation to mycobacterial infection

The similarity of the histological changes of sarcoidosis to those of myco-bacterial tuberculosis, and some observed clinical associations between the two diseases, led some early investigators to the view that sarcoidosis might be an unusual form of tuberculosis. Pinner (1938) held this view strongly enough to propose that sarcoidosis should be called 'non-caseating tubercu-losis'. When the term 'tuberculosis' was first introduced, it was defined, and was definable, only in morbid anatomical terms; but since the time of Koch, it has been definable, and generally is defined, aetiologically, as the disease caused by certain species of mycobacteria. And to state that sarcoidosis is a non-caseating variety of tuberculosis, so defined, is to postulate that myco-bacterial infection is a necessary causal factor in all cases of sarcoidosis. In view of the current inability to demonstrate a causal agent of any sort in most cases of sarcoidosis, this generalization is as unjustified as its opposite, that sarcoidosis cannot be related in any way to mycobacterial infection. It is therefore appropriate to summarize the evidence for and against the possible role of mycobacterial infection in at least some cases of sarcoidosis. In favour of this possibility are the following points:

(a) Observations of the concurrence of sarcoidosis with bacteriologically proved infection with *M. tuberculosis* have been summarized in Chapter 23. Of these cases, those most difficult to explain as coincidental are those in which a clinical picture of mycobacterial tuberculosis merges imperceptibly into one of sarcoidosis; those in which mycobacteria are isolated, sometimes with unusual sorts of evidently mycobacterial lesions, in the course of a disease otherwise characteristic of sarcoidosis; and those in which the discovery of mycobacteria is accompanied by disappearance of specifically sarcoid features.

(b) Non-caseating tubercles may be the most prominent finding in undoubtedly mycobacterial disease. Zettergren (1954) studied 54 lymph-nodes from cases of sarcoidosis and 49 diagnosed as chronic hyperplastic tuberculosis because of the finding of acid-fast bacilli in them, and concluded that the two groups could not be distinguished histologically. It is well recognized that non-caseating granulomas at the periphery of an obviously caseating focus of mycobacterial disease contain very few, possibly no detectable acid-fast bacilli. The agent locally inciting granuloma formation at these sites is unidentified, apart from the presumption that it is derived from the infecting mycobac-teria; it is highly improbable that it is a chemical component of these organisms (Chapter 2, p. 14). Much of the recent information about the cellular immunopathogenesis of the sarcoid granuloma reviewed in Chapter 20 may well be equally relevant to this aspect of the pathogenesis of mycobacterial tuberculosis.

(c) No clear line of demarcation can be drawn between sarcoidosis and certain cases in which a diagnosis of indolent mycobacterial tuberculosis with low tuberculin sensitivity is appropriate. It is, of course, well recognized that patients seriously ill with acutely progressive tuberculosis often have depressed skin sensitivity to tuberculin, and that intercurrent disease of various sorts may cause similar depression (Scadding, 1971b). The cases over which diagnostic difficulty may arise are a smaller group of patients with indolent lung infiltrations, not acutely ill, with persistently negative reactions to tuberculin, in whom mycobacteria, when found, are discoverable only by persistent search and possibly intermittently. Cases of this sort have been described by Mascher (1951), Scadding (1956) and Kent and Schwarz (1967).

In relation to the problem of the relationship between mycobacterial infection and sarcoidosis, cases of proved tuberculosis which present 'sarcoid-like' features with insensitivity to tuberculin are important out of proportion of their rarity. Even failure to respond to antimycobacterial chemotherapy does not distinguish sharply between tuberculosis and sarcoidosis. Occasional cases have been reported in which proved mycobacterial tuberculosis failed to respond to chemotherapy to which the infecting organism was shown to be sensitive *in vitro*, although none of the features such as overwhelming extent of disease were present, responded when corticosteroid was added, as in the case summarized in Chapter 6 (p. 166). In another case under the care of one of us (JGS), the diagnosis of chronic miliary tuberculosis with low tuberculin sensitivity seemed likely, and was supported by the finding of acid-fast bacilli in lesions in a liver biopsy and in the sputum, though they did not grow on culture; but antimycobacterial drugs were ineffective until corticosteroid treatment was added.

(d) The differences, clinical and pathological, between sarcoidosis and indolent forms of tuberculosis are far less than those between these and such acute forms as tuberculous broncho-pneumonia and acute miliary tuberculosis. Even more strikingly, in the rare cases of acute *M. tuberculosis* septicaemia (Ball *et al.*, 1951) there are no formed tubercles, the lesions taking the form of foci of necrosis with very numberous bacilli. The contrast between this picture and that of indolent productive tuberculosis is so great that without the bacteriological evidence it would be difficult to see any connection between them. Nevertheless, they must be accepted as the ends of a range of possible reations to mycobacterial infection. Tuberculin sensitivity may be undetectable at both ends of this range. The possibility that some cases of sarcoidosis are extreme examples of indolent, granulomatous, paucibacillary mycobacterial tuberculosis cannot be rejected *a priori*.

(e) In some epidemiological studies, reviewed in Chapter 4, p. 65 a high proportion of patients with sarcoidosis have been found to have a history of contact with tuberculosis (Parsons, 1960; Ten Have and Orie, 1961; Bunn and Johnston, 1972). Wurm *et al.* (1962) described two sibships in one of which eight cases of sarcoidosis and four of tuberculosis, and in the other four of sarcoidosis three of tuberculosis and two having features of both diseases occured in two generations.

(f) In areas with populations including distinguishable ethnic groups, groups with a higher incidence of tuberculosis generally have a higher incidence of sarcoidosis. In the United States, blacks are more liable to both tuberculosis and sarcoidosis than whites. In London, Brett (1965) studied the changes in prevalance of abnormalities interpreted as due to tuberculosis and sarcoidosis in repeated mass radiographic surveys in an area with considerable proportions of inhabitants of Irish and of West Indian origin. Among persons born in the United Kingdom, the prevalence of both tuberculosis and sarcoidosis remained unchanged; among Irish immigrants the prevalence of both disease diminished, and among West Indians both increased between the times of the two surveys. Thus the prevalence of sarcoidosis showed a change in the same direction as that of tuberculosis in each of three ethnic groups.

(g) Reactions to graded doses of tuberculin were found to be similarly distributed in a series of 133 patients in London with sarcoidosis between 41 in whom there was calcification or other presumptive evidence of mycobacterial infection and 92 with no such evidence (Scadding, 1961), although the deviation of this finding from expectation on the hypothesis that the tuberculous infection was unrelated to the sarcoidosis did not attain statistical significance. Similarly in the observations on the effect of cortisone on tuberculin skin reactions in sarcoidosis mentioned in Chapter 20, p. 426, among the tuberculin-negative sarcoidosis patients, the proportions reacting to tuberculin plus cortisone were the same, whether or not there was calcification or other evidence of old tuberculous infection (Citron and Scadding, 1957).

Arguments against the role of *M. tuberculosis* infection as a necessary factor in the causation of sarcoidosis include:

(a) The proportion of cases of sarcoidosis from which tubercle bacilli are isolated is very small; and in some series has been reported to be zero. The latter statement can of course be interpreted only if the preconceived ideas of the collector of the series are known. If he is one of those who adopts a definition which permits him to diagnose sarcoidosis only if mycobacterial infection has been excluded, the statement simply reiterates his definition and has little factual content. The rejection of the diagnosis of sarcoidosis in a number of cases presenting otherwise characteristic features when intensive investigation led to the isolation of *M. tuberculosis* by Kent *et al.* (1970), quoted in Chapter 23, p.508, is a good example of this.

(b) When tuberculosis was customarily treated in special accommodation in hospitals and sanatoria, patients with sarcoidosis might be admitted for investigation to such units, where they would be liable to be infected with mycobacteria; but this could account for only those cases in which such exposure occurred, and in which the clinical manifestations of overt mycobacterial disease appeared at a considerable interval after the initial presentation.

(c) The fact that tuberculin sensitivity is lower in groups of patients with sarcoidosis than in unselected members of the population from which they are drawn has been regarded as a militating against a mycobacterial aetiology. In view of the occasional occurrence of chronic forms of tuberculosis with negative tuberculin reactions, noted above, this argument has little force.

(d) The common patterns of organ involvement in sarcoidosis differ from those in tuberculosis. The uveal tract, the salivary and lacrimal glands, the heart and skeletal muscle and the small bones of the hands and feet are commonly involved in sarcoidosis, rarely in tuberculosis; conversely the adrenal glands are not infrequently involved in caseating tuberculosis, but almost never in sarcoidosis. It must be admitted, however, that different patterns of organ involvement are well recognized at different stages of, or in different types of reaction to, the same infection: e.g. in tuberculosis itself, in syphilis, and in lepromatous and tuberculoid leprosy.

(e) Epidemiological studies have shown differences between the geographical distributions of sarcoidosis and of tuberculosis (Chapter 4, p. 64). There is evidence from the United States, Denmark and Germany that sarcoidosis is associated with residence in the country, and tuberculosis with residence in towns; and contemporary prevalences of sarcoidosis and of tuberculosis in different parts of the same country show no correlations.

(f) The failure of antituberculosis chemotherapy to influence the course of sarcoidosis is difficult to reconcile with a direct aetiogical role for *M. tuberculosis*. Yet, as noted above, rare cases have been recorded in which a disease undoubtedly due to *M. tuberculosis* sensitive to the drugs in use has failed to respond to chemotherapy alone, responding only after the addition of a corticosteroid to the treatment.

HYPOTHESES RELATING SARCOIDOSIS TO MYCOBACTERIAL INFECTION

Several suggestions about ways in which mycobacterial infection might be related to widespread granulomatous changes without demonstrable acid-fast bacilli or cultivatable mycobacteria have been made.

Mankiewicz (1964) advanced an ingenious hypothesis relating sarcoidosis, mycobacteria and mycobacteriophages. Mankiewicz and van Walbeek (1962) found that a high percentage of patients with tuberculosis and with sarcoidosis were infected with mycobacteriophages. Normal subjects and patients with tuberculosis produced phage-neutralizing antibodies, while those with sarcoidosis showed no appreciable amount of such antibodies either to their own or to another mycobacteriophage. Mycobacteria resembling photochromogens emerged in cultures of virulent tubercle bacilli infected with mycobacteriophage. It was suggested tentatively that sarcoidosis might develop in persons infected with tubercle bacilli and with mycobacteriophage but incapable of producing antibodies to mycobacteriophage; the tubercle bacilli under the influence of the phage assuming unrecognizable forms and eliciting only a non-caseating reaction. In support of this view, Mankiewicz (1964) reported that by serial culture in media enriched with phage-neutralizing rabbit sera, she had isolated from sarcoid tissues mycobacteria resembling the 'anonymous' types. Mankiewicz and Béland (1964) found that in guinea-pigs infected with a small dose of tubercle bacilli, infection with mycobacteriophage DSGA reduced the number of granulomas and made them more discrete, but diminished survival time; from these sarcoid-like lesions, atypical mycobacteria could be isolated. Mankiewicz and Liivak (1967) later confirmed the isolation of mycobacteriophages from stools, tissues and sera of patients with sarcoidosis, from stools and tissues but not from sera of patients with tuberculosis, and only occasionally from stools of healthy subjects.

An objection to this hypothesis is that antibody-production is, if anything, enhanced in sarcoidosis (Chapter 20, p. 419); and the experimental studies to which it led have received little support. Bowman and Daniel (1971) found no difference between the neutralizing activity of sera from patients with sarcoidosis and with tuberculosis against mycobacteriophages D29, Leo and R1; and sera from normal subjects differed only for D29, against which their activity was lower than that of sarcoidosis and tuberculosis sera. Bowman et al. (1972) reported failure of concurrent infection of guinea-pigs with M. tuberculosis and with mycobacteriophage to produce sarcoid-like disease. Rather surprisingly, no attempt appears to have been made to confirm the initial findings of Mankiewicz and van Walbeek (1962) and Mankiewicz (1961) and Mankiewicz and Liivak (1967) that mycobacteriophages are present in the stools of patients with sarcoidosis, which was the starting point of their hypothesis. A brief report by Kozmin-Sokolow and Kostina (1971) mentions the isolation of mycobacteriophage from the stools of patients with sarcoidosis. Cater and Redmond (1963) isolated five strains of bacteriophage with activity against mycobacteria from 17 patients whose sputum yielded tubercle bacilli or Group 3 mycobacteria. Most of the bacteriophages lysed human tubercle bacilli, and one M. kansasii; Group 3, Battey, bacilli which infected many of the patients were insusceptible to the bacteriophages. No patients with sarcoidosis were studied.

Burnet (1959) discussed ways in which mycobacteria might be concerned in the causation of sarcoidosis. The principal suggestion was that they might be present in some form other than that of a cultivatable acid-fast bacillus, possibly in a protoplast or L form, lacking the power to produce the characteristic cell wall, and persisting as an intracellular parasite of mesenchymal cells. It would be necessary to postulate that the protoplast form was not cultivatable and only very rarely liable to revert to bacillary form, that infected cells might migrate to initiate foci of disease in other parts of the body, and that in most cases infected cells would be gradually eliminated, though in unfavourable cases the intracellular virus-like infection might persist and give rise to progressive destructive changes. The affected individual would be expected to show unusually efficient production of humoral antibody, and abnormal cellular immune responses. Epithelioid cells in non-caseating elements of mycobacterial tuberculosis might contain the protoplast form of the bacilli. Burnet's second suggestion was that during the course of a mycobacterial infection, a low-grade virus might infect mesenchymal cells and thereafter behave like the hypothetical protoplast form of tubercle bacillus.

Hanngren *et al.* (1974) reiterated the suggestion that viral and mycobacterial infections might interact in the pathogenesis of sarcoidosis, viral infection depressing T-cell function and mycobacterial infection stimulating B-cell function. Evidence now available that depression of peripheral expression of some aspects of T-cell activity is due to the sequestration of activated T-cells at sites of active sarcoidosis (Chapter 20, p. 443) militates against this hypothesis, and makes it unnecessary to postulate two interactive causal agents.

AETIOLOGY IN THE LIGHT OF THE CELLULAR IMMUNOPATHOGENESIS OF SARCOIDOSIS

Current views of the cellular immunopathogenesis of sarcoidosis, outlined in Chapter 20, p. 442, lead to several questions about aetiology.

Is it possible that no external causal agent is required to initiate and maintain the granulomatous changes of sarcoidosis?

The possibility that sarcoidosis develops as the result of 'an intrinsic biochemical, genetic cellular alteration rather than the stimulation of an external non-host antigen or other substance' was advanced by Silverstein (1976), largely on the grounds that the sarcoid granuloma is biochemically different from other granulomas, principally in its synthesis of ACE. But such differences do not distinguish the sarcoid granuloma unequivocally from other granulomas; granulomatous responses to known agents may show high ACE levels (Farber *et al.*, 1982; Hara *et al.*, 1983). In the original statement of his hypothesis, Silverstein allowed for the possibilities that 'genetic alteration of epithelioid cell precursors might be due to early precursor mutation or to a virus'; and in a later discussion, Silverstein *et al.* (1983) inclined to the view that 'a sarcoidosis agent, perhaps viral' affected epithelioid cell precursors and/or T lymphocytes.

If an external agent is concerned in initiating and maintaining the cellular changes leading to the sarcoid granuloma, what is its character?

Is it related to any already known pathogen?

Is it unique and specific to sarcoidosis? Or is sarcoidosis a response in a person with appropriate immunological reactivity to one of several possible agents?

These questions remain unanswered. Answers to them depend upon the discovery and characterization of an agent or agents that can be identified in the lesions of sarcoidosis. Of the attempts that have been made to find such an agent, most have met with no success, while the agent producing granulomatous changes in mice and transmissible serially in these animals for which evidence was first advanced by Mitchell and Rees (1969) remains uncharacterized.

ATTEMPTS TO ISOLATE CAUSAL AGENTS IN SARCOIDOSIS

Viruses

Löfgren and Lundback (1950) reported the isolation of a virus of the mumps-influenza-Newcastle disease group by serial inoculations into embryonated eggs of gastric lavage material from four and sarcoid tissue from two cases of sarcoidosis. Later (1952) they concluded that this virus must have been a laboratory contamination, since the results could not be repeated in a laboratory where the mumps virus was not handled. Lundback *et al.* (1959) cultured sarcoid lymph-nodes and skin lesions by the plasma clot technique, and observed patchy degeneration of the outgrowing fibroblasts of a type they did not observe in cultures of lymph-nodes of other sorts, but attempts to transfer a cytopathogenic effect to human embryonic lung cultures were unsuccessful.

Steplewski and Israel (1976) tested 28 sarcoid lymph-nodes, four sarcoid lung biopsies, three Kveim test papules and three sarcoid spleen suspensions for evidence of viral infection by co-cultivation of lymphocytes from the sarcoid material with cultured human fibroblasts, and of fibroblasts growing out from sarcoid tissues with human fibroblasts or with monkey Vero cells. Some cytopathic effects were seen in the co-cultivation of nine of the sarcoid lymph-nodes with human fibroblasts, but transfer of supernatant from these to fresh fibroblast cultures did not induce similar changes. All other tests for viral activity were negative, and there was no electron microscopic evidence of viral agents.

Mycoplasmas

Homma *et al.* (1971) reported the isolation of unidentified mycoplasmas from throat swabs of five of 17, and from scalene lymph-node biopsy on one of 17 patients with sarcoidosis. Cultures of granulomatous tissues from lung and hilar lymph-node in two and from liver biopsies showing granulomas in five patients were all negative. Yansson *et al.* (1972) isolated an organism related to *Mycoplasma orale* Type I from four of seven skin biopsy samples and both of two lymph-nodes affected by sarcoidosis. Patients with sarcoidosis had higher indirect haemagglutination titres against the isolated strain of mycoplasma than did controls, but it seems possible that this was due to the generally enhanced humoral antibody response observed in sarcoidosis. *M. orale* Type I is a common commensal; Taylor-Robinson *et al.* (1964) isolated it from 25% of normal subjects, and there is no reason to suppose that in the patients studied by Yansson *et al.* it was pathogenic.

Nocardia-like organisms

Similarly, Uesaka *et al.* (1974) reported briefly the isolation of 17 organisms from 65 tissue samples from 36 patients with sarcoidosis, from cultures in a wide variety of media, incubated at various temperatures and for periods of up to three months. Of these 17 organisms, four cultured from three granulomatous mediastinal or scalene lymph-nodes had the characteristics of *Nocardia*. The characteristics of the other 13 organisms were not described.

ANIMAL INOCULATION STUDIES

Over the years, a number of reports of attempts to transmit sarcoidosis to guinea-pigs or hamsters by inoculation of material from patients have been published (Ravaut *et al.*, 1929; Pautrier and Glasser, 1936; Santoianni, 1938; Grillo, 1939; Amati, 1947, 1948; Rosenthal, 1949; Santoianni and Ayala, 1949; Muratore and Vulpis, 1952). These were uncontrolled, usually based on single patients, and their results must be regarded as inconclusive.

Agent transmissible to mice

Mitchell and Rees (1969, 1970) reported experiments, based on the procedure found useful in the study of leprosy (Shepard, 1960; Rees and Weddell, 1968), in which homogenates of human sarcoid tissues and of control normal tissues were injected into the footpads of 12 week old female CBA strain mice. Initially, both mice made immunodeficient by thymectomy and whole-body irradiation, as used in the leprosy studies, and normal mice were studied, but since closely similar results were obtained in normal and immunodeficient animals, later studies used normal mice only, and early results can be reported without reference to immune status. In later studies, some mice were injected intravenously or intraperitoneally. Findings in this long-term study have been summarized in successive reports (Mitchell and Rees, 1974, 1976, 1980).

Fresh sarcoid lymph-nodes obtained from 26 patients by mediastinoscopy performed for diagnosis and spleens removed for hypersplenism from two patients were the sources of sarcoid splenic tissue. As control tissues, lymph-nodes were obtained from the para-aortic area during the course of vascular surgery in six otherwise healthy individuals, and from the groin at surgery for varicose veins in one other. These nodes showed normal histology apart from some simple inflammatory changes in some. Control splenic tissue was obtained from a Kveim-negative patient whose spleen was removed for gross splenomegaly, but who showed no evidence of sarcoidosis. Homogenates were prepared from the fresh tissues in 1% bovine albumin in saline solution, to yield an approximately 13.5% suspension. For intravenous injection, they were filtered through nylon to remove coarse particles and diluted 1 : 3 or 1 : 4 to reduce toxicity. All were tested by

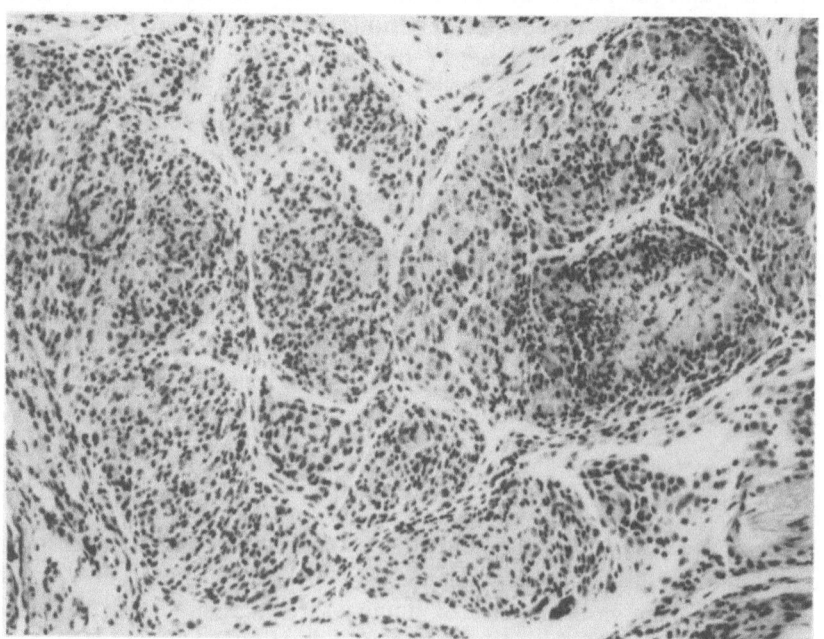

Figure 25.1   Histological of footpad of a normal mouse nine months after inoculation of sarcoid tissue homogenate, showing epithelioid and giant-cell granulomas. H & E. × 160.

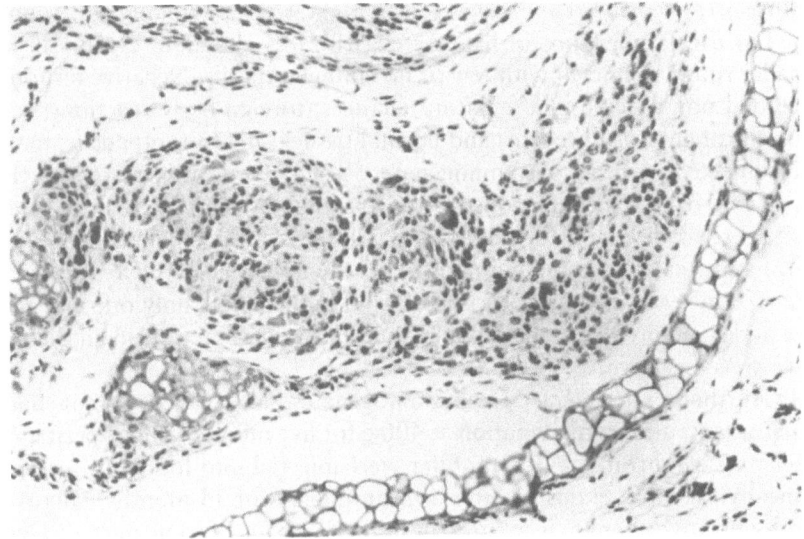

Figure 25.2   Histology of Kveim test given in ear of a mouse 15 months after footpad inoculation with a second-passage homegenate of granulomatous mouse footpad tissue. H & E. × 91.

guinea-pig inoculation and by Löwenstein-Jensen culture for mycobacteria with negative results.

Homogenates were injected into the hind footpads of the mice (0.03 ml), or in some intraperitoneally (0.05 ml) or intravenously (0.1 ml). Full-thickness biopsies, initially of the injected and later of the opposite footpad, were made six to 24 months after injection. Only a proportion of the footpads were sampled at any one time; at least one footpad of all surviving mice injected with sarcoid tissue homogenates and both footpads of all surviving mice injected with nonsarcoid homogenates were examined histologically. Mice becoming sick were killed and their footpads and viscera examined histologically. Histological assessments were made from coded sections that were examined routinely under polarized light to assist in the detection of foreign-body material.

Kveim tests were made in the ears with Lots 0025, 004 and 005 of CSL suspension (Hurley and Bartholomeusz, 1968), usually between nine and 17 weeks after the inoculation of sarcoid or control tissue homogenates. The Kveim tests were assessed microscopically after punch biopsy (4 mm) at intervals of 35–46 days after injection.

Histological responses were categorized as positive, equivocal or negative. In a positive response the essential feature was the presence of one or more granulomas composed principally of epithelioid cells with occasional Langhans-type giant cells. In an equivocal response there was either a diffuse arrangement of epitheliod cells with no true epithelioid-cell granulomas, or focal collections of histiocytes (with less abundant cytoplasm and smaller rounded nuclei) with few or no epithelioid cells. Negative responses included non-specific inflammatory changes, foreign-body reactions, scars with fibroblasts or fibrocytes and normal tissue. Of 193 footpads from 114 mice injected with sarcoid homogenate, 57 showed positive responses (Fig. 25.1) and 46 equivocal responses after a mean interval of 15 months. Kveim tests were made in 111 of these mice; 21 showed a positive response (Fig. 25.2) and were associated with positive footpad histology. Of 173 footpads from 78 mice inoculated with non-sarcoid homogenate only one was positive and six equivocal after the same interval and Kveim tests in all these 78 mice were negative.

In further experiments, fresh homogenates, autoclaved homogenates, supernatants after centrifugation at 400 g for five minutes, and supernatants after passage through a 0.2 μm filter were injected into footpads, intraperitoneally, or intravenously. After a mean interval of 15 months, microscopically positive changes were present in the footpads of some mice receiving each fresh sarcoid homogenate, including the footpads of mice given filtered (0.2μm) supernatant. These positive footpad changes were present in mice inoculated intraperitoneally or intravenously and were again associated with Kveim reactivity. Microscopically the footpads of mice given identically prepared non-sarcoid homogenate were negative and were all associ-

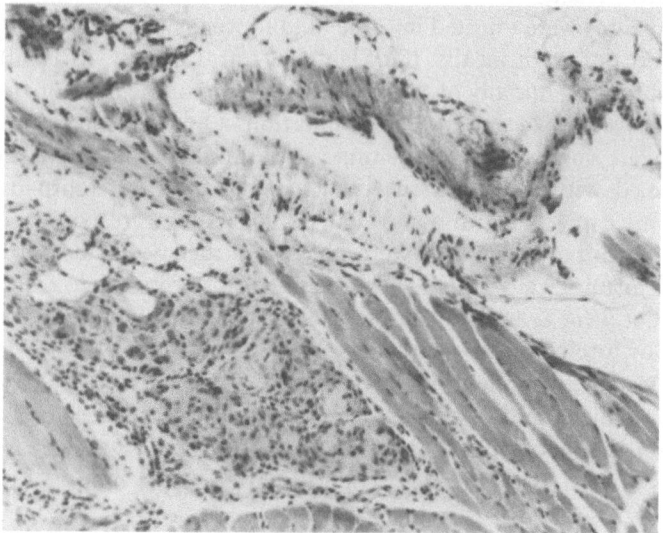

Figure 25.3 Histology of normal mouse 15 months after inoculation of fourth passage homogenate of granulomatous mouse footpads, initiated by intravenous injection of 0.2 μm filtrate of human sarcoid lymph-node homogenate. H & E. × 120.

ated with negative Kveim tests in the ear. No changes were found in mice receiving autoclaved homogenates by any route.

Homogenates of granulomatous tissues of mice injected with sarcoid tissue homogenates were found capable of causing similar changes on injection into normal mice. At the first passage of this sort, fresh homogenates from granulomatous footpads harvested at a mean interval of 15 months after injection of human sarcoid tissue homogenate were injected into the footpads of normal mice, and led to changes interpreted as positive in 24% and as equivocal in 48%; comparable proportions of positive and equivocal histological changes were found in footpads injected with supernatant and with filtrate of supernatant, but autoclaved material produced no response. Up to six successive passages of this sort have been achieved, with granulomatous changes not only in the injected footpad (Fig. 25.3) but also in other footpads and in lungs, liver, spleen and lymph-nodes in a proportion of animals; and intravenous and intraperitoneal injections of granulomatous mouse-tissue homogenate were also found to produce changes in the organs of a proportion of mice.

Sarcoid tissue homogenates retained granuloma-producing capability after storage for one week at $+ 4°C$ or at $- 70°C$ but lost it after storage at $-20°C$, and after irradiation with 2.5 mR. This inactivation by irradiation is in sharp contrast with the retention of selective activity by validated Kveim-test suspensions after similar irradiation (Mitchell *et al.*, 1974a).

Mitchell and Rees (1970) studied Crohn's disease by a similar procedure, using abnormal ileum and mesenteric lymph-nodes obtained from four patients who underwent bowel resection. Homogenates of these tissues were injected into mice, into footpads, intravenously or intraperitoneally. Fifteen to 17 months later, granulomas were found in footpads in a substantial proportion (40% positive, 30% equivocal), and in mesenteric nodes and in bowel in a small proportion of injected mice. No changes were found in other lymph-nodes, liver, spleen or lung. The distribution of changes in internal organs was thus different from that observed in mice injected with sarcoid tissue homogenates; in these, granulomas might be found in lungs, liver and spleen, but not in bowel. Transmission of granulomatous changes serially by injections of granulomatous mouse tissue homogenates originating from human Crohn's tissue homogenates was demonstrated, the changes having similar distributions in successive passages. The effects of storage of homogenates at various temperatures and of irradiation were similar to those found with sarcoid tissue homogenates.

These findings suggested that in both sarcoid and Crohn's disease tissues there is a transmissible agent that can be passaged repeatedly in mice, that is inactivated by autoclaving or by irradiation, and that can pass a 0.2 μm filter. It is presumably viable, and must approximate to the size of a virus or be capable of being deformed so as to pass through 0.2 μm pores.

In further studies, Mitchell and Rees (1983) reported that although all human tissues studied had shown no acid-fast bacilli and had been negative on culture for mycobacteria, acid-fast bacilli had been seen in granulomatous tissues of mice passaged from the sarcoid tissues of six patients. These were found in the lungs of mice, and also in spleen in five, 17 months or more after the injection of fresh homogenate or supernatant filtrate of mouse granulomatous tissue on first to third passage from the original injection of human sarcoid tissue 3–9 years previously. Mycobacteria having the characteristics of human M. *tuberculosis* were grown on Löwenstein-Jensen medium from pooled homogenates of lungs and spleens from mice in two of these serial passages. One of these originated in tissue from a patient with BHL who had a negative tuberculin test and a positive Kveim test; mouse lungs from the second passage and lungs and spleen from third and fourth passages grew M. *tuberculosis*. Two of these passages resulted from supernatant passed through a 0.2 μm filter. The other originated from a patient with BHL, pulmonary infiltration and skin sarcoids, and positive Kveim and negative tuberculin tests; from the second passage, which was with filtered supernatant, a homogenate of lungs and spleen grew M. *tuberculosis*.

In similar studies starting with human Crohn's disease tissues, acid-fast organisms were detected on prolonged subculture of mouse passage tissues originating from each of three patients; these did not have the cultural characteristics of M. *tuberculosis*, and remained unidentified.

Taub and Siltzbach (1974) confirmed the findings of the starting-point of the studies of Mitchell and Rees. No abnormalities were seen in the footpads of 16 mice injected with normal lymph-node homogenates, or in footpads injected with frozen sarcoid homogenates. By contrast, four of 14 mice injected with fresh sarcoid homogenates, and five of 16 with Crohn's disease homogenates showed slowly developing granulomas; lymph-nodes draining the injected sites were hyperplastic, but granulomas were not found in spleen, liver or lung. Kveim tests in the ear were performed 6–8 months after injection in all mice, presumably with a spleen J suspension, as compared with the CSL suspension used by Mitchell and Rees; all were negative.

Other investigators have been unable to repeat these findings. Belcher and Reid (1975) injected homogenates of six sarcoid lymph-nodes and three skin sarcoids into footpads of CBA/J mice; as controls they used three lymph-nodes reported to be either normal or to show 'non-specific lymphadenitis', and, rather surprisingly, skin biopsies from two patients with granuloma annulare and one with 'acute or chronic dermatitis'. Definite or equivocal granulomas were found in 19 of 126 mice injected with sarcoid lymph-node and in five of 51 with non-sarcoid lymph-node homogenates. The corresponding figures for those injected with skin homogenates were seven of 50 and six of 24 respectively; but granuloma annulare seems an odd 'control' for sarcoidosis. In the studies of Iwai and Takhashi (1976), the sources of sarcoid tissues were scalene lymph-nodes from 31 sarcoidosis patients, and of control tissues lymph-nodes from lung hilum, mediastinum or chest wall obtained at thoracotomy in patients with tuberculosis, bronchiectasis or giant bullae. Of mice injected with sarcoid homogenates, 42% showed granulomatous changes in footpads; these were evident three months after injection and persisted without regression for more than one year. Of those injected with the 'control' lymph-node homogenates, 21% showed similar granulomas, generally less well formed. Granuloma-inciting activity persisted after the homogenates had been sterilized, and was present in the sediment but not in the supernatant after centrifugation. The authors concluded that the granulomas were responses to heterotopic protein; they did not specify the strain of mice used. Their control lymph-nodes differed from those used by Mitchell and Rees. Intrathoracic lymph-nodes removed at surgery for bronchiectasis or tuberculosis had almost certainly been draining an area of microbial disease, and were likely to contain particulate matter derived from the respired air, whereas the para-aortic lymph-nodes used by Mitchell and Rees were unlikely to have been affected by the first of these factors, and could not have been affected by the second.

Thus in one study, the initial finding of Mitchell and Rees (1969) that granulomatous changes develop slowly after the injection of homogenates of sarcoid or Crohn's disease homogenates into footpads of mice was confirmed, while in others results were inconclusive, granulomas developing not only in some mice injected with sarcoid tissues but also in a not very different proportion of those receiving the control tissues, which differed in probably important respects from those used by Mitchell and Rees. The long-term serial transmission experiments of Mitchell and Rees have not been repeated by others; and it is probably fair comment that they and suggested interpretations of them have been viewed with some scepticism. Nevertheless, they appear to be complementary to recent work on the cellular immunopathogenesis of sarcoidosis, which leaves open the question of the cause or causes of the activation of immunocompetent cells which leads to the formation of the sarcoid granuloma, and is entirely compatible with the possibility that a replicating viable agent, of a sort difficult (at present) to demonstrate, is the initiator of this process.

The work of Mitchell and Rees suggests that in at least some human sarcoid tissues there is an agent producing in mice granulomatous reactions transmissible in these animals for at least five passages; that this agent is capable of passing a 0.2 μm filter and thus aproximates to the size of a virus or is capable of being deformed sufficiently to pass the filter; and that it is inactivated by autoclaving and by irradiation. The suggestion that the inciting agent may be a tissue component capable, like Kveim-test suspension, of inducing granulomatous reactions in which further production of the active component occurs is refuted by the observation that irradiation inactivates the granuloma-producing capability of homogenates or of filtrates from them, whereas it does not affect the potency of Kveim test suspensions in reactive subjects. There is thus good reason to suppose that it is a replicating and viable agent that is responsible for the serial transmission from human sarcoid tissue of granulomatous changes to mice.

The presumed transmissible agent has not yet been characterized. The finding that after several passages in mice in some instances acid-fast rods appeared in mouse tissue, and in a few eventually became cultivatable as *M. tuberculosis* is compatible with the suggestion of Burnet (1959), outlined above (p. 553) that a protoplast or L form of tubercle bacillus may be an inciting cause of sarcoidosis. It is also compatible with some of the otherwise puzzling associations between sarcoidosis and mycobacterial infection in man (Chapter 23). However, it is highly desirable that the work, of necessity extending over several years, which led to these findings in one laboratory, should be repeated elsewhere.

It cannot be assumed that all cases of sarcoidosis are initiated by the same or one of a closely related group of agents, though of course this seems likely. Other as yet unidentified filter-passing agents, possibly including L forms of other infective agents causing granulomatous inflammation, may remain to be discovered. In the present state of knowledge it is essential to be receptive to, and consider critically, any tenable hypothesis.

Chapter 26

Diagnosis

Some problems in the diagnosis, more especially the differential diagnosis, of sarcoidosis of individual organs have been considered in earlier chapters. In this chapter, more general aspects of the diagnosis of sarcoidosis will be considered.

For the clinician, a diagnosis of sarcoidosis is a statement of belief that the symptoms and signs a patient presents are related to a non-caseating epithelioid-cell granulomatosis. This belief should be based on the summation of all available data, and is most secure if histological comfirmation of compatible granulomatous changes has been obtained from one or more sites. The amount of support required from biopsy varies inversely with the degree of confidence with which the general clinical picture is recognizable as characteristic of sarcoidosis. In most instances, biopsy of one affected organ or from a Kveim test site showing characteristic granulomas is sufficient to establish the probability of the diagnosis. But it must be recognized on the one hand that in some atypical cases, doubt may remain after several biopsies showing granulomas, and certainty be attainable only by necropsy or an unjustifiable number of biopsies; and on the other, that there are some syndromes so characteristic of sarcoidosis, and so likely to proceed in most cases to spontaneous resolution, that it is arguable that the best interests of patients are served by an initial expectant policy without recourse to biopsy.

A number of immunological and biochemical findings, or evidence of asymptomatic involvement of organs liable to be affected in sarcoidosis, may contribute to diagnosis by increasing or diminishing the probability of sarcoidosis, without being conclusive.

PRESUMPTIVE DIAGNOSIS OF SARCOIDOSIS WITHOUT BIOPSY

Although it has become customary to suggest that it is not proper to make a diagnosis of sarcoidosis without biopsy, patients presenting some easily recognizable syndromes associated with bilateral hilar lymphadenopathy (BHL), discussed in Chapter 5, are so likely to be suffering from sarcoidosis that in them, this diagnosis can be accepted without the need for biopsy, provided that there are no discordant features. In a study of 100 patients with BHL, Winterbauer *et al.* (1973) found that all of 34 without symptoms or abnormal findings on physical examination, and all of 13 with erythema nodosum or uveitis, had sarcoidosis; those in whom the hilar lymph-node enlargement was due to lymphoma or metastatic neoplasm all had symptoms or physical signs other than those of erythema nodosum, arthropathy or uveitis. If in a patient with mediastinal lymphadenopathy there is suspicion of caseating tuberculosis, of Hodgkin's or other lymphoma, or of metastatic malignant disease, mediastinoscopy for biopsy of a node is the most direct, and should be the preferred procedure; a Kveim test giving a granulomatous response provides strong evidence favouring sarcoidosis rather than lymphoma or metastatic malignancy, but does not exclude tuberculous lymphadenopathy, and entails a delay of at least four weeks.

SOURCES OF BIOPSY MATERIAL

Because of the wide range of clinical presentations of sarcoidosis, with differing distributions of granulomatous changes, the preferred site for biopsy varies from case to case. If an apparently involved tissue is accessible to a single biopsy procedure – e.g. the skin or a superficial lymph-node – it should be the first choice. In other cases, a number of organs known to be involved asymptomatically in a high proportion of cases of active sarcoidosis have been used. In patients presenting with chronic changes apparently limited to one internal organ, direct biopsy of this organ may be required.

Even though these factors may have been taken into consideration, the choice of site for biopsy is affected by local custom and facilities, and of course by the introduction of new procedures. In a retrospective international review, James *et al.* (1976a) found wide variations in preferred site for biopsy in different centres for cases diagnosed over varying periods of up to 20 years before 1975. For instance, the proportions of histological confirmations by tissue biopsy obtained from lymph-nodes ranged from 13–96%, from skin from less than 1–27%, and from liver from none to 26% in different centres; and from bronchial mucosa from none in London and New York to 67% in Paris. The proportions of cases in which Kveim tests had been performed ranged from only 4% in Naples to all in New York, with an overall average of 60%. Seventy-eight per cent of these tests were interpreted as positive, the diagnosis of sarcoidosis being accepted in the remaining 22% in spite of 'negative' tests. At the time of this review, fibre-optic bronchoscopy with forceps biopsy of bronchial mucosa and lung had only just been adopted for the investigation of sarcoidosis. In a survey of diagnostic methods four years later, Teirstein *et al.* (1980) found that of 209 respondents to a questionnaire, 193 had access to fibre-optic bronchoscopy, and 106 to an acceptable Kveim test suspension. Those using the Kveim test generally chose it in the investigation of hilar adenopathy, though some used fibre-optic bronchoscopy or other procedures; while for pulmonary infiltration with or without hilar lymphadenopathy, choice was about equally divided between the Kveim test and fibre-optic bronchoscopy. Among those who did not use the Kveim test, fibre-optic bronchoscopy was the most commonly chosen procedure irrespective of the radiographic pattern.

Lymph-nodes

As noted in Chapter 10 (p. 257), palpable lymph-nodes are a very favourable source for biopsy confirmation of a diagnosis of sarcoidosis, and should be sought for in all suspected cases; and in cases with intrathoracic changes and no palpable nodes, the Daniels procedure of removing the scalene fat-pad which usually contains small lymph-nodes yields a high proportion of contributory findings. This is now practised in a few centres only (Stjernberg *et al.*, 1980), in others having been displaced by mediastinoscopy.

Mediastinoscopy, a method by which the anterior part of the superior mediastinum can be inspected and lymph-nodes removed for biopsy through an instrument introduced through a small incision in the skin over the suprasternal notch was introduced by Carlens (1959), who in 1964 reported that it had given confirmation of the diagnosis of sarcoidosis in 118 (96%) of 123 cases 'with a reasonable suspicion of sarcoidosis'. There were no complications in Carlens' series, but clearly the procedure should be performed only by an expert and experienced surgeon. Mikhail *et al.* (1979) reported that of 227 patients in whom a diagnosis of sarcoidosis was thought likely and who were investigated by mediastinoscopy, 187 (82%) were found to have lymph-nodes showing sarcoid-type granulomas; the proportion was lower (55%) in those with lung infiltration only than in those with radiologically evident hilar node enlargement, with or without infiltration (88%). Three of seven patients with normal chest radiographs who had changes suggestive of sarcoidosis in extrathoracic sites not readily accessible to biopsy showed granulomatous changes in nodes removed by mediastinoscopy. During the same period, the diagnosis of tuberculous lymphadenitis was confirmed by mediastinoscopy in 48 of 49 patients, and of malignant disease of lymph-nodes in all of 14 patients.

The interpretation of granulomatous changes in lymph-nodes is complicated both by the occurrence of non-caseating changes without discoverable mycobacteria in nodes remote from a focus of caseating mycobacterial tuberculosis, and by sarcoid reactions in nodes draining areas which are the sites of malignant disease, and in association with Hodgkin's and other lymphomas (Chapter 2, p. 33). Welsh and Welsh (1977) reported six patients among about 700 investigated by mediastinoscopy in whom sarcoid-type granulomas were found in lymph-nodes obtained at this procedure, and various forms of malignant disease were or subsequently became apparent. The case-reports suggest that in three of these, generalized sarcoidosis and malignant disease (myeloid leukaemia, carcinoma of the tongue and thyroid carcinoma) were coincidental; while in three there was a local sarcoid reaction in the removed mediastinal nodes to lymphoma in two and to carcinoma of the lung in one.

Liver

Liver biopsy has been widely used in the past in the diagnosis of sarcoidosis, as granulomas are discoverable in a needle biopsy of liver in up to 70% of patients with active sarcoidosis, irrespective of clinical or other evidence of liver dysfunction. Its value is limited by the large number of possible causes of granulomas in the liver, between most of which histology does not discriminate (Chapter 11, p. 265). It may be helpful in cases where the differential diagnosis rests between sarcoidosis and a non-granulomatous disease, e.g. in a patient with chronic lung changes which might be either a late stage of sarcoidosis or fibrosing alveolitis. But lung biopsy would now be preferred by most physicians in such cases.

Skin (Chapter 7)

In patients presenting with skin lesions, biopsy is safe and simple, especially if performed with a punch technique; and since the diagnosis of sarcoid of the skin cannot be sustained in face of an incompatible histological picture, discussion of the percentage of positive findings in such cases is pointless. In all patients suspected of sarcoidosis, a careful search for minor abnormalities of the skin which the patient may not have noticed or mentioned, should be made; old scars, whether traumatic or surgical, should be sought and inspected. Any suspicious abnormality can be submitted to biopsy, with a good prospect of a positive result if the diagnosis of sarcoidosis is correct. Israel and Sones (1964) found that 88% of skin lesions biopsied in 292 cases of sarcoidosis gave typical histological pictures. Subcutaneous nodules, which may be found especially at the early acute stages, are another favourable source of tissue for biopsy.

Bronchi

The available evidence about the proportions of patients at various stages of sarcoidosis in whom biopsy of bronchial mucosa shows granulomas has been reviewed in Chapter 5, p. 92, and Chapter 6, p. 140. Biopsy at the later stages of bronchial involvement, when there may be localized narrowings of main and the proximal parts of segmental bronchi, may show scattered epithelioid and giant-cells with only rare and poorly-formed granulomas in thickened mucosa with round cell and fibroblast infiltration.

The findings in more recent studies in which both bronchial and transbronchial lung biopsy have been performed at fibre-optic bronchoscopy are discussed below.

Lung

Lung biopsy may be performed by thoracotomy, by transcutaneous needle or drill, or transbronchially by forceps at bronchoscopy. Of these, only thoracotomy can be relied upon to produce a large enough sample from a precisely selected part or parts of the lung for critical study in obscure cases; and much information has been obtained by this method about correlations between histology and clinical, functional and radiographic findings (Chapter 6, p. 105). Techniques based on that of Klassen *et al.* (1949) require only a short intercostal incision and constitute an acceptable method of obtaining biopsy material when important decisions depend upon a diagnosis which remains in doubt after simpler methods have been used unsuccessfully. Nevertheless, the procedure is not devoid of discomfort, of complications, or even of some slight risk for the patient, and if all that is required is histological support for a diagnosis of sarcoidosis that seems likely on other grounds, the finding of granulomas in the small and sometimes distorted fragments obtained by transbronchial forceps or percutaneous needle biopsy may be sufficient. If doubt remains after this, and biopsies from other sites, including Kveim tests, have been non-contributory, thoracotomy can be considered.

With the introduction of fibre-optic bronchoscopy, permitting forceps biopsy directed into most broncho-pulmonary segments and the taking of several samples, together with bronchial mucosal biopsies, percutaneous methods, at one time favoured in some centres, are now little used. Koerner *et al.* (1975) described their experience with biopsy during fibre-optic bronchoscopy, with fluoroscopic control to ensure that pleura was not included in the bite of the forceps. Of 26 patients with features suggesting sarcoidosis, the biopsy showed non-caseating granulomas in 21 and normal lung in five. Of these five, two were finally diagnosed as tuberculosis, one as sarcoidosis, and one as multiple pulmonary emboli, one remaining undiagnosed. Teirstein *et al.* (1976a) reported that of 25 patients with sarcoidosis from whom lung and/or bronchial tissue was obtained for biopsy through the fibre-optic bronchoscope, 20 (80%) showed non-caseating granulomas; these were found in all of four with BHL only, five of seven with BHL and pulmonary mottling, and 11 of 14 with pulmonary mottling only. Of the remaining five, histology was normal in three, one had pulmonary fibrosis, and one simple inflammatory changes. Poe *et al.* (1979) performed transbronchial lung biopsy in 41 consecutive patients with suspected sarcoidosis; granulomas were found in 22 of 23 (96%) with radiographic shadowing in the lungs and in eight of 18 (44%) without lung shadowing, of whom 17 had BHL. Roethe *et al.* (1980), taking ten samples from the right lung, five from the upper and five from the lower lobe in each case, obtained granulomas in 36 of 37 patients with presumptive sarcoidosis; the number of samples showing granulomas was lower in the ten with BHL only, ranging from one to three, than in those with lung shadows, in four of whom all ten samples contained them. Mitchell *et al.* (1980) reviewed the procedures by which histological confirmation was obtained in 79 patients with an ultimate diagnosis of sarcoidosis. In 24 there were untypical presenting features, leading to provisional diagnoses other than sarcoidosis in eight. Fibre-optic bronchoscopy was performed in 50, endobronchial changes compatible with sarcoidosis being seen in 19. Bronchial mucosal biopsy was performed in 22, and showed granulomas in 17. Transbronchial lung biopsy performed in 42 cases showed sarcoid-type granulomas in 37. Kveim tests were performed in 44, and were interpreted as positive in 19 and equivocal in 11. Biopsies of lymph-nodes in 12, cervical in ten and mediastinal in two, of liver in two, of skin in one and of parotid gland in one, all showed granulomas.

Broncho-alveolar lavage, showing a high proportion of activated lymphocytes in active sarcoidosis (Chapter 20, p. 435) is of differential diagnostic value in some circumstances, distinguishing sarcoidosis from cryptyogenic fibrosing alveolitis, in which there is a high proportion of neutrophil polymorphs, but not from tuberculosis or extrinsic allergic alveolitis. It can, of course, be combined with biopsy procedures during fibre-optic bronchoscopy.

The finding of granulomas in lung biopsy specimens, especially the small fragments obtained by transbronchial forceps, does not discriminate between the conditions in which granulomas may be present in the lung, though detailed assessment of histology, especially of additional non-granulomatous features, may favour one or more among the possibilities. In particular, lung biopsy, even with the larger samples provided by thoracotomy, may not discriminate reliably between sarcoidosis and mycobacterial tuberculosis. Failure to detect acid-fast bacilli or to culture mycobacteria, or to find caseation in lung biopsies, especially in the small samples obtained by the transbronchial procedure, is no guarantee that mycobacteria are absent from the lung, or that mycobacteria and caseating lesions are not present elsewhere. Andrews and Klassen (1957) referred briefly to two patients in whom the histological diagnosis on open lung biopsy was sarcoidosis, but who subsequently proved to have tuberculosis. In Cases 1 and 3 of Reid and Lorriman (1960) the diagnosis of sarcoidosis suggested by lung biopsy was followed by a clinical course compatible with this diagnosis, including negative tuberculin tests; but cultures both from the biopsy specimen and from gastric contents in one, and from sputum in the other produced *M. tuberculosis*. As mentioned in Chapter 23, p. 508, Kent *et al.* (1970) found mycobacteria on culture of open lung biopsy samples showing non-caseating granulomas from 14 of 30 patients with clinical features otherwise those of sarcoidosis.

As noted in Chapter 6, interpretation of lung biopsies must allow for the facts that in the early acute stages, there may be considerable non-granulomatous cellular infiltration of alveolar walls (alveolitis) (p. 106); while in the late fibrotic stages there may be only nondescript remnants of granulomas, with much hyaline fibrosis, possibly containing residual Schaumann bodies (p. 140).

Conjunctiva

Conjunctival biopsy is discussed in Chapter 8, p. 223. If careful inspection of the conjunctiva shows suspicious abnormalities, especially accompanying uveitis, biopsy, which can be performed simply and safely by an expert, has a fair chance of showing granulomas in a patient with sarcoidosis (Karma, 1979); but random biopsy of a normal-looking conjunctiva is unlikely to be productive.

Skeletal muscle

As noted in Chapter 9 (p. 246), random biopsy of skeletal muscle in patients at the early stage of sarcoidosis with BHL, especially in those with fever, arthropathy or erythema nodosum, shows granulomas in an important proportion of cases; later in the disease, biopsy of muscle is unlikely to show granulomas except in the rare cases with clinical evidence suggesting muscle involvement.

Minor salivary glands

Nessan and Jacoway (1979) took random biopsies of the inner aspect of the lower lip including one or two minor salivary glands in 75 patients with sarcoidosis, already confirmed by other biopsies; granulomas were found in 44 (58%). There is no evidence, however, about the proportion of obscure cases with predominant involvement of one organ in which this procedure is likely to helpful.

Spleen

Selroos (1976b, 1977) performed percutaneous fine-needle aspiration biopsy of the spleen, after confirming a normal platelet count, in 77 patients with verified sarcoidosis. The procedure was performed without local anaesthesia. The aspirated material, spread on slides, air dried, and stained, showed recognizable granulomas in 41 (53%). Five of six with enlarged spleens, 47% with BHL as the only clinical sign of disease, and 67% of those with detected extrathoracic disease showed granulomas. Again, this experience cannot be extrapolated to obscure cases.

THE KVEIM TEST

The background to the use of the Kveim reaction as a diagnostic test, and the procedure by which a sarcoid tissue suspension can be validated for this use are considered in Chapter 21. Here it must be emphasized again that a Kveim test is valuable only if it is performed with a suspension that has been carefully tested both for selectivity and for potency, and that, with an inadequately validated suspension, it may be misleading.

Like random biopsies from sites not symptomatically affected, the Kveim test gives the highest proportion of positive reactions in early active phases of the disease, and a progressively lower proportion in the later stages, when diagnostic help is most likely to be required. Moreover, again like a granulomatous biopsy, a 'positive' test cannot be regarded as establishing a diagnosis of sarcoidosis in a case whose general features include discordant aspects. The difficulties arising from observer variation in the interpretation of the histology of the reaction have been discussed on p. 460. We consider that reports of the results of Kveim tests should be in terms of histology. A 'positive-equivocal-negative' scale misleadingly simplifies a complex situation. A scale of histological appearances ranging from granulomatous, through partially granulomatous and simple inflammatory, to no reaction, is appropriate. This does not exhaust the possible variations, and where appropriate reports should describe mixed reactions, and refer to such features as the number and character of giant cells and the presence of foreign material, especially birefringent, or of necrosis; and the report should be made without knowledge of the clinical features.

The significance of a granulomatous response to a Kveim test should be assessed statistically as increasing or diminishing the probability of the diagnosis of sarcoidosis, after consideration of the clinical picture of the patient tested, and of the proportion of patients with sarcoidosis presenting a similar picture expected to react in this way to the suspension used. If the probability of sarcoidosis is already high, e.g. in a patient with BHL, either symptomless or accompanied by erythema nodosum, a granulomatous response increases this probability slightly; but since 10–15% of such patients in whom the diagnosis is confirmed by other means do not respond, failure to give such a response is almost non-contributory. On the other hand, in patients with chronic sarcoidosis, clinically involving one organ or system predominantly, only a minority react; e.g. about one-third of those with chronic lung changes without BHL. In a patient with this sort of presentation, a granulomatous response considerably increases the probability of the diagnosis of sarcoidosis, while its absence alters the probabilities very little; and direct biopsy of the affected organ, if it is reasonably accessible, is advisable.

The occurrence of granulomatous responses to some well-validated Kveim test suspensions in patients with Crohn's disease and some other bowel diseases (p. 475) should cause no confusion because of the very different clinical features; but the possibility of such reactions in patients with tuberculous lymphadenopathy (though not in Hodgkin's disease) and in patients with indolent granulomatous pulmonary infiltrations from whom *M. tuberculosis* is isolated, mentioned above, must be borne in mind.

In most contexts, the contribution of a granulomatous response to a Kveim test to the diagnosis of sarcoidosis can be regarded as comparable to that of finding granulomas in a biopsy of a site remote from that principally affected. As compared with such biopsies, it has the advantage of being a simple out-patient procedure, and with a carefully validated suspension is sufficiently selective for sarcoidosis to be helpful in cases where confirmation of a probable diagnosis is not urgent. It has the disadvantages that a delay of at least four weeks is inevitable before the result is available, and that since human sarcoid tissue is at present the only source of test-suspensions, and only a proportion of such tissues submitted to the neccesarily prolonged validation process are found to produce acceptable suspensions, difficulties of supply limit its availability. The greatest interest of the Kveim reaction lies in the light it may throw on the pathogenesis and aetiology of sarcoidosis. If the specific substance eliciting the epithelioid cell granuloma in patients with active sarcoidosis were isolated and could be made available without the present limitation of necessary origin from selected human tissues, the test would become both more practicable as a routine procedure and more easy to interpret.

OTHER TESTS CONTRIBUTING TO THE DIAGNOSIS OF SARCOIDOSIS

A number of tests, immunological, biochemical and radiological, may contribute to the diagnosis of sarcoidosis, either generally or in particular contexts, without being specific.

The tuberculin test and other delayed skin reactions

The generally depressed reactivity to agents causing Type IV reactions observed in patients with sarcoidosis (Chapter 20, p. 414) is of limited diagnostic value. The significance of non-reactivity to 'recall' antigens (those of infective agents to which the subject has been exposed previously) depends upon the proportion of reactors to be expected in the general population. When most adults reacted to tuberculin, a negative tuberculin test gave general support to the diagnosis of sarcoidosis, although a positive test was (and is) entirely compatible with it; in communities where the general level of tuberculin sensitivity is now low, the significance of non-reactivity to tuberculin has been reduced to making the diagnosis of caseating tuberculosis very unlikely. Similarly, the significance of skin reactivity to histoplasmin and coccidioidin varies with the local prevalence of the relevant infections.

High proportions of adults are reactive to Candida, Trichophyton and mumps antigens; and failure to respond, especially to more than one of these, supports a diagnosis of sarcoidosis. This support may be useful in a doubtful case, but is not conclusive enough to justify the routine use of these tests.

Deficient capacity to become sensitized to contact antigens, which may be demonstrated by the dinitrochlorobenzene test (p. 418) similarly gives general support to a diagnosis of sarcoidosis; but this test, being itself a sensitizing procedure, cannot be recommended.

Examinations for mycobacteria and other organisms causing granulomatous inflammation

In patients with pulmonary infiltrations, the routine of examinations for mycobacteria and other organisms by microscopy and culture of secretions should be strictly followed, and all biopsy material should be similarly examined. Where the differential diagnosis rests between sarcoidosis and caseating tuberculosis, the finding of tubercle bacilli will of course support the latter diagnosis, especially if it is repeatable. The problem presented by the patient with a syndrome characteristic of sarcoidosis, except that acid-fast bacilli have been seen or tubercle bacilli cultured on one or a few occasions is discussed in Chapter 23, p. 511.

Serum proteins

As noted in Chapter 20, p. 420, changes in serum protein levels, with increase in the total protein and γ-globulin and diminution in albumin may be found in active and extensive sarcoidosis. They are unlikely to be found except in cases with active and extensive disease, in which the diagnosis is likely to be probable on clinical grounds or establishable readily by a suitable biopsy. In such cases, several of the alternative diagnoses to be considered might produce entirely similar serum protein changes. In cases with less extensive and active disease, significant changes in serum protein are unlikely. Thus serum protein changes are of no diagnostic value in sarcoidosis, though they may reflect the activity of the disease.

Serum calcium

Although the serum calcium level and urinary calcium output are elevated in a proportion of patients with sarcoidosis at some stage of the disease (Chapter 19), this finding is rarely of diagnostic value, since it occurs most frequently in patients with active sarcoidosis and multiple manifestations. Although symptoms caused by the abnormal calcium metabolism occasionally lead to the diagnosis of sarcoidosis, routine estimation of the serum calcium level very rarely or never gives diagnostic help in the case of a patient who presents with other manifestations.

Radiography of the hands and feet

Similarly, changes in the bones of the hands and feet rarely occur without active and generally extensive sarcoidosis, most frequently including skin sarcoids. For this reason, radiography of hands and feet in the search for changes characteristic of sarcoidosis in patients in whom the diagnosis is in doubt is only rarely productive; and even if compatible changes are found, the histological confirmation which is desirable is preferably sought from a more easily accessible site or a Kveim test.

Serum angiotensin-converting enzyme and lysozyme levels

Levels of certain enzymes, notably angiotensin-1-converting enzyme (ACE) and lysozyme, have been found to be elevated significantly in the serum of patients with active sarcoidosis, and to be related to the extent and activity of the disease. As noted in Chapter 2 (p.31), ACE and lysozyme have been demonstrated in macrophages, epithelioid cells and giant cells in the sarcoid granuloma. The implications of these findings for the pathogenesis of sarcoidosis are discussed in Chapters 20 (p. 440) and 25 (p. 553). The following discussion concerns the diagnostic value of estimations of these enzymes.

Pascual *et al.* (1973) and Selroos and Klockars (1977) found elevated serum lysozyme levels in patients with sarcoidosis. Those with both BHL and lung infiltration and those with both extra- and intra-thoracic changes showed higher levels than those with BHL only. Khan *et al.* (1973) found similar elevations in pulmonary tuberculosis, levels being related to the activity of the disease, though it correlated poorly with the presence of tubercle bacilli in the sputum. The diagnostic value of serum lysozyme levels in sarcoidosis is thus limited principally to discrimination from non-granulomatous diseases.

Lieberman (1975), using a modification of the spectrophotometric assay described by Cushman and Cheung (1971), found that levels of ACE in the serum of many patients with active sarcoidosis were raised, and fell on resolution or therapeutic suppression of activity with prednisone; even higher levels were found in Gaucher's disease, but raised levels were infrequent in diseases likely to be confused with sarcoidosis. Lieberman *et al.* (1979) extended their observations to 391 patients with sarcoidosis, of whom 58% had levels more than 2 SD above the mean of values in a control group; excluding 91 who were being treated with corticosteroids or whose disease was thought to be inactive, 76% had raised levels. Values tended to be higher in black than in white patients, and in children than in adults. Among patients started on treatment, mean values fell to less than half pretreatment levels. Elevated levels were found in 5% of a group of patients with miscellaneous other pulmonary diseases. Fanburg *et al.* (1976), Silverstein *et al.* (1976) Studdy *et al.* (1978), Turton *et al.* (1979) and Grönhagen-Riska *et al.* (1979) similarly found elevated levels of serum ACE in about half their patients with untreated sarcoidosis. De Remee and Rohrbach (1980) in serial studies found general parallelism between ACE levels and clinical course, including response to corticosteroids. Turton *et al.* (1979) found that both ACE and lysozyme levels fell rapidly towards normal in five sarcoidosis patients after treatment with corticosteroids, but noted falls of 28% and 24% in ACE and lysozyme levels, initially within the normal range in most, in nine patients receiving corticosteroids for other diseases.

In Gaucher's disease, serum ACE levels even higher than those found in some cases of sarcoidosis are usual (Lieberman, 1975). This disease is unlikely to be confused with sarcoidosis; but moderately raised levels have been reported in some patients with pulmonary tuberculosis, leprosy, extrinsic allergic alveolitis (hypersensitivity pneumonitis), primary biliary cirrhosis and pneumoconiosis, all of which in some circumstances might be confused with sarcoidosis. In tuberculosis, Silverstein and Friedland (1979) reported that 6.5% of patients with active and 10.5% of those with inactive disease had raised levels, though generally levels were lower than in sarcoidosis; and Studdy *et al.* (1978) found raised levels in 9% of those with active disease. In some other reports, lower proportions of patients with tuberculosis showed raised levels; but without information about the extent and character of the disease, especially whether it was in an actively granulomatous stage, it is difficult to interpret these findings. Similar considerations apply to the varied reports in leprosy and in chronic beryllium disease, in both of which some have shown a moderate proportion of patients with raised levels and others levels similar to those in control groups. Sprince *et al.* (1980) reported that serum ACE levels in 22 patients with chronic beryllium disease were similar to those in 84 controls, while those of 56 patients with sarcoidosis were very significantly higher. But all those with beryllium disease were old cases, the duration of symptoms ranging from 5–36 years; the duration of illness for the sarcoidosis patients was not stated. In Finland, Grönhagen-Riska *et al.* (1979) found raised ACE levels in three of 18 patients with asbestosis, in eight of 19 with silicosis, and in three of 13 with cryptogenic fibrosing alveolitis. Of patients with primary biliary cirrhosis, 12 of 57 in London and seven of 14 in Rochester, Minnesota, had elevated levels. It is evident that serum ACE levels are of little use in discriminating between sarcoidosis and other diseases in which levels may be raised. However, a high level would favour sarcoidosis in discrimination from diseases in which ACE levels are rarely or never raised; these include Hodgkin's disease, primary lung cancer, chronic lung disease with persistent airflow limitation, and asthma (Studdy *et al.*, 1983). Another complicating factor is that levels may be raised in diabetes mellitus; 18% of 265 diabetic patients in California were found to have raised levels (Lieberman, quoted by Studdy *et al.*, 1983).

The value of serum ACE estimations in diagnosis is thus limited. The association of raised levels in sarcoidosis with extent of granulomatous changes has suggested that changes in serum ACE might be of value in assessment of progress and response to corticosteroid treatment: this is discussed in Chapter 27, p. 586. The combination of gallium-scanning with serum ACE estimation in diagnosis is discussed below.

[67]Gallium scanning

Scanning after intravenous injection of [67]gallium citrate was introduced for detection of the spread of malignant disease (Edwards and Hayes, 1969). [67]Gallium is taken up not only by malignant tumours, including lymphomas, but also by inflammatory processes, including tuberculosis (Lavender *et al.*, 1971; Higasi *et al.*, 1972; Langhammer *et al.*, 1972) and at sites of active sarcoidosis (McKusick *et al.*, 1973). In a study of 29 patients with confirmed sarcoidosis, Heshiki *et al.* (1974) found that radiographically normal lungs showed no abnormal uptake, and that uptake in lungs and hila correlated poorly with clinical activity, although in three patients uptake diminished after corticosteroid treatment. Israel *et al.* (1976) studied

27 patients with sarcoidosis and nine with other pulmonary diseases; they confirmed the avidity of mediastinal and pulmonary sarcoidosis for gallium, but found that gallium scanning did not reveal clinically evident extrapulmonary sarcoidosis in six cases, and concluded that its chief diagnostic value was in the possibility of distinguishing between enlarged hilar bloodvessels and lymphadenopathy. The diagnostic value of [67]gallium scanning in sarcoidosis is thus limited; its possible contribution to the assessment of activity of the disease is discussed in Chapter 27, p. 587.

Nosal *et al.* (1979) investigated 27 patients with clinically active sarcoidosis and 156 patients with other acute and chronic diseases by a combination of [67]gallium scanning and serum ACE measurements. Of the sarcoidosis patients, two had normal ACE levels; one of these had a positive scan, and the other, with a negative scan, was receiving corticosteroid treatment. One with raised ACE had a negative scan. Of the 156 with other diseases, 27 had raised ACE levels; of these 25 had negative scans, only two, one with oat-cell carcinoma of the lung and one with *M. intracellulare* infection, showing abnormal uptake. The combination of raised ACE level and abnormal gallium uptake was thus highly suggestive of sarcoidosis, and in the few patients with other diseases in whom it occurred, confusion with sarcoidosis was unlikely. In view of the many relatively simple procedures by which direct histological evidence to support a diagnosis of sarcoidosis may be obtained, occasion for the use of these indirect procedures in diagnosis must be rare.

SUMMARY

At present, the diagnosis of sarcoidosis is a statement of belief or knowledge that non-caseating epithelioid cell tubercles or their hyalinized remnants are present in a number of affected organs or tissues. This belief is justified in the presence of a combination of clinical, radiological and laboratory findings known to be associated with such changes, and supported by a compatible clinical course. In such cases, corroborative histological evidence from biopsy of an accessible tissue or a Kveim test is usually easy to obtain, and is desirable; but some clinical presentations are so characteristic that for the practical management of the case of a patient presenting them, confirmation by biopsy is not essential, especially if a benign course is probable. In all doubtful cases, and those with symptoms calling for consideration of corticosteroid treatment, support for the diagnosis from biopsy of suitable tissue, or from a Kveim test is required. Easily accessible tissues, such as skin and palpable superficial lymph-nodes, showing clinical signs suggestive of involvement in the disease process present the most favourable and convenient source of material for biopsy. In the early stage of active sarcoidosis, granulomas are in many cases widely disseminated, and 'random' biopsies of a number of tissues, such as liver, salivary glands, skeletal muscle, and impalpable scalene lymph-nodes may show characteristic granulomas. In patients with enlarged hilar lymph-nodes, mediastinoscopy is a favourable procedure by which to obtain histological evidence. In those with lung infiltration, fibre-optic bronchoscopy with biopsy of bronchial mucosa and of lung by flexible forceps under fluoroscopic control will show compatible granulomas in a high proportion of cases of sarcoidosis, but may be non-contributory or inconclusive if changes of other sorts, including normality, are found. The Kveim test depends for its value on availability of a test suspension which has been shown by thorough study to be both potent and selective. It gives the highest proportion of positive results in early active cases where the diagnosis is least in doubt and most easily established by other means. Its greatest contribution to the diagnosis of sarcoidosis is in cases where the clinically evident changes are not readily accessible to biopsy, and in those where an untypical clinical picture is accompanied by a compatible biopsy from a single site; granulomatous changes at a Kveim test site greatly increase the likelihood of sarcoidosis, though their absence does not exclude it. Other tests, ranging from the demonstration of low levels of Type IV hypersensitivity to 'recall' antigens to high levels of serum angiotensin-converting enzyme, may support a diagnosis of sarcoidosis in patients with active and extensive disease, but are unlikely to be helpful in obscure cases. There are some cases where it is wise to reserve judgement, even though there are sarcoid changes in a single biopsy, or a Kveim reaction has been interpreted as positive. Such findings do not establish, though they may suggest, the diagnosis of sarcoidosis in a case presenting discordant elements in the clinical syndrome; multiple biopsies or even a complete necropsy may be required before the diagnosis can be accepted. The need for confirmation by biopsy or Kveim test varies inversely with the confidence with which the clinical syndrome is recognized; this of necessity depends to a large extent upon the experience of the clinician.

Chapter 27

Treatment

Special problems in the treatment of some particular manifestations of sarcoidosis have been discussed in earlier chapters. This chapter is concerned with the general problems of the management of patients with this disease.

Studies of the pathogenesis of sarcoidosis have as yet revealed no specific causal factor which can be eliminated by a therapeutic agent. Symptoms of the early inflammatory changes that occur in association with BHL in some patients can be relieved by non-steroidal anti-inflammatory drugs. Active granulomas and the processes that lead to their formation are susceptible to suppression by corticosteroids, the dosage required to effect this varying from case to case, as does the duration of the active stage of the disease. In many patients, the active stage comes to an end leaving little or no residual changes; but in those following a less favourable course, granulomas become converted into hyalinized connective tissue, which is unlikely to be affected by any form of treatment. These phenomena can be observed directly in sarcoids of the skin (Chapter 7), but these rarely call for corticosteroid treatment. It is in the lungs that sarcoidosis following an unfavourable course most frequently leads to disability and risk to life. While the suppressive effect of corticosteroids on active sarcoidosis of the lungs is generally accepted, opinions differ about whether long-term prognosis can be improved by appropriate use of this suppressive effect; and, if so, whether intensive use of corticosteroids to control 'activity' (variously defined) even in patients with no overt symptoms leads to less residual disability than more limited use to control clinically evident symptoms.

A few other therapeutic agents are currently in use in occasional patients who have not responded to corticosteroids or in whom corticosteroids are contraindicated. These include chloroquine and cytotoxic drugs. A number of drugs that have been used in the past will be reviewed briefly before those in current use are considered.

HISTORICAL

The multiplicity of therapeutic agents that have been used reflects both their ineffectiveness and the very variable course of the disease. The strong tendency to spontaneous regression, partial or complete, of the active stages of the disease is undoubtedly the main reason for the many premature and eventually unconfirmed claims of benefit from a variety of types of treatment. Some of these treatments have been based upon hypotheses about aetiology, and others have been tried because they have been used in other diseases thought to have analogous features. Among these are chaulmoogra oil derivatives, because they had been used in leprosy (Lomholt, 1934), tuberculin (Gougerot and Burnier, 1937; Irgang, 1939) and antituberculosis drugs, to be discussed further below, on the hypothesis of a relationship to tuberculous infection; gold, in part on the same hypothesis (Bureau and Bureau, 1933; Duverne *et al.*, 1948); vitamin D preparations, in part by analogy with lupus vulgaris; chelating agents, probably by analogy with beryllium disease (Rukavina *et al.*, 1958); and radiotherapy, discussed below, possibly by analogy with Hodgkin's disease. Sones and Israel (1961) studied the effects of potassium para-animo-benzoate because of reported favourable results in scleroderma; there was no evidence of benefit. Some agents appear to have been used on a trial and error basis; e.g. arsenic (Boeck, 1916), sodium morrhuate (Barber, 1927), bismuth (Dupont, 1947), and vitamin C in large doses (Joulia *et al.*, 1956; Laugier and Ledoux, 1958; Beurey *et al.*, 1959).

Vitamin D

As noted in Chapter 19, p. 405, treatment with calciferol and other vitamin D preparations was introduced, mainly by dermatologists, after the beneficial effects of such treatment in lupus vulgaris had become apparent (Robertson, 1948). Gilg (1955) reported favourably upon the effect of calciferol upon skin sarcoids, but recognized the danger of hypercalcaemia. In view of this danger, even the tentative use of this agent in sarcoidosis is contra-indicated.

Radiotherapy

It is probable that in the past a number of cases of sarcoid BHL have been treated by radiotherapy under an unconfirmed and mistaken diagnosis of Hodgkin's disease, and of course have appeared to respond favourably because of the usual spontaneous regression. One of us (JGS) has seen two such patients, in whom the diagnosis of sarcoidosis was subsequently established; another had been referred to a radiotherapy department, but fortunately, the diagnosis of sarcoidosis was made before treatment was begun. One of those who had received radiotherapy developed fibrosis in the middle zones of the lungs with considerable disability; it is of course impossible to say how far the radiotherapy contributed to this. Although radiotherapy has been tried for various manifestations of sarcoidosis (Florange, 1910; Jackson, 1925) there is no evidence that it has any beneficial effect (Donlan, 1938).

Antituberculosis chemotherapy

Hoyle *et al.* (1955) reported that in an uncontrolled study treatment of patients with pulmonary sarcoidosis with streptomycin and PAS was followed by improvement in 11 of 29 whose disease was of less than two years' duration, and in one of nine with a longer duration. Because improvement was observed within four months in those improving, the authors suggested that it could be attributed to the treatment; but the proportions improving do not seem to be beyond expectation from the natural course of the disease, and when cortisone was added in 20 cases, radiographic improvement was observed in 17.

Other authors have recorded failure to observe any significant effect in antituberculosis drugs on the course of sarcoidosis (Pulaski and White, 1948; Hedvall, 1950; Gendel *et al.*, 1952; Irael *et al.*, 1953; Holsinger and Dalton, 1954; James and Thomson, 1959). One of us (JGS) treated a number of patients with active sarcoidosis for periods up to one year, without observing evidence of modification of the course of the disease. Moreover, in a few who had shown suppression of various manifestations of sarcoidosis during short periods of cortisone treatment, and had subsequently relapsed, the addition of antituberculosis drugs to a second period of cortisone treatment was tried; most relapsed, and the small proportion not relapsing was no greater than might have been expected from the natural course of the disease.

Currently, antituberculosis chemotherapy is indcated only in those patients with clinical and other features of sarcoidosis who show bacteriological evidence of *M. tuberculosis* (or other mycobacterial) infection (Chapter 23); and prophylactically in those with unequivocally positive tuberculin reactions who are receiving corticosteroid treatment.

CORTICOSTEROIDS

Early observations of the effects of elevation of the level of circulating corticoids either by corticotrophin or by cortisone in patients with sarcoidosis showed that manifestations of activity, both constitutional and local in eyes, skin, lungs, lymph-nodes, salivary glands and liver were favourably affected in the short term (Thorn *et al.*, 1950; Olson *et al.*, 1950; Siltzbach *et al.*, 1951; Lovelock and Stone, 1951; Sones *et al.*, 1951; Small, 1951; Brun *et al.*, 1952; Shulman *et al.*, 1952), and that in those with hypercalcaemia, serum calcuim levels became normal (Shulman *et al.*, 1952). Riley *et al.* (1952) found in three patients with impaired lung function that while ventilatory capacity was improved, severely reduced diffusing capacity was little changed. Repeat biopsies during corticotrophin or cortisone adminis-tration generally showed remission of granulomas (Siltzbach, 1952). All these early observers noted that the cessation of short-term treatment was generally followed by relapse of the active manifestations.

Subsequent reports of uncontrolled series of patients treated for longer periods with oral corticosteroids, usually prednisone or prednisolone, generally confirmed these early findings (Israel *et al.*, 1954; Hoyle *et al.*, 1955; Rudberg-Roos and Roos, 1958; James and Thomson, 1959; Scad-ding, 1961; Hoyle *et al.*, 1967; Turaif *et al.*, 1967; Johns and Ball, 1967; Barber *et al.*, 1971; Refvem, 1974; Johns *et al.*, 1976; Middleton and Douglas, 1980b; Refvem and Refvem, 1980). Extrathoracic manifestations accessible to inspection are usually partially or completely suppressed. Enlarged lymph-nodes in the mediastinum and elsewhere diminish in size to a varying degree. In the lungs, changes that appear non-fibrotic, and especi-ally if they are of short duration, show diminution or clearing of radio-graphic shadows; but functional impairment associated with them usually shows only partial improvement, which is generally more evident in ventila-tory than in gas-exchange tests (Smellie *et al.*, 1961). Older-standing fibrotic lung changes show little objective change, though patients may claim some subjective improvement. Hypercalcaemia and hypercalciuria are controlled, usually by moderate dosage. In some patients, the improvement observed during limited periods of treatment is maintained after its cessation; but in many the condition relapses within a few months towards the former state, or occasionally to a worse one, and this sequence of events may be repeated with further periods of treatment. Occasionally, new manifestations – e.g. skin infiltrations (Scadding, 1972) – appear shortly after the end of a period of corticosteroid treatment. The lability of sarcoidosis in response to corti-costeroid administration is especially easily observed in chronic skin infiltra-tions, in the upper respiratory tract and in the eyes.

These observations suggest that the effect of corticosteroids is no more than suppressive of manifestations of sarcoidosis that are in a labile state, presumably represented pathologically by developing and formed epithe-lioid and giant cell granulomas without fibrosis; but has no effect on the as yet unidentified inciting agent or agents. This suppressive effect benefits patients symptomatically, so that there are clear indications for the use of corticosteroids in the management of those who have troublesome symptoms which cannot be controlled in other ways. Uncontrolled observations show that it can improve long-term prognosis in some cases of ocular sarcoidosis (Chapter 8) in which control of active changes may prevent secondary mechanical effects threatening sight, and in patients with hypercalcaemia in whom irreversible damage by hypercalcaemic nephropathy can be prevented by the control of calcium levels, usually possible with modest doses of corticosteroids (Chapter 19). But opinions differ on the important question whether corticosteroid treatment affects the end-result in those patients with granulomatous infiltrations, especially in the lungs, who initially have no important symptoms or impairment of function (De Remee, 1977).

MANAGEMENT OF PULMONARY SARCOIDOSIS

Both uncontrolled experience and controlled trials have shown that symptoms and signs caused by granulomatous infitrations of the lungs can be relieved by the administration of corticosteroids, though both the dose required to produce this effect, and the duration of treatment required to maintain it, vary from case to case.

Controlled studies

In a number of controlled studies, the progress of patients with pulmonary sarcoidosis receiving specified regimens of corticosteroid treatment has been compared with that of similar groups not receiving corticosteroids. In all of these, treated groups have shown more favourable radiographic changes and some improvement in functional assessments as compared with untreated during the treatment period, but the advantage for the treated group has disappeared on reassessment after the cessation of treatment. In the earlier studies the duration of treatment was unrealistically brief. Hapke and Meek (1971) compared 16 patients treated with prednisolone, 15 mg daily for six months, with 16 matched for age, sex, duration of sarcoidosis and degree of functional impairment. Both groups made satisfactory progress; during the treatment period there was more radiographic clearing in the treated group, but follow-up four years later showed no difference between the two groups. Young *et al.* (1970) treated alternate patients with pulmonary sarcoidosis causing lowered carbon monoxide transfer factor or arterial oxygen pressure with prednisone for at least six months, starting with 60 mg daily; function was marginally better in the treated group at six months, but review one or two years later, and again ten to 15 years later (Harkleroad *et al.*, 1982) showed no difference between treated and untreated groups on clinical, radiological and functional assessments. Israel *et al.*

(1973) enrolled 90 patients with intrathoracic sarcoidosis in a randomized trial of prednisone, 15 mg daily for three months, excluding any with irreversible fibrosis or with uveitis or hypercalcaemia; 83 were followed for at least one year. In 37 with BHL, no difference was found between treated and untreated at any time. In 46 with lung infiltration, improvement was evident at the end of treatment, but after a mean interval of 5.4 years, no difference was found between treated and untreated. Mikami *et al.* (1974) reported a Japanese study in which 50 patients receiving prednisolone for six months, starting with 30 mg daily were compared with 51 receiving placebo tablets; during 'treatment', the group receiving prednisolone showed accelerated subsidence of BHL, and more improvement of pulmonary infiltration, but one year later there was no difference between the two groups. Selroos and Sellergren (1979) randomly allocated 39 patients with pulmonary infiltration due to sarcoidosis to treatment with methylprednisolone or observation for seven months; at the end of this time the radiographic findings, vital capacity and carbon monoxide diffusion capacity were more favourable in the treated group, but at two years and four years, treated and untreated groups were similar. The dosage of methylprednisolone was 24 to 32 mg daily for the first two weeks, and thereafter gradually reduced; half the treated patients received methylprednisolone every other day after the initial two weeks, thus receiving only half the dosage of those on daily treatment. There was no difference in apparent response between the two treated sub-groups. Eule *et al.* (1980) reported a study in which patients with intrathoracic sarcoidosis divided into three groups. Two were treated with predinsolone, initially 40 mg daily and reduced gradually to 10–15 mg, for either six months or one year, and the third observed as controls; 65 and 66 in the two treated, and 78 in the control, groups had been followed for at least three years. The treated patients fared better radiographically during treatment; but 12 and 18 months later, the findings in all groups were similar, and remained so. Yamamoto *et al.* (1983) in a study of matched pairs of patients, 16 with BHL and 21 with BHL and pulmonary infiltration, treated one of each pair with prednisolone, given on alternate days, starting with 60 mg and gradually reducing to 5 mg over 18 months. In the first six months, a higher proportion of treated patients showed radiographic improvement but thereafter treated and untreated fared similarly, the proportions showing resolution at the end of three years being 76% and 74%.

These comparative studies, in which patients with pulmonary sarcoidosis were treated for periods of up to 18 months with corticosteroids, thus confirm that corticosteroids can suppress active granulomas and relieve symptoms; in none was there evidence that this treatment improved long-term prognosis. But these findings can be accepted as valid only for the sorts of patient and the regimens of treatment studied. One criterion for the selection of patients in most of them was the exclusion of any with features that might be regarded as necessary indications for corticosteroid treatment; thus those studied were likely to be a group with a generally favourable prognosis. And it is common experience that the dosage and duration of treatment required to suppress active manifestations vary greatly from case to case, and cannot be forecast for the individual patient; thus protocols specifying dosage and duration in advance may be thought unrealistic in that they do not resemble the procedure which experience has shown to be necessary to maintain an initially favourable response.

Policies of long-term management

In view of uncertainty about long-term effects, it is not surprising that there is no general agreement about the optimal use of corticosteroids in the management of pulmonary sarcoidosis.

Impressed by lack of evidence that prognosis for patients without important symptoms is improved by corticosteroid suppression of clinical evidences of the disease, and reluctant to prescribe treatment which may have undesirable effects without good reason, some physicians have adopted as their indication for the use of corticosteroids the relief of symptoms severe enough to interfere with the patient's normal conduct of life (Scadding, 1961; Mitchell and Scadding, 1974). The assumptions underlying this policy are:

(a) In many patients with pulmonary sarcoidosis, the active stage comes spontaneously to an end, leaving no evident or only trivial changes. There is no evidence that corticosteroid treatment in such cases either reduces the duration of the active stage or diminishes the amount of residual fibrosis.

(b) In those with symptoms restricting their activities, the relief of these is sufficient justification for the use of corticosteroids, provided that the required dose is tolerable for long-term administration.

(c) The severity and pattern of impairment of function in pulmonary sarcoidosis and other diffuse lung diseases reflects the extent and distribution of changes in alveoli, airways and blood vessels in the lungs without necessary implications about the histological character of these changes (Keogh and Crystal, 1980). In sarcoidosis, pre-granulomatous, granulomatous and fibrotic changes may all contribute to impairment of function; and in management, the chief contribution of pulmonary function tests is in following progress. Tests within the normal range are reassuring in a patient with an abnormal chest radiograph. Occasionally results indicating considerable impairment of function may be found in patients who deny symptoms; if this cannot be explained by other disease, it may constitute a valid indication for treatment, especially if serial tests show deterioration. Apart from this, function tests contribute little to decisions about the initiation of corticosteroid treatment.

(d) The various tests of 'activity', discussed below, are certainly of interest for the light they may throw on pathogenesis and the mode of action of corticosteroids, and are of undoubted value in research. They may have a place, to be defined, in assisting decision about duration of treatment in patients with persistently active sarcoidosis; but unless it is found that treatment guided by them leads to better long-term results than that based on simpler criteria, it is inadvisable to advocate their routine use.

(e) It is possible that in some patients with extensive active pre-granulomatous infiltration ('alveolitis') and labile granulomatous changes, in whom corticosteroids produce relief of symptoms and radiographic clearing, prognosis is improved and extent of residual fibrosis diminished. On the suggested criterion for the use of corticosteroids, such patients would of course be treated.

At the other end of the range of opinion, some physicians have thought that the use of corticosteroid treatment on much wider indications to suppress 'activity', variously defined, irrespective of symptoms, is likely to diminish the proportion of patients left with serious disability (Turiaf *et al.*, 1967; De Remee and Anderson, 1974), or have implied that they thought so by advocating prolonged uninterrupted regimens of corticosteroid treatment without feeling the need for a controlled trial to establish their value (Deenstra and Van Ditmars, 1968). The assumptions underlying this view are:

(a) In pulmonary sarcoidosis, the appearance of dyspnoea indicates that fibrosis has developed.

(b) The development of fibrosis can be prevented by the inception of corticosteroid treatment during the pre-fibrotic, possibly asymptomatic stages, and its sufficiently prolonged maintenance.

(c) Either (i) it is possible to establish some criteria by which asymptomatic patients at risk of developing fibrosis can be identified, so that they can be treated; or (ii) all patients with active pulmonary sarcoidosis should receive corticosteroids, and it is possible to establish criteria for the duration of treatment.

The first of these assumptions is doubtful; there is now good evidence – e.g. in the studies of Carrington *et al.* (1976) and Huang *et al.* (1979) reviewed in Chapter 6 – that the profusion of pre-granulomatous cellular infiltration and of granulomas, as well as the extent of fibrosis can be correlated with dyspnoea. The second may be true in some cases, especially those with much pre-granulomatous infiltration, even though none of the controlled studies hitherto reported has produced evidence to support it. It cannot be refuted by reference to past experience, or to the negative results of controlled studies of limited regimens of corticosteroid treatment, since the development of fibrosis in a treated patient can be explained by those who hold these views as due to delayed, inadequate or insufficiently prolonged administration of corticosteroids. This plea can of course be countered by reference to patients with relentlessly progressive sarcoidosis of the lungs (and of other organs) which has led to disability and death in spite of the use of corticosteroids in dosage limited only by side-effects.

Assessment of 'activity'

The practical application of a policy of the second sort depends upon the definition of 'activity', and the specification of the criteria by which it is to be assessed. Activity should properly denote the possibility of change, either favourable or unfavourable, as opposed to inactivity, which implies a stable condition. If criteria of activity are correct, they should define a group of patients some of whom will improve, some deteriorate, and some show no change during limited periods of observation, while all of a group not showing the criteria should remain unchanged. Serial observations are required to show the direction of change in individual active cases, to detect activity in doubtful cases, and to confirm inactivity. The histology of biopsy samples suggests activity if it shows fresh granulomas, especially with pre-granulomatous cellular infiltration, and inactivity if it shows only hyalinizing granulomas and fibrosis, but is subject to sampling error. Clinical features that occur in some cases, such as fever, constitutional symptoms, erythema nodosum, new or worsening respiratory symptoms, or the recent appearance of extrathoracic manifestations are indicants of activity. Some radiographic appearances, especially if they are known to be of recent origin, suggest activity, which may be confirmed by serial observation. Abnormal pulmonary function tests may be due to active or inactive lung disease, changes in serial tests suggesting activity. Response of radiographic changes, of accessible extrathoracic manifestations, and, less convincingly, of symptoms to corticosteroid treatment is evidence of activity. Lymphopenia in the peripheral blood, a changing pattern of serum proteins, and raised erythrocyte sedimentation rate suggest activity.

A number of tests that may be correlated with cellular events in the granulomatous process have been investigated as possible indicants of liability to progress to fibrosis, rather than of unpredictable changeability. These include serum ACE levels, the analysis of cell-types in bronchoalveolar lavage fluid (BAL), and [67]gallium scanning.

Serum ACE levels are elevated in many, but not all patients with active sarcoidosis (Chapter 26, p. 573), and fall with evidence of diminished activity. ACE is present in sarcoid epithelioid cells, but not in macrophages and monocytes (Chapter 2, p. 31), and it has been suggested that serum levels may reflect the number of active granulomas (Silverstein *et al.*, 1976) though alveolar macrophages (Hinman *et al.*, 1978) and circulating monocytes (Friedland *et al.*, 1978) are other possible sources of the enzyme. Elevated levels in patients with sarcoidosis fall with corticosteroid treatment (Baughman *et al.*, 1980), but so do normal levels in patients receiving corticosteroids for other diseases (Turton *et al.*, 1979). ACE levels are less sensitive as evidence of activity than BAL or gallium scanning, being normal in some patients in whom one or both of these indicate activity (Beaumont *et al.*, 1982; Rossman *et al.*, 1982; Schoenberger *et al.*, 1982); thus, a normal level does not exclude activity. Elevated levels in patients with sarcoidosis can be accepted as indicating activity, and changes in serum ACE in untreated patients probably reflect changes in numbers of metabolically active epithelioid cells in granulomas; but the value of ACE estimations in deciding about the need for corticosteroid treatment and in following response to it appears limited.

BAL makes possible the study of effector cells from the pulmonary alveoli. Its contribution to knowledge of the cellular immunology and pathogenesis of pulmonary sarcoidosis is considered in Chapter 20, p. 44. This has led to the concept that granuloma-formation is initiated and maintained by activated T-lymphocytes in the alveoli (Hunninghake *et al.*, 1980; Crystal *et al.*, 1981); these attract monocytes which become converted to macrophages and then to epithelioid cells. The active phase of pulmonary sarcoidosis may be regarded as an alveolitis in which lymphocytes have the leading and macrophages an important role. The proportions of effector cells found by BAL have been found to reflect those found in open lung biopsies (Hunninghake *et al.*, 1981a). In active pulmonary sarcoidosis, the proportion of lymphocytes obtained by BAL is characteristically increased, and many are identifiable as activated T-cells. Though the proportion of macrophages is less than in normal subjects, the absolute numbers are increased, since the total number of cells obtained is much higher. It has been suggested that the proportion of T-lymphocytes in BAL should be regarded as an index of the comtribution of activated lymphocytes to new granuloma-formation, more than 28% indicating a high level of activity of this aspect of the alveolitis of sarcoidosis (Keogh *et al.*,1983; Crystal *et al.*, 1983).

The contribution of gallium-67 scanning to the diagnosis of sarcoidosis is considered in Chapter 26, p. 575. Since ^{67}Ga accumulates selectively at sites of active sarcoidosis, the relationship between indices of lung uptake of ^{67}Ga and clinical, radiological and physiological findings and with other measures of 'activity' have been studied. Line *et al.* (1981) performed scans in 41 patients with sarcoidosis, estimating for each an index of ^{67}Ga uptake in the lungs; 46 (65%) showed high uptake as compared with a control group. Uptake was correlated only weakly with clinical, radiological and physiological findings, but strongly with the percentages of lymphocytes and of T-lymphocytes among cells obtained by BAL. Hunninghake *et al.* (1981b) performed BAL in patients who had just had ^{67}Ga scans; in ten with sarcoidosis, 95% of radioactivity was found to be associated with macrophages and only 5% with lymphocytes; and in eight with cryptogenic fibrosing alveolitis, 66% with macrophages and 34% with neutrophils. *In vitro*, ^{67}Ga was taken up by macrophages from sarcoidosis patients but not by those from normal subjects. It thus appears likely that the correlation between numbers of lymphocytes in BAL and ^{67}Ga uptake is indirect, activated lymphocytes activating macrophages which take up ^{67}Ga. Beaumont *et al.* (1982) performed ^{67}Ga scans in 54 patients with intrathoracic sarcoidosis, repeated in 23. Scans distinguished fibrotic from active lung changes, and detected some previously undetected localizations in mediastinum, spleen and salivary glands. Gallium-67 uptake in the lungs showed rough correlation with serum ACE levels, and was more sensitive than ACE levels to clearing, spontaneous or after corticosteroid treatment. In 29 patients submitted to BAL, there was no correlation between the numbers of lymphocytes per 100 ml of fluid recovered and ^{67}Ga uptake. This discrepancy with the findings of Line *et al.* (1981) may be in part due to technical differences, such as the use of absolute numbers, rather than percentages, of lymphocytes, and different ways of estimating ^{67}Ga uptake; and in part to differences between the groups of patients studied, especially in view of the evidence provided by the study of Hunninghake *et al.* (1981b), mentioned above, that ^{67}Ga uptake reflects activation of macrophages. Thus, while the proportion of T-lymphocytes in BAL is an index of the lymphocytic component, ^{67}Ga uptake in the lungs may be regarded as an index of the macrophage component of active pulmonary sarcoidosis.

Crystal *et al.* (1983) have suggested a grading of activity which takes cognizance of both lymphocyte and macrophage components, by combining the lymphocytic index noted above with a simple assessment of ^{67}Ga uptake in the lungs as 'positive' or 'negative'. If the percentage of lymphocytes in BAL is above 28%, and the ^{67}Ga scan is positive, their overall assessment was 'high intensity alveolitis'; a lymphocyte percentage below 28%, and an negative scan indicated 'low intensity alveolitis'; while a high percentage of lymphocytes with a negative scan, or a low percentage with a positive scan was described as 'split alveolitis'. Keogh *et al.* (1983) performed serial studies in 19 patients with pulmonary sarcoidosis and no evident extrapulmonary localizations. Low intensity alveolitis was found for 80% of the time, but nearly 80% of the patients had either a positive scan or a high proportion of T-cells in BAL at least once. Of observed 'episodes' of high intensity alveolitis, three-quarters spontaneously reverted to low intensity, while 12% of low intensity findings were followed by high intensity. Keogh *et al.* found that of patients with high intensity alveolitis, 85% showed reduction of either lung volumes or diffusing capacity over six months' observation, while of those graded as low intensity, less than 10% showed such deterioration; thus the combination of BAL and ^{67}Ga scanning was of predictive value.

Unsolved problems

The outstanding unsolved problem is aetiological: to what is the complex process that leads to the formation of the sarcoid granuloma a response? The identification of a causal agent or agents would open the way to the possibility of curative treatment aimed at the removal or neutralization of this agent or agents. In the meantime, the principal problem is the optimal use of corticosteroids to suppress some aspects of this response. The short-term effects on symptoms, clinical manifestations accessible to examination, and a variety of tests of 'activity' are not in dispute; but it remains unknown whether a policy of attempting to suppress sarcoid infiltrations of the lungs in all patients throughout the varying duration of 'activity' (however specified) by the administration of corticosteroids for sufficient periods and in sufficient dose would diminish the proportion left eventually with serious, possibly life-threatening impairment of function, as compared with the simpler policy of using corticosteroids to control symptoms as far as possible; and further, if the more vigorous policy were found to give more favourable long-term results, whether the benefit would be of sufficient degree to justify the side-effects of prolonged corticosteroid administration, and the cost and general inconvenience, especially to those who would have progressed favourably without treatment, both of the treatment and of whatever tests of 'activity' were adopted to determine its duration and intensity. Moreover, it should not be assumed, from short-term studies suggesting that during corticosteroid treatment of active pulmonary sarcoidosis evolution towards fibrosis may be delayed, that in those patients who have persistently active disease any practicable scheme of corticosteroid administration can prevent the ultimate development of fibrosis. It is an attractive hypothesis that persistent suppression of activity will necessarily have this effect; but this hypothesis cannot be accepted *a priori*. The reactions being suppressed by corticosteroids are presumably to some as yet unidentified agent or agents that may persist for indeterminate periods, and whose removal is a prerequisite for ultimate cessation of activity. The frequency of recurrences of clinical and other evidences of activity on withdrawal of corticosteroids suggests that they do not hasten removal of this factor. It is possible that they might delay it; if this were so, the effect of prolonged corticosteroid treatment on the amount of residual fibrosis might vary from case to case, depending upon the balance between the favourable effect of suppression of the cellular reaction and the unfavourable effect of impeding the removal of the factor to which it is a response.

It is difficult to see how these doubts can be resolved except by a long-term prospective randomized comparison of two policies for the use of corticosteroids in the management of pulmonary sarcoidosis; one adopting as the principal criterion for their use the relief of symptoms, and the other the control of 'activity' to be defined in terms of whatever tests might be accepted as likely to be best for this purpose, throughout its duration. The definitive comparison would be at the end of an observation-period of at least five years, in terms of symptoms, lung function, radiographic changes, and proportions showing evidence of continued activity. Additionally, it would be desirable to include some assessment of the quality of life during the period of the study for the patients in the two groups. Because differences in end-result between the two groups are likely to be small, the number of patients required is likely to be large, necessitating a multi-centre study. Physicians with strong preconceived ideas about the merits of two policies would regard the study as unethical: only those who admit doubt would be willing to participate. Agreement about the choice of test that should be used to assess activity, and about their frequency might be difficult to attain; this choice would be critical, in view of the possibility that if the final result were equivocal, or favoured the less intensively treated group, it could be claimed that a test not included might have been a better guide to the conduct of corticosteroid treatment. Some patients in both groups would be expected to develop extrathoracic localizations or hypercalcaemia that would call for corticosteroid treatment, irrespective of lung changes, during the study period. Such patients could continue to be included in the study, since the objective would be to compare two policies of management of patients with pulmonary sarcoidosis; in the final assessment it would be informative both to include them in the main analysis and to analyse them separately.

It is doubtful whether such a study is practicable, in view of the many difficulties involved. A less ambitious study is currently being conducted by the British Thoracic Society, although the results are not likely to be available until 1986 or 1987. In this study, a policy of using corticosteroids to control symptoms only is being compared with one of maintaining as far as possible a clear chest radiograph, over a period of five years. In this way, it is hoped to be able to compare the symptomatic, radiographic and functional findings at the end of five years in two initially comparable groups, one of which will have had more intensive corticosteroid treatment than the other. If the more intensively treated group does not fare better, it will be apparent that any advantage from more elaborate procedures for the control of corticosteroid treatment in pulmonary sarcoidosis is likely to be marginal; if it does, search for the optimal procedure in cost-benefit terms will be justified; and it is not impossible that the less intensively treated group will be found to have done at least as well, with fewer corticosteroid side-effects.

Indications for corticosteroid treatment

In view of current uncertainties, indications for corticosteroid treatment in pulmonary sarcoidosis remain largely a matter of clinical judgement, with inevitable variations between physicians, as discussed above. The following comments concern only some special points.

BHL without radiologically evident pulmonary infiltration has a good prognosis, especially if it is accompanied by erythema nodosum, and unless accompanied by some other manifestation does not call for corticosteroid treatment. Initial arthropathy and febrile symptoms can be controlled by non-steroidal anti-inflammatory drugs.

For the patients with pulmonary infiltration, with or without BHL, we incline to the view that the indication for the use of corticosteroids is the presence of symptoms troublesome enough to warrrant relief by what may prove to be indefinitely prolonged treatment with hormones which may have important side-effects, and themselves cause symptoms. This view is, of course, open to revision should a comparative study show that better long-term results are produced by a policy of using corticosteroids to suppress 'activity' as assessed by such criteria as radio-isotope scanning, enumeration of cell-types in BAL, serum ACE levels or other tests, individually or in combination. In the meantime, we consider that the simpler policy has the advantage of not interfering with the lives of the majority of patients who have no important symptoms, and in whom the disease resolves leaving little or no detectable fibrosis, while helping the minority in whom it follows a less favourable course by alleviating symptoms, irrespective of any effect corticosteroid treatment may have on the development and extent of fibrosis. It seems probable that the proportions of patients with pulmonary sarcoidosis who require corticosteroid treatment on these, or any other, criteria vary between populations; in both North America and Europe, it is the general impression that more blacks than whites with pulmonary sarcoidosis have symptoms caused by it, as well as by accompanying extrathoracic localizations of sarcoidosis, requiring control by corticosteroids.

Stenosing sarcoidosis of the bronchi (Chapter 6, p. 143) responds well to corticosteroid treatment, and represents a situation in which suppression of active sarcoidosis is likely to diminish the probability of permanent lung damage due to the non-specific consequences of bronchostenosis. In patients who have developed the proximal bronchostenoses characteristic of this condition, corticosteroid treatment may need to be continued indefinitely to maintain improvement initially attained.

In the presence of irreversible fibrotic changes in the lungs, the symptoms such as dyspnoea and paroxysmal cough may be diminished in variable degree in a few patients by corticosteroid treatment. There are probably two elements in the causation of such relief: suppression of such residues of active sarcoid granuloma as remain, and diminution of airway obstruction by reduction of bronchial mucosal swelling. The correct policy in such a case is an empirical one; in the minority of patients in whom symptoms are found to be alleviated by a dose of a corticosteroid that is tolerable for prolonged administration, the treatment is worth continuing; in others in whom it is tried and found ineffective, it should be withdrawn.

Hypercalcaemia

Hypercalcaemia that cannot be controlled by limitation of calcium intake and avoidance of vitamin D preparations constitutes an absolute indication for corticosteroid treatment. Fortunately, it is usually controllable by modest dosage (Chapter 19, p. 412).

Uveitis

If not controlled by local treatment, uveitis requires systemic corticosteroid treatment (Chapter 8, p. 215.

Skin sarcoids

These call for corticosteroid treatment only if they are disfiguring to a degree causing distress to the patient; and whether the improvement produced is worth while can be determined only by trial. It may be found that any improvement is outweighed by the changes in appearance caused by the side-effects of the high doses that may be required to suppress persistent infiltrations of the lupus pernio type. Moreover, such infiltrations are likely to recur after cessation of treatment (Chapter 7, p. 204). The behaviour of persistent skin infiltrations in response to corticosteroids illustrates both the ability of corticosteroids to suppress formed granulomas, of which such infiltrations are composed, and their inability to remove whatever it is that incites the formation of granulomas.

Nervous system

The response of sarcoidosis involving the central nervous system is unpredictable. In the presence of a diffuse meningeal infiltration or a local deposit within the brain of spinal cord, corticosteroid treatment is advisable, since suppression of the active granuloma may be expected to relieve symptoms; however, focal epilepsy may be aggravated (Chapter 14, p. 326).

Other organs

If myocardial sarcoidosis can be diagnosed during life, a trial of corticosteroid treatment is clearly indicated, though its results cannot be predicted (Chapter 15, p. 347).

Similarly, if sarcoidosis of other internal organs – e.g. liver, spleen alimentary tract – is causing symptoms, the effect of corticosteroid treatment should be tried.

The foregoing views are in general agreement with the recommendations of the Committee on Therapy of the American Thoracic Society (1971) with some minor differences of emphasis.

Procedure in corticosteroid treatment

In view of the many uncertainties, only general guidelines to the use of corticosteroids in the management of sarcoidosis can be given. The purpose of corticosteroid treatment is to suppress some features of the active stage of the disease. The dosage required to attain this varies from case to case, and the duration of the active stage cannot be predicted. Hence the duration of the treatment can be determined only by trial, and it is not possible to prescribe any predetermined 'course' of treatment. Once the decision has been made that it is in the patient's best interest to attempt to suppress some manifestation of the disease, be it a symptom, a localization accessible to examination, or a test of 'activity', the rational procedure is to determine what dose will effect this; if this is tolerable for long-term administration, to continue it, with periodic gradual reductions of dosage during which careful watch is kept for recrudescence of the feature which has been suppressed or other evidences of activity; and to reinstitute suppressive dosage should such evidence appear.

The usual procedure is to start with a relatively large dose until maximal improvement has been attained. In most cases of pulmonary sarcoidosis, 30 mg daily of prednisolone is appropriate, though if initial response is poor, it is advisable to increase it before the conclusion is reached that the disease is in an unresponsive stage. In some patients with extensive and active disease, and in those with severe involvement of some extrapulmonary sites – e.g. the central nervous system – doses of the order of 60 mg daily may be needed to obtain optimal suppressive effects. After six to 12 months of the maintenance dose, very gradual reduction with careful observation of symptoms, clinical and other assessments appropriate to the chief sites of involvement, and whatever tests of activity may be thought appropriate, is the only means by which it can be decided whether corticosteroid administration should be continued. In this decision, any side-effects of corticosteroids that have been observed should be given due weight, as should the possibility that indefinitely prolonged treatment may be required to maintain the level of improvement that has been attained.

At the corticosteroid dosages required in most cases, side-effects are not serious, and problems of pituitary-adrenal suppression are rarely observed. Alternate-day treatment may diminish these, while maintaining anti-inflammatory effects (Harter *et al.*, 1963; MacGregor *et al.*, 1969). Selroos and Sellergren (1979), as noted above, found that alternate-day administration of methylprednisolone in dosage diminishing from 20 mg to 4 mg was as effective in maintenance of improvement attained by initial daily dosage as was daily administration. With the very gradual reduction of dosage that is advisable when withdrawal of corticosteroid treatment in sarcoidosis is being attempted, pituitary-adrenal suppression is generally not a problem. Westerhof *et al.* (1970) studied adrenocortical function in patients on two prolonged regimens of daily prednisone for sarcoidosis reported by Deenstra and van Ditmars (1968). These started with 40 mg daily and reduced gradually to 2.5 mg daily at the end of three years and four years respectively, with a final few months of 2.5 mg on alternate days. When the daily dose had been reduced to 7.5 mg, plasma corticosteroid levels showed a diurnal rhythm, and low dosages of prednisone at the end of these regimens were additive to the returning function of the adrenals.

Antimalarial drugs

The use of antimalarial drugs, especially chloroquine, in skin sarcoidosis, and the ocular and other complications of such treatment have been discussed in Chapter 8, p. 205. A few reports have appeared on the effects of chloroquine on lung changes. Morse *et al.* (1961) thought that the response of lung changes to 500 mg of chloroquine sulphate daily for six months was less striking than that of skin changes, a response regarded as definite being observed in only one of six cases; mucosal lesions in two cases treated both responded. Davies (1963) treated five patients with pulmonary sarcoidosis with chloroquine for periods up to one year, the initial dose being 400–600 mg daily, with diminution in radiographic shadows and relief of symptoms in most; in two improvement initiated by prednisolone was maintained. All patients showed bleaching of the hair as a side-effect; one complained of misty vision but no objective change could be found in this or any other of the treated patients' eyes. Siltzbach and Teirstein (1964) treated 43 patients with 500 mg of chloroquine daily for periods ranging from four to 17 months. Of 14 with hilar lymphadenopathy alone, 11 improved during treatment and six relapsed afterwards; and of 29 with pulmonary infiltration with or without hilar lymphadenopathy, 20 improved and five relapsed. Fourteen of their patients had skin sarcoids; all improved under treatment, and nine relapsed afterwards. In some patients treatment caused minor discomforts, not requiring cessation of treatment; only one developed corneal changes after ten months of treatment and these cleared three weeks after it was stopped. The British Tuberculosis Association (1967) conducted a controlled study in which patients with pulmonary sarcoidosis were randomly allocated to treatment with chloroquine sulphate, 600 mg daily for eight weeks and 400 mg daily for a further eight weeks. Assessments at four and six months showed significant radiological improvement in the treated group, with some improvement in dyspnoea and ventilatory function, but eight months after the end of treatment there was no difference between treated and control groups. Morse (1967) carried out, in 30 patients with pulmonary and mediastinal lymph-node sarcoidosis, a cross-over study, in which six months of treatment with chloroquine phosphate 250 mg twice daily and six months of placebo tablets were given, half the patients starting with chloroquine and half with the placebo. Continuous improvement was observed in nine, of whom four received placebo and five chloroquine during the first six months: these were regarded as spontaneous improvements. Chloroquine was regarded as having had a beneficial effect if improvement occurred during the first six months in those then receiving chloroquine and was followed by relapse during the following six months on placebo, or during the second six months in those then receiving chloroquine, followed by relapse during subsequent observation. On these criteria, intrathoracic sarcoidosis was judged to have been favourably affected in 14 of the 21 not showing spontaneous improvment. Among 55 patients treated with 500 mg of chloroquine daily for four months or more, including the 30 in the cross-over study, nine could not tolerate the drug because of nausea and vomiting, and two developed a presumably drug-related rash; one developed corneal changes which resolved after cessation of treatment; none showed retinal changes.

Occasions for considering the use of chloroquine, to which its derivative hydroxychloroquine may be preferred since it is said to cause less gastrointestinal upset, in sarcoidosis are rare. These drugs have a suppressive effect on granulomas but this is less reliable and slower in onset than that of corticosteroids; and their value is reduced by the frequency of gastric discomfort in patients taking them, and by the risk of retinal damage in patients taking them for more than six months, which calls for careful ophthalmological supervision if treatment is prolonged. Thus they should be considered only if there is an urgent indication for suppression of an active granulomatous change, and a contraindication to the use of corticosteroids. Recrudescence of persistently active sarcoidosis after cessation of chloroquine which has had a suppressive effect on it is to be expected, just as after cessation of corticosteroid treatment.

Immunosuppressive and cytotoxic drugs

Lacher (1968) reported a single case in which the addition of methotrexate, 20 mg twice weekly, to prednisone, 75 mg three times weekly, which had failed to control florid sarcoidosis of five years' duration in a young black woman, involving lymph-nodes, skin, lungs, liver, spleen and joints, with fever, was followed by remission of all manifestations; this was maintained during 18 months' further observation, during which prednisone was withdrawn and a reducing dosage of methotrexate continued. The temporal relationship of remission to the administration of methotrexate was striking, but coincidental spontaneous improvement could not be excluded.

Israel (1971) treated 25 patients with active progressive sarcoidosis in whom corticosteroids were not effective or not tolerated with chlorambucil, 2 mg four times daily, or methotrexate, 20 mg twice weekly, five being treated with both these drugs. In six, 'dramatic' clinical and radiological improvement was observed, but relapse occurred three to 12 months later; in some others there was symptomatic improvement only. No ill effects were observed.

Sharma *et al.* (1971a) reported observations on ten patients who had sarcoidosis of two to 20 years' duration, which was said not to have responded to corticosteroids or chloroquine, and who were treated with azathioprine 100 mg daily for six to 30 weeks. All had intrathoracic changes and six uveitis. Improvement in clinical findings, including uveitis, and in radiographic appearances were noted in three, but no long-term observations were reported.

As noted in Chapter 7, p. 206, Veien and Brodthagen (1977) reported suppressive effects of methotrexate, 25 mg once weekly, on skin sarcoids in 12 of 16 patients, with relapse on cessation of treatment, and on uveitis in three of four who also showed this localization.

Kataria (1980) treated ten patients with progressive sarcoidosis with chlorambucil, either because they had not responded to corticosteroids, or because there was a contraindication to corticosteroid treatment. Eight showed some clinical improvement, but effects on radiographic changes in lungs and on lung function were variable, and one patient with severe central nervous system sarcoidosis died. In patients showing improvement, it became evident within three months.

The mode of action of these drugs in sarcoidosis is uncertain. Israel (1971) considered that because of the rapid onset of improvement in responsive patients, and of relapse after cessation of treatment, and of inconstant changes in immunoglobulin levels, the effect was anti-inflammatory, like that of corticosteroids, rather than cytotoxic or immunosuppressive. However, the possibility of effects of the latter sorts demands close surveillance of patients treated in this way, and these drugs can have only a very limited place, on an admittedly empirical basis, in patients with extensive active sarcoidosis causing severe symptoms which has failed to respond to corticosteroids. We are aware of one patient with intractable and life-threatening sarcoidosis of the central nervous system in whom as a last resort treatment with methotrexate was started; in spite of careful surveillance, he developed generalized herpes virus infection of which he died.

Levamisole

The observation that levamisole, introduced as an antihelminthic, might restore skin reactivity in anergic patients with malignant disease, and stimulate some aspects of lymphocyte activity *in vitro* (Tripodi *et al.*, 1973; Binianimov and Ramot, 1975) has led to a few trials of its use in sarcoidosis (Rosenthal *et al.*, 1976; Veien, 1977; Cole *et al.* 1979). These all showed no benefit, and side-effects preventing the completion of the trial therapy in many patients; effects on immunological findings were variable. The lack of clinical response is not surprising, since the immunological abnormality in sarcoidosis is in most respects over-activity, only the ability to develop and express Type IV hypersensitivity reactions being depressed.

CONCLUSION

No therapeutic measure so far studied appears to affect the agent or agents inciting the development of sarcoid granulomas. The measure most reliably affecting sarcoidosis is increase in corticosteroid levels, usually effected by oral corticosteroids. The effect of this is to suppress active granulomas and some aspects of the processes that lead to the formation of granulomas. Clinical manifestations of active sarcoidosis can in many instances be suppressed by corticosteroids, but the dosage required varies, and there is no evidence that the duration of the active stage of the disease can be diminished, and recrudescence is frequent after limited periods of treatment. Two indications for the long-term use of corticosteroids in sufficient dosage to suppress manifestations that cannot be controlled in other ways are uveitis and hypercalcaemia, in both of which serious secondary effects may be prevented by such treatment. For other localizations of sarcoidosis, opinion is divided about whether prolonged corticosteroid treatment of persistently active infiltrations can prevent the ultimate development of irreversible hyaline fibrosis. In none of the controlled studies of corticosteroid treatment of pulmonary sarcoidosis with 'courses' of corticosteroid treatment which have been published has there been any long-term advantage for the treated groups, although during treatment they have fared better in various clinical and other assessments than the untreated. Currently, the question whether corticosteroid treatment directed by various objective tests of 'activity' might produce better long-term results is being investigated. Fortunately, the natural course of many cases of sarcoidosis is towards spontaneous remission. Symptoms may be controllable during the active stage by moderate dosage causing no serious side-effects, and this constitutes a useful guide-line to the sensible use of corticosteroids in pulmonary sarcoidosis. For some of the less common clinical presentations of sarcoidosis, e.g. in the central nervous system or in the heart, which may be immediately life-threatening, a trial of corticosteroid treatment is indicated; the effect is unpredictable, but only by trial can those patients who respond favourably be identified.

The physician's responsibility in the management of sarcoidosis is not only to recognize those cases in which intervention of this sort is required, but also, and perhaps of greater importance, so to explain the situation to patients, the majority of whom present no indication for active treatment, that the disease interferes as little as possible with their lives.

References

Aaronson, H.G., Meir, J.H. and Ulin, A.W. (1957) A case of sarcoidosis of the colon. *J. Albert Einstein Med. Cent.*, **6**, 14–16.

Abeler, V. (1979) Sarcoidosis of the cardiac conducting system. *Am. Heart J.*, **97**, 701–7.

Aberg, H. (1964) Tuberculosis and sarcoidosis. *Acta Tuberc. Pneumol. Scand.*, **45**, 84–8.

Adams, R., Denny-Brown, D. and Pearson, C. (1962) *Diseases of Muscle*, 2nd Ed., Hoeber, New York, p. 453.

Adamson, C.A., Ehrner, L., Lindstedt, J.A. and Nordenstam, H. (1960) Intrapulmonary cavities in chronical pulmonary sarcoidosis. *Acta Tuberc. Pneumol. Scand.*, **38**, 131–9.

Addrizzo, J.R., Minkowitz, S. and Lyons, H.A. (1971) Triple biopsy in the diagnosis of sarcoidosis. In *Proc. 5th International Conference on Sarcoidosis, Prague, 1969* (eds. L. Levinsky and F. Macholda), Universita Karlova, Prague, pp. 476–9.

Adickes, G.C., Zimmerman, S.L. and Cardwell, E.S., Jr (1951) Sarcoidosis with fatal cardiac involvement. *Ann. Intern. Med.*, **35**, 898–909.

Agate, J.N. (1948) Delayed pneumonitis in a beryllium worker. *Lancet*, **2**, 530–3.

Agner, E. and Larsen, J.H. (1979) Yersinia enterocolitica infection and sarcoidosis. *Scand. J. Respir. Dis.*, **5**, 230–4.

Ahmed, S.S., Rozefort, R., Taclob, L.T. and Brancato, R.W. (1971) Development of ventricular aneurysm in cardiac sarcoidosis. *Angiology*, **28**, 323–9.

Ahvonen, P. (1972) Yersiniosis in Finland. *Ann. Clin. Res.*, **4**, 30–48.

Ainslie, D. and James, D.G. (1956) Ocular sarcoidosis. *Br. Med. J.*, **1**, 954–7.

Akokan, G., Celikoglu, S., Goksel, F. and Demirci, S. (1977) HLA antigens in Turkish patients with sarcoidosis. *N. Engl. J. Med.*, **296**, 759 (c).

Alajouanine, T., Bertrand, I., Degos, R., Contamin, F. and Escourolle, R. (1958) Sarcoidose ganglionnaire, cutanée et oculaire avec attenite secondaire diffuse, périphérique et centrale, du système nerveux. *Rev. Neurol.*, **99**, 421–47.

Al Arif, L., Goldstein, R.A., Affronti, L.F., Janicki, B.W. and Foellmer, J.W. (1980) HLA antigens and sarcoidosis in a North American black population. In *Proc. 8th International Conference on Sarcoidosis, Cardiff, 1978* (eds. W. Jones-Williams and B.H. Davies), Alpha Omega, Cardiff, pp. 206–12.

Alario, A., Viac, J. and Thivolet, J. (1977) Evidence for a T-cell reaction in the cutaneous sarcoid granuloma. *Arch. Dermatol. Res.* **259**, 135–40.

Albright, F. (1956) The cause of hypercalciuria in sarcoid and its treatment with cortisone and sodium phytate. *J. Clin. Invest.*, **35**, 1229–42.

Albright, F. and Reifenstein, E.C., Jr (1948) *Parathyroid glands and metabolic bone disease. Selected studies*, Williams and Wilkins, Baltimore.

Algvere, P. (1970) Fluorescein studies of retinal vasculitis in sarcoidosis: report of a case. *Acta Ophthalmol.*, **48**, 1129–39.

Allen, A.W., Donaldson, G., Sniffen, R.C. and Goodale, F., Jr (1954) Primary malignant lymphoma of the gastro-intestinal tract. *Ann. Surg.*, **140**, 428–38.

Allen, B.R. (1979) Sarcoid of the nose with collapse of nasal cartilage. *Br. J. Dermatol.*, **100**, 54–6.

Allen, D.C., Biggart, J.D. (1983) Granulomatous disease in the vermiform appendix. *J. Clin. Pathol.*, **36**, 632–8.

Allen, E.H., Batten, J.C., and Jefferson, K. (1956) Sarcoidosis of the alimentary tract. *Br. J. Radiol.*, **29**, 56–61.

Allison, J.R. and Mikell, P.V. (1932) Sarcoid associated with tuberculosis of the larynx; report of case. *Arch. Dermatol. Syphilol, Chicago*, **25**, 334–43.

Altchek, A., Gaines, J.A., and Siltzbach, L.E. (1955) Sarcoidosis of the uterus. *Am. J. Obstet. Gynecol.*, **70**, 540–7.

Amati, G. (1947) Ricerche sperimentali nella malattia di Besnier–Boeck–Schaumann. (Experimental research in Besnier–Boeck–Schaumann disease.) *Boll. Soc. Ital. Biol. Sper.*, **23**, 377–9.

Amati, G. (1948) Esperienze bioloche sulla malattia di Besnier–Boeck–Schaumann. Risultati batteriologici ed istologici nella prova intraganglionare secondo Ninni. *Rev. Ist. Sieroter Hol.*, **23**, 229–46.

American Thoracic Society (1971) Treatment of sarcoidosis. A statement by the Committee on Therapy. *Am. Rev. Respir. Dis.*, **103**, 433–4.

Amman, A.J. and Hong, R. (1971) Selective IgA deficiency: presentation of 30 cases and a review of the literature. *Medicine (Baltimore)*, **50**, 223–36.

Ammitzbøll, F. (1956) A case of Boeck's sarcoid with isolated localization in the musculature. *Acta Rheumatol., Scand.*, **2**, 3–10.

Ampikaipakan, K., Prathap, G. and Mitchell, D.N. (1983) Sarcoidosis in Malaysia. In *Proc. 9th International Conference on Sarcoidosis, Paris*, Pergamon Press, Oxford, pp. 626–8.

Andersen, K.E. (1977) Systemic sarcoidosis with necrobiosis-lipoidica-like scalp lesions. *Acta Derm.-Venereol.*, **57**, 367–9.

Anderson, J., Dent, C.E., Harper, C. and Philpot, G.R. (1954) Effect of cortisone on calcium metabolism in sarcoidosis with hypercalcaemia: possibly antagonistic actions of cortisone and vitamin D. *Lancet*, **2**, 720–4.

Anderson, R., Brett, G.Z., James, D.G., and Siltzbach, L.E. (1963a) The prevalence of intrathoracic sarcoidosis. *Med. Thorac.*, **20**, 152–62.

Anderson, R., James, D.G., Peters, P.M., and Thomson, A.D. (1963a) The Kveim test in sarcoidosis, *Lancet*, **2**, 650–3.

Anderson, W.B., Parker, J.J. and Sondheimer, F.K. (1966) Optic foramen enlargement caused by sarcoid granuloma. *Radiology*, **86**, 319–22.

Anderson, W.M. (1942) Bronchial adenoma with metastasis to the liver. *J. Thorac. Surg.*, **12**, 351–60.

Andrews, N.C., and Klassen, K.P. (1957) Eight years' experience with pulmonary biopsy. *J. Am. Med. Assoc.*, **164**, 1061–9.

Anning, S.T., Dawson, J., Dolby, D.E. and Ingram, J.T. (1948) The toxic effects of calciferol. *Q. J. Med.*, **17**, 203–28.

Appel, B. (1941) Sarcoid. *Arch. Dermatol. Syph., NY*, **43**, 172–3.

Appell, A.A., Pritzker, H.S. and Klotz, P.G. (1951) Pyloric obstruction due to sarcoid of the stomach. *Arch. Surg. (Chicago)*, 62, 140–4.

Appelmans, M. and Horenbeeck, A. van (1941) Sur l'origine de la fievre uveo-parotidienne. *Opthalmologica*, 102, 65–79.

Arbuse, D. and Madonick, M. (1938) Uveo-parotid fever (Heerfordt's syndrome); neurologic manifestations. *Am. J. Med. Sci.*, 196, 222–32.

Arkless, H.A., Gokcebay, T.M. and Mendell, T.H. (1958) Sarcoidosis of the heart. *Am. J. Cardiol.*, 1, 648–51.

Arnoux, A., Morcamp, C., Tonnel, A.B., Aerts, C., Marsac, J., Huchon, G., Saltiel, J.C., Martin, J.P., Voisin, C., Chretien, J. and Laval, A.M. (1980) Bronchopulmonary cellular and protein studies in sarcoidosis and hypersensitivity pneumonitis. In *Proc. 8th International Conference on Sarcoidosis, Cardiff, 1978* (eds W. Jones-Williams and B.H. Davies), Alpha Omega, Cardiff, pp. 409–16.

Aronson, S.M. and Perl, D.P. (1973) Clinical neuropathological conference. *Dis. Nerv. Syst.*, 34, 392–5.

Arova, Y.R. (1963) Sarcoidosis of the larynx *J. Laryngol. Otol.*, 77, 714–9.

Arzt, L. (1955) Foreign body granuloma and Boeck's sarcoid. *J. Invest. Dermatol.*, 24, 155–6.

Asdourian, G.K. and Goldberg, M.F. (1975) Peripheral retinal neovascularization in sarcoidosis. *Arch. Ophthalmol.* 93, 787–91.

Ashutosh, K. and Keighley, J.F.H. (1976) Diagnostic value of serum angiotension converting enzyme activity in lung diseases. *Thorax*, 31, 552–7.

Askenazy, C.L. (1952) Sarcoidosis of the central nervous system. *J. Neuropathol. Exp. Neurol.*, 11, 392–400.

Attwood, W.G., Miller, R.C. and Nelson, C.T. (1966) Sarcoidosis and the malignant lymphoreticular diseases. *Arch. Dermatol.*, 94, 144–51.

Avioli, L.V., Birge, S.J. and Lee, S.W. (1968) Effect of prednisone on vitamin D metabolism in man. *Endocrinology*, 28, 1341–6.

Avioli L.V. and Haddad, J.G. (1973) Vitamin D: current concepts. *Metab. Clin. Exp.*, 22, 507–31.

Ayres, W.W., Ober, W.B. and Hamilton, P.K. (1951) Post-traumatic subcutaneous granulomas associated with a crystalline material. *Am. J. Pathol.*, 27, 303–15.

Azar, H. (1968) Amyloidosis. *Pathobiol. Ann.*, 3, 104–22.

Azzopardi, J.G. and Menzies, T. (1960) Primary malignant lymphoma of the alimentary tract. *Br. J. Surg.*, 47, 358–66.

Babu, V.S., Eisen, H. and Pataki, K. (1979) Sarcoidosis of the central nervous system. *J. Computer Assisted Tomography*, 3, 396–7.

Bacharach, T., and Zalis, E.G. (1963) Sarcoid syndrome associated with coccidioidomycosis. *Am. Rev. Respir. Dis.*, 88, 248–51.

Bachmann, E. (1947) Über Morbus Boeck mit Übergang in gewöhnliche Tuberkulose. *Schweiz. Z. Tuberk. Pneumonol.*, 4, 210–17.

Baden, H.P. and Holcomb, F.D. (1968) Erythema nodosum from oral contraceptives. *Arch. Dermatol.*, 98, 634–5.

Bäfverstedt, B. (1968) Erythema nodosum migrans. *Acta Derm.-Venereol.*, 48, 381–4.

Bagley, C.M., Roth, J.A., Thomas, L.B. and Devita, V.T. (1972) Liver biopsy in Hodgkin's disease. *Ann. Intern. Med.*, 76, 219–25.

Bahr, A.L., Krumholz, A., Kristt, D. and Hodges, F.J. (1978) Neuroradiological manifestations of intracranial sarcoidosis. *Radiology*, 127, 713–7.

von Bahr, G. (1938) A case of uveo-parotitis with perivasculitis and other rare symptoms. *Acta Ophthalmol.*, **16**, 101–8.

Bailey, R.R. (1966) Systemic sarcoidosis with pericarditis and pericardial effusion. *NZ Med. J.*, **65**, 704–8.

Baldwin, D.M., Roberts, J.G. and Croft, H.E. (1974) Vertebral sarcoidosis. *J. Bone Jt Surg.*, **56**, 629–32.

Ball, K.P., Joules, H. and Pagel, W. (1951) Acute tuberculous septicaemia with leucopenia. *Br. Med. J.*, **2**, 869–73.

Bammer, H. (1958) Ein Fall von Sarcoid der Skelett-muskulatur unter dem bilde einer progressiven Muskeldystrophie. *Nervenarzt*, **29**, 422–5.

Banaszak, E.F., Thiede, W.H. and Fink, J.N. (1970) Hypersensitivity pneumonitis due to contamination of an air conditioner. *Engl. J. Med.*, **283**, 271–6.

Banerjee, T. and Hunt, W.E. (1972) Spinal cord sarcoidosis. *J. Neurosurg.*, **36**, 490–3.

Barber, H.W. (1927) Boeck's sarcoid (benign lymphogranuloma of Schaumann) treated by intramuscular injection of sodium morrhuate. *Br. J. Dermatol.*, **39**, 156–9.

Barber, H.W. (1945) Benign lymphogranuloma of Schaumann with apparent involvement of anterior pituitary. *Proc. R. Soc. Med.*, **39**, 92–3.

Barbolini, G., Bisetti, A., Saltini, C. and Zaneone, N.A. (1977) Histological and histochemical pattern of phytohemagglutinin (PHA) skin test in patients with sarcoidosis. *Z. Erkr. Atmungsorgane*, **149**, 259–64.

Barbolini, G. and Mastronardi, V. (1976) Sarcoïdose primitive du nerf optique avec test à la métopirone très positif documentation anatomo-clinique. *Poumon Coeur*, **23**, 453–65.

Barbour, G.L., Coburn, J.W., Slatopolsky, E., Norman, A.W. and Horst, R.L. (1981) Hypercalcemia in an anephric patient with sarcoidosis: evidence for extrarenal generation of 1,25-dihydroxyvitamin D. *Engl. J. Med.*, **305**, 440–3.

Barbu Z., Barbu, E. and Alexa, M. (1971) Later results of ACTH and corticosteroid treatment in sarcoidosis. In *Proc. 5th International Conference on Sarcoidosis*, University Kavlova, Prague, pp. 626–8.

Bar-Meir, S., Topilsky, M., Kessler, H., Pinkhas, J. and de Vries, A. (1977) Coincidence of sarcoidosis and amyloidosis. *Chest*, **71**, 542–4.

Barmwater, K. (1936) Über Boeck's Sarkoid auf den Schleimnäuten. *Hals-Nas. u. Ohrenarz*, **27**, 259–64.

Baro, C. and Butt, C.G. (1969) Hamazaki-Wesenberg bodies in sarcoidosis. *Lab. Med.*, *Bull. Pathol.*, p. 281. Cited by Doyle *et al.* (1973).

Barrett, G.M. and Rickards, A.G. (1953) Chronic brucellisis. *J. Med.*, **22**, 23–42.

Baruah, J.K., Glasaner, F.E., Sil, R. and Smith, B.H. (1978) Sarcoidosis of the cervical cord. *Neurosurgery*, **3**, 216–18.

Bass, N.M., Burroughs, A.K., Scheuer, P.J., James, D.G. and Sherlock, S. (1982) Chronic intrahepatic cholestasis due to sarcoidosis. *Gut*, **23**, 417–21.

Basset, F., Corrin, B., Spencer, H., Lacronique, J., Roth, C., Soler, P., Battesti, J.P., Georges, R. and Chrétian, J. (1978) Pulmonary histiocytosis 'X'. *Am. Rev. Respir. Dis.*, **118**, 811–20.

Basset, F., Soler, P., Jaurand, M.C. and Bignon, J. (1977) Ultrastructural examination of bronchoaveolar lavage for diagnosis of histiocytosis 'X'. *Thorax*, **32**, 303–6.

Bast, G., Bostelmann, W. and Schünemann, G. (1964) Klinischpathologische Studie zum Krankheitsbild des Morbus Boeck mit hypophysär-dien-zephaler Beteiligung. *Z. Tuberk.*, **121**, 294–309.

Bates, D.V., Varvis, C.J., Donevan, R.E. and Christie, R.V. (1960) Variations in the pulmonary capillary blood volume and membrane diffusion component in health and disease. *J. Clin. Invest.*, **39**, 1401–12.

Bates, G.S. and Walsh, J.M. (1948) Boeck's sarcoid: observations on seven patients, one autopsy. *Ann. Intern. Med.*, **29**, 306–17.

Batson, J.M. (1961) Calcification of the ear cartilage associated with hypercalcaemia of sarcoidosis. *N. Engl. J. Med.*, **265**, 876–7.

Battesti, J.P., Georges, R., Basset, Faud, Saumon, G. (1978) Chronic cor pulmonale in pulmonary sarcoidosis. *Thorax*, **33**, 76–84.

Battesti, J.P., Saumon, G., Valeyre, D., Amouroux. J., Pechnick, B., Sandron, D. and Georges, R. (1982) Pulmonary sarcoidosis with an alveolar radiographic pattern. *Thorax*, **37**, 448–52.

Bauer, H.J. and Löfgren, S. (1964). International study of pulmonary sarcoidosis in mass chest radiography. *Acta Med. Scand.*, Suppl. **425**, 102–5.

Bauer, H.J. and Wijkström, S. (1964) The prevalence of pulmonary sarcoidosis in Swedish mass radiographic surveys. *Acta Med. Scand.*, Suppl. **425**, 112–14.

Bauer, J.T. (1951) Granuloma (sarcoid) of the stomach; report of a case associated with carcinoma. *Bull. Ayer Clin. Lab. P. Hosp.*, **4**, 35–43.

Baughman, R.P., Roberts, R.D. and Ploy-Song-Sang, Y. (1980) Relationship between serum angiotensin-converting enzyme and sarcoid activity during steroid therapy. *Am. Rev. Respir. Dis.*, **121**, 110A.

Baum, G.L., Schwarz, J. and Barlow, P.B. (1973) Sarcoidosis and specific etiologic agents: a continuing enigma. *Chest*, **63**, 488–94.

Bazex, A., Dupré, A., Christol, B., Cantala, P. and Bazex, J. (1970) Sarcoidosis with atrophic lesions and ulcers. *Br. J. Dermatol.*, **83**, 255–62.

Bazex, A., Dupré, A., Lassère, J. and Bazex, J. (1972) Les formes cutanées ulcereuses de la maladie de Besnier–Boeck–Schaumann. *J. Med. Lyon.*, **53**, 1027–33.

Bear, R.A., Handelsman, s., Lang, A., Cattran, D., Wilson, D., Johnson, M., Lee, K.Y. and Cole, E.H. (1979) Clinical and pathological features of six cases of sarcoidosis presenting with renal failure. *Can. Med. Assoc. J.*, **121,**, 1367–71.

Beaumont, D., Herry, J.Y., Sapene, M., Bourguet, P., Larzul, J.J. and de Labarthe, B. (1982) Gallium-67 in the evaluation of sarcoidosis: correlation with serum angiotensin-converting enzyme and broncho-alveolar lavage. *Thorax*, **37**, 11–18.

Becker, W.F., and Coleman, W.D. (1961) Surgical significance of abdominal sarcoidosis. *Ann. Surg.*, **153**, 987–95.

Becker, W.F., Krull, P., Deicher, H. and Kalden, J.R. (1972) The direct migration inhibition test in sarcoidosis patients using a Kveim antigen preparation. *Praxis*, **26** (43–8 of Proceedings).

Van Beek, C. and Haex, A.J.Ch. (1943) Aspiration biopsy of the liver in mononucleosis infectiosa and in Besnier–Boeck–Schaumann's disease. *Acta Med. Scand.*, **113**, 125–34.

Van Beek, C. and Haex, A.J.Ch., and Smit, A. (1948) Specifieke afwijkingen in de lever bij likjders aan erythema nodosum. *Ned. Tijdschr. Geneeskd.*, **92**, 4171–81.

Van Beek, C., Haex, A.J.Ch. and Smit, A. (1949) De diagnostiek van acute haematgene tuberculose. *Ned. Tijdschr. Geneesk*, **93**, 3465–9.

Beekman, J.F., Zimmet, S.M., Chun, B.K., Miranda, A.A. and Katz, S. (1975) Spectrum of pleural involvement in sarcoidosis. *Arch. Intern. Med.*, **136**, 323–30.

Belcher, R.W., Palazij, R. and Wolinsky, E. (1975) Immunologic studies in patients with sarcoidosis and cryoptococcosis. *Arch. Dermatol.*, 111, 711–16.

Belcher, R.W. and Reid, J.C. (1975) Sarcoid granulomas in CBA/J mice, histological response after inoculation with sarcoid and non-sarcoid tissue homegenates. *Arch. Pathol.*, 99, 283–5.

Belitsos, N.J., Merz, W.G., Bowersox, D.W. and Hutchings, G.M. (1974) *Allescheria boydii* mycetoma complicating pulmonary sarcoid. *Johns Hopkins Med. J.*, 135, 259–67.

Bell, N.H. and Bartter, F.C. (1967) Studies of ^{47}Ca metabolism in sarcoidosis; evidence for increased sensitivity of bone to vitamin D. *Acta Endocrinol. (Copenhagen)*, 54, 173–80.

Bell, N.N., Gill, J.R., Bartter, F.C., Diller, E. and Smith, H. (1964) On the abnormal calcium absorption in sarcoidosis: evidence for increased sensitivity to vitamin D. *Am. J. Med.*, 36, 500–13.

Bell, N.H., Stern, P.H., Pantzer, E., Sinha, T.K. and Deluca, H.F. (1979) Evidence that increased circulating 1α, 25-dihydorxy-vitamin D is the probable cause for abnormal calcium metabolism in sarcoidosis. *J. Clin. Invest.*, 64, 218–25.

Benatar, S.R. (1978) Sarcoidosis in South Africa. *S. Afr. Med. J.*, 52, 602–6.

Benatar, S.R. (1980) A comparative study of sarcoidosis in white, black and coloured South Africans. In *Proc. 8th International Conference on Sarcoidosis , Cardiff, 1978* (eds W. Jones-Williams and B.H. Davies), Alpha Omega, Cardiff, pp. 508–12.

Benda, R., Orinstein, E. and Morelec, R. (1955) Aller et retour entre une maladie de Besnier–Boeck–Schaumann et une tuberculose pulmonaire. *J. Fr. Med. Chir. Thorac.*, 10, 49–53.

Bendixen, G., Søborg, M. (1969) A leucocyte migration technique for *in vitro* detection of cellular (delayed type) hypersensitivity in man. *Dan. Med. Bull.*, 16, 1–6.

Benedetto, R. Di and Lefrak, S. (1970) *Am. Rev. Respir. Dis.*, 102, 801–7.

Benedict, E.B., Castleman, B. (1941). Sarcoidosis with bronchial involvement. *N. Engl. J. Med.*, 224, 186–9.

Benedict, W.L. (1949) Sarcoidosis involving the orbit: report of two cases. *Arch. Ophthalmol., NY*, 42, 546–50.

Bennington, J.L., Porus, R., Ferguson, B., Hannon, G. (1968) Cytology of gastric sarcoid: report of a case. *Acta Cytol.*, 12, 30–6.

Berblinger, W. (1939) Zur Zenntnis der atypischen Tuberkulose. *Acta Davos.*, 5, 1–11.

Berg, S. and Bergstrand, H. (1937) Beitrag zur Klinik und Pathologie der benignen Lymphogranulomatose. *Beitr. Klin. Tuberk. SpezifischenTuberk.-Forsch..*, 90, 536–56.

Berger, H.W., Zaldivar, C., Chusid, E.L. (1968) Anonymous mycobacteria in the etiology of sarcoidosis. *Ann. Intern. Med.*, 68, 872–4.

Berger K.W. and Relman, A.S. (1955) Renal impairment due to sarcoid infiltration of the kidney: report of a case proved by renal biopsies before and after treatment with cortisone. *N. Engl. J. Med.*, 252, 44–9.

Berger, R.L., Boyd, T.F. and Strieder, J.W. (1963) Complications of scalene lymph-node biopsy. *J. Thorac. Cardiovasc. Surg.*, 45, 307–11.

Bergman, K.C., Kirschnick, A.M., Djuric, B. (1979) Demonstration of an antigenic component in Kveim antigen. *Allergol. Immunopath.*, 7, 249–52.

Bergmann, A. (1958) Zur Klinik und Pathologie der Boeckschen Lungenkrankheit. *Beitr. Klin. Tuberk. Spezifischen Tuberk.-Forsch.*, 92, 581.

Bergmann, K.C., Zaumsell, J. and Lachmann, B. (1973) Quantitative IgE – Bestimmung bei sarkoidose. *Z. Erkr. Atmungsorgane, 37*, 351–2.

Bering, P. (1910) Zur Kentnis des Boeckschen Sarkoids. *Dermatol. Z., 17*, 404–12.

Berk, R.N. and Brower, T.D. (1964) Vertebral sarcoidosis. *Radiology, 82*, 660.

Berkman, Y.M. and Javors, B.R. (1976) Anterior mediastinal lymphadenopathy in sarcoidosis. *Am. J. Roentgenol., 983–7.*

Bernard, L.A. and Owens, J.C. (1960) Isolated cryptococcosis associated with Boeck's sarcoidosis. *Arch. Intern. Med., 106*, 101–11.

Bernaudin, J.F., Soler, P., Basset, F. and Chretien, J. (1975) La cellule épithélioïde: données ultrastructurales au cours de diverses entités pathologiques humaines. *Pathol. et Biol., 23*, 494–8.

Bernstein, A. (1935) Tularaemia: report of three fatal cases with autopsies. *Arch. Interim. Med., 56*, 117–35.

Bernstein, E.T. and Spoor, H.J. (1952) Study of the diagnostic value of the BCG vaccination reaction. *J. Invest. Dermatol., 18*, 385.

Bernstein, D.S., Thorn, G.W. and Jackson, J. (1965) Hypercalceamia associated with sarcoidosis, hypernephroma and parathyroid adenoma. *J. Clin. Endocrinol., 25*, 1436–40.

Bernstein, J. and Rival, J. (1978) Sarcoidosis of the spinal cord as the presenting manifestation of the disease. *South. Med. J., 71*, 1571–3.

Bernstein, S.S. and Oppenheimer, B.S. (1942) Boeck's sarcoid: report of six cases with one necropsy. *J. Mt Sinai Hosp., NY, 9*, 329–43.

Berte, S.J. and Pfotenhauer, M.A. (1962) Massive pleural effusion in sarcoidosis. *Am. Rev. Respir. Dis., 86*, 261–4.

Bertino, J. and Myerson, R.M. (1960) The role of splenectomy in sarcoidosis. *Arch. Intern. Med., 106*, 213–17.

Besnier, E. (1889) Lupus pernio de la face. *Ann. Dermatol. Syphiligr., 10*, 333–6.

Bethlem, N.M., de Figueiredo, S. and Bethlem, E.P. (1983) The epidemiology of sarcoidosis in Brazil. In *Proc. 9th International Conference on Sarcoidosis, Paris*, Pergamon Press, Oxford, p. 628.

Beurey, J., Rousselot, R., Mougerolle, J.M. and Finale, R. (1959) Maladie de Schaumann à éléments ulcéronécrotiques: action de la vitamine C. *Bull. Soc. Fr. Dermatol. Syphiligr., 66*, 361.

Bianchi, F.A. and Keech, M.K. (1964) Sarcoidosis with arthritis. *Ann. Rheum. Dis., 23*, 463–79.

Biberfeld, P. and Hedfors, E. (1974) Atypical blood lymphocytes in sarcoidosis: morphology, cytochemistry and membrane properties. *Scand. J. Immunol. 23*, 615–25.

Billings, F.T. and Shapiro, J.L. (1954) The induction of sarcoid-like lesions by the injection of tuberculin. *Bull. Johns Hopkins Hosp., 94*, 139–47.

Biniaminov, M. and Ramot, B. (1975) *In vitro* restoration of thymus-derived lymphocyte function in Hodgkin's disease. *Lancet, 1*, 464.

Birchall, G. (1966) Sarcoidosis and thyroiditis. *Br. J. Clin. Pract., 20*, 586–7.

Birkhäuser, H. (1957) Funf weiterer Fälle von Morbus Boeck-artigen Läsionen nach BCG.-Impfung. *Schweiz Med. Wochenschr., 87*, 1434–9.

Biro, L., Hill, A.C. and Kuflik, E.G. (1968) Secondary syphilis with unusual clinical and laboratory findings. *J. Am. Med. Assoc., 206*, 889–91.

Bisetti, A. and Livi, E. (1977) Fréquence et caractères de la sarcoïdose pulmonaire familiale. *Z. Erkr. Atmungsorgane, 149*, 212–18.

Bistrong, H.W., Tenney, R.D. and Sheffer, A.L. Asymptomatic cavitary sarcoidosis. *J. Am. Med. Assoc., 1970, 213*, 1030–2.

Bitterman, P.B. and Crystal, R.B. (1981) Alveolar macrophages in idiopathic pulmonary fibrosis and sarcoidosis are spontaneously secreting a growth factor causing human lung fibroblasts to replicate. *Clin. Res.,* **49,** 443A.

Bjarnason, D.F., Forrester, D.M. and Swezey, R.L. (1973) Destructive arthritis of large joints: a rare manifestation of sarcoidosis. *J. Bone Joint Surg.,* **55,** 618–22.

Bjørnstad, R. (1950) Tuberculin sensitivity in Boeck's sarcoid. *Acta Tuberc. Scand.,* **24,** 15–29.

Bjørnstad, R.B. (1949) Intracutaneous tests with killed tubercle bacilli in patients with sarcoid. *Acta Derm.-Venereol.,* **28,** 174–85.

Bjørnstad, R.T. (1948) Progressive Boeck's sarcoid associated with protracted destructive tuberculosis. *Acta Tuberc. Pneumol. Scand.,* **22,** 142–53.

Black, T.I. (1966) Sarcoidosis of the nose. *J. Laryngol. Otol.,* **80,** 1065–8.

Blackburn, G., Hadfield, G. and Hunt, A.H. (1939) Regional ileitis. *St Bart's Hosp. Rep.,* **72,** 181–224.

Blackstone, M.O., Dhar, G.J., Mizuno, H. and Para, M.F. (1976) Gastric sarcoidosis presenting as antral scarring. *Gastroenterology,* **22,** 211–12.

Blaese, R.M., Weiden, J., Oppenheim, J. and Waldman, T.A. (1973) Phytohaemagglutinin as a skin test for the evaluation of cellular immune competence in man. *J. Labor. and Clin. Med.,* **81,** 538–48.

Blain, J.G., Riley, W. and Logothetis, J. (1965) Optic nerve manifestations of sarcoidosis. *Arch. Neurol.,* **13,** 307–9.

Blair, A.W. (1967) Indolent non-caseating mycobacterial tuberculosis. *Arch. Dis. Child.,* **42,** 294–7.

Blasi *et al.* (1974) On the incidence of sarcoidosis in Italy. In *Proc. 6th International Conference on Sarcoidosis, Tokyo.* (eds K. Iwai and Y. Hosoda), University of Tokyo Press, Tokyo, p. 317.

Blegvad, O. (1931) Boeck's Sarcoid der Conjunctiva. *Acta Opthalmol.,* **9,** 180–99.

Bleisch, V.R. and Robbins, S.L. (1952) Sarcoid-like granulomata of the pituitary gland. *Arch. Intern. Med.,* **89,** 877–92.

Bloch, B. (1907) Beitrag zur Kenntnis des Lupus pernio. *Monatsschr. Prakt. Derm.,* **45,** 177–84.

Bloch, S., Morison, I.J. and Seedat, Y.K. (1968) Unusual skeletal manifestations in case of sarcoidosis. *Clin. Radiol.,* **19,** 226–8.

Bloom, R., Sybert, A. and Mascatello, V.J. (1978) Granulomatous biliary tract obstruction due to sarcoidosis. *Am. Rev. Respir. Dis.,* **117,** 783–7.

Blum, E.B. and Mitchell, N. (1952) Massive gastro-intestinal hemorrhage in a case of Boeck's sarcoid. *Ann. Intern. Med.,* **36,** 185–95.

Bodian, M. and Lasky, M.A. (1950) Sarcoidosis of the orbit. *Am. J. Ophthalmol.,* **33,** 343–53.

Boeck, C. (1899) Multiple benign sarcoid of the skin. *J. Cutan. Dis.,* **17,** 543–50.

   (1905) Forgesetzte untersuchugen über des multiple benigne Sarkoid. *Arch. Dermatol. Syph., Wien,* **73,** 71, 301–32.

   (1916) Nochmals zur klinik und zur Stellung des 'benignen Miliarlupods'. *Arch Dermatol. Syph., Wien,* **121,** 707–41.

Boelen, L.J. (1941) De ziekte van Besnier–Boeck. *Ned. Tijdschr. Geneeskol.,* **85,** 4164–7.

Bohnen, R.F., Jubiz, W., Rallinson, M., Stevens, L.E. and Tyler, F.H. (1971) Sarcoidosis and autonomous parathyroid hyperplasia. *J. Am. Med., Assoc.,* **217,** 1385–7.

Boller, R. and Goedel, A. (1935) Zur Kenntnis der Klinik und pathologischen Anatomie der multiplen Blutdrüsensklerose. *Wien. Arch. Inn. Med.,* **27**, 41–74.

Bolton, W.K., Atuk, N.O., Rametta, C., Sturgill, B.C. and Spargo, B.H. (1976) Reversible renal failure from isolated granulomatous renal sarcoidosis. *Clin. Nephrol.,* **5**, 88–92.

Boman, A. (1952) Diabetes insipidus vid lymphogranulomatosis benigna. *Nord. Med.,* **47**, 675.

Bonakdarpour, A., Levy, W. and Aegerter, E.E. (1971) Osteosclerotic changes in sarcoidosis. *Am. J. Roentgenol.,* **113**, 646–9.

Bonnevie, P. and With, T.K. (1937) Ein Fall von Sarkoid Boeck (Lymphogranulo matosis benigna) zur Heilung gekommen unter Entwicklung einer aktiven multiplen Tuberkulose und unter Änderung der Tuberkulinreaktivität. *Arch. Dermatol. Syph., Wien,* **175**, 407–11.

Bordley, J.E. and Proctor, D.F. (1942) Destructive lesion in paranasal sinuses associated with Boeck's sarcoid. *Arch. Otolaryngol.,* **36**, 740–2.

Bornstein, J.S., Frank, M.I. and Radner, D.B. (1962) Conjunctival biopsy in the diagnosis of sarcoidosis. *N. Engl. J. Med.,* **267**, 60–4.

Borrie, P. (1952) BCG vaccination as a method of research. *Br. J. Dermatol.,* **64**, 357–60.

Borrie, P.F. (1957) Sarcoidosis with skin lesions simulating necrobiosis lipoidica. *Proc. R. Soc. Med.,* **50**, 391–2.

Bottcher, E. (1959) Disseminated sarcoidosis with a marked granulomatous arteritis. *Arch. Pathol.,* **68**, 419–23.

Böttger, D. (1971) The blood picture in pulmonary sarcoidosis – prognostic aspects. In *Proc. 5th International Conference on Sarcoidosis, Prague, 1969* (eds L. Levinsky and F. Macholda), Universita Karlova, Prague, p. 535.

Böttger, D. (1977) Prognostic significance of lymphopenia in pulmonary sarcoidosis. *Z. Erkr. Atmungsorgane,* **149**, 197–201.

Botti, R.E. and Young, F.E. (1959) Myocardial sarcoid, complete heart block and aortic stenosis. *Ann. Intern. Med.,* **51**, 811–20.

Bour, D.J.H., (1942) Over de ziekte van Besnier–Boeck. Diss. Amsterdam, cited by van Rijssel (1947).

Bourke, E. and Barniville, H. (1973) Granulomatous sarcoid nephritis. *Ir. J. Med. Sci.,* **142**, 127–34.

Boushy, S.F., Kurtzman, R.S., Martin, N.D. and Lewis, B.M. (1965) The course of pulmonary function in sarcoidosis. *Ann. Intern. Med.,* **62**, 939–55.

Bouza, E., Burgaleta, C. and Golde, D.W. (1978) Infections in hairy cell leukaemia. *Blood,* **51**, 851–9.

Bovornkitti, S. (1974) Sarcoidosis in Thailand. In *Proc. 6th International Conference on Sarcoidosis, Tokyo* (eds. K. Iwai and Y. Hosoda, University of Tokyo Press, Tokyo, pp. 311–14.

Bowman, B.U., Amos, W.T. and Geer, J.C. (1972) Failure to produce experimental sarcoidosis in guinea-pigs with *Mycobacterium tuberculosis* and mycobacteriophage DS6A. *Am. Rev. Respir. Dis.,* **105**, 85–94.

Bowman, B.U. and Daniel, T.M. (1971) Further evidence against the concept of decreased phage neutralizing ability of serum of patients with sarcoidosis. *Am. Rev. Respir. Dis.,* **104**, 908–14.

Bowry, S., Chan, C.H., Weiss, H., Katz, S. and Zimmerman, H.J. (1970) Hepatic involvement in pulmonary tuberculosis. *Am. Rev. Respir. Dis.,* **101**, 941–8.

Boyd, J.F. and Valentine, J.C. (1970) Unidentified yellow bodies in human lymphnodes. *J. Pathol.,* **102**, 59–60.

Bradstreet, C.M.P., Dighero, M.W. and Mitchell, D.N. (1980) The Kveim test: analysis of results of tests using K 19 materials. In *Proc. 8th International Conference of Sarcoidosis, Cardiff, 1978* (eds W. Jones-Williams and B.H. Davies), Alpha Omega, Cardiff, pp. 674–7.

Brandt, N.J. and Stürup, H. (1959) Kryptokokmeningitis behandelt med amphotericin B. *Ugeskr. Laeg.*, **121**, 1132–4.

Branson, J.H. and Park, J.H. (1954) Sarcoidosis: hepatic involvement. *Ann. Intern. Med.*, **40**, 111–45.

Brashear, R.E. and Carman, C.T. (1969) Sarcoidosis and malakoplakia. *Dis. Chest*, **56**, 360–3.

Brett, G.Z. (1964) Prevalence of intrathoracic sarcoidosis among ethnic groups in north London during 1958–1967. In *Proc. 5th International Conference on Sarcoidosis, Prague, 1969* (eds. L. Levinsky and F. Macholda), Universita Karlova, Prague, p. 238.

Brett, G.Z. (1965) Epidemiological trends in tuberculosis and sarcoidosis in a district of London between 1958 and 1963. *Tubercle*, **46**, 412–6.

Bretza, J. and Mayfield, J.D. (1978) *Mycobacterium intracellulare* presenting as a sarcoid-like illness. *South. Med. J.*, **71**, 872–4.

Brewerton, D.A. (1975) HLA 27 and acute anterior uveitis. *Ann. Rheum. Dis.*, **34**, Suppl. 1, 33–5.

Brewerton, D.A., Cockburn, C., James, D.C.O., James, D.G. and Neville, E. (1977) HLA antigens in sarcoidosis. *Clin. Exp. Immunol.*, **27**, 227–9.

Brincker, H. (1972) Sarcoid reactions and sarcoidosis in Hodgkin's disease and other malignant lymphomata. *Br. J. Cancer*, **26**, 120–8.

Brincker, H. and Wilbek, E. (1974) The incidence of malignant tumours in patients with respiratory sarcoidosis. *Br. J. Cancer*, **29**, 247–51.

Briner, J. and Gartmann, J. (1978) Glomerulonephritis bei Sarkoidose. *Schweiz. Med. Wochenschr.*, **108**, 401–6.

Bringel, C., Ripe, E., Björkhem, I. and Holmberg, I. (1980) Plasma concentration of 25-OH-D3 in patients with hypercalcaemia due to sarcoidosis: the effect of corticosteroids after vitamin D2 and D3. In *Proc. 8th International Conference on Sarcoidosis, Cardiff, 1978* (eds. W. Jones-Williams and B. H. Davies), Alpha Omega, Cardiff, pp. 220–4.

British Thoracic and Tuberculosis Association (1969) Geographical variations in the incidence of sarcoidosis in Great Britain: a comparative study of four areas. *Tubercle*, **50**, 211–32.

British Thoracic and Tuberculosis Association (1973) Familial associations in sarcoidosis. *Tubercle*, **54**, 87–97.

British Tuberculosis Association (1967) Chloroquine in the treatment of sarcoidosis. *Tubercle*, **47**, 252–72.

British Tuberculosis Association (1968) Aspergillosis in persistent lung cavities after tuberculosis. *Tubercle*, **49**, 1–11.

British Tuberculosis Association (1970) Aspergilloma and residual tuberculous cavities – a re-survey *Tubercle*, **51**, 227–45.

Brock, D.J. and Grieco, M.H. (1972) Cryptococcal prostatitis in a patient with sarcoidosis. *J. Urol.*, **107**, 1017–21.

Brodkin, R.H. (1969) Leg ulcers: a report of two cases caused by sarcoidosis. *Acta Derm.-Venereol.* **49**, 584–7.

Brody, P.A., Pripstein, S., Strange, G. and Kohout, N.D. (1976) Vertebral sarcoidosis. *Am. J. Roentgenol.*, **126**, 900–2.

Bronsky, D. and Dunn, Y.O.L. (1965) Sarcoidosis and hypogammaglobulinaemia. *Am. J. Med. Sci.,* **250,** 11–8.

Brooks, J., Strickland, M.C., Williams, J.P., Vulpe, M. and Fowler, H.L. (1979) Computed tomography changes in neurosarcoidosis clearing with steroid treatment. *J. Computer Assisted Tomography,* **3,** 398–9.

Brostoff, J. and Walker, J.G. (1971) Leucocyte migration inhibition with Kveim antigen in Crohn's disease. *Clin. Exp. Immunol.,* **9,** 707–11.

Brownstein, S. and Jannotta, F.S. (1974) Sarcoid granulomas of the optic nerve and retina. *Can. J. Ophthalmol.,* **9,** 372–8.

Bruins Slot, W.J. (1936) Ziekte van Besnier–Boeck en Febris uveo-parotidea (Heerfordt) *Ned. Tijdschr. Geneeskd.,* **80,** 2859–63.

Bruins Slot, W.J., Goedbloed, J. and Goshings, J. (1938) Die Besnier–Boeck–Schaumann–sche Krankheit und die uveo-parotitis (Heerfordt). *Acta Med. Scan.,* **94,** 74–97.

Brun, A. (1961) Chronic polymyositis on the basis of sarcoidosis. *Acta Psychiat. Neurol. Scand.,* **36,** 515–23.

Brun, J., Mouriquand, C., Combey, P. and Vauzelle, J.L. (1959) Thyroidite scléreuse d'origine sarcoïdosique avec myxoedême et fibrose pulmonaire diffuse. Lyon Méd., **201,** 177.

Brun, J., Perrin-Fayolle, M. and Biot, N. (1963) La pleurésie intarissable de la sarcoidose de Besnier–Boeck–Schaumann. *Pr. Méd.,* **71,** 607–9.

Brun, J., Revol, A. and Perrin-Fayolle, M. (1964) Un nouveau test de la sarcoidose ganglio-pulmonaire: le test à la Metopirone. *Poumon Coeur,* **20,** 1015–30.
(1965) Metyrapone ditartrate (Metopirone) test during ganglio-pulmonary sarcoidosis of Besnier–Boeck–Schaumann. *Dis. Chest* , **48,** 337–46.

Brun, J. and Viallier, J. (1948) Sarcoidose avec troubles pulmonaires pseudo-cystiques. *J. Fr. Med. Chir. Thorac.,* **2,** 273–6.

Brun, J. Viallier, J. and Augagneur, J. (1964) Sarcoidose et mycobactéries atypiques. *Rev. Tuberc. Pneumol.,* **28,** 178–82.

Brun, J., Viaillier, J. and Perrin, M. (1952) Maladie de Besnier–Boeck–Schaumann: formes infiltratives et emphysémateuses: leur traitement par la cortisone. *J. Fr. Med. Chir. Thorac.,* **6,** 278–83.

Bruschi, M. and Howe, J.S. (1950) Classification of the hematologic variations and abnormalities associated with Boeck's sarcoid: review of the literature. Report of a case of thrombocytopenic purpura associated with sarcoidosis with recovery following splenectomy. *Blood,* **5,** 478–89.

Buchem, F.S.P. Van (1946) On morbid conditions of the liver and diagnosis of Besnier–Boeck–Schaumann disease. *Acta Med. Scand.,* **124,** 168–84.

Buck, A.A. and McKusick, V.A. (1961) Epidemiologic investigations of sarcoidosis: III Serum proteins; syphilis; association with tuberculosis; familial aggregation. *Am. J. Hyg.,* **74,** 174–88.

Buck, A.A. and Sartwell, P.E. (1961) Epidemioligic investigations of sarcoidosis. II Skin sensitivity and environmental factors. *Am. J. Hyg.,* **74,** 152–73.

Buckle, R.M. (1960) Reticulosarcoma complicating sarcoidosis. *Tubercle,* **41,** 213–5.

Buckle, R.M. (1963) Sarcoid goitre. *Proc. R. Soc. Med.,* **56,** 611–2.

Buckley, C.E. and Dorsey, F.C. (1970) A comparison of serum immunoglobin concentrations in sarcoidosis and tuberculosis *Ann. Intern. Med.,* **72,** 37–42.

Buckley, C.E., Nagaya, H. and Sicker, H.O. (1966) Altered immunologic activity in sarcoidosis. *Ann. Intern. Med.,* **64,** 508–20.

Buckley, C.E. and Trayer, H.R. (1972) Serum IgD concentrations in sarcoidosis and tuberculosis. *Clin. Exp. Immunol.,* 10, 257–65.

Bulkley, B.H., Rouleau, J.R., Whitaker, J.Q., Strauss, H.W. and Pitt, B. (1977) The use of [201]thallium for myocardial perfusion imaging in sarcoid heart disease. *Chest,* 72, 27–32.

Bullock, J.B. and Ray, E.S. (1961) Histoplasmosis simulating sarcoidosis. *Virginia. Med. Mon.,* 88, 153.

Bunforte, R.J., Topolsky, M., Siltzbach, L.E. and Glade, P.R. (1972) Phytohaemo-glutinin skin test: a possible *in vitro* measure of cell-mediated immunity. *J. Pediatr.,* 81, 775–80.

Bunim, J.J., Kimberg, D.V., Thomas, L.B., Scott, J.V. and Klatskin, G. (1962) The syndrome of sarcoidosis, psoriasis and gout. Combined clinical staff conference at the National Institutes of Health. *Ann. Intern. Med.,* 57, 1018–40.

Bunn, D.T. and Johnston, R.N. (1972) A ten-year study of sarcoidosis. *Br. J. Dis. Chest.,* 66, 45–52.

Bureau, G. and Bureau, Y. (1933) Sarcoïdes disseminées du thorax: guérison par les sels d'or. *Bull. Soc. Fr. Dermatol. Syphiligr.,* 40, 84–6.

Burgoyne, J.S. and Wood, M.G. (1972) Psoriasiform sarcoidosis. *Arch. Dermatol.,* 106, 896–8.

Burman, M.S. and Mayer, L. (1936)Arthroscopic examination of knee joint: report of cases observed in course of arthroscopic examination, including instances of sarcoid and multiple polypoid fibromatosis. *Arch. Surg.,* 32, 846–74.

Burnell, C.H., Connors, E.R., Albright, F. and Howard, J.E. (1949) Hypercalcaemia without hypercalciuria or hypophosphataemia, calcinosis, and renal insuffici-ency: syndrome following prolonged intake of milk and alkali. *N. Engl. J. Med.,* 240, 787–94.

Burnet, F.M. (1959) *The Clonal Selection Theory of Acquired Immunity,* Cam-bridge University Press, Cambridge, pp. 160–3.

Burns, D.A. and Sarkany, I. (1976) Tuberculous ulceration of the penis. *Proc. R. Soc. Med.,* 69, 883–4.

Burr, J.M., Farrell, J.J. and Hills, A.G. (1960) Sarcoidosis and hyperparathyroidism with hypercalcaemia: special usefulness of the cortisone test. *N. Engl. J. Med.,* 261, 1271–5.

Burt, R.W. and Kuhl, D.E. (1971) Giant splenomegaly in sarcoidosis demonstrated by radionuclide scintiphotography. *J. Am. Med. Assoc.,* 215, 2111–9.

Buss, J. and Dörken, H. (1975) Epidemiology of intrathoracic sarcoidosis in the Federal Republic of Germany. *Pneumonology,* 153, 1–20.

Bybee, J.D., Bahar, D., Greenberg, S.D. and Jenkins, D.E. (1968) Bronchoscopy and bronchial mucosal biopsy in the diagnosis of sarcoidosis. *Am. Rev. Respir. Dis.,* 97, 232–9.

Byrne, B.B., Evans, A.S., Fouts, D.N. and Israel, H.L. (1973) A seroepidemological study of Epstein-Barr virus and other viral antigens in sarcoidosis. *Am. J. Epidemiol.,* 97, 355–63.

Byström, J. (1968) Localized sarcoidosis of the appendix simulating mb. Crohn. *Act Chir. Scand.,* 134, 163–5.

Cain, H. and Kraus, B. (1977) Entwicklungsstörungen den Leber und Leberkarzi-nom in Säuglings - und kindesalter. *Dscg Med. Wochenrschr,* 102, 505–9.

Cain, H. and Kraus, B. (1980) Mehrkernige Riesenzellen in Granulomen. *virchows Arch. (Patu, Anat.),* 385, 309–33.

Callen, J.P. (1979) Sarcoidosis appearing initially as polymyositis. *Arch. Dermatol.*, **115**, 1336–7.

Cameron, C. and Dawson, E.K. (1942) Sarcoidosis: review based on case of the disease, *Edinburgh Med. J.*, **49**, 737–56.

Camp, W.A. and Frierson, J.G. (1962) Sarcoidosis of the central nervous system. *Arch. Neurol.*, **7**, 432–41.

Campbell, E.J.M., Scadding, J.G. and Roberts, R.S. (1979) The concept of disease. *Br. Med. J.*, **2**, 757–62.

Campbell, I.W., Short, A.I.K. and Douglas, A.C. (1980) Hypothalamic manifestations of sarcoidosis, with particular reference to hypothalamic hypopituitarism. In *Proc. 8th International Conference on Sarcoidosis, Cardiff, 1978* (eds. W. Jones-Williams and B.H. Davies), Alpha Omega, Cardiff, pp. 579–86.

Campbell, M.J. and Clayton, Y.M. (1964) Broncho-pulmonary aspergillosis. *Am. Rev. Respir. Dis.*, **89**, 186–96.

Campbell, P.B. (1977). Defective monocyte leukotaxis in sarcoidosis. *Am. Rev. Respir. Dis.*, **116**, 251–9.

Cantin, A., Bégin, R., Rola-Pleszcynski, M. and Boileau, R. (1983) Heterogeneity of bronchoalveolar lavage cellularity in Stage III pulmonary sarcoidosis. *Chest*, **83**, 485–6.

Carasso, B. (1974) Sarcoidosis of the larynx causing airway obstruction. *Chest*, **65**, 693–5.

Carlens, E. (1959) Mediastinoscopy: a method for inspection and tissue biopsy in the superior mediastinum. *Dis. Chest.*, **36**, 343–52.

Carlens, E. (1964) Biopsies in connection with bronchoscopy and mediastinoscopy in sarcoidosis: a comparison. *Acta Med. Scand.*, Suppl. **425**, 237–8.

Carlens, E., Hanngren, Å. and Ivemark, B. (1974) The concomitance of feverish onset of sarcoidosis and necrosis formation in the lymph-nodes. In *Proc. 6th International Conference on Sarcoidosis, Tokyo* (eds. K. Iwai and Y. Hosoda), University of Tokyo Press, Tokyo, pp. 409–12.

Carli, G. (1955) Sarcoide di Boeck–Schaumann del solco balano prepuziale. *Minerva Dermatol*, **30**, 178–80.

Carnes, W.H. and Raffel, S. (1949) Comparison of sarcoidosis and tuberculosis with respect to complement fixation with antigens derived from the tubercle bacillus. *Bull. Johns Hopkins Hosp.*, **85**, 204–20.

Caro, J.F., Glennon, J.A. and Israel, H.L. (1980) Neuroendocrine studies in sarcoidosis. In *Proc. 8th International Conference on Sarcoidosis, Cardiff, 1978* (eds. W. Jones-Williams and B.H. Davies), Alpha Omega, Cardiff, pp. 587–94.

Carr, I. (1980) Sarcoid macrophage giant cells. Ultrastructure and lysozyme content. *Virchows Arch. B.*, **32**, 147–55.

Carr, D.T. and Gage, R.P. (1954) Prognosis of sarcoidosis. *Am. Rev. Tuberc.*, **69**, 78–83.

Carr, I., Carr, J., Lobo, A. and Malcolm, D. (1978) The secretion of lysosyme *in vivo* by macrophages into lymph and blood in a rat granuloma. *J. Reticuloendoth. Soc.*, **24**, 41–8.

Carr, I. and Norris, P. (1977) The fine structure of human macrophage granules in sarcoidosis. *J. Pathol.*, **122**, 29–33.

Carrington, C.B., Gaensler, E.A., Mikus, J.P., Schachter, A.W., Burke, G.W. and Goff, A.M. (1976) Structure and function in sarcoidosis. *Ann. NY Acad. Sci.*, **278**, 265–83.

Carrington, C.B., Gaensler, E.A., Coutu, R.E., Fitzgerald, M.X. and Gupta, R.G. (1978) Natural history and treated course of usual and desquamative inter stitial pneumonia. *N. Engl. J. Med.,* **298,** 801–9.

Carrington, C.B. and Liebow, A.A. (1966) Limited forms of angiitis and granulomatosis of Wegener's type. *Am. J. Med.,* **41,** 497–527.

Carstensen, B., Odelberg, A. and Wahlgren, F. (1956) Retroclavicular block dissection in the diagnosis of sarcoidosis of the lung. *Lancet,* **1,** 265–6.

Carter, C.J., Gross, M.A. and Johnson, F.B. (1969) The selective staining of curious bodies in lymph-nodes of patients as a means for diagnosis of sarcoid. *Stain Technol.,* **44,** 1–4.

Caspary, E.A. and Field, E.J. (1971) Lymphocyte sensitization in sarcoidosis. *Brit. Med. J.,* **2,** 143–5.

Castellanos, A. and Galan, E. (1946) Sarcoidosis: report of a case in child simulating Still's disease. *Am. J. Dis. Child.,* **71,** 513–29.

Castells, H.R., Rey, J.C., Dimier, H.G. and Valli, E.F. (1970) Encuesta sobre sarcoidosis en la republica Argentina. *Torax,* **19,** 236–7.

Castoldi, P. and Giudici, E. (1955) Granuloma di Besnier–Boeck–Schaumann con localizzazioni alle salpingi. *Minerva Ginecol.,* **7,** 627–30.

Cater, J.C. and Redmond, W.B. (1963) Mycobacterial phages isolated from stool specimens of patients with pulmonary disease. *Am. Rev. Respir. Dis.,* **87,** 726–9.

Cattell, R.B. and Wilson, R.D. (1951) Sarcoidosis of the spleen: report of two cases. *Lahey Clin. Found. Bull.,* **7,** 66–71.

Cavara, V. (1928) Sopra un caso di febris uveo-parotidea di Heerfordt. *Boll. Oculist.,* **7,** 925 (abstr. in *Klin Monatsbl. Augenheilkd.* **82,** 416.)

Cavioto, H. and Feigin, I. (1959) Non-infectious granulomatous angiitis with a predilection for the nervous system. *Neurology,* **9,** 599–609.

Celikoglu, S. and Siltzbach, L.E. (1969) A study of sarcoidosis and leprosy in Turkey employing the Kveim reaction. *Dis. Chest.,* **55,** 400–4.

Celikoglu, S., Vieira, L.O.D.B. and Siltzbach, L.E. (1971) Serum immunoglobin levels in sarcoidosis. In *5th International Conference on Sarcoidosis* (eds. L. Levinsky and F. Macholda), University Karlova, Prague, pp. 168–70.

Chalvardjian, A. (1978) Sarcoidosis of the female genital tract. *Am. J. Obstet, Gynecol.,* **132,** 78–80.

Chamberlain, M.A. (1962) A case of sarcoidosis of the nervous system. *Guy's Hosp. Rep.,* **111,** 25–32.

Chamberlin, G.W., Jennings, W.P. and Lieben, J. (1957) Chronic pulmonary disease associated with beryllium dust. *Penn. Med. J.,* **60,** 497–503.

Chang, T.W., Kung, P.C., Gingras, P.C. Goldstein, G. (1981) Does OKT$_3$ monoclonal antibody react with an antigen-recognition structure on human T cells? *Proc. Nat. Acad. Sci. USA,* **78,** 1805–8.

Chanial, G. (1937) *Etiologie du Syndrome de Besnier–Boeck,* Thèse de Médecine, Lyon (quoted by Brun and others, 1964).

Chapman, J. (1961) Report of International Conference on Sarcoidosis, Washington, 1960. *Am. Rev. Respir. Dir.,* **84,** 169–70.

Chapman, J.S. (1960) *The Anonymous Mycobacteria in Human Disease,* Thomas, Springfield.

Chapman, J.S. and Speight, M. (1967) Sequential studies of mycobacterial antibodies in sarcoidosis serum. In *4th International Conference on Sarcoidosis* (eds. J. Turiaf and J. Chabot), Masson, Paris, p. 265.

Chase, M.W. (1961) The preparation and standardization of Kveim testing antigen. *Am. Rev. Respir. Dis.*, **84**, 86–8.

Chase, M.W. and Siltzbach, L.E. (1961) Further studies on the fractionation of materials used in the intracutaneous diagnosis test for sarcoidosis. *Excerpta Med., Int. Congr. Ser.*, **42**, 58.

Chase, M.W. and Siltzbach, L.E. (1967) Concentration of the active principle responsible for the Kveim reaction. In *Proc. 4th International Conference on Sarcoidosis, Paris* (eds. J. Turiaf and J. Chabot), Masson, Paris, pp. 151–3.

Cheitlin, M.D., Sullivan, B.H., Meyers, J.E., Jr and Hench, R.F. (1960) Portal hypertension in hepatic sarcoidosis. *Gastroenterology*, **38**, 60–9.

Chesner, C. (1950) Chronic pulmonary granulomatosis in residents of a community near a beryllium plant: three autopsied cases. *Ann. Intern. Med.*, **32**, 1028–48.

Chevrant-Breton, J., Revillon, L., Pony, J.C. and Huguenin, A. (1977) Sarcoidose à manifestations cutanées extensives ulcéreuses et atrophiantes. *Ann. Dermatol. Venereol., Paris*, **104**, 805–10.

Chrisholm, J.C. and Lang, G.R. (1966) Solitary circumscribed pulmonary nodule: an unusual manifestation of sarcoidosis. *Arch. Intern. Med.*, **118**, 376–8.

Chumbley, L.C. and Kearns, T.P. (1972) Retinopathy of sarcoidosis. *Am. J. Ophthalmol.* **73**, 123–31.

Chun, S.K., Andy, J.J., Jilly, P. and Currey, C.L. (1975) Ventricular aneurysm in sarcoidosis. *Chest*, **68**, 392–3.

Churg, A., Carrington, C.B. and Gupta, R. (1979) Necrotizing sarcoid granulomatosis. *Chest*, **76**, 406–13.

Churg, J. and Strauss, L. (1951) Allergic granulomatosis, allergic angiitis and periarteritis nodosa. *Am. J. Pathol.*, **27**, 277–94.

Chusid, E.L., Shah, R. and Siltzbach, L.E. (1971). Tuberculin tests during the course of sarcoidosis in 350 patients. *Am. Rev. Respir. Dis.*, **104**, 13–21.

Chusid, E. and Siltzbach, L.E. (1974) Sarcoidosis of the pleura. *Ann. Intern. Med.*, **81**, 190–4.

Chusid, E.L. (1980) Clubbing of the fingers in sarcoidosis. In *Proc. 8th International Conference on Sarcoidosis, Cardiff, 1978* (eds. W. Jones-Williams and B.H. Davies), Alpha Omega, Cardiff, pp. 543–6.

Citron, K.M. (1954) Sarcoidosis, hypercalcaemia, calcinosis and renal impairment. *Proc. R. Soc. Med.*, **47**, 507–9.

Citron, K.M. (1955) Renal impairment in sarcoidosis, with special reference to nephrocalcinosis. *Postgrad. Med. J.*, **31**, 516–24.

Citron, K.M. (1957) Skin tests in sarcoidosis *Tubercle*, **38**, 33–41.

Citron, K.M. and Scadding, J.G. (1957a) Stenosing non-caseating tuberculosis (sarcoidosis) of the bronchi. *Thorax*, **12**, 10–7.

Citron, K.M. and Scadding, J.G. (1957b) The effect of cortisone upon the reaction of the skin to tuberculin in tuberculosis and sarcoidosis. *Q. J. Med.*, **26**, 277–289.

Citron, K.M. (1958) Tissue culture studies of tuberculin sensitivity in man. *Tubercle, Lond.*, **39**, 65–75.

Clague, R.B. (1972) Sarcoidosis or Crohn's disease? *Br. Med. J.*, **3**, 804.

Claman, H.N. (1972) Corticosteroids and lymphoid cells. *N. Engl. J. Med.*, **287**, 388–97.

Clark, E.J. and Blount, A.W. (1966) A fatal case of myocardial sarcoidosis. *Lancet*, **86**, 568–70.

Clausen, J.E. (1973) Migration inhibitory effect of cell-free supernatants from tuberculin-stimulated cultures of human mononuclear leucocytes demonstrated by two-step MIF agarose assay. *J. Immol.*, **110**, 546–51.

Clayton, R., Breathnach, A., Martin, B. and Feiwel, M. (1977) Hypopigmented sarcoidosis in the Negro. *Br. J. Dermatol.,* **96,** 119–25.

Clayton, R. and Wood, P. (1974) Subcutaneous nodular sarcoid. *Dermatologica.* **149,** 51–4.

Clinicopathological Conference (1950) Sarcoidosis with lung cavitation. *Postgrad. Med. J.,* **26,** 494–503.

Clinicopathological Conference, US Naval Hospital, Portsmouth, Va (1957) *US Armed Forces Med. J.,* **8,** 855.

Clinicopathological Conference (1969) A case of sarcoidosis with cryptococcal meningitis. *Brit. Med. J.,* **4,** 729–32.

Clinicopathological Conference, Case 39–1978 (1978) *N. Engl. J. Med.,* **299,** 765–9.

Clot, J., Andary, J., Bousquet, J., Godart, P. and Michel, F.B. (1979) Sous populations lymphocytaires des liquides de lavage broncho-alvéolaire. *Bull. Eur. Physiopathol. Resp.,* **36,** 27–8.

Coburn, A.F. and Moore, L.V. (1936) Experimental induction of erythema nodosum. *J. Clin. Invest.,* **15,** 509–11.

Coburn, J.W., Hobbs, C., Johnston, G.S., Richert, J.H., Shinaberger, J.H. and Rosen, S. (1967) Granulomatous sarcoid nephritis. *Am. J. Med.,* **42,** 273–83.

Cochrane, C.G. and Hawkins, O.J. (1968) Studies on circulating immune complexes. *J. Exp. Med.,* **127,** 137–54.

Coers, C., Durant, J., Malmendier, G. and Witwer, M. (1956) Un cas de sarcoïdose avec insuffisance renal et envahissement musculaire généralise. *Acta Clin. Belg.,* **11,** 348–64.

Cogan, D.G., Albright, F. and Bartter, F.C. (1948) Hypercalcaemia and band keratopathy. *Arch. Ophthalmol.,* **40,** 624–38.

Cohen, J.D. and Clarke, S.W. (1974) Sarcoidosis and thyrotoxicosis. *Proc. R. Soc. Med.,* **67,** 220–1.

Cohn, Z.A. and Benson, B. (1965) The differentiation of mononuclear phagocytes. Morphology, cyto-chemistry and biochemistry. *J. Exp. Med.,* **121,** 153–70.

Cohn, Z.A., Fedorko, M.E., Hirsch, J.G., Morse, S.I. and Siltzbach, L.E. (1967) The distribution of Kveim activity in subcellular fractions from sarcoid lymphnodes. In *Proc. 9th International Conference on Sarcoidosis, Paris* (eds. J.A. Chetien, J. Marsac and J.C. Saltiel), Pergamon Press, Oxford, pp. 141–9.

Cole, P.J., Citron, K.M., Plowman, P.N., Evans, T.G.J.R. and Vick, R.M. (1979) The treatment of sarcoidosis by levamisole. *Br. J. Dis. Chest,* **73,** 367–72.

Coleman, C.C. and Meredith, J.M. (1940) Diffuse tuberculosis of pituitary gland simulating tumor with post-operative recovery. *Arch. Neurol. Psychiatry,* **44,** 1076–85.

Coleman, S.L., Brull, S. and Green, W.R. (1972) Sarcoid of the lacrimal sac and surrounding area. *Arch. Opthalmol.,* **88,** 645–6.

Collins, D. (1955) A study of 50 000 specimens of human veriform appendix. *Surg. Gynecol. Obstet.,* **101,** 437–45.

Collis, W.R.F. (1932) A new conception of the aetiology of erythema nodosum. *Q. J. Med.,* **1,** 141–56.

Collyns, J.A.H. (1959) Isolated granulomatous myocarditis. *Am. Heart J.,* **58,** 630–6.

Colover, J. (1948) Sarcoidosis with involvement of the nervous system. *Brain,* **71,** 451–75.

Colp, C. (1977) Sarcoidosis: course and treatment. *Med. Clin. North Am.,* **61,** 1267–78.

Comfort, M.W., Weber, H.M., Baggenstoss, A.H. and Kiely, W.F. (1950) Non specific granulomatous inflammation of the stomach and duodenum: its relation to regional ileitis. *Am. J. Med. Sci.,* **220**, 616–32.

Coni, N.K. (1968) Sarcoidosis in the British Army. A ten year survey. *Br. J. Dis. Chest,* **62**, 100–6.

Connor, T.B., Thomas, W.C. Jr and Howard, J.E. (1956) The etiology of hypercalcaemia associated with lung carcinoma. *J. Clin. Invest.,* **35**, 697–8.

Cooch, J.W. (1961) Sarcoidosis in the United States Army, 1952 through 1956. *Am. Rev. Respir. Dis.,* **84** (5 pt. 2) 103–8.

Cook, D.M., Dines, D.E. and Dycus, D.S. (1970) Sarcoidosis presenting as dysphagia. *Chest,* **57**, 84–6.

Cook, G.C. and Carter, R.A. (1966) Sarcoidosis in the West African: a report of three cases. *Br. J. Dis. Chest,* **60**, 23–7.

Cook, J.R., Brubaker, R.F., Savell, J. and Sheagren, J. (1972) Lacrimal sarcoidosis treated with corticosteroids. *Arch. Ophthalmol.,* **88**, 513–17.

Cornelius, C.E., Stein, K.M., Hanshaw, W.J. and Sprott, D.A. (1973) Hypopigmentation and sarcoidosis. *Arch. Dermatol.,* **108**, 249–51.

Correa, P. (1954) Sarcoidosis associated with glomerulonephritis. *Arch. Pathol.,* **57**, 523–9.

Costello, M.J. (1961) Sarcoidosis with folliculopapular lesions. *Arch. Dermatol.,* **84**, 536–7.

Cottenot, F., Beer, F., Théodore, A. and Duterque, M. (1977) Sarcoïdose à lésions hypertrophiques et ulerées chez un Antillais. *Ann. Dermatol. Venéréol. (Paris),* **104**, 62–3.

Cotter, E.F. (1939) Boeck's sarcoid: autopsy in a case with visceral lesions. *Arch. Intern. Med.,* **64**, 286–95.

Coup, A.J. and Hopper, I.P. (1980) Granulomatous lesions in nasal biopsies. *Histopathology,* **4**, 293–308.

Cowdell, R.H. (1954) Sarcoidosis with special reference to diagnosis and prognosis. *Q. J. Med.,* **23**, 29–55.

Cowling, D.G., Quaglino, D., and Barrett P.K.M. (1964) Effect of Kveim antigen and old tuberculin on lymphocytes in culture from sarcoid patients. *Br. Med. J.,* **1**, 1481–2.

Cox, W.L. and Donald, J.M. (1964) Acquired haemolytic anaemia and Boeck's sarcoidosis. *Am. Surg.,* **30**, 199–202.

Crane, A.R. and Zetlin, A.M. (1945) Haemolytic anaemia, hypoglobulinema and Boeck's sarcoid. *Ann. Intern. Med.,* **23**, 882–9.

Creston, J.E. and Dibble, P.A. (1961) Nasal sarcoidosis. *Arch. Otolaryngol.,* **74**, 210–2.

Creveld, S. Van (1941) Disturbances of metabolism in Besnier–Boeck's disease. *Ann. Paediatr.,* **157**, 1–16.

Crick, R., Hoyle, C. and Mather, G. (1955) Conjunctival biopsy in sarcoidosis. *Br. Med. J.,* **2**, 1180–1.

Crick, R., Hoyle, C. and Smellie, H. (1961) The eyes in sarcoidosis. *Br. J. Ophthalmol.,* **45**, 461–81.

Critchley, M. and Philips, P. (1924) Uveo-parotitic paralysis. *Lancet,* **2**, 906–7.

Crispell, K.R., Parson, W., Hamlin, J. and Hollifield, G. (1956) Addison's disease associated with histoplasmosis. Report of four cases and review of the literature. *Am. J. Med.,* **20**, 23–9.

Crohn, B.B., Ginsburg, J. and Oppenheimer, G.D. (1932) Regional ileitis: a pathologic and clinical entity. *J. Am. Med. Assoc.,* **99**, 1323–9.

Crohn, G.C. and Yarnis, H. (1958) *Regional Ileitis,* 2nd Edn., Grune and Stratton, New York, p. 239.

Crompton, M.R. and MacDermott, V. (1961) Sarcoidosis associated with progressive muscular wasting and weakness. *Brain,* **84,** 62–74.

Crystal, R.G., Hunninghake, G.W., Gadek, J.E., Keogh, B.A., Rennard, S.I. and Bitterman, P.B. (1983) State of the art: the pathogenesis of sarcoidosis. In *Proc. 9th International Conference on Sarcoidosis, Paris,* Pergamon Press, Oxford, pp. 13–35.

Crystal, R.G., Roberts, W.C., Hunninghake, G.W., Gadek, J.E., Fulmer, J.D. and Line, B.R. (1981) Pulmonary sarcoidosis: a disease characterized and perpetuated by activated T-lymphocytes. *Ann. Intern. Med.,* **94,** 73–94.

Cudkowicz, L. (1956) Rhesus (D) factor in sarcoidosis. *Lancet,* **1,** 480.

Culligan, J.M. and Snoddy, W.T. (1945) Sarcoid of spleen. *Minn. Med.,* **28,** 568–9.

Cummings, M.M. (1964) An evaluation of the possible relationship of pine pollen to sarcoidosis (a critical summary). *Acta Med. Scand.,* Suppl. **425,** 48–50.

Cummings, M.M., Dunner, E., Schmidt, R.H., Jr and Barnwell J.B. (1956) Concepts of epidemiology of sarcoidosis: preliminary report of 1194 cases reviewed with special reference to geographic ecology. *Postgrad. Med.,* **19,** 437–46.

Cummings, M.M. and Hudgins, P.C. (1958) Chemical constituents of pine pollens and their possible relationship to sarcoidosis. *Am. J. Med. Sci.,* **236,** 311–17.

Cummins, S.D., Clark, D.H. and Gandy, T.H. (1951) Boeck's sarcoid of the thyroid gland. *Arch. Pathol.,* **51,** 68–71.

Cummiskey, J. and Dean, G. (1979) The frequency of sarcoidosis in Ireland. *J. Ir. Med. Assoc.,* **72,** 500–5.

Curran, J.F. Jr and Curran, J.F. Snr (1950) Boeck's sarcoid of the pancreas. *Surgery,* **28,** 574–8.

Curtis, A.C., Taylor, H. and Grekin, R.H. (1947) Sarcoidosis: results of treatment with varying amounts of calciferol and dihydrotachysterol. *J. Invest. Dermatol.,* **9,** 131–50.

Curtis, G.H. (1951) Cutaneous hypersensitivity to beryllium: study of 13 cases. *Arch. Dermatol. Syphilol., NY,* **64,** 470–82.

Curtis, G.H. (1959) The diagnosis of beryllium disease, with special reference to the patch test. *Arch. Ind. Health,* **19,** 150–3.

Curtis, G.T. (1964) Sarcoidosis of the nasal bones. *Br. J. Radiol.,* **37,** 68–70.

Cushard, W.G., Simon, A.B. Canterbury, J.M. and Reiss, E. (1972) Parathyroid function in sarcoidosis. *N. Engl. J. Med.,* **286,** 395–8.

Cushman, D.W., Cheung, H.S. (1971) Spectrophotometric assay and properties of angiotensin-converting enzyme of rabbit lung. *Biochem. Pharmacol.,* **20,** 1637–48.

Cutler, S.S., Sankaranarayanan, G. (1978) Vertebral sarcoidosis. *J. Am. Med. Assoc.,* **240,** 557–8.

Da Costa, J.L. (1973) Geographic epidemiology of sarcoidosis in SE Asia. *Am. Rev. Respir. Dis.,* **108,** 1269–72.

Dagradi, A.E., Sollod, N. and Friedlander, J.H. (1952) Sarcoidosis with marked hepatosplenomegaly and jaundice: case report. *Ann. Intern. Med.,* **36,** 1317–23.

Dall, J.L.C. and Keane, J.A. (1959) Disturbances of pigmentation with chloroquine. *Br. Med. J.,* **1,** 1387–9.

Dalmark, G. (1942) Lymphogranulomatose benigne: un cas avec des altérations mammaires comme seul symptome. *Acta Chir. Scand.*, 86, 168–78.

Danbolt, N. (1943) On Kveim's reaction in Boeck's sarcoid. *Acta Med. Scand.*, 114, 143–60.

Danbolt, N. (1947) Re-examination of Caesar Boeck's first patient with multiple benign sarcoid of the skin. *Schweiz. Med. Wochenschr.*, 77, 1149–50.

Danbolt, N. (1948) On the antigenic properties of tissue suspensions prepared from Boeck's sarcoid. *Acta Derm.-Venereol.*, 28, 151–7.

Danbolt, N. (1951a) On the skin test with sarcoid tissue suspension (Kveim's reaction). *Acta Derm.-Venereol.*, 31, 184–93.

Danbolt, N. (1951b) Progressive papule caused by injection of sarcoid tissue suspension (Kveim's test) in a patient with Boeck's sarcoid. *Acta Derm.-Venereol.*, 31, 446–8.

Danbolt, N. and Nilssen, R.W. (1945) Investigations on the course of Kveim's reaction and its clinical value. *Acta Derm.-Venereol.*, 25, 489–502.

Danel, C., Dewar, A., Corrin, B., Turner-Warwick, M. and Chrétien, J. (1983) Ultrastructural changes in bronchoalveolar lavage cells in sarcoidosis and comparison with the tissue granuloma. *Am. J. Pathol.*, 112, 7–17.

Daniel, T.M. and Schneider, G.W. (1962) Positive Kveim tests in patients without sarcoidosis. *Am. Rev. Respir. Dis.*, 86, 98–9.

Daniele, R.P., McMillan, L.J., Dauber, J.H. and Rossman, M.D. (1978) Immune complexes in sarcoidosis. *Chest*, 74, 261–4.

Daniele, R.P. and Rowlands D.T. (1976a) Lymphocyte subpopulations in sarcoidosis: correlation with disease activity and duration. *Ann. Intern. Med.*, 85, 593–600.

Daniele, R. P. and Rowlands, D.T. (1976b) Antibodies to T cells in sarcoidosis *Ann. NY Acad. Sci.*, 278, 88–100.

Daniels, A.C. (1949) a method of biopsy useful in diagnosing certain intrathoracic diseases. *Dis. Chest*, 16, 360–7.

Daniels, M., Ridehalgh, F. and Springett, V.H. (1948) *Tuberculosis in young Adults*, H.R. Lewis, London.

Daniels, W.B. and MacMurray, F.G. (1954) Cat scratch disease: report of 160 cases. *J. Am. Med. Assoc.*, 154, 1247–51.

Darier, J. and Roussy, G. (1906) Des sarcoïdes sous-cutanées. *Arch. Med. Exp.*, 18, 1–50.

Dattoli, J.A., Lieben, J. and Bisbing, J. (1964) Chronic beryllium disease: a follow-up study. *J. Occup. Med.*, 6, 189–94.

Dauber, J.H., Rossman, M.D. and Daniele, R.P. (1979) Bronchoalveolar cell population in acute sarcoidosis: observations on smoking and non-smoking patients. *J. Lab. Clin. Med.*, 94, 862–71.

Daum, J.J., Canter, H.G. and Katz, S. (1965) Central nervous system sarcoidosis with alveolar hypoventilation. *Am. J. Med.*, 38, 893–8.

Davidson, C.N., Dennis, J.M., McNinch, E.R., Wilson, J.K.V. and Brown, W.H. (1954) Nephrocalcinosis associated with sarcoidosis: a presentation and discussion of 7 cases. *Radiology*, 62, 203–14.

Davies, B.H., Williams, J.D., Smith, M.D., Jones-Williams, W. and Jones, K. (1982) Peripheral blood lymphocytes in sarcoidosis. *Path. Res. Pract.*, 175, 97–109.

Davies, D. (1963) Sarcoidosis treated with chloroquine. *Br. J. Dis. Chest*, 57, 30–6.

Davies, J., Nellen, M. and Goodwin, J.F. (1982) Reversible pulmonary hypertension in sarcoidosis. *Postgrad. Med. J.*, 58, 282–5.

Davies, M.J., Pomerance, A. and Teare, R.D. (1975) Idiopathic giant cell myocarditis. *Br. Heart J.*, 37, 192–5.

Davies, R.J. (1972) Dysphagia, abdominal pain and sarcoid granulomata. *Br. Med. J.*, 2, 564–5.

Davis, A.E., Belber, J.P. and Movitt, E.R. (1954) Association of haemolytic anaemia with sarcoidosis. *Blood*, 9, 379–83.

Davis, M.W. and Crotty, R.Q. (1952) Sarcoidosis associated with polyarthritis. *Ann. Intern. Med.*, 36, 1098–106.

Davis, S.D., Eidelman, S. and Loop, J.W. (1970) Nodular lymphoid hyperplasia of the small intestine and sarcoidosis. Arch. Intern. Med., 126, 668–72.

Dawson, J. (1954) Pulmonary tuberous sclerosis and its relationship to other forms of the disease. *Q. J. Med.*, 23, 113–45.

Day, A.L., Sypert, G.W. (1977) Spinal cord sarcoidosis. *Ann. Neurol.*, 1, 79–85.

Debray, C., Darnaud, C., Voisin, R., Martin, E. and Moreau, G. (1967) Les localisations sur le tube digestif de la maladie de Besnier–Boeck–Schaumann. *Arch. Fr. Mal. Appar. Dig.*, 56, 254–73.

Decker R.E., Mardayat, M., Marc, J., Rasool, A. (1979) Neurosarcoidosis with computerized tomographic visualization and transphenoidal exicision of a supra- and intrasellar granuloma. *J. Neurosurg.*, 50, 814–16.

Deenstra, H. and Van Ditmars, M.J. (1968) Sarcoidosis. *Dis. Chest*, 53, 57–61.

De Haas, E.B.H. (1952) Deux complications oculaires rares de la maladie de Besnier–Boeck chez un même sujet: kérato-conjonctivite sèche et calcification de la cornée. *Ophthalmologica, Basel*, 123, 65–7.

Delaney, P. (1977) Neurologic manifestations of sarcoidosis. *Ann. Intern. Med.*, 87, 336–45.

Delaney, P., Henkin, R.I., Manz, H., Satterley, R.A. and Bauer, H. (1977) Olfactory sarcoidosis. *Arch. Otolaryngol.*, 103, 717–24.

Delgado, T.E., Lee, S.H. and Kumar, V. (1981) Sarcoidosis of the foramen magnum. *Penn. Med.*, 84, 62–3.

De Lor, C.J. (1962) Sarcoidosis and collagen diseases of the gastro- intestinal tract. *Am. J. Gastroenterol.*, 38, 547–54.

De Nardi, J.M., Van Ordstrand, H.S. and Carmody, M.G. (1949) Chronic pulmonary granulomatosis: report of 10 cases. *Am. J. Med.*, 7, 345–55.

Deneberg, M. (1965) Sarcoidosis of the myocardium and aorta. *Am. J. Clin. Path.*, 43, 445–9.

Dent, C.E. (1956) Cortisone test for hyperparathyroidism. *Br. Med. J.*, 1, 230.

Dent, C.E. (1970) Calcium metabolism in sarcoidosis. *Postgrad. Med. J.*, 46, 471–3.

Dent, C.E., Flynn, F.V. and Nabarro, J.D.N. (1953) Hypercalcaemia and impairment of renal function in generalized sarcoidosis. *Br. Med. J.*, 2, 808–10.

Dent, C.E. and Watson, L. (1966) Hyperparathyroidism and sarcoidosis. *Br. Med. J.*, 1, 646–9.

Dent, C.E. and Watson, L. (1968) The hydrocortisone test in primary and tertiary hyperparathyroidism. *Lancet*, 2, 662–5.

Deodhar, S.D., Barna, B. and van Ordstrand, H.S. (1973) A study of the immunological aspects of chronic berylliosis. *Chest*, 63, 309–13.

De Remee, R.A. (1977) The present status of treatment of pulmonary sarcoidosis: a house divided. *Chest*, 71, 388–92.

De Remee, R.A. and Anderson, H.A. (1974) Sarcoidosis: a correlation of dyspnoea with roentgenographic stage and pulmonary function changes. *Mayo Clin. Proc.*, 49, 742–5.

De Remee, R.A. and Rohrbach, M.S. (1980) Serum angiotensin-converting enzyme activity in evaluating the clinical course of sarcoidosis. *Ann. Intern. Med.,* **92,** 361–5.

Deshayes, P., Desseauve, J., Hubert, J., Lemercier, J.P. and Geffroy, Y. (1965) Un cas de polyarthrite au cours d'une sarcoïdose. Un cas de spondylarthrite anhylosante au cours d'une sarcoïdose. *Rev. Rhum.,* **32,** 671–4.

De Tribolet, N. and Zander, E. (1978) Intracranial sarcoidosis presenting angiographically as a sub-dural haematoma. *Surg. Neurol.,* **9,** 169–71.

Devic, M., Masson, R. and Bonnefoy, J. (1955) A propos d'une observation de myosite à nodules de Besnier–Boeck. *Rev. Neurol.,* **92,** 563–7.

Devine, K.D. (1965) Sarcoidosis and sarcoidosis of the larynx. *Laryngoscope,* **75,** 533–69.

De Vuyst, P., de Troyer, A. and Yernault, J.C. (1979) Bloody pleural effusion in a patient with sarcoidosis. *Chest,* **76,** 607–9.

Dhakhwa, R.B., Harman, E. and Safirstein, B.H. (1976) Sarcoidosis presenting as multiple pulmonary nodules. *J. Am. Med. Assoc.,* **236,** 2529–30.

Di Benedetto, R. and Lefrak, S. (1970) Systemic sarcoidosis with severe involvement of the upper respiratory tract. *Am. Rev. Respir. Dis.,* **102,** 801–7.

Di Benedetto, R.J. and Ribaudo, C. (1966) Bronchopulmonary sarcoidosis. *Am. Rev. Respir. Dis.,* **94,** 952–5.

Dicken, C.H., Carrington, S.G. and Winkelmann, R.K. (1969) Generalized granuloma annulare. *Arch. Dermatol.,* **99,** 556–63.

Dickerman, J.D., Holbrook, P.R. and Zinkman, W.H. (1972) Etiology and therapy of thrombocytopenia associated with sarcoidosis. *J. Pediatr.,* **31,** 758–64.

Dickie, H.A. and Rankin, J.R. (1958) Farmer's lung: an acute granulomatous interstitial pneumonitis occurring in agricultural workers. *J. Am. Med. Ass.,* **167,** 1069–76.

Dickinson, E. (1971) Sarcoid meningoencephalitis. *Dis. Nerv. Syst.,* **32,** 118–24.

Dickinson, J.A. (1969) Sarcoidal reaction in tattoos. *Arch. Dermatol.,* **100,** 315–9.

Dickson, E.C. (1938) Primary coccidioidomycosis. *Am. Rev. Tuberc.,* **38,** 722–9.

Didion, H. (1943) Uber einen Fall von isolierter produktiver Riesenzellmyokarditis. *Virchows Arch.,* **310,** 85.

Dilling, N.V. (1956) Giant-cell myocarditits. *J. Path. Bacteriol.,* **71,** 295–300.

Dines, D.E., De Remee, R.A. and Green, P.A. (1971) Sarcoidosis associated with regional enteritis (Crohn's disease). *Minn. Med.,* **54,** 617–20.

Dines, D.E., Stubbs, S.E. and McDougall, J.C. (1978) Obstructive disease of the airways associated with Stage I sarcoidosis. *Mayo Clin. Proc.,* **53,** 788–91.

Dittrich, O. (1931) Uber den direkten tuberkelbazillen nachweis beim Lupus pernio und beim Sarcoid Boeck. *Dermatol. Z.,* **60,** 395–403.

Doniach, I. and Wright, E.A. (1951) Two cases of giant-cell granuloma of the pituitary gland. *J. Path. Bacteriol.* **63,** 69–79.

Donlan, C.P. (1938) X-ray therapy of Boeck's sarcoid. *Radiology,* **51,** 237–40.

Doub, H.P. and Menagh, F.R. (1929) Bone lesions in sarcoid: a roentgen and clinical study. *Am. J. Roentgenol.,* **21,** 149–55.

Douglas, A. (1974) Sarcoidosis of the central nervous system. In *Proc. 6th International Conference on Sarcoidosis, Tokyo* (eds. K. Iwai and Y. Hosoda), University of Tokyo Press, Tokyo, pp. 340–3.

Douglas, A.C. (1961) Sarcoidosis in Scotland. *Am. Rev. Respir. Dis.,* **84,** 143–7.

Douglas, A.C. and Moloney, A.F.J. (1973) Sarcoidosis of the central nervous system. *J. Neurol., Neurosurg., Psychiatry,* **36,** 1024–33.

Douglas, A.C., MacLeod, J.C. and Matthews, J.D. (1973) Symptomatic sarcoidosis of skeletal muscle. *J. Neurol. Psychiatry*, **36**, 1034–40.

Douglas, A.C., Wallace, A., Clark, J., Stephens, J.H., Smith, I.E. and Allan, N.C. (1976) The Edinburgh Spleen: source of a validated Kveim-Siltzbach test material. *Ann. NY Acad. Sci.*, **278**, 670–9.

Douglas, S.D., Daughaday, C.C., Schmidt, M.E. and Siltzbach, L.E. (1976) Kinetics of monocyte receptor activity for immuno-proteins in patients with sarcoidosis. *Ann. NY Acad, Sci.*, **278**, 190–200.

Douglas, S.D. and Siltzbach, L.E. (1974) Electron microscopy of Kveim biopsies in sarcoidosis. In *Proc. 6th International Conference on Sarcoidosis, Tokyo* (eds. K. Iwai and Y. Hosoda), University of Tokyo Press, Tokyo, pp. 54–6.

Dowie, L.N. (1964) A short review of sarcoidosis with a report of three cases with involvement of the nasal mucosa. *J. Laryngol. Otol.*, **78**, 931–6.

Doyle, W.F., Brahman, H.D. and Burgess, J.H. (1973) The nature of yellow- brown bodies in peritoneal lymph-nodes. *Arch. Pathol.*, **96**, 320–6.

Dressler, M. (1938) Uber einen Fall von Splenomegalie durch Sternal punktion als Boecksche Krankheit verifiziert. *Klin. Wochenschr.*, **17**, 1467–71.

Du Bois, R.M., Townsend, P.J., Cole, P.J., Haslam, P.J. and Turner- Warwick, M. (1981) Bronchoalveolar macrophages in sarcoidosis and cryptogenic fibrosing alveolitis. *Clin. Allergy*, **11**, 409–19.

Dumas, R., Bady, B. and Tommasi, M. (1971) Problémes posés par les formes amyotrophiques de la sarcoïdose (les localisations musculaires de la sarcoïdose). *Lyon Med.*, **225**, 975–81.

Dunlap, R W. and Hallenbeck, G.A. (1952) Portal hypertension associated with sarcoidosis and with haemochromatosis: report of 2 cases with splenectomy and splenorenal anastomosis. *Proc. Staff Meet. Mayo Clin.*, **27**, 266–72.

Dupont, A. (1947) Le traitement de la maladie de Besnier–Boeck par le bismuth. *Arch. Belg. Dermatol. Syphiligr.*, **3**, 73–9.

Duverne, J., Bonnayme, R. and Perrot, A.J. (1948) Maladie de Besnier–Boeck–Schaumann chez un syphilitique non modifiée par le bismuth, tres améliorée par la chrysothérapie. *Lyon Méd.*, **180**, 507–8.

Duvernoy, W.F.C. and Garcia, R. (1971) Sarcoidosis of the heart presenting with ventricular tachycardia and atrioventricular block. *Am. J. Cardiol.*, **28**, 348–52.

Dyer, N.H., Cook, P.L. and Kemp-Harper, R.A. (1969) Oesophageal stricture associated with Crohn's disease. *Gut*, **10**, 549–54.

Dyken, P.R. (1962) Sarcoidosis of skeletal muscle. *Neurology*, **12**, 643–51.

Eckstein, H.B. and Parker, R.A. (1958) Giant-cell granulomatous thickening of the gastric pylorus of probable sarcoid origin. *Br. J. Surg.*, **45**, 659–61.

Edwards, C.L. and Hayes, R.L. (1969) Tumour scanning with [67]gallium citrate. *J. Nucl. Med.*, **10**, 103–5.

Edwards, M.H., Wagner, J.A. and Krause, L.A.M. (1952) Sarcoidosis with thrombocytopenia. *Am. Intern. Med.*, **37**, 803–12.

Ehrlich, L. and Schwartz, S.O. (1951) Splenomegaly in thrombocytosis purpura. *Am. J. Med. Sci.*, **221**, 158–68.

Ehrner, L. (1946) A case of lymphogranulomatosis benigna (Schaumann) complicated by miliary tuberculosis in a BCG-vaccinated patient. *Acta Tuberc. Scand.*, **20**, 138–57.

Eiseman, B., Seelig, M.G. and Womack, N. (1947) Talcum powder granuloma. *Ann. Surg.*, **126**, 820–32.

Eisenberg, H., Terasaki, P.I., Sharma, D.P. and Mickey, M.R. (1978) HLA association studies in black sarcoidosis patients. *Tissue Antigens*, **11**, 484–6.

Elling, P. and Wanstrup, J. (1969) Immunohistochemical demonstration of immunoglobulin IgD in sarcoid lymph-nodes. *Acta Path. Microbiol. Scand.,* 77, 326–8.

Elliott, R.H.E. and Turner, J.C. (1951) Splenectomy for purpura haemorrhagica. *Surg. Gynecol. Obstet.,* 92, 539–44.

Ellis, F.W. (1955) Coexistent arrested disseminated coccidioidomycosis and Boeck's sarcoid. *Calif. Med.,* 82, 400–4.

Ellman, P. and Andrews, L.G. (1959) BCG sarcoidosis. *Br. Med. J.,* 1, 1433–5.

Ellman, P. and Hanson, A. (1958) The co-existence of bronchial carcinoma and sarcoidosis. *Br. J. Tuberc.,* 52, 218–21.

Emanuel, D.A., Lawton, B.R. and Wenzel, F.J. (1964) Histopathology and immunology of farmers' lung. *Am. Rev. Resp. Dis.,* 90, 287.

Emerson, P.A. and Young F.H. (1956) Sarcoidosis following tuberculosis. *Tubercle,* 37, 116–9.

Emirgil, C., Sobel, B.J. and Williams, M.H. (1969) Long-term study of pulmonary sarcoidosis: the effects of steroid therapy as evaluated by pulmonary function studies. *J. Chronic Dis.,* 22, 69–86.

Engberg, J. and Jepsen, O. (1963) Hearing impairment and dizziness in sarcoidosis. *Danish Med. Bull.,* 9, 28–32.

Engel, A. (1935) Fall ov hiluslymfom och erythema nodosum med negativ tuberkulin-reaktion. *Nord. Med. Tidskr.,*9, 679–82.

Engelbreth-Holm, J. (1938) A study of tuberculous splenomegaly and splenogenic controlling of cell emission from the bone marrow. *Am. J. Med. Sci.,* 195, 32–47.

Engelhard, J.L.B. (1946) Aufwiskingen in den uterus bij de ziekte van Besnier–Boeck–Schaumann. *Ned Tijdschr. Verlosk.,* 47, 41–5.

Engle, R.L. (1953) Sarcoid and sarcoid-like granulomas: a study of 27 post-mortem examinations. *Am. J. Pathol.,* 29, 53–69.

Enzer, N. (1946) Generalised Boeck's sarcoidosis with thrombocytopenic purpura. *Am. J. Pathol.,* 22, 663–4.

Epstein, W.L. and Maycock, R.L. (1957) Induction of allergic contact dermatitis in patients with sarcoidosis, *Proc. Soc. Exp. Biol. Med.,* 96, 786–7.

Erickson, T.C., Odom, G.L. and Stern, K. (1942) Boeck's disease (Sarcoid) of the central nervous system: report of case with complete clinical and pathological study. *Arch. Neurol. Psychiatry, Chicago,* 48, 613–21.

Etienne-Martin, P., Klepping, C., Guerrin, J., Barthes, H., Binet, J. and Dusserre, L. (1962) Syndrome nephrotique au cours d'une maladie de Besnier–Boeck–Schaumann à localisation pulmonaire, osseuse et hépatique. *J. Méd. Lyon,* 43, 193–8.

Eule, H. (1971) Findings by lung biopsy in patients with Löfgren's syndrome. In *Proc. 5th International Conference on Sarcoidosis, Prague, 1969* (eds. L. Levinsky and F. Macholda), Universita Karlova, Prague, pp. 469–72.

Eule, H., Roth, I. and Weide, W. (1980) Clinical and functional results of a controlled clinical trial of the value of prednisolone therapy in sarcoidosis, Stage I and II. In *Proc. 8th International Conference on Sarcoidosis, Cardiff, 1978* (eds. W. Jones-Williams and B.H. Davies), Alpha Omega, Cardiff, pp. 624–8.

Everts, W.H. (1947) Sarcoidosis with brain tumour. *Trans. Am. Neurol. Assoc.,* 72, 128–30.

Fagan, E.A., Moore-Gillon, J.C. and Turner-Warwick, M. (1983) Multiorgan granulomas and mitochondrial antibodies. *N. Engl. J. Med.,* 308, 572–5.

Faguet, G.B. (1978) Cellular immunity in sarcoidosis: evidence for an intrinsic defect of effector cell function. *Am. Rev. Respir. Dis.* **118**, 89–96.

Fahimi, H.D., Deren, J.J., Gottlieb, L.S. and Zamcheck, N. (1963) Isolated granulomatous gastritis: its relationship disseminated sarcoidosis and regional ileitis. *Gastroenterology,* **45**, 161–75.

Fairley, G.H. and Matthias, J.Q. (1960) Cortisone and skin sensitivity to tuberculin in reticuloses. *Br. Med. J.,* **2**, 433–6.

Faivre, G., Rauber, G., Lamy, P. and Larcan, A. (1956) Sarcoidose de Besnier–Boeck–Schaumann avec endocardite mitro-aortique; étude anatomoclinique. *Arch. Mal. Coeur Vaiss.,* **49**, 1147–53.

Falls, W.F., Randall, R.E., Sommers, S.C., Stacy, W.K., Larkin, E.G. and Still, W.J.S. (1972) Non-hypercalcaemic sarcoid nephropathy. *Arch. Intern. Med.,* **130**, 285–91.

Fanburg, B.L., Schoenberger, M.D., Bachus, B. and Snider, G.L. (1976) Elevated serum angiotensin I converting enzyme in sarcoidosis. *Am. Rev. Respir. Dis.,* **114**, 525–8.

Farber, H.W., Fairoan, R.P. and Glayser, F.L. (1982) Talc granulomatosis: laboratory findings similar to sarcoidosis. *Am. Rev. Respir. Dis.,* **125**, 258-61.

Farmer, J.L. and Winkelmann, R.K. (1960) Psoriasis in association with sarcoidosis. *Arch. Dermatol.,* **81**, 983–6.

Farzan, S. (1977) Sarcoidal reaction in tattoos. *NY State J. Med.,* **77**, 1477–9.

Faunce, H.F., Ramsey, G.C. and Sy., W., (1976) Protracted yet variable major pulmonary artery compression in sarcoidosis. *Radiology,* **119**, 313–4.

Favez, G. (1963) Association momentanée de sarcoïdose et de tuberculose respiratoire. *Med. Thorac.,* **20**, suppl. 60–2.

Favez, G. and Leuenberger, P. (1971) Circulating antibodies directed against Kveim antigen and a human normal spleen extract in sarcoidosis. *Am. Rev. Respir. Dis.,* **104**, 1599–601.

Fein, A., Gupta, R. and Goodman, P. (1980) Spontaneous pneumothorax as a presenting pulmonary manifestation of sarcoidosis. *Chest,* **77**, 455–6.

Felson, B. (1967) The roentgen diagnosis of disseminated pulmonary alveolar diseases. *Semin. Roentgenol.,* **2**, 3–21.

Ferguson, E.H. and Paris, J. (1958) Sarcoidosis: study of 29 cases, with review of splenic, hepatic, mucous membrane, retinal and joint manifestations. *Arch. Intern. Med.,* **101**, 1065–84.

Ferrans, V.J., Hibbs, R.G., Black, W.C., Walsh, J.J. and Burch, G.E. (1965) Myocardial degeneration in cardiac sarcoidosis: histochemical and electron microscopic studies. *Am. Heart J.,* **69**, 159 – 72.

Fiechtner, J., Reinecker, M. and Hansotia, P. (1978) Sarcoidosis in the nervous system (correspondence). *Ann. Intern. Med.,* **88**, 131.

Field, E.J., Caspary, E.A., Hall, R. and Clark, F. (1970) Circulating sensitized lymphocytes in Graves' disease. Observations on its pathogenesis. *Lancet,* **1**, 1144–7.

Fine, M., Flocks, M. (1953) Bilateral optic neuroretinitis with sarcoidosis treated with corticotrophin and cortisone. *Arch. Ophthalmol.,* **50**, 358–62.

Fine, R.D., Gaylor, J.B. and Adams, J.H. (1963) Sarcoid granuloma of brain. *Med. J. Aust.,* **1**, 856–60.

Firooznia, H., Young, R. and Lee, T. (1970) Sarcoidosis of the larynx. *Radiology,* **95**, 425–8.

Fischer, D., Lebeau, B. and Rochemaure, J. (1979) Association chronologique sarcoidose–tuberculose. *Sem. Hôp. Paris,* **55**, 1371–6.

Fischer, A.M. (1959) The clinical picture associated with infections due to Crypto-coccus neoformans (Torula histolytica). *Bull. Johns Hopkins Hosp.*, **86**, 383–414.

Fisher, A.M. and Davis, B.D. (1942) The serum proteins in sarcoid: electrophoretic studies. *Bull. Johns Hopkins Hosp.*, **71**, 364–74.

Fisher, O.E., Burton, G.G. and Bryan, W.F. (1971) Sarcoidosis involving the lacrim-al sac. *Am. Rev. Respir. Dis.*, **103**, 708–10.

Fishman, S.M. and Canalis, R.F. (1979) Nasopharyngeal sarcoidosis. *Ear, Nose and Throat.* **58**, 4–9.

Fitzgerald, M.X, Fitzgerald, O. and Towers, R.P.(1971) Granulomatous hepatitis of obscure aetiology. *Q. J. Med.*, **50**, 371–83.

Fitzpatrick, D.P. and Ewart, G.E. (1957) Central nervous system sarcoidosis success-fully treated with prednisone. *Arch. Intern. Med.* **100**, 139–42.

Flandin, C., Parat, M. and Paumeau-Delille, G. (1936) Sarcoîdes noueuses dissemi-nées avec diabète insipide associé. *Bull. Soc. Med. Hôp., Paris,* **52**, 1423–6.

Fleischner, F. (1924) Die Erkrankung der Knochen bei Lupus pernio und Boeck's Miliarlupoid. *Fortschr. Geb. Rontgenstr.*, **32**, 193–218.

Fleming, H.A. (1974) Sarcoid heart disease. *Br. Heart J.*, **36**, 54–68.

Fleming, H.A. (1980) Sarcoid heart disease. *Thorax,* **35**, 641–3.

Fletcher, G.H. (1966) Sarcoidosis in miners in the republic of Zambia. *Cent. Afr. J. Med.*, **12**, 29–30.

Florange, A. (1910) Uber einem Fall von Lupus pernio und seine Reaktion auf Rötgenbestrahlung. *Dermatol. Z.*, **17**, 558–64.

Fog, J. and Wilbek, E. (1974) Sarkoidosens epidemiologic i Danmark. *Ugeskr. Laeg.*, **136**, 2183–91.

Folger, H.P. (196) uveoparotitis (Heerfordt): report of a case *Arch. Ophthalmol. Chicago,* **15**, 1098–116.

Fong, Y. W. and Sharma, O.P. (1975) Pruritic maculo-papular skin lesions in sarcoidosis. *Arch. Dermatol.*, **111**, 362–4.

Fouts, D.W., Byrne, E. B. and Israel, H. L. (1970) Hepatitis-associated antigen and sarcoidosis (correspondence) *Lancet*, **2**, 1257.

Forbes, G. and Usher, A. (1962) Fatal myocardial sarcoidosis. *Br. Med. J.*, **2**, 771–3.

Fordtran, J.S. (1956) Immunological studies in sarcoidosis. *Bull. Tulane Univ. Med. Fac.*, **15**, 143–64.

Forgacs, P., McDonald, C.K. and Skelton, M.O. (1957) The B.C.G. lesion in sarcoidosis. *Lancet*, **1**, 188–90.

Forgan-Smith, R. and Newton, D. (1974) Sarcoidosis, tuberculous meningitis and visual disturbance. *Tubercle,* **55**, 309–12.

Fox, V.A., James, D.G., Scheuer, P.J., Sharma, O.P. and Sherlock, S. (1969) Im-paired delayed hypersensitivity in primary biliary cirrhosis. *Lancet,* **1**, 959–62.

Foxworthy, D.T. and Freeman, S. (1952) Biliary cirrhosis and cutaneous xanthoma-tosis due to sarcoidosis. *J. Lab. Clin. Med.*, **40**, 799.

Fraimow, W. and Myerson, R.M. (1957) Portal hypertension and bleeding oesophageal varices secondary to sarcoidosis of the liver. *Am. J. Med.*, **23**, 995–8.

Franceschetti, A. and Babel, J. (1949) La chorio-retinite en 'traches de bougie'; manifestations de la maladie de Besnier–Boeck. *Ophthalmologica*, **118**, 701–10.

Franceschetti, A. and De Morsier, G. (1941) La neuro-uvéo-parotidite (syndrome de Heerfordt). *Rev. Med. Suisse Romande*, **61**, 129–49.

Franco-Saenz, R., Ludwig, G.D. and Henderson, L.W. (1970) Sarcoidosis of the skull. *Ann. Intern. Med.* **72**, 929–31.

François, J., Lentini, F. and Kooner-Singh, K. (1977) Les manifestations ophthalmoscopiques de la sarcoîdose de Besnier–Boeck. *Ann. Ocul.*, **210**, 751–6.

Frank, B.B., Raffensperger, E.C (1965) Hepatic granulomata. *Arch. Intern. Med.*, **115**, 223–34.

Franz, G. and Wurm, K. (1962) Einfluss der Graviditat auf den verlauf der Lungensarkoidose. *Tuberkulosearzt*, 696–713.

Freiman, D.G. and Hardy, H.L. (1970) The relation of pulmonary pathology to clinical course and prognosis based on a study of 130 cases from the U.S. Beryllium Case Registry. *Hum. Pathol.*, **1**, 25–44.

Freimow, W. and Myerson, R.M. (1957) Portal hypertension and bleeding oesophageal varices secondary to sarcoidosis of the liver. *Am. J. Med.*, **23**, 995–8.

French, A.J. and Mason, J.T. (1951) Malakoplakia of urinary bladder and sarcoidosis. *J. Urol.*, **66**, 229–33.

Fresko, D. and Lazarus, S.S. (1982) Reactive systemic amyloidosis complicating long-standing sarcoidosis. *NY State J. Med.*, 232–4.

Freundlich, I.M., Lipshitz, H.I., Glassman, L.M. and Israel, H.L. (1970) Sarcoidosis. Typical and atypical thoracic manifestations and complications. *Clin. Radiol.*, **21**, 376–83.

Frey, U. (1948) Ubergang von Boeckscher Krankheit in Miliartuberkulose. *Helvet. Med. Acta*, **15**, 129–151.

Fried, K.H. and Genz, H. (1958) Sarkoidose (Morbus Besnier–Boeck– Schaumann) bei B.C.G.-geimpften. *Tuberk. Arzt.*, **12**, 558–69.

Friedland, J., Selton, C. and Silverstein, E. (1978) Induction of angiotensin converting enzyme in human monocytes in culture. *Biochem. Boipsys. Res. Commun.*, **83**, 843–9.

Friedman, M. (1944) Sarcoidosis of spleen: report of case with autopsy and study on intracellular 'asteroid bodies'. *Am. J. Path*, **20**, 621–35.

Friedman, O.H., Blaugrund, S.M. and Siltzbach, L.E. (1963) Biopsy of the bronchial wall as an aid in diagnosis of sarcoidosis. *J. Am. Med. Assoc.*, **183**, 646–50.

Friedman, S.M., Hunter, S.B., Irigoyen, Kung, P.C., Goldstein, G. and Chess, L. (1981) Functional analysis of human T-cell subsets defined by monoclonal antibodies. II Collaborative T–T interactions in the generation of TNP-altered self-reactive cytotoxic T-lymphocytes. *J. Immunol.*, **126**, 1702–5.

Friou, G.J. (1952) Delayed cutaneous hypersensitivity in sarcoidosis, *J. Clin. Invest.*, **31**, 630–5.

Fromantin, M., Gautier, D., Quercy, E. and Kamalodine, T. (1975) Hyperthyroidie, Sarcoîdose, syndrome aménorrhée-galactorrhae d'apparition simultanée chez une même malade. *Ann. Med. Interne*, **126**, 853–6.

Fujita, N., Torres A. and Sharma, O.P. (1974) Ectopic calcification in sarcoidosis (correspondence). *J. Am. Med. Assoc.*, **227**, 556.

Fuld, H. (1960) Sarcoidosis treated with chloroquine. *Lancet*, **2**, 1029–30.

Fuller, C.J. (1953) Farmer's lung: a review of present knowledge. *Thorax*, **8**, 59–64.

Fulton, A., Jampol, L. and Albert, D.M. (1976) Gastrointestinal sarcoidosis diagnosed by conjunctival biopsy. *Am. J. Ophthalmol.* **82**, 102–4.

Fung, W.P., Foo, K.T. and Lee, Y.S. (1975) Gastric sarcoidosis presenting with haematemesis. *Med. J. Aust.*, **2**, 47–9.

Funk, C.F. (1933)Boecksches Sarkoid – Lupus pernio – und Lungenbeteiligung. *Arch. Dermatol. Syph.*, Wien, **167**, 560–77.

Furtado, D. and Carvalho, O. (1947) Une nouvelle forme de tuberculose musculaire. *Monatsschr. Psychiatr. Neurol.*, **114**, 54–71.

Gaines, J.D., Eckman, P.B. and Remington, J.S. (1970) Low CSF glucose level in sarcoidosis involving the central nervous system. *Arch. Intern. Med.*, **125**, 336–6.

Gallily, K. and Ben-Ishay, Z. (1975) Immune cytolysis of mono-macrophages *in vitro. J. Reticuloendothelial Soc.*, **18**, 44–52.

Galvin, C. (1967) Intra-abdominal sarcoidosis. *J. Ir. Med. Assoc.*, **60**, 253–5.

Gandy, W.M. (1950) Primary cutaneous cryptococcosis. *Arch. Dermatol. Syphilol.*, **621**, 97–104.

Gange, R.W. (1979) Sarcoidosis in husband and wife. *Clin. Exp. Dermatol.*, **4**, 107–9.

Gange, R.W., Black, M.M. and Carrington, P. (1979) Defective neutrophil migration in granuloma annulare, necrobiosis lipoidica and sarcoidosis *Arch. Dermatol.* **115**, 32–5.

Gange, R.W., Smith, N.P. and Fox, E.D. (1978) Eruptive cutaneous sarcoidosis of unusual type. *Clin. Exp. Dermatol.*, **3**, 299–306.

Gange, R.W., Black, M.M., Carrington, P. and McKerron, R. (1977) Defective neutrophil migration in sarcoidosis. *Lancet*, **2**, 379–81.

Ganguin, H.G. (1956) Ein Beitrag zur Ätiologie und Pathogenese des Morbus Boeck. *Allerg. Asthma*, **2**, 88–94.

Garcia, E.L., Garrido, T.A., Lorenzo, E.M. and Guedes, J.R. (1959) Sarcoidosis con anemia hemolitica sintomática. *Rev. Clin. Esp.*, **72**, 183–6.

García Morán, J. (1948) Enfermedad de Besnier–Boeck–Schaumann con localisaction gastrica. *Rev. Clin. Esp.*, **28**, 187–90.

Garcin, R. and Lapresle, J. (1958) Sur un cas de sarcoïdose musculaire ayant simulé une polymyosite. *Rev. Neurol.*, **99**, 322–6.

Gardiner, I.T., Uff, J.S. (1978) Acute pleurisy in sarcoidosis. *Thorax*, **33**, 124–7.

Gardner, L.U. (1937) The similarity of the lesions produced by silica and by the tubercle bacillus. *Am. J. Pathol.*, **13**, 13–14.

Gardner-Thorpe, C. (1972) Muscle weakness due to sarcoid myopathy. *Neurology*, **22**, 917–28.

Garland, H.G. and Thompson, J.G. (1953) Uveo-parotid tuberculosis (Febris uveoparotidea of Heerfordt). *Q. J. Med.*, **26**, 157–50.

Gass, J.D.M. and Olson, C.L. (1973) Sarcoidosis with optic nerve and retinal involvement. *Trans. Am. Acad. Opthalmol. Otolaryngol.*, **77**, 739–50.

Gebsattel, E. Von (1920) Beitrag zum Verständnis atypischer Tuberkulose-formen. *Beitr. Klin. Tuberk.*, **43**, 1.

Gee, J.B.L., Bodel, P.T., Zorn, S.K., Hinman, L.M., Stevens, C.A. and Matthay, R.A. (1978) Sarcoidosis and mononuclear phagocytes. *Lung*, **155**, 243–53.

Gee, J.B.L. and Fisk, R.B. (1980) Bronchoalveolar lavage. *Thorax*, **35**, 1–8.

Geeraerts, W.J., McNear, K.W., Maxey, E.F. and Guerry, D. (1962 Retinopathy in sarcoidosis. *Acta Ophthalmol*, **40**, 429–514.

Geller, R.A., Kuremsky, D.A., Copeland, J.S. and Stept, R. (1977). Sarcoidosis and testicular neoplasm: an unusual association *J. Urol.* **118**, 487–8.

Gendel, B.R., Young, J.M. And Greimer, D.J. (1952) Sarcoidosis: a review of 24 additional cases. *Am. J. Med.*, **12**, 205–8.

Gentry, J., Nitowsky, H.M. and Michael, M., Jr. (1955) Studies on the epidemiology of sarcoidosis in the United States: the relationship to soil areas and to urban-rural residence. *J. Clin. Invest.*, **34**, 1839–56.

Gentzen, G. (1937) Ueber Riesenzellgranulome bei zwei Fällen von Endocardfibrose. *Beitr. Pathol. Anat. Allg. Pathol.* **98**, 375–98.

Géraud, J. Rascol, A. and Jorda, P. (1965) La sarcoidose cérébrale à propos d'une observation anatomo-clinique.*Rev. Neurol. (Paris)*, **112**, 85–98.

German, W.M. (1940). Lupoid-sarcoid reaction induced by foreign body. *Am. J. Clin. Pathol.*, 19, 245–50.

Gherardi, G.J. (1950) Localised lymph-node sarcoidosis associated with carcinoma of bile ducts. *Arch. Pathol.*, 49, 103–8.

Ghose, T., Landrigan, P. and Asif, A. (1974) Localisation of immunoglobulin and complement in pulmonary sarcoid granulomas. *Chest*, 66, 264–8.

Ghosh, P., Flemming, H.A., Gresham, G.A. and Stovin, P.G.I. (1972) Myocardial sarcoidosis. *Br. Heart J.*, 34, 796–73.

Gilchrist, T.C. and Stokes, R. (1903) The presence of peculiar calcified bodies in lupus-like tissue. *J. Cutan. Dis.*, 21, 463.

Gilg, I. (1955) Kliniske Undersøgelser over Boeck's Sarcoid. Copenhagen.

Gilg, I. and Brodthagen, H. (1967) Hydroxchloroquine in the treatment of sarcoidosis. In *Proc. 4th International Conference of Sarcoidosis, Paris* (eds. J. Turiaf and J. Chabot), Masson, Paris, pp. 764–6.

Gilliland, I.C., Johnston, R.N., Stradling, P. and Abdel-Wahab, E.M (1956) Serum proteins in pulmonary tuberculosis. *Br. Med. J.*, 1, 1460–4.

Gilroy, J. (1971) Kveim Test (correspondence). *Br. Med. J.*, 3, 369.

Ginns, L.C., Goldenheim, P.D., Burton, R.C., Colvin, R.B., Miller, L.G., Goldstein, G., Hurwitz, C. and Kazemi, H. (1982) T-cell subsets in peripheral blood and lung lavage in idiopathic pulmonary fibrosis and sarcoidosis: analysis by monoclonal antibodies and flow cytometry. *Clin. Immunol. Immunopathol.*, 25, 11–20.

Gjersøe, A. and Kjerulf-Jensen, K. (1950) Hypothalamic lesion caused by Boeck's sarcoid. *J. Clin. Endocrinol*, 10, 1602–8.

Gjessing, H.G.A. (1916) Über iridozyklitis als Teilerscheinung bei der Mikulischen Erkrankung. *Klin. Monatsbl. Augenheilkd.*, 56, 252–85.

Glass, S.J. and Davis, S. (1944) Granuloma of the pituitary associated with panhypopituitarism. *J. Clin. Endocrinol.*, 4, 489–92.

Glenner, C.G. and Page, D.L. (1976) Amyloid amyloidosis and amyloidogenesis. *Int. Rev. Exp. Pathol.*, 15, 1–92.

Goeckerman, W.H. (1928) Sarcoids and related lesions: report of 17 cases. *Arch. Dermatol. Syphilol., Chicago*, 18, 237–62.

Goldberg, M.S. and Newell, L.F.W. (1944) Sarcoidosis with retinal involvement. *Arch. Ophthalmol.*, 32, 93–6.

Goldfarb, B.L. and Cohen, S.S. (1970) Coexistent disseminated sarcoidosis and Hodgkin's disease. *J. Am. Med, Assoc.*, 211, 1525–8.

Goldman, S., Djurić, B. and Behrend, H. (1974) Further epidemiologic study of sarcoidosis in Yugoslavia. In *Proc. 6th International Conference on Sarcoidosis. Tokyo.* (eds K.Iwai and Y. Hosoda) University of Tokyo Press, Tokyo, pp. 315–6.

Goldschmidt., W.N. (1925) Uber circinär-verrucöse Umwandlung bei einem Sarkoid Boeck und eine ähnliche Form bei Lupus vulgaris. *Arch. Dermatol. Syph.*, 149, 331–8.

Goldsmith, R.S. and Ingbar, S.H. (1966) Inorganic phosphate treatment of hypercalcaemia of diverse etiologics. *N. Engl. J. Med.*, 274, 1–7.

Goldstein, R.A., Israel, H.L., Becker, K.L. and Moore, C.F. (1971) The infrequency of hypercalcaemia in sarcoidosis. *Am. J. Med.*, 51, 21–9.

Goldstein, R.A., Israel, H.L., Becker, K.L. and Royan, J.J. (1974a) Hypercalciurea and sarcoidosis. In *Proc. 6th International Conference on sarcoidosis, Tokyo* (eds. K. Iwai and Y. Hosoda), University of Tokyo Press, Tokyo, pp. 413–4.

Goldstein, R.A., Israel, H.L., Janicki, B.W. and Yokoyami, M. (1974b) Serum immunoglobulin D levels in sarcoidosis. In *Proc. 6th International Conference on Sarcoidosis, Tokyo* (eds. K. Iwai and Y. Hosoda) University of Tokyo Press, Tokyo, pp. 196–8.

Goldstein, R.A., Israel, H.L. and Rawnsley, H.M. (1969) Effect of race and stage of disease on the serum immunoglobulins in sarcoidosis. *J. Am. Med. Ass.,* 208, 1153–5.

Goldstein, R.A., Janicki, B.W., Mirro, J. and Foellmer, J.W. (1968) Cell- mediated immune response in sarcoidosis. *Am. Rev. Respir. Dis.* 1176, 55–62.

Golitz, L.E., Shapiro, L., Hurwitz, E. and Stritzler, R. (1973) Cicatrial alopecia of sarcoidosis. *Arch. Dermatol.,* 107, 758–60.

Golomb, H.M., Catovsky, D. and Golde, D.W. (1978) Hairy cell leukaemia: a clinical review based on 71 cases. *Ann. Intern. Med.,* 89, 677–83.

Goobar, J.E., Gilmer, W.S., Jr., Carroll, D.S. and Clark, G.M. (1961) Vertebral sarcoidosis. *J. Am. Med. Assoc.* 178, 1162–3.

Goodbody, R.A. and Taylor, A.J. (1957) Sarcoidosis and bronchial carcinoma. *Tubercle,* 38, 419–21.

Goodman, S.S. and Margulies, M.E. (1959) Boeck's sarcoid simulating a brain tumour. *Arch. Neurol. Psychiaty,* 81, 419–23

Goodwin, J.S., Bankhurst, A.D. and Messner, R.P. (1977) Suppression of human T-cell mitogenesis by prostaglandin: existence of a prostaglandin-producing suppressor cell. *J. Exp. Med.,* 146, 1719–34.

Goodwin, J.S., Dettoratius, R., Israel, H.E., Peake. G.T. and Messner, R.P. (1979) Suppressor cell function in sarcoidosis. *Ann. Intern. Med.,* 90, 169–73.

Gordon, H. (1961) Erythema nodosum: a review of 115 cases. *Br. J. Dermatol,* 73, 393–409.

Gordon, W.W., Cohn, A.M., Greenberg, S.D. and Komorn, R.M. (1976) Nasal sarcoidosis. *AMA Arch. Otolaryngol.,* 102, 11–4.

Gore, I. and McCarthy, A.M. (1944) Boeck's sarcoid: report of a case involving the stomach. *Surgery,* 16, 865–73.

Gormsen, H. (1948) The occurrence of epithelioid cell granulomas in human bone marrow. *Acta Med. Scand. Suppl.,* f20213, 154–64.

Gormsen, H. (1956) On the occurrence of epithelioid cell granulomas in the organs of BCG-vaccinated human beings. *Acta Path. Microbiol. Scand.,* Suppl. 111, 117–20.

Gorton, G. and Linell, A.G. (1957) Malignant tumours and sarcoid reactions in regional lymph-nodes. *Acta Radiol.,* 47, 381–92.

Gougerot, H. and Burnier, A. (1937) Sarcoïdes nodulaires disseminées: Guérison par la tuberculine. *Bull. Soc. Fr. Dermatol. Syphiligr.,* 44, 635–7.

Gould, H. and Kaufman, H.E. (1961) Sarcoid of the fundus. *Arch. ophthalmol.,* 65, 453–6.

Gould, S.R., Handley, A.J. and Barnardo, D.E. (1973) Rectal and gastric involvement in a case of sarcoidosis. *Gut,* 14, 971–3.

Gourevitch, A. and Cunningham, I.J. (1959) Sarcoidosis of the sigmoid colon. *Postgrad. Med. J.,* 35, 689–91.

Gozo, A.G., Cusnow, I., Cohen, H.C. and Okun, L. (1971) The heart in sarcoidosis. *Chest,* 60, 379–388.

Granström, K.O., Gripwall, E., Kristofferson, C.E. and Lindgren, A.G.H. (1946) A case of uveo-parotid fever (Heerfordt) with autopsy findings. *Acta Med. Scand.,* 126, 307–18.

Grant, I.W.B., Hillis, B.R. and Davidson, J. (1956) Diffuse interstitial fibrosis of the lungs (Hamman–Rich syndrome). *Am. Rev. Tuberc.,* 74, 485–510.

Grant, L.J. and Ginsburg, J. (1955) Eosinophilic granuloma (honeycomb lung) with diabetes insipidus. *Lancet,* **2**, 529–32.

Gravesen, P.B. (1942) *Lymphogranulomatosis benigna.* Odense.

Greenberg, G., Anderson, R., Sharpstone, P. and James, D.G. (1964) Enlargement of parotid gland due to sarcoidosis. *Br. Med. J.* **2**, 861–2.

Greenberg, S.D., Györkey, F., Weg, J.G., Jenkins, D.E. and Györkey, P. (1970) The ultrastructure of the pulmonary granuloma in sarcoidosis. *Am. Rev. Respir. Dis.,* **102**, 648–52.

Greenberg, S.R., Atwater, J. and Israel, H.L. (1965) Frequency of hemoglobino-pathies in sarcoidosis. *Ann. Intern. Med.,* **62**, 125–8.

Greenwood, R., Smellie, H., Barr, M. and Cunliffe, A.C. (1958) Circulating anti-bodies in sarcoidosis. *Bri. Med. J.,* **1**, 1388–91.

Greer, K.E., Harman, L.E. and Kayne, A.L. (1977) Unusual cutaneous manifesta-tions of sarcoidosis. *South. Med. J.,* **70**, 666–8.

Grier, R.S., Nash, P. and Freiman, D.G. (1948) Skin lesions in persons exposed to beryllium compounds. *J. Ind. Hyg.,* **30**, 228–37.

Griffiths, J.C. (1969) Skeletal sarcoidosis. *Br. J. Clin. Pract.,* **23**, 296–8.

Grigor, R.R. and Hughes, G.R.V. (1976) Chronic sarcoid arthritis. Br. Med. J., **2**, 1044.

Griggs, R.C., Markesbery, W.R. and Condemi, J.J. (1973) Cerebral mass due to sarcoidosis. *Neurology,* **23**, 981–9.

Grillo, V. (1938) Contributo alla malattia di Besnier–Boeck: Una fase sarcoidea della infezione tubercolare? *G. Ital. Dermatol. Sifiol.,* **79**, 547–69.

Grillo, V. (1939) Riproduzione delle lesioni istologiche della malattia di Besnier–Boeck–Schaumann in gangli linfatici di cavie inoculate in peritoneo acon spap-polato di tessuto 'sarcoideo'. *Arch. Ital. Med. Sper.,* **4**, 515–22.

Grimminger, A. (1955) Uber Bronchial veranderungen beim Morbus Boeck Bron-choskopisches Bild und Verlauf. *Tuberkulosearzt,* **9**, 539–45.

Gristwood, R.E. (1958) Nerve deafness associated with sarcoidosis. *J. Laryngol. Otol.,* **72**, 479–91.

Grönhagen-Riska, C., Fyhrquist, F., Hortling, L. and Koskimies, S. (1983) Familial occurrence of sarcoidosis and Crohn's disease. *Lancet,* **1**, 1287–8.

Grönhagen-Riska, C., Selroos, O., Wäger, G.and Fyhrquist, F. (1979) Angiotensin-converting enzyme. *Scand. J. Respir. Dis.,* **60**, 94–101.

Groslambert, R., Chateau, R., Martin, H. and Gras, F. (1971) 'Myopathie tardive' à nodules granulomateux présumée d'étiologic sarcoïdosique. *Lyon Méd.,* **225**, 983–7.

Gross, N.J. (1973) The paradoxical skin response in sarcoidosis: a hypothesis. *Am. Rev. Respir. Dis.,* **107**, 798–801.

Gross, N.J. and Holt, P.J. (1977) Cell-mediated immunity in sarcoidosis: effect of corticosteroids. *Br. J. Dis. Chest.* **71**, 25–35.

Groth-Petersen, E., Knudsen, J. and Wilbek, E. (1959) Epidemiological basis of tuberculosis eradication in an advanced country. *Bull. W. H. O.,* **21**, 5.

Gruber, E. (1956) Sarcoidosis of the lacrimal glands associated with Sjögren's syndrome. *Arch. ophthalmol.,* **55**, 42–7.

Gruenfeld, G.E. (1950) Granuloma of large size caused by implantation of talcum (talcum sarcoids). *Arch. Surg. (Chicago),* **59**, 917–24.

Grufferman, S., Cole, P., Smith, P.G. and Lukes, R.J. (1977) Hodgkin's disease in siblings. *N. Engl. J. Med.,* **296**, 248–50.

Guédon, J., Mattieu, F., Chomé, J., Chebat, J., Safar, M. and Kuss, R. (1967) Sarcoïdose rénale à forme pseudo-tumorale révélatrice de l'affection. *Presse Med.*, 75, 265–8.

Guibert, H.L. (1947) Maladie de Besnier–Boeck– Schauman à localisation gastro-ganglionnaire pure *Ann. Anat. Pathol. Anat. Normale Med.-Chir.*, 17, 295–300.

Gumpel, J.M., Johns, C.J. and Shulman, L.E. (1967) The joint disease of sarcoidosis. *Ann. Rheum. Dis.*, 26, 194–205.

Gundelfinger, B.F. and Britten, S.A. (1961) Sarcoidosis in the United States Navy. Report of International Conference on Sarcoidosis, Washington, 1960. *Am. Rev. Respir. Dis.*, 84, 109–15.

Gupta, R.C., Kueppers, F., DeRemee, R.A., Huston, K.A. and McDuffie, F.C. (1977) Pulmonary and extrapulmonary sarcoidosis in relation to circulating immune conplexes. *Am. Rev. Respir. Dis.* 116, 261–6.

Gupta, R.G., Sicilian, L., Catchatourian, R., Bekerman, C., Oparil, S. and Szidon, J.P. (1982) Angiotensin-converting enzyme in serum and in bronchoalveolar lavage in sarcoidosis. *Respiration*, 43, 153–7.

Gupta, S.K., Chatterjee, S. and Roy, M (1982) Clinical profile of sarcoidosis in India. *Lung, India*, 1, 5–10.

Güthert, H. and Hübner, O. (1944) Epithelioidzelliger sklerosierende Miliartuberkulose. *Virchows Arch.*, 313, 182.

Gutman, A.B. and Gutman, E.B. (1937) Relation of serum calcium to serum albumin and globulin. *J. Clin. Invest.*, 16, 903–19.

Haas, G. and Joseph, H. (1908) Un cas d'infantilisme avec syndrome de Miculicz fruste, accompagné d'iridochoroidite. *Ann. Ocul., Paris*, 139, 130.

Hadfield, G. (1939) The primary histological lesion of regional ileitis. *Lancet*, 2, 773–5.

Hadfield, J.W., Page, R.L., Flower, C.D.R. and Stark, J.E. (1982) Localised airway narrowing in sarcoidosis. *.Thorax*, 37, 443–7.

Hagerstrand, I. and Linell, F. (1964) The prevalence of sarcoidosis in the autopsy material from a Swedish town. *Acta Med. Scand., Suppl.* 425, 171–3.

Hagn-Meincke, F. (1944) Boeck's sarcoid and its relation to tuberculosis. *Acta Tuberc. Scand.*, 18, 1—19.

Hahnemann, S., Transbøl, I. and Hornum, I. (1967) The serum calcium fractions in hypercalcaemic sarcoidosis with and without hyperparathyroidism. In *Proc. 4th International Conference on Sarcoidosis, Paris.* (eds J. Turiaf and J. Chabot), Masson, Paris, pp. 605–9.

Haines, M. and Stallworthy, J.A. (1952) Genital tuberculosis in the female. *J. Obstet. Gynecol. Br. Emp.*, 59, 721–47.

Haldimann, C. (1941) Hornhant- und Bindehautveranderung bei Boeckscher Krankheit. *Ophthalmologica*, 102, 137–45.

Hall, G., Naish, P., Sharma, O.P., Doe, W. and James, D.G. (1969) The epidemiology of sarcoidosis. *Postgrad. Med. J.*, 45, 241–50.

Hällström, K., Sairenen, E. and Ohela, K. (1972) A pilot study on Yersiniosis in south-eastern Finland. *Acta Med. Scand.*, 191, 485–91.

Hamazaki, Y. (1938) Uber ein neues, säurefeste Substanz führendes Spindelkörperchen der menschlichen Lymphdrüsen. *Virchows Arch. A.*, 301, 490–522.

Hamilton, R., Petty, T.L. and Haiby, G. (1965) Cavitary sarcoidosis of the lung. *Arch. Intern. Med.*, 116, 428–30.

Hamman, L., and Rich, A.R. (1944) Acute diffuse interstitial fibrosis of the lungs. *Bull. Johns Hopkins Hosp.*, **74**, 177–212.

Hammond B. L. and Kataria, Y.P. (1980) Nasal sarcoidosis with septal perforation. *J. Otolaryngol.*, **9**, 31–4.

Handslip, P.D., Bone, M., Woodhead, J.S. and Davies, B.H. (1980) Calcium and phosphate metabolism in sarcoidosis with particular reference to parathyroid function. In *Proc. 8th International conference on Sarcoidosis, Cardiff, 1978* (eds. W. Jones-Williams and B.H. Davies), Alpha Omega, Cardiff, pp. 225–32.

Hanifin, J.M., Epstein, W.L. and Cline, M.J . (1970) *In vitro* studies of granulomatous hypersensitivity to beryllium. *J. Invest. Dermatol.*, **55**, 284–8.

Hann, F. Von (1913) Über die bedcutung der Hypophysenveränderungen bei Diabetes insipidus. *Frankf. Z. Pathol.*, **21**, 337.

Hanngren, A., Biberfeldt, G., Carlens, E., Hedfors, E., Nilsson, B.S., Ripe, E. and Wahren, B. (1974) Is sarcoidosis due to an infectious interaction between virus and mycobacterium? In *Proc. 6th International Conference on Sarcoidosis, Tokyo*, (eds. K. Iwai and Y. Hosoda), University of Tokyo Press, Tokyo pp. 8–11.

Hannuksela, M. (1971) Erythema nodosum: with special reference to sarcoidosis. *Ann. Clin. Res.*, **3**, Suppl. 7.

Hannuksela, M. and Ahvonene, P. (1969) Erythema nodosum due to *Yersinia enterocolitica*. *Scand. J. Infect. Dis.*, **1**, 17–19.

Hannuksela, M. and Salo, D.P. (1969) The significance of the quantitative Mantoux test in sarcoidosis. *Scand. J. Respir. Dis.*, **50**, 259–64.

Hapke, E.J. and Meek, J.C. (1971) Steroid treatment in pulmonary sarcoidosis. In *Proc. 5th International Conference on Sarcoidosis, Prague, 1969* (eds. L. Levinsky and F. Macholda), Universita Karlova, Prague, pp. 621–5.

Hapke, E.J., Seal, R.M.E., Thomas, G.O., Hayes, M. and Meek, J.C. (1968) Farmer's lung: a clinical, radiographic, functional and serological correlation of acute and chronic stages. *Thorax*, **23**, 451–68.

Hara, A. Sawada, H., Fukuyama, K. and Epstein, W.L. (1983) Tissue angiotensin-converting enzyme(ACE) in sarcoid and hypersensitivity granulomas. In *Proc. 9th International Conference on Sarcoidosis, Paris*, Pergamon Press, Oxford, pp. 351–5.

Hardebeck, H. (1953) Boecksches Sarkoid der Prostata. *Z. Urol.*, **46**, 202–3.

Hardt, F., Veien, N., Bendixen, G., Brodthagen, H., Faber, V., Genner, J., Heckscher, T., Ringstad, J., Sorensen, S.F., Wanstrup, J. and Wijk, A. (1976) Immunological studies in sarcoidosis: a comparison of *in vivo* and *in vitro* Kveim tests. *Ann. NY Acad. Med.*, **278**, 711–6.

Hardt, F., Wanstrup, J. (1969) Sarcoidosis: an *in vitro* Kveim reaction based on the leucocyte migration test. *Acta Pathol. Microbiol. Scand.*, **76**, 493–4.

Hardy, H.L. (1951) The character and distribution of disease in American industries using beryllium compounds. *Proc. R. Soc. Med.*, **44**, 257–62.

Hardy, H.L. (1956) Differential diagnosis between beryllium poisoning and sarcoidosis. *Am. Rev. Tuberc.*, **74**, 885–96

Hardy, H.L. and Tabershaw, I.R. (1946) Delayed chemical pneumonitis occurring in workers exposed to beryllium compounds. *J. Ind. Hyg.*, **28**, 197–211.

Hardy, W.E., Tugan, H., Haidak, G. and Budnitz, J. (1967) Sarcoidosis: a case presenting with dysphagia and dysphonia. *Ann. Intern. Med.*, **66**, 353–7.

Hargreave, F.E., Pepys, J. (1972) Allergic respiratory reactions in bird fanciers provoked by allergen inhalation provocation tests. *J. Allergy Clin. Immunol.* **50**, 157–73.

Hargreave, F.E., Pepys, J., Longbottom, J.L. and Wraith, D.G. (1966) Bird-breeder's (fancier's lung. *Lancet*, **1**, 445–9.

Harkleroad, L.E., Young, R.L., Savage, P.J., Jenkins, D.W. and London, R.E. (1982) Pulmonary sarcoidosis: long term follow up of the effects of steroid therapy. *Chest,* **82**, 84–7.

Harontunian, L.M., Fisher, A.M. and Smith, E.W. (1964) Tuberculosis and sarcoidosis. *Bull. Johns Hopkins Hosp.,* **115**, 1–28.

Harrell, G.T. (1940) Generalised sarcoidosis of Boeck; a clinical report on 11 cases with studies of the blood and the etiologic factors. *Arch. Intern. Med.,* **65**, 1003–34.

Harrell, G.T. and Fisher, S. (1939) Blood chemical studies in Boeck's sarcoid, with particular reference to protein, calcium and phosphatase values. *J. Clin. Pathol.,* **18**, 687–93.

Harrell, G.T. and Horne, S.F. (1945) The reaction to lepromin of patients with sarcoid or tuberculosis compared with that of patients in general hospitals with a discussion of the mechanism of the reaction. *Am. J. Trop. Med.,* **25**, 523–35.

Harris, T.R., Blumenfeld, H.B., Gruthirds, T.P. and McCall, C.B. (1965) Coexisting sarcoidosis and cryptococcosis. *Arch. Intern. Med.,* **115**, 637–43.

Harris, U.S. and Shore, C. (1952) Boeck's sarcoid: observations on the use of B.C.G. vaccine. *Dis. Chest,* **22**, 159–62.

Harrison, G.N., Lipham, M., Elguindi, A.S. and Loebl, D.H. (1979) Acute sarcoidosis occurring during the course of systemic lupus erythematosus. *South. Med. J.,* **72**, 1387–8.

Harrison, H.E. and Harrison, H.C. (1960) Transfer of Ca^{45} across intestinal wall *in vitro* in relation to action of vitamin D and calciferol. *Am. J. Physiol.,* **199**, 265–71.

Harrison, P.V. and Ive, F.A. (1978) Sarcoidosis in husband and wife. *NY State J. Med.,* **78**, 2130.

D'Arcy Hart, P., Mitchell D.N. and Sutherland, I. (1964) Associations between Kveim test results, previous B.C.G. vaccination, and tuberculin sensitivity in healthy young adults. *Br. Med. J.,* **1**, 795–804.

Hart, W.M. (1979) Optic disc oedema in sarcoidosis. *Am. J. Ophthalmol.,* **88**, 769–71.

Harter, J.G., Reddy, W.J. and Torn, G.W. (1963) Studies on an intermittent corticosteroid dosage regimen. *N. Engl. J. Med.,* **269**, 591–6.

Harthorne, J.W. and Freiman, D.G. (1975) Clinico-pathological conference case 46–1975. *N. Engl. J. Med.,* **293**, 1138–45.

Harvey, J.C. (1959) A myopathy of Boeck's sarcoid. *Am. J. Med.,* **26**, 356–63.

Harvier, P., Turiaf, J., Claisse, R. and Rose, J. (1950). Maladie de Besnier–Boeck–Schaumann fébrile à localisation multiples. *Bull. Soc. Méd. Hôp., Paris,* **66**, 192–7.

Hasan, F. M. and Kazemi, H. (1974) Chronic beryllium disease: a continuing epidemiologic hazard. *Chest,* **65**, 289–93.

Haslam, P. (1978) in Turner-Warwick, M. *Immunology of the Lung,* Edward Arnold, London, p. 153.

Haslam, P.L., Turton, C.W.G., Heard, B., Lukoszek, A., Collins, J.V., Salsbury, A.J. and Turner-Warwick, M. (1980a) Bronchoalveolar lavage in pulmonary fibrosis: comparison of cells obtained with lung biopsy and clinical features. *Thorax,* **35**, 9–18.

Haslam, P.L., Turton C.W.G., Lukoszek, A., Salsbury, A.J., Deward, A., Collins, J.V. and Turner-Warwick, M. (1980b) Bronchoalveolar lavage fluid cell counts in cryptogenic fibrosing alveolitis and their relation to therapy. *Thorax,* **35**, 328–9.

Hasselt, J.A. Van (1935) Nog een geval van ziekte van Mylius-Schürmann. *Ned. Tijdschr. Geneeskd.*, 79, 5384.

Hausfeld, K.F. (1961) Primary sarcoidosis of the scrotum: case report. *J. Urol.*, 86, 269–72.

Haushalter, P. and Lucien, M. (1908) Polyurie simple et tubercle de phypophyse. *Rev. Neurol.*, 12, 1.

Hautschmann, L. (1939) Über torpide sklerosierende Tuberkulosen mit eigenartigem grosszelligem histologischem Befund. *Ergeb. Gesamten Lungen-Tuberkuloseforsch.*, 9, 1.

Hawley, R.J., Beaman, B.L., Williams, M.C. and Yeager, H. (1979) The ultrastructure of bronchial macrophages and lymphocytes in sarcoidosis. *Hum. Pathol.* 10, 155–63.

Headings, V.E., Weston, D., Young, R.C. and Hackney, R.L. (1976) Familial sarcoidosis with multiple occurrences in eleven families. *Ann. NY Acad. Sci.*, 278, 377–85.

Hebert, L.A., Lemann, J., Petersen, J.R. and Lennon, E.J. (1966) Studies of the mechanism by which phosphate lowers serum calcium concentration. *J. Clin. Invest.*, 45, 1886–94.

Hedfors, E. and Möller, E. (1972) HLA antigens in sarcoidosis. *Tissue Antigens*, 3, 95–8.

Hedfors, E. (1974) Activation of peripheral T-cells of sarcoidosis patients and healthy controls. *Clin. Exp. Immunol.*, 18, 379–90.

Hedfors, E. (1975) Immunological aspects of sarcoidosis. *Scand. J. Respir. Dis.*, 565, 1–19.

Hedfors, E., Holm, G. and Pettersson, D. (1974) Lymphocyte subpopulations in sarcoidosis. *Clin. Exp. Immunol.*, 17, 219–26.

Hedfors, E. and Lindström, F. (1983) HLA-B8/DR3 in sarcoidosis. *Tissue Antigens*, 22, 200–3.

Hedfors, E., and Norberg, R. (1974) Evidence for circulating immune complexes in sarcoidosis. *Clin. Exp. Immunol.*, 16, 493–6.

Hedvall, E. (1950) Streptomycin therapy in lymphogranuloma benignum. *Arch. Tisiol.*, 5, 5–14.

Heerfordt, C.F. (1909) Uber eine 'Febris uveo-parotidea subchronica. *Graefes Arch. Ophthalmol.*, 70, 254–73.

Heffernan, J.C. and Blenkinsop, W.K. (1978) Epididymal sarcoidosis. *Br. J. Urol.*, 50, 211.

Heilman, D.H., Bernton, H.W. and Higgins, G.A. (1970) Cultures of human tissues for studies on delayed allergy with observations on sarcoidosis. *J. Lab. Clin. Med.*, 75, 488–98.

Heimbeck, J. (1950) The significance of erythema nodosum tuberculosum. *Acta Tuberc. Scand.*, 24, 388–96.

Heller, S., McLean, R.A., Campbell, C.G. and Jones, I.H. (1957) A case of co-existent non-meningitic cryptococcosis and Boeck's sarcoid. *Am. J. Med.*, 22, 986–94.

Hellerström, S. (1941) Das Erythema nodosum – Problem im Licht des Lymphogranuloma inguinale. *Acta Med. Scand.*, 109, 131–3.

Hemmings, I.L. and McLean, D.C. (1971) Thyroid involvement in systemic sarcoidosis. *J. Pediatr.*, 78, 131–3.

Hendrix, J.Z. (1963) The remission of hypercalcaemia and hypercalciuria in sarcoidosis by vitamin D depletion. *Clin. Res.* 11, 220.

Hendrix, J.Z. (1964) Sarcoidosis and bone mineral metabolism. *Clin. Res.* 12, 457.

Hendrix, J.Z. (1966) Abnormal skeletal mineral metabolism in sarcoidosis. *Ann. Intern. Med.,* **64,** 797–805.

Henkind, P. and Gottlieb, M.B. (1973) Bilateral internal ophthalmoplegia in a patient with sarcoidosis. *Br. J. Ophthalmol.,* **57,** 792–6.

Henneman, P.H., Carroll, E.L. and Dempsey, E.F. (1954) Mechanism responsible for hypercalciuria in sarcoid. *J. Clin. Invest.,* **33,** 941–2.

Herring, A.B. and Urich, H. (1969) Sarcoidosis of the central nervous system. *J. Neurol. Sci.,* **9,** 405–22.

Hertzberg, O. (1948) *The Achievements of B.C.G. Vaccination,* Johan Grundt Tanum, Oslo.

Heshiki, A., Schatz, S.L., McKusick, K.A., Bowersox, D.W., Soin, J.S. and Wagner, H.N. (1974) Gallium 67 citrate scanning in patients with pulmonary sarcoidosis. *Am. J. Roentgenol.,* **122,** 744–9.

Hess, C.E., Ayers, C.R., Wetzel, R.A., Mohler, D.N. and Sandusky, W.R. (1971). Dilutional anaemia of splenectomy. *Ann. Surg.,* **173,** 693–7.

Hetherington, S. (1982) Sarcoidosis in young children. *Am. J. Dis. Child.,* **136,** 13–5.

Hewlett, R.H. and Brownell, B. (1975) Granulomatous myopathy: its relationship to sarcoidosis and polymyositis. *J. Neurol. Neurosurg. Psychiatry.,* **38,** 1090–9.

Hiatt, J.C. and Lide, J.N. (1949) Blastomycosis complicating Boeck's sarcoid. *N. C. Med. J.,* **10,** 650–6.

Hiatt, J.S. Jr. (1948) Sarcoidosis following primary tuberculosis. *Am. Rev. Tuberc.,* **58,** 98–101.

Hickling, R. A. (1938) Tuberculous splenomegaly with miliary tuberculosis of the lungs. *Q. J. Med.,* **7,** 263–9.

Hietala, S.O., Stinnett, R.G., Fanuce, H.F., Sharpe, A.R., Scoggins, W.G. and Smith, R.H. (1977) Pulmonary artery narrowing in sarcoidosis. *J. Am. Med. Ass.,* **237,** 572–3.

Higasi, T., Nakayama, Y., Murata, A., Nakamura, K., Sugiyama, M., Kawaguchi, T. and Suzuki, S. (1972) Clinical evaluation of ^{67}Ga-citrate scannning. *J. Nucl. Med.,* **13,** 196–201.

Higgins, G. A. and Moore, C.F. (1969) Sarcoidosis and hyperparathyroidism. *Am. J. Med.,* **46,** 305–11.

Hillerdal, O., Hultquist, G. and Linder, L. (1965) A case of sarcoidosis, syphilis and rheumatoid arthritis. *Acta Tuberc. Scand.,* **46,** 65–70.

Hines, H.L., Elgart, M.L. and MacKenzie, A.R. (1961) Sarcoidosis: case presentation and discussion. *J. Urol.,* **85,** 71–4.

Hines, J.D. and Sancetta, S.M. (1963) Myocardial sarcoidosis simulating healed myocardial infarction. *Ohio Med. J.,* **59,** 689–92.

Hinman, L.M., Stevens, C., Matthay, R.A. and Gee, J.B.L. (1979) Angiotensin convertase activities in human alveolar macrophages: effects of cigarette smoking and sarcoidosis. *Science,* **205,** 202–3.

Hinman, L.M., Stevens, C.A., Matthay, R.A., Reynolds, H.Y. and Gee, J.B.L. (1978) Lysozyme and angiotensin convertase activity in human alveolar macrophages: the effects of cigarette smoking and pulmonary sarcoidosis. *Am. Rev. Respir. Dis.,* **117,** 67A.

Hinson, K.W.F., Moon, A.J. and Plummer, N.S. (1952) Broncho-pulmonary aspergillosis. *Thorax,* **7,** 317–33.

Hinterbuchner, L.P. (1964) Myopathic syndrome in muscular sarcoidosis. *Brain,* **87,** 355–66.

Hiraga, Y. *et al.* (1974) Epidemiology of sarcoidosis in a Japanese working group – a ten year study. In *Proc. 6th International Conference, on Sarcoidosis, Tokyo* (eds, K. Iwai and Y. Hosoda), University of Tokyo, pp. 303–6.

Hiraga, Y., Hosoda, Y. and Zenda, I. (1977) A local outbreak of sarcoidosis in northern Japan. *Z. Erkr. Atmungsorgane* 149, 38–43.

Hirayama, J. (1939) Ein Fall von diffuser spezifischer Myocarditis mit zahlreichen Riesenzellen. *Trans. Soc. Pathol. Jpn.,.29*, 261–5.

Hirsch, J.G., Cohn, Z.A., Morse, S.I., Schaedler, R.W., Siltzbach, L.E., Ellis, J.T. and Chase, M.W. (1961) Evaluation of the Kveim reaction as a diagnostic test for sarcoidosis. *N. Engl. J. Med.,* 265, 827–30.

Hirsch, J.G., Fedorko, M.E. and Dwyer, C.M. (1967) The ultrastructure of epithelioid and giant cells in positive Kveim test sites and sarcoid granulomata. In *Proc. 4th International Conference on Sarcoidosis, Paris* (eds. J. Turiaf and J. Chabot), Masson, Paris, pp., 59–70.

Hirschhorn, K., Schreibman, R.R., Bach, R.H. and Siltzbach, L.E. (1964) In vitro studies of lymphocytes from patients with sarcoidosis and lymphoproliferative diseases. *Lancet,* 2, 842–3.

Hirschman, R.J. and Johns, C.J. (1965) Hemoglobin studies in sarcoidosis. *Ann. Intern. Med.,* 62, 129–32.

Hirsh, E.F. (1935) Radial inclusions of giant cells. *Arch. Pathol,* 20, 665–82.

Hirshant, Y., Glade, P., Vieira, L., Ainbender, E., Dvorak, B. and Siltzbach, L.E. (1970). Sarcoidosis, another disease associated with serologic evidence for herpes-like virus infection, *New Engl. J. Med.,* 283, 502–506.

Ho, K - L (1979) Sarcoidosis of the uterus. *Hum. Pathol.,* 10, 219–72.

Ho, S.U., Berenberg, R.A., Kim, K.S. arid Dal Canto, M.C. (1979) Sarcoid encephalopathy with diffuse inflammation and focal hydrocephalus shown by sequential CT. *Neurology,* 29, 1161–5.

Hobbs, H.E. and Calnan, C.D. (1958) The ocular complications of chloroquine therapy. *Lancet,* 1, 1207–9.

Hobbs, H.E., Sorsby, A. and Freedman, A. (1959) Retinopathy following chloroquine therapy. *Lancet,* 2, 478–80.

Hoffbrand, B.I. (1963) B.C.G. and sarcoidosis. *Br. Med. J.* 1, 658–9.

Hoffbrand, B.I. (1968) Occurrence and significance of lymphopenia in sarcoidosis. *Am. Rev. Respir. Dis.,* 98, 107–10.

Holcomb, F.D. (1965) Erythema nodosum associated with the use of an oral contraceptive. *Obstet. Gynecol.,* 25, 156–7.

Holdstock, G., Millward-Sadler, G.H. and Wright, R. (1979) Granulomatous hepatitis. *In Liver and Biliary Disease* (eds. R. Wright, K. Alberti, S. Karran and G.H. Millward-Sadler). W.B. Saunders.

Hollister, W.F. and Harrell, G.T. (1941) Generalised sarcoidosis of Boeck accompanied with tuberculosis and streptococcic bacteremia. *Arch. Pathol.,* 31, 178–88.

Holsinger, R.E. and Dalton, J.E. (1954) Isoniazid therapy in cutaneous tuberculosis and sarcoidosis. *J. Am. Med. Assoc.,* 154, 475–81.

Holt, J.F. and Owens, W.I. (1949) Osseous lesions of sarcoidosis. *Radiology,* 53, 11–30.

Holtzman, I.N. (1961) Sarcoidosis followed by biliary cirrhosis and xanthomatoses. *NY J. Med.,* 61, 1757–64.

Homans, J. and Hass, G.M. (1933) Regional ileitis: a clinical, not pathological entity. *N. Engl. J. Med.,* 209, 1315–24.

Homma, H., Okano, H. and Motchuzuki, H. (1971) An attempt to isolate mycoplasmas from patients with sarcoidosis. In *Proc. 5th International Conference on Sarcoidosis, Prague, 1969* (eds. L. Levinsky and F. Macholda), Universita Karlova, Prague, 101.

Honey, M. and Jepson, E. (1957) Multiple bronchostenoses due to sarcoidosis: report of 2 cases. *Br. Med. J.*, **2**, 1330–4.

Honeybourne, D. (1980) Ethnic differences in the clinical features of sarcoidosis in south-east London. *Br. J. Dis. Chest*, **74**, 63–9.

Höök, O. (1954) Sarcoidosis with involvement of the nervous system: report of 9 cases. *Arch. Neurol. Psychiatry*, Chicago. **71**, 554–75.

Hooper, R. and Holden, H. (1970) Acoustic and vestibular problems in sarcoidosis. *Arch. Otalaryngol.*, **92**, 386–91.

Hopf, B. and Krebs, A. (1974) 'Ulcera cruris' als seltene form einer Sarkoidose. *Dermatologica*, **149**, 55–62.

Hopkins, A. (1974) Tuberculous meningitis as a complication of sarcoidosis. *J. Neurol. Neurosurg. Psychiatry,* **37**, 644–6.

Hornum, I. and Transbøl, I. (1976) Observations on the different calcium metabolic patterns in sarcoidosis. *Acta Med. Scand.*, **200**, 341–9.

Horsmanheimo, M. (1974a) Correlation of tuberculin-induced lymphocyte transformation with skin test sensitivity and with clinical manifestations of sarcoidosis. *Cell. Immunol.*, **10**, 329–37.

Horsmanheimo, M. (1974b) Lymphocyte transforming factor in sarcoidosis. *Cell. Immunol.*, **10**, 338–43.

Horsmanheimo, M., Horsmanheimo, A., Fundenberg, H.H., Siltzbach, L.E. and McKee, K.T. (1980) Kveim test reactivity with leucocyte migration in agarose and lymphocyte transformation tests. In *Proc. 8th International Conference on Sarcoidosis, Cardiff* (eds. W. Jones-Williams and B.H. Davies), Alpha Omega, Cardiff, pp. 186–90.

Horsmanheimo, M. and Virolainen, M. (1974) Enhancement of tuberculin-induced lymphocyte transformation by precultivated macrophages from patients with sarcoidosis. *Scand. J. Immunol.*, **3**, 21–7.

Horsmanheimo, M. and Virolainen, M. (1976) Transfer of tuberculin sensitivity by transfer factor in sarcoidosis. *Clin. Immunol. Immunopathol.* **6**, 231–7.

Horton, R., Lincoln, N.S. and Pinner, M. (1939) Non-caseating tuberculosis: case reports. *Am. Rev. Tuberc.*, **39**, 187–203.

Horwitz, O. (1961) Geographic epidemiology of sarcoidosis in Denmark, 1954–1957. *Am. Rev. Respir. Dis*, **84**, (5 pt. 2), 135–42.

Horwitz, O. (1971) Epidemiology of sarcoidosis in Demnark. In *Proc. 5th International Conference on Sarcoidosis, Prague, 1969* (eds. L. Levinsky and F. Macholda), Universita Karlova, Prague, 254.

Horwitz, O., Payne, P.G. and Wilbek, E. (1967) Epidemiology of sarcoidosis in Denmark. *Dan. Med. Bull.*, **14**, 178–82.

Hosoda, Y., Oka, H., Chiba, Y. and Kitamura, K. (1967) Long term observations on tuberculin sensitivity in sarcoidosis. In: *Sarcoïdose, Proc. 4th International conference on Sarcoidosis 1967* Masson, Paris, 308–12.

Hosoda, Y. *et al.* (1971) Sarcoidosis and pregnancy. *Jpn. J. Chest. Dis.*, **30**, 305–13.

Hosoda, Y. *et al.* (1974) Epidemiology of sarcoidosis in Japan. In *Proc. 6th International Conference on Sarcoidosis, Tokyo,* eds. K. Iwai and Y. Hosoda), University of Tokyo Press, Tokyo, pp. 297–302.

Howard, J.E., Cary, R.A., Rubin, P.S. and Levin, M.D. (1949) Diagnostic problems in patients with hypercalcaemia. *Trans. Assoc. Am. Physicians,* **62**, 624–9.

Howell, R.G. (1954) Sarcoidosis with involvement of the central nervous system. *Proc. R. Soc. Med.,* **47**, 1065–6.

Hoyle, C., Dawson, J. and Mather, G. (1954) Skin sensitivity in sarcoidosis. *Lancet,* **2**, 164–8.

Hoyle, C., Dawson, J. and Mather, G. (1955) Treatment of pulmonary sarcoidosis with streptomycin and cortisone. *Lancet,* **1**, 638–43.

Hoyle, C., Smyllie, H. and Leak, D. (1967) Prolonged treatment of pulmonary sarcoidosis with corticosteroids. *Thorax,* **22**, 519–24.

Hsing, C.T., Han, F.C., Liu, H.C. and Chu, B.Y. (1964) Sarcoidosis among Chinese. *Am. Rev. Respir. Dis.,* **89**, 917–22.

Huang, C.T., Henrich, A.E., Rosen, Y., Moon, S. and Lyons, H.A. (1979) Pulmonary sarcoidosis: roentgenographic, functional and pathologic correlations. *Respiration,* **37**, 337–45.

Hudelo, Montlaur and Laforestier (1925) Lymphogranulomatose de Schaumann (Lupus pernio) à forme anormale. *Bull. Soc. Fr. Dermatol. Syphiligr.,* **32**, 109–12.

Humber, D.P., Nsanzumuhire, H., Alnoch, J.A., Webster, A.D.B., Aber, V.R., Mitchison, D.A., Girling D.J. and Nunn, A.J. (1980) Controlled double-blind study of the effect of rifampin on humoral and cellular immune responses in patients with pulmonary tuberculosis and in tuberculosis contacts. *Am. Rev. Respir. Dis.,* **122**, 425–36.

Hunninghake, G.W., Broska, P., Haber, R., Keogh, B.A., Line, B.R. and Crystal, R.G. (1981) Correlation of lung T-cell and macrophage function with disease activity in pulmonary sarcoid. *Clin. Res.,* **49**, 550A.

Hunninghake, G.W. and Crystal. R.G. (1981a) Mechanisms of hypergammaglobulinaemia in pulmonary sarcoidosis: site of increased antibody production and role of T-lymphocytes. *J. Clin. Invest.,* **67**, 86–92.

Hunninghake, G.W. and Crystal, R.G. (1981b) Pulmonary sarcoidosis: a disorder mediated by excess helper T-lymphocyte activity at sites of disease activity. *N. Eng. J. Med.,* **305**, 429–34.

Hunninghake, G.W. and Crystal, R.G. (1982) Chemotactic inactivator in leprosy and in acute illness. *N. Engl. J. Med.,* **305**, 429–34.

Hunninghake, G.W., Fulmer, J.D., Young, R.C. and Crystal, R.G. (1980a) Comparison of lung and peripheral lymphocyte sub-populations in pulmonary sarcoidosis. In *Proc. 8th International Conference on Sarcoidosis, Cardiff, 1978* (eds. W. Jones-Williams and B.H. Davies), Alpha Omega, Cardiff, pp. 426–35.

Hunninghake, G.W., Fulmer, J.D., Young, R.C., Gadek, J.E. and Crystal, R.G. (1979b) Localisation of the immune response in sarcoidosis. *Am. Rev. Respir. Dis.,* **120**, 49–57.

Hunninghake, G.W., Gadek, J.E., Kawanami, O., Ferrans, V.J. and Crystal, R.G. (1979a) Inflammatory and immune processes in the human lung in health and disease: evaluation by bronchoalveolar lavage. *Am. J. Pathol.,* **97**, 149–206.

Hunninghake, G.W., Gadek, J.E., Lawley, T.J. and Crystal, R.G. (1981) Mechanisms of neutrophil accumulation in the lungs of patients with idiopathic pulmonary fibrosis. *J. Clin. Invest.,* **68**, 259–69.

Hunninghake, G.W., Gadek, J.E., Young, R.C. Jr., Kawanami, O., Ferrans, V.J. and Crystal, R.G. (1980b) Maintenance of granuloma formation in pulmonary sarcoidosis by T-lymphocytes within the lung. *N. Engl. J. Med.,* **302**, 594–8.

Hunninghake, G.W., Kawanami, O., Ferrans, V.J., Young, R.C., Roberts, E.V. and Crystal, R.G. (1981c) Characterization of the inflammatory and immune effector cells in the lung parenchyma of patients with interstitial lung disease. *Am. Rev. Respir. Dis.,* **123,** 407–12.

Hunninghake, G.W., Line, B.R., Szapiel, S.V. and Crystal, R.G. (1981d) Activation of inflammatory cells increases the localisation of gallium-67 at sites of disease. *Clin. Res.,* **49,** 171A.

Hunt, B.J. and Yendt, E.R. (1963) The response of hypercalcemia in sarcoidosis to chloroquine. *Ann. Intern. Med.,* **59,** 554–64.

Hunter, F.T. (1936) Hutchinson-Boeck's disease (generalised sarcoidosis). *N. Engl. J. Med.,* **214,** 346–52.

Hunter, T., Arnott, J.E. and McCarthy, D.S. (1980) Features of systemic lupus erythematosus and sarcoidosis occurring together. *Arthritis Rheum.,* **23,** 364–66.

Hurley, H.J. and Shelley, W.B. (1959) Comparison of the granuloma producing capacity of normals and sarcoid granuloma patients: experimental analysis of the sarcoid diathesis theory. *Am. J. Med. Sci.,* **237,** 685–92.

Hurley, H.J. and Shelley, W.B. (1960) Sarcoid granulomas after intradermal tuberculin in normal human skin. *Arch. Dermatol. Syphilol. NY,* **82,** 65–72.

Hurley, T.H. and Bartholomeusz, C.L. (1968) The Kveim test in sarcoidosis. *Med. J. Aust.,* **2,** 947–9.

Hurley, T.H. and Bartholomeusz, C.L. (1971) An international Siltzbach-Kveim test study using an Australian (C.S.L.) test material. In *Proc. 5th International Conference on Sarcoidosis, Prague, 1969,* eds. L. Levinsky and F. Macholda, Universita Karlova, Prague, pp. 343–348.

Hurley, T.H. and Sullivan, J.R. (1974) Results obtained with Australian Kveim test material, 1966–1972. In *Proc. 6th International Conference on Sarcoidosis, Tokyo,* (eds. K. Iwai and Y. Hosoda), University of Tokyo Press, Tokyo, pp. 73–6.

Hurley, T.H. Sullivan, J.R. and Hurley, J.V. (1975) Reaction to Kveim test material in sarcoidosis and other diseases. *Lancet,* **1,** 494–6.

Hutchinson, J. (1877) *Illustrations of Clinical Surgery,* J. and A. Churchill, London, 42–3.

Hutchinson, J. (1895) *Smaller Atlas of Illustrations of Clinical Surgery,* West Newman, London.

Hutchinson, J. (1898) Cases of Mortimer's malady. *Arch. Surg., Lond.,* **9,** 307–14.

Hutchinson, J. (1900) Mortimer's malady (a form of lupus). *Arch. Surg.,* **11,** 290–7.

Huzly, A., Hoffmans, A., Seidel, H., Grimminger, A., Hausser, R., Arnold, C. and Forschbach, G. (1963) Les bronches dans la sarcoidosie. *Bronches,* **13,** 531–58.

Ingerstad, R. and Stigmar, G. (1971) Sarcoidosis with ocular and hypothalamic manifestations. *Acta Ophthalmol.,* **49,** 1–10.

Irgang, S. (1939) Sarcoid of Boeck: report of a case of generalised cutaneous distribution and involvement with clinical cure with tuberculin. *Arch. Dermatol. Syphiol., Chicago,* **40,** 35–44.

Irgang, S. (1952) Verrucous and papillomatous types of sarcoid. *Arch. Dermatol.,* **62,** 105–8.

Irgang, S. (1955) Ulcerative cutaneous lesions in sarcoidosis: report of a case with clinical resemblance to papulo-necrotic tuberculide. *Br. J. Dermatol. Syph.,* **67,** 255–60.

Israel, H.L. (1969) Influence of race and geographic origin on incidence of sarcoidosis in the United States. In *Proc. 5th International Conference on Sarcoicosis, Prague, 1969* (eds. L. Levinsky and F. Macholda), Universita Karlova, Prague, 235–7.

Israel, H.L. (1970) Influence of race and geographical origin on sarcoidosis. *Arch. Environ. Health,* **20**, 608–9.

Israel, H.L. (1971) Effects of chlorambucil and methotrexate in sarcoidosis. In *Proc. 5th International Conference on Sarcoidosis, Prague, 1969* (eds. L. Levinsky and F. Macholda), Universita Karlova, Prague, pp. 632–4.

Israel, H.L., De Lamater, E., Sones, M., Willis, W.D. and Mirmelstein, A. (1952) Chronic disseminated histoplasmosis: an investigation of its relationship to sarcoidosis. *Am. J. Med.,* **12**, 252–60.

Israel, H.L., Fonts, D.W. and Beggs, R.A. (1973) A controlled trial of prednisone treatment of sarcoidosis. *Am. Rev. Respir. Dis.,* **107**, 609–14.

Israel, H.L. and Goldstein, R.A. (1968) Metyrapone test in sarcoidosis. *Am. Rev. Respir. Dis.,* **98**, 713–6.

Israel, H.L. (1971) Relation of Kveim-antigen reaction to lymphadenopathy. *N. Engl. J. Med.,* **284**, 345–9.

Israel, H.L. and Goldstein, R.A. (1973) Hepatic granulomatosis and sarcoidosis. *Ann. Intern. Med.,* **79**, 669–78.

Israel, H. L., Hetherington, H.W. and Ord, J.G. (1941) a study of tuberculosis among students of nursing. *J. Am. Med. Assoc.* **117**, 839–43.

Israel, H.L., Lenchner, G. and Steiner, R.M. (1981) Late development of mediastinal calcification in sarcoidosis. *Am. Rev. Respir. Dis.* **124**, 302–5.

Israel, H.L., Lenchner, G.S. and Atkinson, G.W. (1982) Sarcoidosis and aspergilloma: the role of surgery. *Chest,* **32**, 430–2.

Israel, H.L. and Ostrow, A. (1969) Sarcoidosis and aspergilloma. *Am. J. Med.,* **47**, 243–50.

Israel, H.L., Park, C.H. and Mansfield, C.M. (1976) Gallium scanning in sarcoidosis. *Ann. NY Acad. Sci.,* **278**, 514–6.

Israel, H.L., Patterson, J.R. and Smukler, N.M. (1964) Latex fixation tests in sarcoidosis. *Acta Med. Scand.* Suppl. **425**, 40–42.

Israel, H.L. and Sones, M. (1955) The diagnosis of sarcoidosis with special reference to the Kveim reaction. *Ann. Intern. Med.,* **43**, 1269–82.

Israel, H.L. and Sones, M. (1958) Sarcoidosis: clinical observations on 160 cases. *Arch. Intern. Med.,* **102**, 766–76.

Israel, H.L. and Sones, M. (1959) The differentiation of sarcoidosis and beryllium disease. *Arch. Ind. Health.,* **19**, 160–163.

Israel, H.L. and Sones, M. (1964) Selection of biopsy procedures for diagnosis of sarcoidosis. *Acta Med. Scand.,* Suppl. **425**, 222–4.

Israel, H.L. and Sones, M. (1964) Selection of biopsy procedures for sarcoidosis diagnosis. *Arch. Intern. Med.,* **113**, 255–60.

Israel, H.L. and Sones, M. (1965) Immunologic defect in patients recovered from sarcoidosis. *N. Engl. J. Med.,* **273**, 1003–6.

Israel, H.L. and Sones, M. (1966) A study of bacillus Calmette-Guerin vaccination and the Kveim reaction. *Ann. Intern. Med.,* **64**, 87–91.

Israel, H.L., Sones, M., Beerman, H. and Pastras, T. (1958) A further study of the Kveim reaction in sarcoidosis and tuberculosis. *N. Engl. J. Med.,* **259**, 365–9.

Israel, H.L., Sones, M. and Harrell, D. (1953) Ineffectiveness of isoniazid and iproniazid in therapy of sarcoidosis. . *Am. Rev. Tuberc.,* **67**, 671–3.

Israel, H.L., Sones, N. and Harrell, D. (1954) Cortisone treatment of sarcoidosis: experience with 36 cases. *J. Am. Med. Assoc.,* **156**, 461 –6.

Israel, H.L., Sones, M., Roy, R.L. and Stein, G.N. (1961) The occurrence of intrathoracic calcification in sarcoidosis. *Am. Rev. Respir. Dis.*, **84**, 1–11.

Israel, H.L., Sones, M., Stein, S.C. and Aronson, J.D. (1950) B.C.G. vaccination in sarcoidosis. *Am. Rev. Tuberc.*, **62**, 408–17.

Israel, H.L. and Washburne, J.D. (1980) Characteristics of sarcoidosis in black and white patients. In *Proc. 8th International Conference on Sarcoidosis, Cardiff, 1978* (eds. W. Jones-Williams and B.H. Davies), Alpha Omega, Cardiff, pp. 497–507.

Ito, Y., Morikawa, S., Hirano, T., Kioi, S., Hirasawa, K. and Kinoshita, Y. (1977) Gastric sarcoidosis in Japan. *Z. Erkr. Atmungsorgane*, **149**, 134–6.

Ito, Y., Ogima, I. and Kinoshita, Y. (1974) Familial sarcoidosis in Japan. In *Proc. 6th International Conference on Sarcoidosis*, Tokyo Press, Tokyo, pp. 30–3.

Iversen, K., Christoffersen, P. and Poulsen, H. (1970) Epithelioid cell granulomas in liver biopsies. *Scand. J. Gastroenterol.*, Suppl. 7, 61–7.

Iveson, J.M.I., Cotterill, J.A. and Wright, V. (1975) Sarcoidosis presenting with multiple tattoo granulomata. *Postgrad. Med. J.*, **51**, 670–7.

Iwai, K. and Takahashi, S. (1976) Transmissibility of sarcoid specific granulomas in the footpads of mice. *Ann. NY Acad. Sci.*, **276**, 249–9.

Izumi, T., Kobara, Y., Morioka, S., Sato, A. and Tsuji, S. (1974) False-positive reaction in the Kveim test using the CSL Kveim material. In *Proc. 6th International Coference on Sarcoidosis, Tokyo*, (eds. K. Iwai and Y. Hosoda), University of Tokyo Press, Tokyo, pp. 77–8.

Jackson, A. and Hood, T.R. (1958) Sarcoidosis with involvement of the pituitary gland. *Ann. Intern. Med.*, **49**, 467–71.

Jackson, A.I. (1957) Splenectomy in sarcoidosis. *Am. J. Surg.*, **94**, 802–5.

Jackson, B.H. (1925) Use of X-ray in uveoparotitis. *Am. J. Ophthalmol.*, **8**, 361.

James, D.G. and Thomson, A.D. (1959) The course of sarcoidosis and its modification by treatment. *Lancet*, **1**, 1057–61.

Jackson, G.A. (1957) Correspondence. *Lancet*, **1**, 637.

Jackson, W.P.U. and Dancaster, C. (1959) A consideration of the hypercalciuria in sarcoidosis, idiopathic hypercalciuria and that produced by vitamin D. *J. Clin. Endocrinol.* **19**, 658–80.

Jacobs, D.S. (1963) Primary gastric malignant lymphoma and pseudolymphoma. *Am. J. Clin. Pathol.*, **40**, 379–94.

Jacobsen, A.W. (1937) Generalised tuberculosis of the lymph-nodes and multiple cystic tuberculosis of the bones. *J. Pediatr.* **8**, 292–307.

Jadassohn, J. (1913) Die Tuberkulide. *Arch Dermatol. Syph., Wein*, **119**, 10.

Jadassohn, W. (1932) Immunobiologie der Haut. *Handbuch der Haut und Geschlechtskrankheiten*, Julius Springer, Berlin, vol. 2, 367.

Jalan, K.N., MacLean, N., Ross, J.M., Sircus, W. and Butterworth, S.T.G. (1969) Carcinoma of the terminal ileum and sarcoidosis in a case of ulcerative colitis. *Gastroenterology*, **56**, 583–8.

James. D.G. (1956) Diagnosis and treatment of sarcoidosis. *Lancet*, **2**, 900–4.

James, D.G. (1959) Ocular sarcoidosis. *Am. J. Med.*, **26**, 331–9.

James, D.G. (1959) Dermatological aspects of sarcoidosis. *Q. J.Med.*, **28**, 109–24.

James, D.G. (1961) Erythema nodosum. *Br. Med. J.*, **1**, 853–7.

James, D.G. (1966) Immunology of sarcoidosis. *Lancet*, **2**, 633–5.

James, D.G. (1974) Multi-system ocular syndromes. *J. R. Coll. Physicians, London*, **9**, 63–78.

James, D.G., Anderson, R., Langley, D. and Ainslie, D. (1964) Ocular sarcoidosis. *Br. J. Ophthalmol.*, **48**, 461–70.

James, D.G. and Brett, G.Z. (1964) Prevalence of intrathoracic sarcoidosis in Britain. *Acta Med. Scand.,* Suppl. **425**, 115–7.

James, D.G., Neville, E. and Langley, D.A. (1976) Ocular sarcoidosis *Trans. Ophthalmol. Soc. UK,* **79**, 133–9.

James, D.G., Neville, E., Piyasena, K.H.G., Walker, A.N., and Hamlyn, A.N. (1974) Possible genetic influences in familial sarcoidosis. *Postgrad. Med. J.,* 664–70.

James, D.G. and Pepys, J. (1956) Tuberculin in aqueous and oily solutions: skin test reactions in normal subjects and in patients with sarcoidosis. *Lancet,* **1**, 602.

James, D.G. and Sharma, O.P. (1967) Neurological complications of sarcoidosis. *Proc. R. Soc. Med.,* **62**, 1169–70.

James, D.G. and Thompson, A.D. (1959) The course of sarcoidosis and its modification by treatment. *Lancet,* **1**, 1057–61.

James, D.G. and Thomson, A.D. (1955) The Kveim test in sarcoidosis. *Q. J. Med.,* **24**, 49–60.

James, D.G., Thomson, A.D. and Wilcox, A. (1956) Erythema nodosum as a manifestation of sarcoidosis. *Lancet,* **2**, 218–21.

James, D.G., Zatouroff, M.A., Trowell, J. and Rose, J.C. (1967) Papilloedema in sarcoidosis. *Br, J. Ophthalmol.,* **51**, 526–9.

James, D.G. *et al.* (1976a) A world-wide review of sarcoidosis. *Ann. NY Acad. Med.,* **278**, 321–34.

James, D.G. *et al* (1976b) Description of sarcoidosis: Report of the Subcommittee on classification and definition. *Ann. NY Acad. Sci.,* **278**, 742.

James, E.F. (1961) Transition from pulmonary tuberculosis to sarcoidosis. *Am. Rev. Respir. Dis.,* **84**, 78–83.

James, I., and Wilson, A.J. (1945) Spontaneous rupture of spleen in sarcoidosis. *Br. J. Surg.,* **33**, 280–2.

James, T.N. (1977) Sarcoid heart disease. *Circulation,* **56**, 320–6.

Jampol, L.M., Woodfin, W. and McLean, E.B. (1972) Optic nerve sarcoidosis. *Arch. Ophthalmol.,* **87**, 355–60.

Jansson, E., Hannuksela, M., Eklund, H., Halme, H. and Tuuri, S. (1972) Isolation of a mycoplasma from sarcoid tissue. *J. Clin. Pathol.,* **25**, 837–42.

Jasper, P.L., and Denny, F.W. (1968) Sarcoidosis in children with special emphasis on the history and treatment. *J Paediatr.* **73**, 499–512.

Jaumandreu, C.A., Navarrete, E. and Casinelli, J.F. (1964) Sarcoidosis de endometrio. *Torax,* **13**, 320–5.

Javitt, N.B. and Daniels, R.A. (1959) Myasthenia gravis with sarcoidosis. *J. Mt Sinai Hosp., NY,* **26**, 177–87.

Jawali, M.H., Hanson, T.J., Schemmel, J.E., Beck, P. and Katz, F.H. (1980) Hypothalamic sarcoidosis and hypopituitarism. *Horm. Res.,* **12**, 1–9.

Jefferson, M. (1957) Sarcoidosis of the nervous system. *Brain,* **80**, 540–56.

Jefferson, M., Smith, W.T., Taylor, A.B. and Valteris, K. (1954) Bronchial carcinoma and sarcoidosis. *Thorax,* **9**, 291–8.

Jencks, W.P., Smith, E.R.B. and Durram, E.L. (1956)The clinical significance of the analysis of serum protein distribution by filter paper electrophoresis. *Am. J. Med.,* **21**, 387–405.

Jersild, M. (1938) The syndrome of Heerfordt (uveo-parotid fever): a manifestation of Boeck's sarcoid. *Acta Med. Scand.,* **97**, 322–8.

Jersild, P.M. (1939) Diabète insipide au cours de sarcoïdes de Boeck. *Ann. Dermatol. Syphiligr., Paris,* **10**, 641–3.

Jessing, A. (1943) Lymphogranulomatosis benigna i ventriklen. *Nord. Med.,* **17**, 161–2.

Johansson, R. (1958) Sarkoidos (morbus Schaumann) och hemolytisk anemi. *Nord. Med.*, **60**, 1746–9.

Johns, C.J. and Ball, W.C. (1967) Steroids in pulmonary parenchymal sarcoidosis. In *Proc. 4th International Conference on Sarcoidosis, Paris*, (eds. J. Turiaf and J. Chabot), Masson, Paris, pp. 742–8.

Johns, C.J., Macgregor, M.I., Zachary, J.B. and Ball, W.C. (1976) Extended experience in the long-term corticosteroid treatment of pulmonary sarcoidosis. *Ann. NY Acad. Med.*, **278**, 722–31.

Johns, C.J., Macgregor, M.I., Zachary, J.B., Kaplan, J. and Silverstein, K.J. (1980) Chronic sarcoidosis: outcome, unusual features and complications. In *Proc. 8th International Conference on Sarcoidosis, Cardiff, 1978* (eds. W. Jones-Williams and B. H. Davies), Alpha Omega, Cardiff, pp. 558–566.

Johnson, J.E., De Remee, R.A., Kneppers, F. and Roberts, G.D. (1977) Prevalence of fungal complement-fixing antibodies in sarcoidosis. *Am. Rev. Respir. Dis.*, **116**, 145–7.

Johnson, N. McI., Brostoff, J., Hudspith, B.N., Boot, J.R. and McNicol, M.W. (1981) Ty Cells in sarcoidosis: E rosetting monocytes suppress lymphocyte transformation. *Clin. Exp. Immunol.*, **43**, 491–6.

Johnson, R.L. Jr., Lawson, W.H. and Wilcox, W.C.N. (1961) Alveolar-capillary block in sarcoidosis. *Clin. Res.*, **9**, 196.

Jonas, A.F. Jr. (1939) Granulomatous myocarditis. *Bull. Johns Hopkins Hosp.*, **64**, 45–65.

Jones-Williams, W. (1958) A histological study of the lungs in 52 cases of chronic beryllium disease. *Br. J. Industr. Med.*, **15**, 84–91.

Jones-Williams, W. (1960a) The beryllium granuloma. *Proc. R. Soc. Med.*, **64**, 946–8.

Jones-Williams, W. (1960b) The nature and origin of Schaumann bodies. *J. Path. Bact.*, **79**, 193–201.

Jones-Williams, W., Erasmus, D.A., James, E.M.V. and Davies, T. (1970) The fine structure of sarcoid and tuberculous granulomas. *Postgrad. Med. J.*, **46** 496–500.

Jones-Williams, W., Erasmus, D.A., Jenkins, D., James E.M.V. and Davies, T. (1971) A comparative study of the ultrastructure and histochemistry of sarcoid and tuberculous granulomas. In *Proc. 5th International Conference on Sarcoidosis* (eds. L. Levinsky and A. Macholda), Universita Karlova, Prague, pp. 115–23.

Jones-Williams, W., Pioli, E., Jones, D.J., Calcraft, B., Johnson, A.J. and Dighero, M. (1974) *In vitro* Kveim-induced macrophage inhibition factor in sarcoidosis, Crohn's disease and tuberculosis. In *Proc. 6th International Conference on Sarcoidosis, Tokyo*, (eds. K. Iwai and Y. Hosoda), University of Tokyo Press, Tokyo, pp. 44–50.

Jones-Williams, W., Pioli, E., Jones, D.J. and Dighero, M.(1972) The Kmif (Kveim-induced macrophage migration inhibition factor) test in sarcoidosis. *J. Clin. Pathol.*, **25**, 951–3.

Jones-Williams, W., Seal, R.E.M., Davies, K.J. and Chapman, J.S. (1976) International Kveim histology trial. *Ann. NY Acad. Sci*, **278**, 687–99.

Jones-Williams, W. and Williams, D. (1967) Residual bodies in sarcoid and sarcoid-like granulomas. *J. Clin. Pathol.*, **20**, 574–7.

Jordan, J.W. and Darke, C.S. (1958) Chronic beryllium poisoning. *Thorax*, **13**, 69–71.

Jordon, J.W. and Osborne, E.D. (1937) Besnier–Boeck's disease: report of two cases with extensive involvement. *Arch. Dermatol. Syphilol., NY,* **35**, 663–84.

Jörgensen, G. (1963a) Sarkoidose und Bronchialkarzinom. *Tuberkulosearzt,* **17**, 708–12.

Jörgensen, G. (1963b) Sarkoidose und Schwangerschaft. *Beitr. Klin. Tuberk. Spezifischen Tuberk-Forsch.,* **127**, 605–8.

Jörgensen, G. (1964a) Sarkoidose und B.C.G.-Impfung. *Prax. Pneumol.,* **18**, 25–8.

Jörgensen, G. (1964b) Die genetik der Sarkoidose. *Acta Med. Scand.,* Suppl. **425**, 213–5.

Jörgensen, G. and Wurm, K. (1964) Die Blutgruppen bei der Sarkoidose. *Acta Med. Scand.,* Suppl. **425**, 213–5.

Joulia, P., Lecoulant, P., Petges, A., Texier, L. and Fruchard, J. (1956) Maladie de Besnier–Boeck–Schaumann à type de sarcoïdes à petits éléments trés profus: régression presque compléte après un mois de traitment par la vitamine C à hautes doses. *Bull. Soc. Fr. Dermatol. Syphiligr.,* **63**, 495.

Jüngling, O. (1920) Ostitis tuberculosa multiplex cystica (eine eigenartige Form der Knochentuberkulose). *Fortschr. Geb. Roentgenstr.,* **27**, 375–83.

Jüngling, O. (1928) Über Ostitis tuberculosa multiplex cystoides, zugleich ein Beitrag zur Lehre von der Tuberkuliden des Knochens. *Beitr. Klin. Chirug.,* **143**, 401–75.

Kadin, M.E., Donaldson, S.S. and Dorfman, R.F. (1970) Isolated granulomas in Hodgkin's disease. *N. Engl. J. Med.,* **283**, 859–61.

Kahan, A., (1952) Sarcoidosis with involvement of the central nervous system. *Proc. R. Soc. Med.,* **45**, 509.

Kahn, L.B. Gordon, W. and Camp, R. (1974) Florid sarcoid reaction associated with lymphoma of the skin. *Cancer,* **33**, 1117–22.

Kalbian, V.V. (1957) Bronchial involvement in pulmonary sarcoidosis. *Thorax,* **12**, 18–23.

Kalden, J.R., Becker, F.W., Krull, P. and Deicher, H. (1974) The *in vitro* Kveim reaction in sarcoidosis and other diseases. In *Proc. 6th International Conference on Sarcoidosos, Tokyo,* (eds. K. Iwai and Y. Hosoda), University of Tokyo Press, Tokyo, pp. 39–41.

Kalkoff, K.W. and Ehring, F. (1948) Zur Rückbildung tuberkulöser Hauterscheinungen bei progredienter Lungentuberkulose. *Strahlentherapie,* **77**, 359–70.

Kämpfer, R. (1964) Über extrapulmonale Organmanifestationen des Morbus Boeck unter besonderer Berucksichtigung der Schleimhaut der oberen Luftwege. *Prax. Pneumol.,* **18**, 204–17.

Kantor, F.S., Dwyer, J.M. and Mangi, R.J. (1976) Sarcoid. *J. Invest. Dermatol.* **67**, 470–6.

Kaplan, H. and Klatskin, G. (1960) Sarcoidosis, psoriasis and gout: syndrome or coincidence? *Yale J. Biol. Med.,* **32**, 335–52.

Kaplan, J., Johns, C.J. (1979) Mycetomas in pulmonary sarcoidosis: non-surgical management. *Johns Hopkins Med. J.,* **145**, 157–61.

Karlish, A.J. (1967) Measurements of Kveim specific nodules in sarcoidosis. In *Proc. 9th Interntational Conference on Sarcoidosis, Paris,* (eds. J.A. Chetien, J. Marcac and J.C. Saltiel), Pergamon Press, Oxford, pp. 176–80.

Karlish, A.J. (1971) The effect of steroids on the development of the Kveim reaction. In *Proc. 5th International Conference on Sarcoidosis, Prague, 1969,* (eds. L. Levinsky and F. Macholda), Universita Karlova, Prague, pp. 357–70.

Karlish, A.J., Cox, E.V., Hampson, F. and Hemsted, E.H. (1970) Kveim test in Crohn's disease. *Lancet*, 2, 977–8.

Karlish, A.J. and MacGregor, G.A. (1970) Sarcoidosis, thyroiditis and Addison's disease. *Lancet*, 2, 330–3.

Karlish, A.J., Thompson, R.P.H., Williams, R. (1969) A case of sarcoidosis and primary biliary cirrhosis. *Lancet*, 2, 599.

Karma, A. (1979) Ophthalmic changes in sarcoidosis. *Acta. Ophthalmol.*, Suppl. 141, 1–94.

Kataria, Y. P. (1980) Chlorambucil in sarcoidosis. *Chest*, 78, 36–43.

Kataria, Y.P. and Glauss, K.R. (1978) Sarcoidosis: phytohaemagglutinin response of lymphocyte fractions isolated by velocity sedimentation and enhanced helper-cell activity. *Am. Rev. Respir. Dis.* 117, 519–26.

Kataria, Y.P., LoBuglio, A.F. Helentjaris, T. and Bromberg, P.A. (1975) Phyto-haemagglutin skin test in patients with sarcoidosis. *Am. Rev. Respir. Dis.*, 112, 575–8.

Kataria, Y.P., Sagoni, A.L., LoBuglio, A.F. and Bromberg, P.A. (1973) *In vitro* observations of sarcoid lymphoytes and their correlation with cutaneous anergy and clinical severity. *Am. Rev. Respir. Dis.*, 108, 767–76.

Kataria, Y.P., Sharma, O.M., Israel, H. and Rogers, M. (1980) Kveim antigen CRI. In *Proc. 8th International Conference on Sarcoidosis, Cardiff, 1978* (eds. W. Jones-Williams and B.H. Davies), Alpha Omega, Cardiff, pp. 660–7.

Kataria, Y.P. and Whitcomb, M.E. (1980) Splenomegaly in sarcoidosis. *Arch. Intern. Med.*, 140, 35–7.

Kataria, Y.P., Zafranas, A. and Sharma, H.M. (1978) Immunohistochemistry of human cutaneous sarcoidosis: a study of 9 cases. *Hum. Pathol.*, 9, 517–22.

Kater, R.M.H. and Stening, G.F.H. (1967) Gastric sarcoidosis. *Aust. NZ J. Surg.*, 37, 174–6.

Katsouros, T. (1971) Mittellappenatelktase bei Sarkoidose. *Prx. Pneumol.*, 25, 478–82.

Katz, D.H. and Benacerrat, B. (1972) The regulatory influence of activated T- cells on B-cell responsiveness to antigen. *Adv. Immunol.*, 15, 1–94.

Katz, P. and Fauci, A.S. (1978) Ingibition of polyclonal B-cell activation by suppres-sor monocytes in patients with sarcoidosis. *Clin. Exp. Immunol.*, 32, 554–62.

Katz, P. and Fauci, A.S. (1979) The effect of corticosteroids on immunoregulation in sarcoidosis. *Cell. Immunol.*, 42, 308–18.

Katz, P., Haynes, B.F. and Fauci, A. (1978) Alteration of T. lymphocyte subpopula-tions in sarcoidosis. *Clin. Immunol. Innunopathol.*, 10, 350–4.

Kaugh, Y.C., Goody, H.E. and Luscombe, H.A. (1978) Ichthyosiform sarcoidosis. *Arch. Dermatol.*, 114, 100–1.

Kay, S. (1950) Sarcoidosis of spleen: report of 4 cases with 23-year follow-up in one case. *Am. J. Pathol.*, 26, 427–43.

Kay, S. (1956) Sarcoidosis of the Fallopian tubes: report of a case. *J. Obstet. Gynaecol. Br. Emp.*, 63, 871–4.

Kean, B.H. and Koekenga, M.T. (1952) Giant-cell myocarditis. *Am. J. Pathol.*, 28, 1095–105.

Keating, J.P., Weissbluth, M., Ratzaan, S.K. and Barton, L.L. (1973) Familial sarcoidosis. *Am. J. Dis. Child.*, 126, 644–7.

Kelemen, J.T. and Mandi, L. (1969) Sarcoidose in der Placenta. *Zentralbl. Allg. Pathol., Pathol. Anat.*, 112, 18–21.

Keller, A.Z. (1971) Hospital, age, racial, occupational, geographical, clinical and survivorship characteristics in the epidemiology of sarcoidosis. *Am. J. Epide-miol.*, 94, 222–30.

Keller, A.Z. (1973) Anatomic sties, age attributes and rates of sarcoidosis in US veterans. *Am. Rev. Respir. Dis.,* 107, 615–20.

Keller, A.Z. and Dunner, E., (1967) Inquiry into the epidemiologica aspects of sarcoidosis. In *Proc. 4th International Conference on Sarcoidosis, Paris* (eds. J. Turiaf and J. Chabot), Masson, Paris, pp. 319–25.

Kelley, J.S. and Green, W.R. (1973) Sarcoidosis involving the optic nerve head. *Arch. Ophthalmol.,* 89, 486–8.

Kelley, M.L., Jr. and McHardy, R.J. (1955) An unusual case of fatal hepatic sarcoidosis. *Am. J. Med.,* 18, 842–50.

Kelly, A.P. (1978) Ichthyosiform sarcoid. *Arch. Dermatol.,* 114, 1551–2.

Kendig, E.L. (1974) The clinical picture of sarcoidosis in children. *Pediatrics,* 54, 289–92.

Kendig, E.L. and Brummer, D.L. (1976) The prognosis of sarcoidosis in children. *Chest,* 70, 351–3.

Kennedy, C. (1976) Sarcoidosis presenting in tattoos. *Clin. Exp. Dermatol.,* 1, 395–9.

Kennedy, W.P.U. (1967) An evaluation of freeze-dried Kveim reagent. *Br. J. Dis Chest,* 61, 40–4.

Kenney, M. and Stone, D.J. (1963) Objective evaluation of the Kveim test in a 'double-blind' study. *Am. Rev. Respir. Dis.,* 87, 504–8.

Kent, D.C. (1965) Recurrent unilateral hilar adenopathy in sarcoidosis. *Am. Rev. Respir. Dis.,* 91, 272–6.

Kent, D.C., Houk, V.N., Elliott, R.C., Sokolowski, J.W., Baker, J.H. and Sorensen, K. (1970) The definitive evaluation of sarcoidosis. *Am. Rev. Respir. Dis.,* 101, 721–7.

Kent, D.C. and Schwarz, R. (1967) Active pulmonary tuberculosis with negative tuberculin skin reactions. *Am. Rev. Respir. Dis.,* 95, 411–8.

Keogh, B.A. and Crystal, R.G. (1980) Clinical significance of pulmonary function testing in interstitial pulmonary disease. *Chest,* 78, 857–65.

Keogh, B.A. and Crystal, R.G. (1982) Alveolitis: the key to the interstitial lung disorders. *Thorax,* 37, 1–10.

Keogh, B.A., Hunninghake, G.W., Line, B.R. and Crystal, R.G. (1983) The alveolitis of pulmonary sarcoidosis: evaluation of natural history and alveolitis dependent changes in lung function. *Am. Rev. Respir. Dis.,* 128, 256–65.

Kerbrat, G. and Cellerier, R. (1954) Altérnance d'une tubérculose pulmonaire et d'une maladie de Besnier–Boeck–Schaumann. *J. Fr. Med. Chir. Thorac.,*8, 266–70.

Kerley, P. (1942) The significance of the radiological manifestations of erythema nodosum. *Br. J. Radiol.,* 15, 155–65.

Kerley, P. (1943) The aetiology of erythema nodosum. *Br. J. Radiol.* 16, 199–204.

Kerley, P. and Twining, E.W. (1951) *A Textbook of X-ray Diagnosis,* 2nd Edn, Lewis, London, vol. 2, 526.

Khan, K., Perillie, P.E. and Finch, S.C. (1973) Serum lysozyme in pulmonary tuberculosis. *Am. J. Med. Sci.,* 265, 297–302.

Khan, L.B., Gordon, W. and Camp, R. (1974) Florid sarcoid reaction associated with lymphoma of the skin. *Cancer,* 33, 1117–122.

Khan, M.M. Gill, D.S. and McConkey, B. (1981) Myopathy and external pulmonary artery compression caused by sarcoidosis. *Thorax,* 36, 703–4.

Khoury, F., Teasdale, P.R., Smith, L., Jones, O.G. and Carter, J.R. (1979) Angiotensin-converting enzyme in sarcoidosis: a British study. *Br. J. Dis. Chest,* 73, 382–8.

Kienböck, R. (1901) Zur radiographischen Anatomie und Klinik der syphilitischen Knochenerkrankengen an Extremitaten. *Z. Heilk. (Chirurg),* 23, 103–85.

Kimberg, D.V. (1969) Effects of vitamin D and steroid hormones on the active transport of calcium by the intestine. *N. Engl. J. Med.*, 280, 1936–45.

Kimberg, D.V., Baerg, R.D., Gershon, E. and Grandusius B.T. (1971) Effect of cortisone treatment on the active transport of calcium by the small intestine. *J. Clin. Invest.*, 50, 1309–21.

Kimbrell, O.C., Jr. (1957) Sarcoidosis of the spleen. *N. Engl. J. Med.*, 257–61.

King, B.P., Esparza, A.R., Kahn, S.I. and Garella, S. (1976) Sarcoid granulomatous nephritis occurring as isolated renal failure. *Arch. Intern. Med.*, 136, 241–5.

Kinney, E.L., Jackson, G.L., Rceves, W.C., Zeiss, R. and Beers, E. (1980) Thallium-scan myocardial defects and echocardiographic abnormalities in patients with sarcoidosis without clinical cardiac dysfunction. *Am. J. Med.*, 68, 497–503.

Kirkham, T.H. (1973) Neuro-ophthalmic presentations of sarcoidosis. *Proc. R. Soc. Med.*, 66, 167–9.

Kirks, D.R., McCormick, V.D. and Greenspan, R.H., (1973) Pulmonary sarcoidosis: roentgenologic analysis of 150 patients. *Am. J. Roentgenol.*, 117, 777–86.

Kirschner, B.S. and Holinger, P.H. (1976) Laryngeal obstruction in childhood sarcoidosis. *J. Pediatr.* 88, 263–5.

Kirshbaum, J.D. and Levy, H.A. (1941) Tuberculoma of hypophysis with insufficiency of anterior lobe: study of 2 cases. *Arch. Intern. Med.*, 68, 1095–104.

Klassen, K.P., Anlyan, A.J. and Curtis, G.M. (1949) Biopsy of diffuse pulmonary lesions. *Arch. Surg.*, 59, 694–704.

Klatskin, G. (1976) Hepatic granulomata problems in interpretation. *Ann. NY. Acad. Sci.* 278, 427–32.

Klatskin, G. and Gordon, M. (1953) Renal complications of sarcoidosis and their relationship to hypercalcemia; with a report of 2 cases simulating hyperparathyroidism. *Am. J. Med.*, 15, 484–98.

Klatskin, G. and Yesner, R. (1950) Hepatic manifestations of sarcoidosis and other granulomatous disease. *Yale J. Biol. Med.*, 23, 207–48.

Klauder, J.V. (1953) Sarcoid of the eyelids, conjunctiva, and uveal tract treated with quinacrine hydrochlorine. *Arch. Dermatol. Syphilol.*, NY 68, 474.

Klein, K. and Lehotan, A. (1952) Thrombopenische Purpura und Sarkoidose der Milz. *Schweiz. Med. Wochenschr.*, 82, 927–8.

Kleinberg, D.L., Noel, G.L. and Franz, A.G. (1977) Galactorrhoea: a study of 235 cases. including 48 with pituitary tumours. *N. Engl. J. Med.*, 296, 589–600.

Klinefelter, H.F., Jr. and Salley, S.M. (1946) Sarcoidosis simulating glomerulonephrits. *Bull. Johns Hopkins Hosp.*, 89, 333–41.

Klockars, M. and Selroos, O. (1977) Immunohistochemical demonstration of lysozyme in the lymph nodes and Kveim reaction papules in sarcoidosis. *Acta Pathol. Microbiol Scand., Sect. A.*, 85, 169–73.

Knapp, F.N. and Knott, W.W. (1949) Sarcoid involving the orbit. *Trans. Am. Ophthalmol. Soc.*, 47, 147–57.

Kneppers, F., Mueller-Eekhardt, C., Heinrich, O., Schawb, B. and Boachertz, D. (1979) HLA antigens of patients with sarcoidosis. *Tissue Antigens*, 4, 56–8.

Knodel, A.R. and Beekman, J.F. (1980) Severe thrombocytopenia and sarcoidosis. *J. Am. Med. Assoc.*, 243, 258–9.

Knoop, R. (1958) Malakoplakia: oversigt og beskrivaeke af det forste tilfaeldgei Danmark. *Ugeskr. Laeg.*, 120, 498–504.

Kobayashi, F. (1974) The incidence and course of ocular lesion in sarcoidosis. In *Proc. 6th International Conference on Sarcoidosis, Tokyo* (eds. K. Iwai and Y. Hosoda), University of Tokyo Press, Tokyo, pp. 349–53.

Koch, M.L., Cote, R.H. (1965) Comparison of fluorescence acid-fast bacilli in smear preparations and tissue sections. *Am. Rev. Respir. Dis.*, 91, 283–4.

Koerner, S.K., Sakowitz, A.J., Appleman, R.I., Becker, N.H. and Schoenbaum, S.W. (1975) Transbronchial lung biopsy for the diagnosis of sarcoidosis. *N. Engl. J. Med.,* **223,** 268–70.

Kohn, N.N. (1980) Sarcoidosis of the colon. *J. Med. Soc. N. J.* **77,** 517–8.

Kohout, J. (1976a) Passive transfer of tuberculin sensitivity in sarcoidosis. *Pneumologie,* **153,** 217–21.

Kohout, J. (1976b) Macrophage reactivity in skin window of sarcoidosis patients. *Ann. NY Acad. Sci.* **278,** 201–3.

Kolodny, E.H., Rebeiz, J.J. Caviness, V.S. and Richardson, E.P. (1968) Granulomatous angiitis of the central nervous system. *Arch. Neurol.,* **19,** 510–24.

Kömpf, D., Neudörfer, B., Kayser-Gatachalin, C., Meyer-Wahl, L. and Ranft, K. (1976) Mononeuritis multiplex bei Boeckscher sarkoidose. *Nervenarzt,* **47,** 687–9.

Konda, J., Ruth, M., Sassaris, M. and Hunter, F.M. (1980) Sarcoidosis of the stomach and rectum. *Am. J. Gastroenterol.,* **73,** 516–8.

Konstantin-Hansen, K.K. and Arentsen, J. (1981) Cerebral sarcoidosis and fresh toxoplasmosis in the same case. *Ugeskr. Laeg.,* **143,** 344–5.

Kooij, R. (1958) On the nature of the Kveim reaction and the pathogenesis of sarcoidosis. *Dermatologica,* **117,** 336–54.

Kooij, R. (1964) The nature of the Kveim reaction (1959) *Acta Med. Scand.,* Suppl. **425,** 79–82.

Kooij, R. and Gerritsen, T. (1958) On the nature of the Mitsuda and the Kveim reaction. *Dermatologica,* **116,** 1–27.

Kooij, R., Ruitenberg, E.J., Sirks, J.L., Stam, J. and Meyer, S. (1976) Experience with a Dutch Kveim suspension in men and guinea pigs. *Ann. NY Acad. Med.,* **276,** 717–21.

Korn, R.J., Kellow, W.F., Heller, P., Chomet, B. and Zimmerman, H.J. (1959) Hepatic involvement in extrapulmonary tuberculosis. *Am. J. Med.* **27,** 60–71.

Kossmann, F. (1959) Morbus Besnier–Boeck–Schaumann des Magens, *Med. Klin. Munich,* **54,** 1011–3.

Kovnat, P.J. and Donohue, R.F. (1965) Sarcoidosis involving the pleura, *Ann. Intern. Med.,* **62,** 120–4.

Kozmin-Sokolow, B.N. and Kostina, Z.I. (1971) Discovery of myocobacteriophages in patients with tuberculosis and sarcoidosis. *Probl. Tuberk.,* **49,** 74–5.

Krabbe, K.H. (1949) Muscular localisation of benign lymphogranulomatosis. *Acta Med. Scand.,* Suppl. **234,** 193–8.

Kraus, E.J. (1942) Sarcoidosis (Besnier–Boeck–Schaumann disease) as cause of pituitary syndrome. *J. Lab. Clin. Med.,* **28,** 104–6.

Krauss, L. (1958) Genital sarcoidosis: case report and review of the literature. *J. Urol.,* **80,** 367–70.

Kreibich, K. (1904) Über Lupus pernio. *Arch. Dermatol. Syph., Wien,* **71,** 3–16.

Kreibich, K. and Kraus, A. (1908) Beitrage zur Kenntnis des Boeckschen benignen Miliarlupoid. *Arch. Dermatol. Syph., Wien,* **92,** 173–204.

Kremer, H., Schucharnd, J., Zonnchen, B. and Prechtel, K. (1975) Extreme Thrombzytopenie bei Sakoidose. *Muench. Med. Wochenschr.,* **117,** 1479–82.

Kremer, R.M. and Williams, J.S. (1970). Gastric sarcoidosis. *Ann. Surg.,* **36,** 686–90.

Kroll, J.J., Shapiro, L., Koplan, B.S. and Feldman, F. (1972) Subcutaneous sarcoidosis with calcification. *Arch. Dermatol.,* **106,** 894–5.

Kryger, J. and Ronnov-Jensen, X. (1959) Myopathy in Boeck's sarcoid. *Acta. Rheum. Scand.,* **5,** 314–22.

Kueppers, F., Mueller-Eckhardt, C., Heinrich, D., Schwab, B. and Brachertz, D. (1974) HLA antigens of patients with sarcoidosis. *Tissue Antigens,* 4, 56–8.

Kulka, W.E. (1950) Sarcoidosis of the heart: a cause of sudden and unexpected death. *Circulation,* 1, 772–6.

Kumpe, D.A., Rao, C.V.G.K., Garcia, J.H. and Heck, A.F.(1979) Intracranial neurosarcoidosis. *J. Computer Assisted Tomography,* 3, 329–30.

Kung, P.C., Goldstein, G. (1980) Functional and developmental compartments of human T-lymphocytes. *Vox Sang.,* 39, 121–7.

Kung, P.C., Goldstein, G., Reinherz, E.L. and Schlossman, S.F. (1979) Monoclonal antibodies defining distincive human T-cell surface antigens. *Science,* 206, 347–9.

Kunkel, H.G., Simon, H.J. and Fudenberg, H. (1958) Observations concerning positive serologic reactions for rheumatoid factor in certain patients with sarcoidosis and other hyperglobulinemic states. *Arthritis and Rheum.* 1, 289–96.

Kunkel, P. C. and Yesner, R. (1950) Thrombocytopenic purpura associated with sarcoid granulomas of spleen. *Arch. Pathol.,* 50, 778–86.

Kurn, R.J., Kellow, W.F., Heller, P., Chomet, B. and Zimmerman, H.J., (1959) Hepatic involvement in extrapulmonary tuberculosis. *Am. J. Med.,* 27, 60–71.

Kurti, V. and Mankiewicz, E. (1972) *In vitro* study of macrophages from patients with sarcoidosis. *Can. Med. Assoc. J.* 107, 509–15.

Kuzel, W.C., Schaffarzick, R.W., Naugler, W.E. Koets, P., Mankle, E.A., Brown, B. and Camplin, B. (1955) Some observations on 520 gouty patients. *J. Chron. Dis.,* 2, 645–69.

Kuznitzky, E. and Bittorf, A. (1915) Boecksches Sarkoid mit Beteiligung innerer Organe. *Müench. Med. Wochenschr.,* 62, 1349–53.

Kveim, A. (1941) En ny og specifikk kutan-reaksjon ved Boecks sarcoid. *Nord. Med.,* 9, 169–72.

Kyrle, J. (1921) Die Anfangsstadien des Boeckschen Lupoids: Beitrag zur Frage der tuberkulösen Aetiologie dieser Dermatose. *Arch. Dermatol. Syph., Berlin,* 131, 33–68.

Lacher, M.J. (1968) Spontaneous remission or response to methotrexate in sarcoidosis. *Ann. Intern. Med.,* 69, 1247–8.

Lacronique, J., Bernaudin, J.F., Soler, P., Lange, F., Kawanami, O., Saumon, G., Georges, R. and Basset, F. (1983) Alveolitis and granulomas: sequential course in pulmonary sarcoidosis. In *Proc. 9th International Conference on Sarcoidosis, Paris,* Pergamon Press, Oxford, pp. 36–42.

Lafou, R., Pages, P., Passouant, P., Labauge, R., Minvielle, J. and Pages, A. (1955) Localisations musculaires de la maladie de Besnier–Boeck–Schaumann. A propos de 3 observations. *Rev. Neurol.,* 92, 557–63.

Landers, P.H. (1949) Vitreous lesions observed in Boeck's sarcoid. *Am. J. Ophthalmol.* 32, 1740–1.

Langhammer, H., Glaubitt, G., Grebc, S.F., Hampe, J.F., Haubold, U., Hör, G., Kaul, A., Koeppe, P., Koppenhagen, J., Roedler, H.D. and van der Schoot, J.B. (1972) ^{67}Ga for tumour scanning. *J. Nucl. Med.,* 13, 25–30.

Larbaqui, D. and Lazib, A. (1977) La sarcoïdose médiastinopulmonaire existe-t-elle dans les pays á haute prévalence tuberculeuse? *Z. Erkr. Atmungsorgane,* 149, 67–74

Laroche, C., Gennes, J.L., de, Hazard, J. and Samarcqu, P. (1955) Maladie de Besnier–Boeck–Schaumann avec manifestations polyarticulaires et localisations endomyopéricadiarques mortelles. *Bull. Soc. Med. Hôp., Paris,* 71, 908–13.

Larsen, A.K. (1950) Kan dobbetsidig hilusadenitis framkaldes af Calmette-vaccination? *Nord. Med.*, 43, 170.

Larsson, L.G. (1951) Nasopharyngeal lesions in sarcoidosis. *Acta. Radiol.*, 36, 361–73.

Larsson, L.G., Liljestrand, A. and Wahlund, H. (1952) Treatment of sarcoidosis with calciferol. *Acta. Med. Scand.*, 143, 380–7.

Lash, R., Coker, J. and Wong., B.Y.S. (1979) Treatment of heart block due to sarcoid heart disease. *J. Electrocardiol.* (San Diego), 12, 325–9.

Lathan, S.R., Block, R.A. and McLean, R.L. (1968) Sarcoidosis with metastatic calcification. *Am. J. Med.*, 44, 1000–4.

Laties, A.M. and Scheie, H.G. (1972) Evolution of multiple small tumours in sarcoid granuloma of the optic disc. *Am. J. Ophthalmol.* 74, 60–7.

Laugier, P. and Ledoux, A. (1958) Maladies de Besnier–Boeck–Schaumann, avec manifestations cutanées et pulmonaires, rapidement améliorées par la vitamine C à haute dose. *Bull. Soc. Fr. Dermatol. Syphiligr.* 65, 201–3.

Laval, J. (1952) Ocular sarcoidosis. *Am. J. Ophthalmol.*, 35, 551–4.

Lavender, J.P., Lower, J., Barker, J.R., Burn, J.I. and Chaudri, M.A., (1971) Gallium-67 citrate scanning in neoplastic and inflammatory lesions. *Br. J. Radiol.*, 45, 361–6.

Lawrence, H.S. (1949) The cellular transfer of cutaneous hypersensitivity to tuberculin in man. *Proc. Soc. Exp. Biol.*, 71, 516.

Lawrence, H.S. (1959) Homograft sensitivity. An expression of the immunologic origins and consequences of individuality. *Physiol. Rev.* 39, 811–59.

Lawrence, H.S. (1969) Transfer factor. *Adv. Immunol.*, 11, 195–266.

Lawrence, H.S. (1970) Transfer factor and cellular immune deficiency disease. *N. Engl. J. Med.*, 283, 411–9.

Lawrence, H.S. and Zweiman, B. (1968) Transfer factor deficiency response: a mechanism of anergy in Boeck's sarcoid. *Trans. Assoc. Am. Physicians.*, 81, 240–8.

Lawrence, W.P., El Gammal, T., Pool, W.H. and Apter, L. (1974) Radiological manifestations of neurosarcoidosis: report of 3 cases. *Clin. Radiol.*, 25, 343–8.

Leake, E.S. and Myrvik, Q.N. (1971) Osmiophilic structures in granulomatous macrophages and the problem of intracellular mycobacteria. *Am. Rev. Respir. Dis.*, 104, 132–3.

Lebacq, E. (1964) *La Sarcoidose de Besnier–Boeck–Schaumann:* Brussels, Editions Arscia; Libraire Maloine, Paris, pp. 132–40.

Lebacq, E. (1970) Perturbations du métabolisme calcique dans la sarcoïdose. *Poumon Coeur*, 36, 799–813.

Lebacq, E., Desmet, G., and Verhaegen, H. (1970) Renal involvement in sarcoidosis. *Postgrad. Med. J.*, 46, 526–9.

Lebacq, E.G., Henrion, J. and Meyeur, S. (1977) Hypercalciuria in sarcoidosis. *Z. Erkr. Atmungsorgane*, 219–23.

Lebacq, E.G., Henrion, J., Mayeur, S. and Lambert, M, (1980) Hypercalciuria in sarcoidosis patients with normocalcaemia: pathogenesis and treatment. In *Proc. 8th International Conference on Sarcoidosis, Cardiff, 1978,* (eds. W. Jones-Williams and B.H. Davies), Alpha Omega, Cardiff, pp. 215–9.

Lebacq, E., Pluygers, E. and Tirzmalis, A. (1956a) Sarcoïdose de foie et de la rate. *Rev. Med. -Chir. Mal. Foie*, 31, 31–54.

Lebacq, E., Tirzmalis, A., Mairiaux, E. and Pluygers, E. (1956b) Sarcoidose de Besnier–Boeck–Schauman avec anémie hémolytique par auto-immunisation. *Bull. Soc. Med. Hôp.*, Paris, 72, 614–20.

Lee, J.Q. and Lee, W.K. (1974) The search for sarcoidosis in Korea. In *Proc. 6th International Conference on Sarcoidosis, Tokyo* (eds. K. Iwai and Y. Hosoda), Unversity of Tokyo Press, Tokyo, pp. 307–8.

Lee, S.M. and Michael, A.F. (1978) Focal glomerular sclerosis and sarcoidosis. *Arch. Pathol. Lab. Med.*, 102, 572–5.

Lees, A.W. (1956) Tuberculin-negative tuberculosis presenting as sarcoidosis. *Lancet*, 2, 56–8.

Lehmuskallio, E., Hannuksela, M. and Halme, H. (1977) The liver in sarcoidosis. *Acta Med. Scand.*, 202, 289–93.

Leider, M. and Sulzberger, M.B. (1949) Studies in the allergy of infections: responses of the skin to BCG vaccination in various categories of tuberculin sensitivity. *J. Invest. Dermatol.*, 13, 249–64.

Leider, M. and Hyman, A.B. (1950) Histological responses of the skin to BCG vaccination in various categories of tuberculin sensitivity. *J. Invest. Dermatol.* 14, 459–470.

Leithold, S.L., Reeder, P.S. and Baker, L.A. (1957) Crytococcal infection treated with 2-hydroxystilbamidine in a patient with Boeck's sarcoid. *Arch. Intern. Med.*, 99, 736–43.

Leitner, S.J. (1946) Neue Untersuchungen beim Morbus Besnier–Boeck–Schaumann (epithelioidzellige Granulomatose), *Schweiz. Z. Tuberk. Pneumonol.*, 3, 108.

Leitner, S.J. (1949) *Der Morbus Besnier–Boeck–Schaumann, Basel*, 2nd edn., Pitman, London, 76.

Leitner, S.J. (1950) Boeck's sarcoidosis. *Tubercle*, 31, 174–83.

Lemming, R. (1940a) An attempt to analyse the tuberculin anergy of Schaumann's disease and uveo-parotid fever by means of BCG vaccination. *Acta Med. Scand.*, 103, 400–29.

Lemming, R. (1940b) Morbus Schaumann-liknanade fall med larynxforundringar och med overgang i en egendomlig form av tuberculos. *Nord. Med.*, 8, 2750.

Lemming, R. (1942) Development of Boeck's sarcoid at the place of the skin where BCG vaccination has been made in a case of Schaumann's disease. *Acta Med. Scand.*, 110, 151–60.

Lenartowicz, J. and Rothfeld, J. (1930) Ein Fall von Hautsarkoiden (Darier-Roussy) mit identischen Veranderungen im Gehirn und den inneren Organen. *Arch. Dermatol. Syph., Wien*, 161, 504–19.

Lender, M. and Dallberg, L. (1974) Coincidence of sarcoidosis and Hashimoto's thyroiditis. *Am. Rev. Respir. Dis.*, 112, 113–7.

Leng-Levy, J., David-Chaussé, J., Martin-Dupont, C., Aparicio, M. and Milliez, P. (1965) Maladie de Besnier–Boeck–Schaumann à localisation rénale. *Bull. Soc. Med. Hôp., Paris*, 116, 907–11.

Lenzini, L., Heather, C.J. and Rottoli, L. (1980) Bronchoalveolar cells in humans: II General morphology and ultrastructure of pulmonary macrophages and small mononuclear cells in sarcoidosis. *Respiration*, 40, 81–93.

Lenzini, L., Heather, C.J., Rottoli, L. and Rottoli, P. (1978) Studies on bronchoalveolar cells in humans: I Preliminary morphological studies in various respiratory diseases. *Respiration*, 36, 145–52.

Leophante, P., Dutau, G., Boissou, H., Durroux, R. and Delaude, A. (1972) Sarcoïdose et phéochromocytome surrénalien. *Poumon Coeur*, 28, 333–7.

Lepow, H., Rubenstein, L., Chu, F. and Shandra, J. (1957) A case of Cryptococcus neoformans meningoencephalitis complicating Boeck's sarcoid. *Pediatrics*, 19, 377–86.

Leppard (1971) Sarcoidosis and hyperthyroidism. *Proc. R. Soc. Med.,* **64,** 396.

Lesné, E., Launay, C. and Sée, G. (1935) Diabète insipide au cours d'une maladie de Besnier–Boeck. *Bull. Soc. Med. Hôp., Paris,* **51,** 1137–46.

Leuke, E.S. and Myrvik, Q.N. (1972) Rosette arrangement of electron dense structures in granulomatous alveolar macrophages. *J. Reticuloendothel. Soc.* **12,** 305–13.

Letocha, C.E., Shields, J.A. and Goldberg, R.E. (1975) Retinal changes in sarcoidosis. *Can. J. Ophthalmol.,* **10,** 184–92.

Levin, P.N. (1935) The neurological aspects of uveo-parotid fever. *J.Nerv. Ment. Dis.,* **81,** 176–91.

Levine, B.W., Saldena, M. and Hutter, A.M. (1971) Pulmonary hypertension in sarcoidosis. *Am. Rev. Respir. Dis.,* **103,** 413–7.

Levinsky, L., Cummiskey, J., Rømer, F.K., Wurm, K., Buss, J., Dövken, H., Steinbrüek, P., Zaumseil, P., Jaroszewiez, W., Mándi, L., Szegdy, G., Centea, A., Burilkov, T., Blasi, A., Olivieri, D., Maviani, B., Bisetti, A., Goodman, S., Djuriě, B., Lazaroo, P. and Celikoǧlu, S.I, (1976) Sarcoidosis in Europe. *Ann. NY Acad. Med.,* **278,** 335–46.

Levinson, R.S., Metzger, L.F., Stanley, N.N., Kelsen, S.G., Altose, M.D., Cherniak, N.S. and Brody, J.S. (1977) Airway function in sarcoidosis. *Am. J. Med.,* **62,** 51–9.

Levitt, J.M. (1941) Boeck's sarcoid with ocular localisation. *Arch. Ophthalmol.,* **26,** 358–88.

Lewis, J.G. (1961) The evolution of sarcoidosis into caseating tuberculosis of the lungs and skin. *Tubercle,* **42,** 95–100.

Lewis, J.G. (1964a) Distribution of O and A blood groups in sarcoidosis. *Postgrad. Med. J.,* **40,** 722–4.

Lewis, J.G. (1964b) Eosinophilic granuloma and its variants with special reference to lung involvement. *Q. J. Med.,* **33,** 337–58.

Lewis, J.G. and Woods, A.C. (1961) The ABO and rhesus blood groups in patients with respiratory disease. *Tubercle,* **42,** 362–5.

Licharew, W. (1908) Moskauer venereologische und dermatologische Gesellschaft. 8 December 1907. *Derm. Zbl.,* **11,** 235.

Lichtenstein, E. (1953) Histiocytosis X. *Arch. Pathol.,* **56,** 84–102.

Lichtman, A.L., McDonald, J.R., Dixon, C.F. and Mann, F.C. (1946) Talc granuloma. *Surg. Gynecol., Obstet.,* **83,** 531–46.

Liddle, G.W., Estep, H.L., Kendall, J.W., Jr. and Townes, A.W. (1959) Clinical application of a new test of pituitary reserve. *J. Clin. Endocrinol.,* **19,** 875.

Lieberman, J. (1975) Elevation of serum angiotensin converting enzyme (ACE) level in sarcoidosis. *Am. J. Med.,* **59,** 365–72.

Lieberman, J., Nosal, A., Schlessner, L.A. and Sastre-Foker, A. (1979) Serum angiotensin-converting enzyme for diagnosis and therapeutic evaluation of sarcoidosis. *Am. Rev. Respir. Dis.,* **120,** 392–35.

Liebow, A.A. (1973) Pulmonary angiitis and granulomatosis. *Am. Rev. Respir. Dis.,* **108,** 1–18.

Liebow, A.A., Carrington, C.R.B. and Friedman, P.J. (1972) Lymphomatoid granulomatosis. *Hum. Pathol.,* **3,** 457–558.

Liebow, A.A., Steer, A. and Billingsley, J.G. (1965) Desquamative interstitial pneumonia. *Am. J. Med.,* **39,** 369–407.

Lief, P.D., Bogartz, L.J., Loerner, S.K. and Buchberg, A.S., (1969) Sarcoidosis and primary hyperparathyroidism. *Am. J. Med.,* **47,** 825–30.

Lillington, G.A. and Jamlis, R.W. (1963) Scalene node biopsy. *Ann. Intern. Med.*, **59**, 101–10.

Lim, K.H. (1961) Four episodes of sarcoidosis after pulmonary tuberculosis. *Tubercle*, **42**, 350–4.

Lin, S.R., Levy, W., Go, E.B., Lee, I. and Wong, W.K. (1973) Unusual osteosclerotic changes in sarcoidosis, simulating osteoblastic metastases. *Radiology*, **106**, 311–2.

Lindig, W. (1951) Ein Beitrag zur Frage der klinisch isolierten Boeckschen Lungenerkrangkungen und ihrer Prognose. *Z. Tuberk.*, **98**, 141–52.

Lindsay, J.R. and Perlman, H.B. (1951) Sarcoidosis of the upper respiratiory tract. *Ann. Otol. Rhinol. Laryngol.* **69**, 549–66.

Lindvall, K., Edhag, O., Erhardt, L.R., Sjögren, A. and Swahn, A. (1978) Complete heart block due to granulomatous giant cell myocarditis: report of 3 cases. *Eur. J. Cardiol.* **8**, 349–58.

Line, B.R., Hunninghake, G.W., Keogh, B.A., Jones, E.J., Johnston, G.S. and Crystal, R.G. (1981) Gallium-67 scanning to stage the alveolitis of sarcoidosis: correlation with clinical studies, pulmonary function studies, and broncho alveolar lavage. *Am. Rev. Respir. Dis.*, **123**, 440–6.

Liot, F., Lemoine, J.M. and Chretien, J. (1963) Etude endoscopique et histologique des bronches principales dans la sarcoïdose. *Bronches*, **13**, 611–26.

Little, J.A. and Steigman, A.J. (1960) Erythema nodosum in primary histoplasmosis. *J. Am. Med. Assoc.*, **173**, 875–7.

Littman, M.L. and Zimmerman, L.E. (1956) *Cryptococcosis (Torulosis or European blastomycosis)*, Grune and Stratton, New York.

Littner, M.R., Schachter, E.N., Putnam, C.E., Odero, D.O. and Gee, J.B.L. (1977) The clinical assessment of radiographically atypical pulmonary sarcoidosis. *Am. J. Med.*, **62**, 361–7.

Livingstone, G. (1956) Sarcoidosis of maxillary antrum. *J. Laryngol.*, **70**, 426–7.

Lloyd-Davies, R.W. and Forbes, G.B. (1965) Sarcoidosis of the gall-bladder. *Gastroenterology*, **49**, 287–90.

Lobo, A., Carr, I. and Malcolm, D. (1978) The EM immunocytochemical demonstration of lysozyme in macrophage giant cells in sarcoidosis. *Experientia*, **34**, 1088–9.

Lockman, D.S. (1980) Porphyria cutanea tarda and sarcoidosis. *J. Am. Acad. Dermatol.*, **2**, 62–5.

Löfgren, S. (1945) Erythema nodosum following treatment with sulphanilamide compounds. *Acta Med. Scand.*, **122**, 175–91.

Löfgren, S. (1946) Erythema nodosum: studies on etiology and pathogenesis of 185 adult cases. *Acta Med. Scand.*, Suppl. 174, 124, 1–197.

Löfgren, S. (1950) Age distribution of erythema nodosum. *Acta Med. Scand.*, **136**, 241–9.

Löfgren, S. (1953) Primary pulmonary sarcoidosis. *Acta Med. Scand.*, **145**, 424–31, 465–74.

Löfgren, S. (1957) Diagnosis and incidence of sarcoidosis. *Br. J. Tuberc.*, **51**, 8–13.

Löfgren, S. and Lindgren, A.G.H. (1959) Cavern formation in pulmonary sarcoidosis. *Acta Chir. Scand.*, Suppl. 245, 113–8.

Löfgren, S. and Lundback, H. (1950) Isolation of virus from 6 cases of sarcoidosis: preliminary report. *Acta Med. Scand.* **138**, 71–5.

Löfgren, S. and Lundback, H. (1952) The bilateral hilar lymphoma syndrome: a study of the relation to tuberculosis and sarcoidosis in 212 cases. *Acta Med. Scand.*, **142**, 265–73.

Löfgren, S., Snellman, B. and Lindgren, A.G.H. (1957) Renal complications in sarcoidosis: functional and biopsy studies. *Acta Med. Scand.*, **159**, 295–305.

Löfgren, S., Snellman, B. and Nordenstam, H. (1955) Foreign-body granulomas and sarcoidosis. *Acta Chir. Scand.*, **108**, 405–18.

Löfgren, S. and Snellman, B. (1964) Principles and procedures for obtaining biopsies in sarcoidosis. In *Proc. 3rd International Conference of Sarcoidosis, Stockholm, 1983*, (ed. Sven Löfgren) Svenska Boleförlaget, Norstedts.

Löfgren, S. and Stavenow, S. (1961) Course and prognosis of sarcoidosis: Stockholm, in the Proceedings of the International Conference on Sarcoidosis, Washington. *Am. Rev. Respir. Dis.*, **84**, 71–3.

Löfgren, S., Strøm, L. and Widstrom, G. (1953) Tuberculosis immunity in sarcoidosis studied with the aid of radioactive BCG vaccine. *Acta Paediat.*, **43**, suppl. 100, 160–6.

Löfgren, S.and Wahlgren, F. (1949) On the histopathology of erythema nodosum. *Acta Derm.-Venereol.*, **29**, 1–13.

Lombardo, C. (1905) I corpi inclusi nelle cellulé giganti. *Giorn. Ital. Mal. Vener.* **40**, 478.

Lomholt, S. (1934) Douze cas de sarcoïdes de Boeck traités a l'antileprol. *Bull. Soc. Fr. Dermatol. Syphiligr.* **41**, 1354–62.

Lomholt, S. (1937) Sarkoid (Boeck) oder Lymphogranulomatosis benigna (Schaumann): ein kurzer Übersichtauf dem Grundlage von 60 Fällen. *Acta Derm.-Venereol.*, **18**, 137–49.

Lomholt, S. (1943) Beitrag zur Kveimreaktion bei Lymphogranulomatosis benigna. *Acta Derm.-Venereol.*, **24**, 447–56.

Long, W.H. (1961) Granulomatous (Fiedler's) myocarditis with extra-cardiac involvement. *J. Am. Med. Assoc.*, **177**, 184–6.

Longcope, W.T., Fisher, A.M. (1942) Involvement of the heart in sarcoidosis of Besnier–Boeck–Schaumann. *J. Mt Sinai Hosp.*, **8**, 784–97.

Longcope, W.T., Freiman, D.G. (1952) A study of sarcoidosis. *Medicine, Baltimore*, **31**, 1–132.

Lorber, S.H., Shay, H., Woloshin, H. (1954) A Roentgen study of the gastrointestinal tract in proven cases of sarcoidosis. *Gastroenterology*, **26**, 451–61.

Lordon, R.E., Young, R.L., Shapiro, S.S., Smith, R.E. and Weg, J.G. (1968) Sarcoidosis. II A clinical evaluation of the alteration in delayed hypersensitivity. *Am. Rev. Respir. Dis.*, **97**, 1009.

Lovelock, F.J., and Stone, D.J. (1951) Cortisone therapy of Boeck's sarcoid. *J. Am. Med. Assoc.*, **147**, 930–2.

Lovelock, F.J., and Stone, D.J. (1953) The therapy of sarcoidosis. *Am. J. Med.*, **15**, 477–83.

Lowe, M.V. (1980) Sarcoidosis in Jamaica. In *Proc. 8th International Conference on Sarcoidosis, Cardiff* (eds. W. Jones-Williams and B.H. Davies), Alpha Omega, Cardiff, pp. 514–8.

Lucas, P.F. Acute hypercalcaemia from carcinomatosis without bone metastases. (1960) *Br. Med. J.*, **1**, 1350.

Lucia, S.P., and Aggeler, P.M. (1940) Sarcoidosis (Boeck) lymphogranulomatosis benigna (Schaumann); observations on the bone marrow obtained by sternal puncture. *Acta Med. Scand.*, **104**, 351–65.

Lühe, V.D. (1958) Ubergangsfälle der Sarkoidose (Morbus Besnier–Boeck–Schaumann), in eine banal tuberkulose. *Dermatol. Wochenschr.*, **138**, 1077–91.

Lukin, R.R., Chambers, A.A., Soleimapour, M. (1975) Outlet obstruction of the fourth ventricle in sarcoidosis. *Neuroradiology*, **10**, 65–8.

Lull, R.J., Dunn, B.E., Gregoratos, G., Cox, W.A., Fisher, G.W., (1972) Ventricular aneurysm due to cardiac sarcoidosis with surgical cure of refractory ventricular tachycardia. *Amer. J. Cardiol.*, **30**, 282–7.

Lundback, H., and Löfgren, S. (1952) Attempts at isolation of virus strains from cases of sarcoidosis and malignant lymphoma. I. Statistical evaluation of results previously reported. *Acta Med. Scand.*, **143**, 98–104. II. Further isolation and control experiments, *Acta Med. Scand.*, **143**, 105–9.

Lundback, H., Löfgren, S. and Nordenstamm, M. (1959) Cultivation of sarcoidotic tissue from lymph-nodes and skin. *Br. J. Exp. Pathol.* **40**, 61–5.

Lussier, L., Chandler, D.K.F., Sybart, A., Yeager, H. (1978) Human alveolar macrophages: antigen-independent binding of lymphocytes. *J. Appl. Physiol.* **45**, 933–8.

Lutz, W. (1919) Zur Kenntnis der Boeckschen Miliarlupoïde. *Arch. Dermatol. Syph., Wien*, **126**, 947–64.

MacBride, H.J. (1923) Uveo-parotic parotic paralysis. *J. Neurol. Psychopathol.*, **4**, 242.

MacFarlane, D.A. (1955) Intestinal sarcoidosis. *Br. J. Surg.*, **42**, 639–42.

MacFarlane, J.T. (1981) Recurrent erythema nodosum and pulmonary sarcoidosis. *Postgrad. Med. J.*, **57**, 525–7.

MacGregor, R.R., Sheagren, J.N., Lipsett, M.B. and Wolff, S.M. (1969) Alternate day prednisone therapy, *New Engl. J. Med.*, **208**, 1427–31.

MacKay, G. (1921) A case of uveoparotitis with iridocycloplegia. *Trans. Ophthalm. Soc. UK*, **37**, 208–220.

MacKay, J.B., Laing, M.C. and Reid, J.D. (1964) Sarcoidosis: some observations on present status, prevalence and treatment. *NZ Med. J.*, **63**, 264–71.

Mackensen, G. (1952) Veränderungen am Angenhintergrund bei Besnier–Boeck–Schaumannscher Erkrankung. *Klin. Monatsbl. Augenheilkd.*, **121**, 51–63.

Mackenzie, S. (1886) Erythema nodosum, especially dealing with its connection with rheumatism. *Br. Med. J.* **1**, 744.

MacLeod, I.B., Jenkins, A.M. and Gill, W. (1965) Sarcoidosis involving the vermiform appendix. *J. R. Coll. Surg. Edinburgh*, **10**, 319–23.

Macpherson, P. (1961) Erythema nodosum in Scotland. *Tubercle*, **42**, 341–9.

Macpherson, P. (1967) The changing pattern of erythema nodosum in the Western Highlands. *Tubercle*, **48**, 54–7.

Macpherson, P. (1970) A survey of erythema nodosum in a rural community between 1954 and 1968. *Tubercle*, **51**, 324–7.

Macquet, V., Leduc, M. and Lafitte, P. (1965) Pleurésie chronique par sarcoïdosie pleurale. *Lille Med.*, **10**, 207–10.

MacSearraigh, E.T., Doyle, C.T., Twomey, M. and O'Sullivan, D.J. (1978) Sarcoidosis with renal involvement. *Postgrad. Med. J.* **54**, 528–32.

McCallum, R.I., Rannie, I. and Verity, C. (1961) Chronic pulmonary berylliosis in a female chemist. *Br. J. Ind. Med.*, **18**, 133–42.

McCartney, W.H., Lindner, L.E., Prather, J.L. and Nusynowitz, M.L. (1979) Brain scan abnormalities in intracerebral sarcoidosis. *Clin. Nuclear Med.* **4**, 32–4.

McClelland, D.B. and Van Furth, R. (1975) *In vitro* synthesis of lysozyme by human and mouse tissues and leucocytes. *Immunology*, **28**, 1099–114.

McClement, J., Renzetti, A.D., Himmelstein, A. and Cournand, A. (1953) Cardiopulmonary function in the pulmonary form of Boeck's sarcoid and its modification by cortisone therapy. *Am. Rev. Tuberc.*, **67**, 154–72.

McConkey, B. (1958) Muscular distrophy in sarcoidosis. *Arch. Intern. Med.*, **102**, 443–6.

McCort, J.J., Wood, R.H., Hamilton, J.B. and Ehrlich, D.E. (1947) Sarcoidosis: a clinical and roentgenographic study of 28 proven cases. *Arch. Intern. Med.,* **80,** 293–321.

McCoy, R.C., and Tisher, C.C. (1972) Glomerulonephritis associated with sarcoidosis. *Am. J. Pathol.,* **68,** 339–53.

McCullough, N.B., Louria, D.B., Hilbish, T.F., Thomas, L.B. and Emmons, C. (1958) Cryptococcosis: Clinical Staff Conference. *Nat. Inst. Health. Ann. Intern. Med.,* 49, 642–61.

McDonald, S. and Sewell, W.T. (1913–14) Malakoplakia of the bladder and kidneys. *J. Pathol. Bacteriol.,* **18,** 306.

McFarlane, D.A. (1955) Intestinal sarcoidosis. *Br. J. Surg.,* **42,** 639–642.

McFarland, R.B., and Goodman, S.B. (1963) Sporotrichosis and sarcoidosis. Report of a case with comments upon possible relationships between sarcoidosis and fungus infections, *Arch. Intern. Med.,* **112,** 760–5.

McGovern, J.P. and Merritt, D.H. (1953) Sarcoidosis in childhood. *Adv. Pediatr.,* **8,** 97–135.

McGowan, A.J. and Smith, E. (1967) Urological implications of sarcoidosis. *J. Urol.,* **97,** 1090–3.

McGregor, I. (1961) *The two-year mass radiography campaign in Scotland 1957– 1958.* HMSO, Edinburgh.

McIntyre, J.A., McKee, K.T., Loadholt, C.B., Mercurio, L. and Lin, I. (1977) Increased HLA-B7 antigen frequency in South Carolina blacks in association with sarcoidosis. *Transplant. Proc.,* Suppl. 1, **9,** 173–6.

McKelvie, P., Goesson, C., Pokhrel, R.P. and Jackson, P. (1968) Sarcoidosis of the upper air passages. *Br. J. Dis. Chest,* **62,** 200–5.

McKusick, K.A., Soin, J.S., Ghiladi, A. and Wagner, H.N. (1973) Gallium[67] accumulation in pulmonary sarcoidosis. *J. Am. Med. Assoc.,* **223,** 688.

McKusick, V.A. (1953) Boeck's sarcoid of stomach with comments on etiology of regional ileitis. *Gastroenterology,* **23,** 103–13.

McLaughlin, J.S., Eck, W. van, Thayer, W., Albrink, W.S. and Hayes, M.A. (1961) Gastric sarcoidosis. *Ann. Surg.,* **153,** 283–8.

McLoud, T.C., Putnam, C.E., Pascual, R. (1974) Eggshell calcifications with systemic sarcoidosis. *Chest,* **66,** 515–7.

McNeill, R.S., Rankin, J., and Forster, R.E. (1958) The diffusing capacity of the pulmonary membrane and the pulmonary capillary blood volume in cardiopulmonary disease. *Clin. Sci.,* **17,** 465–82.

Maddrey, W.C., Johns, C.J., Boitnott, J.K. and Iber, F.L. (1970) Sarcoidosis and chronic hepatic disease: a clinical and pathologic study of 20 patients. *Medicine Baltimore,* **49,** 375–95.

Maderazo, E.G., Ward, P.A., Wjronick, C.L., Kubik, J. and DeGraff, A.C. (1976) Leukotactic dysfunction in sarcoidosis. *Ann. Intern. Med.,* **84,** 414–9.

Madigan, J.C., Gragondas, E.S., Schwartz, P.L. and Lapus, J.V. (1977) Peripheral retinal neovascularisation in sarcoidosis and sickle cell anaemia. *Am. J. Ophthalmol.* **83,** 210–4.

Magnus. E.M. (1956) Two cases of sarcoidosis involving the hypophysis treated with corticotrophin and cortisone. *Acta Endocrinol.,* **22,** 1–8.

Magnusson, B. (1956) The effect of sarcoidosis sera on the tuberculin response. *Acta Derm. -Venereol.,* **36,** Suppl. 35.

Mahé, C., Amouroux, J., Turbie, P. and Battesti, J.P. (1979) Données de la cytologie du liquide de lavage broncho-alveolaire dans la sarcoidose mediastino-pulmonaire. *Poumon Coeur,* **35,** 241–4.

Maher-Loughnan, G.P. (1953) Sarcoidosis proceeding to open pulmonary tuberculosis with subsequent recovery. *Br. J. Tuberc.,* **47**, 162–5.

Maillard, A.A. and Goepfert, H. (1978) Nasal and paranasal sarcoidosis. *Arch. Otolaryngol.,* **104**, 197–201.

Malecki, S. (1965) Der Übergang einer aktiven Lungentuberkulose in Sarkoidose. *Z. Tuberk.,* **124**, 377–9.

Malmros, H. (1947) Late primary infection and B.C.G. vaccination. *Am. Rev. Tuberc.,* **56**, 267–78.

Mandi, L. (1964) Thoracic sarcoidosis in childhood. *Acta Tuberc. Scand.,* **45**, 256–70.

Mangi, R.J., Dwyer, J.M., Gee, B. and Kantor, F.S. (1974a) The immunological competence of subjects with sarcoidosis. *Clin. Exp. Immunol.,* **18**, 519–28.

Mangi, R.J., Dwyer, J.M. and Kantor, F.S. (1974b) The effect of plasma upon lymphocyte response *in vitro* – demonstration of a humoral inhibitor in patients with sarcoidosis. *Clin. Exp. Immunol.,* **18**, 519–28.

Mankiewicz, E. (1961) Mycobacteriophages isolated from persons with tuberculous and non-tuberculous conditions. *Nature, London,* **191**, 1416–7.

Mankiewicz, E. (1964) The relationship of sarcoidosis to anonymous bacteria. *Acta Med. Scand.,* Suppl. **425**, 68–73.

Mankiewicz, E. and Béland, J. (1964) The role of mycobacteriophages and of cortisone in experimental tuberculosis and sarcoidosis. *Am. Rev. Respir. Dis.,* **89**, 717–20.

Mankiewicz, E. and Liivak, M. (1967) Mycobacteriophages isolated from human sources. *Nature, London,* **216**, 485–6.

Mankiewicz, E. and van Walbeek, M. (1962) Mycobacteriophages: their role in tuberculosis and sarcoidosis. *Arch. Environ. Health.* **5**, 122–8.

Mariani, A.F., Clifton, S., Davies, D.J., Dawborn, J. K., Fitzgerald, J.E., Ihle, B.U., Niall, J.F. and Ryan, G.B. (1978) Membranous glomerulonephritis associated with sarcoidosis. *Aust. NZ J. Med.,* **8**, 420–5.

Mariani, B. (1977) Epidemiological data on sarcoidosis in Italy. *Z. Erkr. Atmungsorgane,* **149**, 47–9.

Mariano, M. and Spector, W.G. (1974) The formation and properties of macrophage polykaryons (inflammatory giant-cells) *J. Pathol.,* **113**, 1–19.

Markoff, N. (1951) Kalkschrumfniere bei Morbus Boeck. *Helv. Med. Acta,* **18**, 389–94.

Marlarkey, W.B. and Kataria, Y.P. (1974) Sarcoidosis and hyperprolactinaemia. *Ann. Intern. Med.,* **81**, 116.

Marshall, R. and Karlish, A.J. (1971) Lung function in sarcoidosis. An investigation of the disease seen at a clinic in England and a comparison of the value of various lung function tests. *Thorax,* **26**, 402–5.

Marshall, R., Smellie, H.C., Baylis, J.H., Hoyle, C. and Bates, D.V. (1958) Pulmonary function in sarcoidosis. *Thorax,* **13**, 48–58.

Marten, R.H. and Warner, J. (1971) Lung function in sarcoidosis. An investigation of the disease seen at a clinic in England and a comparison of the value of various lung function tests. *Thorax,* **26**, 402–5.

Martenstein, H. (1921) Wirkung das Serums von Sarkoid-Boeck und Lupus-pernio-Kranken auf Tuberkulin. *Arch. Dermatol. Syph. Wien,* **136**, 17–24.

Martenstein, H. (1924) Sarkoid Boeck und Lupus pernio. *Arch. Dermatol. Syph., Berlin,* **147**, 70–99.

Martin, D.S. and Smith, D.T. (1939) Blastomycosis: a report of 13 new cases. *Am. Rev. Tuberc.,* **39**, 275, 488–515.

Martin, F.R.R. and Carr, R.J. (1953) Crohn's disease involving the stomach: a report of 2 cases. *Br. Med. J.*, 1, 700–2.

Martini, A. (1949) Beiträge zur Klinik der atypischen Tuberkulose. *Beitr. Klin. Tuberk.*, 101, 212–8.

Martland, H.S., Brodkin, H.A. and Martland, H.S., Jr. (1948) Occupational beryllium poisoning in New Jersey. *J. Med. Soc., N. J.*, 45, 5–14.

Mascher, W. (1951) Tuberculin-negative tuberculosis. *Am. Rev. Tuberc.*, 63, 501–25.

Mather, G. (1957) Calcium metabolism and bone changes in sarcoidosis. *Br. Med. J.*, 1, 428–53.

Mather, G., Dawson, J. and Hoyle, C. (1955) Liver biopsy in sarcoidosis. *Q. J. Med.*, 24, 331–53.

Matsui, Y., Iwai, K. Tachihana, T., Fruie, T., Shigematsu, N., Izumi, T., Homma, A.H., Mikami, R., Hongo, O., Hiraga, Y. and Yamamoto, M. (1976) Clinicopathological study on fatal myocardial sarcoidosis. *Ann. NY Acad. Sci.*, 278, 455–69.

Matsuoka, L.Y., Levine, M., Glasser, S. and Barsky, S. (1980) Ichthyosiform sarcoid. *Cutis*, 25, 188–89.

Matthews, W.B. (1959) Sarcoidosis of the nervous system. *Br. Med. J.*, 1, 267–70.

Matthews, W.B. (1975) Sarcoid neuropathy. In *Peripheral Neuropathy* (eds. P.J. Dyck, P.K. Thomas and E.H. Lambert) W.B. Sauders, Philadelphia, Chapter 59.

Maurice, P.A. (1955) La participation de la musculature à la maladie de Besnier–Boeck–Schaumann. *Helv. Med. Act.*, 22, 16–42.

Mawer, E.B., Backhouse, J., Lumb, G.A., Stanbury, S.W. (1971) Evidence for the formation of 1,25 dihydrocholecalciferol during metabolism of vitamin D in man. *Nature London, New Biol.*, 232, 188–9.

Mayock, R.L., Bertrand, D., Morrison, C.E., and Scott, J.H. (1963) Manifestations of sarcoidosis: analysis of 145 patients , with a review of 9 series selected from literature. *Am. J. Med.*, 35, 67–89.

Mayock, R.L., Sullivan, R.D., Greening, R.R., and Jones, R., Jr. (1957) Sarcoidosis and pregnancy. *J. Am. Med. Assoc.* 164, 158–63.

Mazza, G. (1908) Über das multiple benigne Sarkoid der Haut (Boeck). *Arch. Dermatol. Syph., Wien*, 91, 57–78.

Meachim, G., and Young, M.H. (1963) De Quervains subacute granulomatous thyroiditis: histological identification and incidence. *J. Clin. Pathol.*, 16, 189–99.

Medeiros, A.A., Marty, S.D., Tosh, F.E., and Chin, T.D.Y. (1966) Erythema nodosum and erythema multiforme as clinical manifestations of histoplasmosis in a community outbreak. *N. Engl. J. Med.*, 274, 415–20.

Megalif, N.I. and Brencsone, R.B. (1977) Betrachten zur Sarkoidose-Inzidenz in der Lettischen SSR. *Z. Erkr. Atmungsorgane*, 149, 44–6.

Meira, J.A., Ferreira, J.M. and Jamra, M. (1949) Sarcoidose (molestia de Besnier–Boeck–Schaumann) *Rev. Med. Cir. Sao Paulo.*, 9, 1–60.

Melmon, K.L. and Goldberg, J.S. (1962) Sarcoidosis with bilateral exophthalmos as the presenting symptom. *Am. J. Med.*, 33, 158–60.

Melsom, H., Sannev, T. and Seljelid, R. (1975) Macrophage cytolytic factor: some observations on its physicochemical properties and mode of action. *Exp. Cell Research*, 94, 221–6.

Mendes, E., Hepner Levy, L. and DeUlhoa Cintra, A.B. (1976) Kveim test in patients suspected of sarcoidosis and in leprosy patients in a geographical area not yet investigated. *Allergolog. Immunopathol.*, 4, 45–50.

Merrill, H.G. and Oaks, L.W. (1931) Uveo-parotitis (Heerfordt): with case report. *Am. J. Ophthalmol.*, **14**, 15–21.

Metchnikoff, E. (1893) *Lectures on the Comparative Pathology of Inflammation* (trans. F.A. and E. H. Starling), London, 163.

Meyer, A., Nico, J.P. and Guize, L. (1967) La reaction de Kveim chez de jeunes adults ou des enfants dont les réactions tuberculiniques sont restées négatives malgré deux vaccinations. In *Proc. 4th International Conference on Sarcoidosis, Paris,* (eds. J.Turiaf and J. Chabot, Masson, Paris, pp. 67–71.

Meyer, J.S., Foley, J.M. and Campagna-Pinto, D. (1953) Granulomatous angiitis of the meninges in sarcoidosis. *Arch. Neurol. Psychiatry Chicago,* **69**, 587–600.

Meyers, M. and Barsky, S. (1978) Ulcerative sarcoidosis. *Arch. Dermatol.,* **114**, 447.

Michael, M., Jr., Cole, R.M., Beeson, P.B. and Olson, B. (1950) Sarcoidosis: preliminary report on a study of 350 cases with special reference to epidemiology. *Am. Rev. Tuberc.,* **62**, 403–7.

Michaels, L., Brown, N.G. and Cory-Wright, M. (1960) Arterial changes in pulmonary sarcoidosis. *Arch. Pathol.,* **69**, 741–9.

Michel, P.J., Cretin, J. and Sellem, G. (1968) Sarcoidose cutanée de Besnier–Boeck–Schaumann atrophocicatricielle. *Bull. Soc. Fr. Dermatol. Syphiligr.,* **75**, 398–500.

Michon, P., Dornier, R., Kling, C., Larcan, A. and Huriet, C. (1957) Anémie hémolytique avec anticorps et maladie de Besnier–Boeck–Schaumann. *Bull. Soc. Med. Hôp., Paris,* **73**, 903–8.

Mlczoch, F. and Kohout, J. (1962) Das 'Gewebsbild' vei verschiedenen erkrankugen: eine Anwendung der Deckglasmethode in der Klinik. *Klin. Wochenschr.,* **40**, 99–105.

Middleton, W.G. and Douglas, A.C. (1980a) Further experience with Edinburgh-prepared Kveim-Siltzbach test suspensions. In *Proc. International Conference on Sarcoidosis, Cardiff, 1978* (eds. W. Jones-Williams and B.H. Davies), Alpha Omega, Cardiff, pp. 655–9.

Middleton, W.G. and Douglas, A.C. (1980b) Prolonged corticosteroid therapy in pulmonary sarcoidosis. In *Proc. 8th International Conference on Sarcoidosis, Cardiff, 1978* (eds. W. Jones-Williams and B.H. Davies), Alpha Omega, Cardiff, pp. 632–47.

Mikami, R., Hiraga, Y., Iwai, K., Kosuda, T., Mochizuki, H., Homma, H., Osada, H., Chiba, Y., Soejima, R., Odaka, M., Hosada, Y., Hashimoto, T., Yanagawa, H., Shigemutsu, I. and Nakao, K. (1974) A double-blind controlled trial on the effect of corticosteroid therapy in sarcoidosis. In *Proc. 6th International Conference on Sarcoidosis, Tokyo,* (eds. K. Iwai and Y. Hosoda), University of Tokyo Press, Tokyo, pp. 533–8.

Mikhail, J.R. (1970) Identical twins, one presenting as sarcoidosis, the other as tuberculosis. *Postgrad. Med. J.,* **46**, 521–5.

Mikhail, J.R., Lovell, D., McGhee, K.J. and Mitchell, D.N. (1976) Sarcoidosis presenting with a pleural effusion. *Tubercle,* **57**, 123–5.

Mikhail, J.R. and Mitchell, D.N. (1971) Mediastinoscopy; a diagnostic procedure in hilar and paratracheal lymphadenopathy. *Postgrad. Med. J.* **47**, 698–704.

Mikhail, J.R., Mitchell, D.N. and Ball, K.P. (1974) Abnormal electrocardiographic findings in sarcoidosis. In *Proc. 6th International Conference on Sarcoidosis, Tokyo* (eds. K. Iwai and Y. Hosoda), University of Tokyo Press, Tokyo, pp. 365–72.

Mikhail, J.R., Mitchell, D.N. and Drury, R.A.B. (1970) Identical twins, one presenting with tuberculosis, and the other with sarcoidosis. *Am. Rev. Respir. Dis.,* **102**, 636–40.

Mikhail, J.R., Mitchell, D.N., Dyson, J.L., Jones-Williams, W., Ogunlesi, T.O.O. and van Hein-Wallace, S.E. (1972) Sarcoidosis with genital involvement. *Am. Rev. Respir. Dis.,* 106, 465–8.

Mikhail, J.R., Mitchell, D.N., Sutherland, I. and McNicol, M.W. (1980) Sarcoidosis presenting in a district general hospital. In *Proç. 8th International Conference on Sarcoidosis, Cardiff, 1978* (eds W. Jones-Williams and B.H. Davies), Alpha Omega, Cardiff, pp. 532–42.

Mikhail, J.R., Shepherd, M. and Mitchell, D.N. (1979) Mediastinal lymph-node biopsy in sarcoidosis. *Endoscopy,* 1, 5–8.

Millbourne, E. (1950) Splenektomie bei einen Fall von Lymphogranulomatosis benigna (Schaumann). *Acta Med. Scand.,* 137, 20–6.

Miller, A., Chuang, M., Teirstein, A.S. and Siltzbach, L.E. (1976) Pulmonary function in stage I and II sarcoidosis. *Ann. NY Acad. Sci.,* 278, 292–300.

Miller, A., Teirstein, A.S., Jackler, I. and Siltzbach, L.E. (1974) Evidence of airway involvement in late pulmonary sarcoidosis using flow-volume curves and N_2 washout. In *Proc. 6th International conference on Sarcoidosis, Tokyo* (eds. K. Iwai and Y. Hosoda), University of Tokyo Press, Tokyo, pp. 421–4.

Miller, L.K., Rochester, D. and Miller, J.W. (1981) Extensive abdominal lymphadenopathy in sarcoidosis. *Am. J. Gastroenterol.,* 75, 367–9.

Ministry of Health (1961) *Report for the Year 1960,* London, HMSO, Tables 21 and 22.

Mino, R.A., Frelick, R.W., Murphy, A.I., Jr., and Hooker, J.W. (1948) Severe systemic sarcoidosis with ascites and splenomegaly. *Del. Med. J.,* 20, 65–75.

Mistilis, S.P., Green, J.R. and Schiff, L. (1964) Hepatic sarcoidosis with portal hypertension. *Am. J. Med.,* 36, 470–5.

Mitchell, D.N., Bradstreet, C.M.P., Dighero, M.W., Hinson, K.F.W. and Rees, R.J.W. (1974a) Irradiated Kveim suspensions. *Lancet,* 1, 734.

Mitchell, D.N., Cannon, P., Dyer, N.H. Hinson, K.F.W. and Willoughby, J.M.T. (1969) The Kveim test in Crohn's disease. *Lancet,* 2, 571–3.

Mitchell, D.N., Cannon, P., Dyer, N.H. and Willoughby, J.M.T., (1970) Further observations on the Kveim test in Crohn's disease. *Lancet,* 2, 496–8.

Mitchell, D.N. (1983) The Kveim test: analysis of results using K41 materials. In *Proc. 9th International Conference on Sarcoidosis, 1981, and other granulomatous disorders* (eds. J. Chrétien, J. Marsac and J.C. Saltiel) Pergamon Press, Oxford, pp. 615–6.

Mitchell, D.N., Hinson, K.F.W., Dyer, N.H., Willoughby, J.M.T. and Cannon, P. (1974b) Some recent observations on the Kveim reaction. In *Proc. 6th International Conference on Sarcoidosis, tokyo* (eds K. Iwai and Y. Hosoda), University of Tokyo Press, pp. 90–5.

Mitchell, D.N., McSwiggan, D.A., Mikhail, J.R., Heimer, G.V. and Sutherland, I. (1975) Antibody to herpes-like virus in sarcoidosis. *Am. Rev. Respir. Dis.,* 111, 880–2.

Mitchell, D.N., Mikhail, J.R. Turner-Warwick, M. and Sutherland, I. (1977a). Immunoglobulin levels in patients with sarcoidosis. 149, 247–52.

Mitchell, D.M., Mitchell, D.N., Collins, J.V. and Emerson, C.J. (1980) Transbronchial lung biopsy through fibreoptic bronchoscope in diagnosis of sarcoidosis. *Br. Med. J.,* 1, 679–81.

Mitchell, D.N. and Rees, R.J.W. (1969) A transmissible agent from sarcoid tissue. *Lancet,* 2, 81–4.

Mitchell, D.N. and Rees, R.J.W. (1970) A transmissible agent from Crohn's disease tissue. *Lancet,* 2, 168–171.

Mitchell, D.N. and Rees, R.J.W. (1974) The production of granulomas in mice by sarcoid tissue suspension. In *Proc. 6th International Conference on Sarcoidosis, Tokyo* (eds. K. Iwai and Y. Hosoda), University of Tokyo Press, Tokyo, pp. 12–9.

Mitchell, D.N. and Rees, R.J.W. (1976) The nature and physical characteristics of a transmissible agent from human sarcoid tissue. *Ann. NY Acad. Sci.,* **278,** 88–100.

Mitchell, D.N. and Rees, R.J.W. (1980) Further observations on the nature and physical characterisitics of transmissible agents from human sarcoid and Crohn's disease tissues. In *Proc. 8th International Conference on Sarcoidosis, Cardiff,* pp. 121–32.

Mitchell, D.N. and Rees, R.J.W. (1983) The nature and physical characteristics of transmissible agents from human sarcoid and Crohn's disease tissues. In *Proc. 9th International Conference on Sarcoidosis, Paris,* Pergamon Press, Oxford, pp. 132–41.

Mitchell, D.N., Rees, R.J.W. and Goswami, K.K.A. (1976) Transmissible agents from human sarcoid and Crohn's disease tissues, *Lancet,* **2,** 761–5.

Mitchell, D.N. and Scadding, J.G. (1974) Sarcoidosis: state of the art. *Am. Rev. Respir. Dis.,* **110,** 774–802.

Mitchell, D.N., Scadding, J.G., Heard, B.E. and Hinson, K.F.W. (1977b) Sarcoidosis: histopathological definition and clinical diagnosis. *J. Clin. Pathol.* **30,** 395–408.

Mitchell, D.N., Siltzbach, L.E., Sutherland, I. and D'Arcy Hart, P. (1967) Some further observations on the Kveim test in relation to B.C.G. vaccination and tuberculin sensitivity. In *Proc. 9th International Conference on Sarcoidosis, Paris* (eds. J.A. Chrétien, J. Marsac and J.C. Saltiel), Pergamon Press, Oxford, pp. 154–61.

Mitchell, D.N., Sutherland, I., Bradstreet, C.M.P. and Dighero, M.W., (1976) Validation and standardization of Kveim test suspensions prepared from two human spleens. *J. Clin. Pathol.,* **29,** 203–10.

Mitchell, T.H., Stamp, T.C.B. and Jenkins, J.L. (1983) Hypercalcaemic sarcoidosis in hypoparathyroidism . *Br. Med. J.,* **1,** 764–5.

Miyamoto, C., Nomura, S., Kudo, E. and Hamamoto, Y. (1962) An autopsy case of sarcoidosis in the intestinal canal. *Bull. Osaka Med. Sch.,* **18,** 48–55.

Moldover, A. (1958) Sarcoidosis of the spinal cord: report of a case with remission associated with cortisone therapy. *Arch. Intern. Med.,* **102,** 414–7.

Mollaret, H.H. (1971) L' infection humaine à Yersinia enterocolitica en 1970 à la lumière de 642 cas recents. *Pathol. Biol. (Paris),* **19,** 189–205.

Möller, E., Hedford, E. and Wiman, L.G. (1974) HLA genotypes and MLR in familial sarcoidosis. *Tissue Antigens.* **4,** 299–305.

Møller, P. (1952) Case of Boeck's sarcoid with Kveim reactions persisting through nine years. *Acta Derm.-Venereol.,* **32,** 435–6.

Mora, R.G. (1980) Sarcoidosis: a case with unusual manifestations. *South. Med. J.,* **73,** 1063–5.

Morales, A.R., Levy, S., Davies, J. and Fine, G. (1974) Sarcoidosis and the heart *Pathol. Ann.,* **9,** 139–55.

Morax, P.V. (1956) Les localisations neuro-oculaires de la reticulo-endotheliose de Besnier-Boeck-Schaumann. *Ann. Ocul.* **189,** 73–91.

Moreau, M.R. (1949) Formes articulaires de la maladie de Besnier–Boeck–Schaumann. *Bull. Acad. Nat. Med., Paris,* **133,** 89–91.

Morera Prat, J., Aranda Torres, A., Vancells, B.V., (1983) Sarcoidosis in Spain. In *Proc. 9th International Conference on Sarcoidosis, Paris*, Pergamon Press, Oxford, 625.

Moretta, L., Ferrarini, M., Mingari, M.C., Moretta, A. and Webb, S.R. (1976) Subpopulations of human T-cells identified by receptors for immunoglobulins and mitogen responsiveness. *Immunology*, 117, 2171–4.

Moretta, L., Webb, S.R., Grossi, C.E., Lydyard, P.M. and Cooper, M.D., (1971) Functional analysis of two human T-cell sub-populations. *J. Exp. Med.*, 146, 184–200.

Morgan, T., Coupland, W.G., Vanderfield, G.K. and Church, D. (1965) Hypothalamic-pituitary sarcoidosis. *Australas. Ann. Med.*, 14, 250–6.

Morland, A. (1947) A case of sarcoidosis of the lung with regional ileitis. *Tubercle*, 28, 32–3.

Morrison, W.L. (1975) Wart immunity, autoantibodies, and Australia antigen in sarcoidosis. *Br. J. Derm.*, 93, 717–8.

Morrison, J.G.L. (1974) Bantu sarcoidosis. *Br. J. Dermatol.*, 90, 649–55.

Morrison, J.G.L. (1976) Sarcoidosis in a child, presenting as an erytheroderma with keratotic spines and palmar pits. *Br. J. Dermatol.*, 95, 93–7.

Morse, S.I. (1967) The therapeutic effect of chloroquine in sarcoidosis. In *Proc. 9th International Conference on Sarcoidosis, Paris* Pergamon Press, Oxford, pp. 755–63.

Morse, S.I., Cohn, Z.A., Hirsch, J.G. and Shaedler, R.W. (1961) The treatment of sarcoidosis with chloroquine. *Am. J. Med.*, 30, 779–84.

Morsier, G. de, Maurice, P. and Martin, F. (1954) Besnier–Boeck diffus des muscles et lésions du système nerveux centrale: deux observaxtions anatomo-cliniques. *Acta Neurol. Psychiatr. Belg.*, 54, 34–51.

Moscovic, E.A. (1978) Sarcoidosis and mycobacterial L forms. *Pathology Ann.*, 13, 69–164.

Moyer, J.H. and Ackerman, A.J. (1950) Sarcoidosis: a clinical and roentgenological study of 28 cases. *Am. Rev. Tuberc.*, 61, 299–312.

Mucha, V. and Obzechowski, K. (1919) Ein Fall von Tuberkulöser Dermatomyositis (Typus Boeck). *Wien. Klin. Wochenschr.*, 32, 25–30.

Müller, J. and Pedrazzini, A. (1948): Morbus Besnier–Boeck–Schaumann mit Übergang in Miliartuberkilose, *Schweiz. Med. Wochenschr.*, 78, 126.

Müller, W., Wurm, K. and Franz, G. (1961) Das vorkommen einer Rheumafactor analogen Serumsubstanz bei Sarkoidose (Morbus Boeck). *Beitr. Klin. Tuberk.*, 124, 462–70.

Müller, W., Wurm, K. and Reindell, H. (1958) Tuberkulose-Antikörper bei Morbus Boeck. *Beitr. Klin. Tuberk. Spezifischen Tuberk-Forsch.*, 118, 229.

Munt, P.W. (1974) Sarcoidosis of the appendix presenting as appendiceal perforation and abscess. *Chest*, 66, 295–7.

Munt, P.W., Marshall, R.N. and Underwood, I.E. (1975) Hyperprolactinaemia in sarcoidosis. *Am. Rev. Respir. Dis.* 112, 269–72.

Muratore, R. and Vulpis, N. (1952) Modificazioni prodotte nelle cavie dalla iniezione di liquido preparato da materiale sarcoidosico secondo la technica di Löfgren e Lundbäck. I. Ricerche anatomistologiche. *Boll. Soc. Ital. Biol. Sper.*, 28, 169–72.

Murphy, G.P. and Schirmer, H.K. (1961) Nephrocalcinosis urolithiasis and renal insufficiency in sarcoidosis. *J. Urol.*, 86, 702–6.

Mustakallio, K.K., Vuopio, P., Videman, T., Venesman, P. and Putkonen, T. (1967). Immunoglobulins, haptoglobin and transferrin in sarcoidosis. *Ann. Med. Intern. Fenn.*, 56, 19–21.

Myers, G.B., Gottlieb, A.M., Mattman, P.E., Eckley, G.M. and Chason, J.L. (1952) Joint and skeletal muscle manifestations in sarcoidosis. *Am. J. Med.,* **12,** 161–9.

Myers, J.J., Granville, N.B. and Witter, B.A. (1979) Hairy cell leukaemia and sarcoidosis. *Cancer,* **43,** 1777–81.

Myers, W.P.L. (1956) Hypercalcaemia in neoplastic disease *Cancer,* **9,** 1135–40.

Mylius, K. and Schürmann, P. (1929) Universelle sklerosierende tuberkulöse grosszellige Hyperplasie, eine besondere Form atypischer Tuberkulose. *Beitr. Klin. Tuber. Spezifischen Tuberk.-Forsch.,* **73,** 166–209.

Nadel, E.M. and Ackermann, L.V. (1950) Lesions resembling Boeck's sarcoid in lymph-nodes draining an area containing a malignant neoplasm. *Am. J. Clin. Pathol.,* **20,** 952–7.

Nathan, M.H., Newman, A., Ochsner, J.L. and Blum, L. (1960) Sarcoidosis of the upper gastro-intestinal tract. *Am. J. Roentgenol.,* **84,** 275–80.

Nathan, M.P.R., Chase, P.H., Elguezabel, A. and Weinstein, M. (1976) Spinal cord sarcoidosis. *NY State J. Med.* **76,** 748–52.

Naumann, O. (1938) Kasuistischer Beitrag zur Kenntnis der Schaummannnschen 'Benignen Granulomatose' (Morbus Besnier–Boeck–Schaumann). *Z. Kinderheilkd.,* **60,** 1–8.

Neault, R.W., Riley, F.C. (1970) Report of a case of dacryocystitis secondary to Boeck's sarcoid. *Am. J. Ophthalmol.,* **70,** 1011–3.

Needleman, S.W., Siber, R.A., von Brecht, J.H., Goeken, J.A. (1982) Systemic lupus erythematosus complicated by disseminated sarcoidosis. *Am. J. Clin. Pathol.,* **78,** 105–7.

Negus, D. (1966) Giant-cell granuloma of the stomach. *Br. J. Surg.,* **53,** 475–7.

Nelson, C.T. (1948) Observations on the Kveim reaction in sarcoidosis of the American negro. *J. Invest. Dermatol.,* **10,** 15–26.

(1949) Kveim reaction in sarcoidosis, *Arch. Dermatol. Syphilol. NY,* **60,** 377–89.

(1957) The Kveim reaction in sarcoidosis, *J. Chronic Dis.,* **6,** 158–77.

Nelson, C.T., and Schwimmer, B. (1957) The specificity of the Kveim reaction. *J. Invest. Dermatol.,* **28,** 55–61.

Nelson, S., Schwabe, A.D. (1966) Progressive hepatic decompensation with terminal hepatic coma in sarcoidosis. *Am. J. Dig. Dis.,* **11,** 495–501.

Nelson, S., Sears, M.E. (1968) Massive sarcoidosis of the liver. *Am. J. Dig. Dis.,* **13,** 95–106.

Nessan, V.J., Jacoway, J.R. (1979) Biopsy of minor salivary glands in the diagnosis of sarcoidosis. *N. Engl. J. Med.,* **301,** 922–4.

Nestman, R.H., (1949) Sarcoidosis: a review of 11 cases including 2 autopsies. *W. V. Med. J.,* **45,** 240–6.

Neubert, F.R. (1946) Posterior uveitis in a case of sarcoidosis. *Br. J. Ophthalmol.,* **30,** 24–8.

Neville, E. (1977) HLA antigens and disease. *J. Mt Sinai Hosp.,* **44,** 772–7.

Neville, E., Carstairs, L.S. and James, D.G. (1977) Sarcoidosis of bone. *Q. J. Med.,* **46,** 215–27.

Neville, E., James, D.G., Brewerton, D.A., James, D.C.O., Cockburn, C. and Fenichal, B. (1980) HLA antigens and clinical features of sarcoidosis. In *Proc. 8th International Conference on Sarcoidosis, Cardiff, 1978* (eds. W. Jones-Williams and B.H. Davies), Alpha Omega, Cardiff, pp. 201–5.

Neville, E., Mills, R.G.S., Jash, D.G. (1976) Sarcoidosis of the upper respiratory tract and its assocation with lupus pernio. *Thorax,* **31,** 660–4.

Newill, C.A., Johns, C.J., Cohen, B.H., Diamond, E.L., Bias, W.B. (1983) Sarcoidosis, HLA and immunoglobulin markers in Baltimore blacks. In *Proc. 9th International Conference on Sarcoidosis, Paris,* Pergamon Press, Oxford, pp. 253–6.

Nickerson, D.A. (1937) Boeck's sarcoid: report of 6 cases in which autopsies were made. *Arch. Pathol.,* 24, 19–29.

Nickol, H.J. (1961) Ein Beitrag zum Morbus Besnier–Boeck–Schaumann der oberen Luftwege. *HNO,* 9, 108–110.

Nielsen, E.G. (1968) Metyrapone test during gangliopulmonary sarcoidosis. *Dis. Chest,* 53, 722–25.

Nielsen, J. (1934) Recherches radiologiques sur les lésions des os et des poumons dans les sarcoïdes de Boeck. *Bull. Soc. Fr. Dermatol. Syphiligr.,* 41, 1187–1218.

Niitu, Y., Horikawa, M., Hasgawa, S., Kubota, H., Komatsu, S. and Suetake, T. (1974a) Electroencephalography in patients with intrathoracic sarcoidosis. In *Proc. 6th International Conference on Sarcoidosis, Tokyo* (eds. K. Iwai and Y. Hosoda), University of Tokyo Press, Tokyo, pp. 344–8.

Niitu, Y., Horikawa, M., Suetake, T., Hasegawa, S., Kubota, H. and Komatsu, S. (1974b). Intrathoracic sarcoidosis in children. In *Proc. 6th International Conference on Sarcoidosis, Tokyo,* (eds. K. Iwai and Y. Hosoda), University of Tokyo Press, Tokyo, pp. 512–4.

Niitu, Y., Horikawa, M., Sakagnchi, M., Ikeno, N., Hasegawa, S., Komatsu, S., Kubota, H. and Suetake, T. (1974c) Serum immunoglobulins and EB virus antibody in intrathoracic sarcoidosis. In *Proc. 6th International Conference on Sarcoidosis, Tokyo,* pp. 226–230.

Niitu, Y., Watanabe, M., Suetake, T. Handa, T., Munakata, K. and Shiroisha, K. (1965) Sixteen cases of intrathoracic sarcoidosis found among school children in Sendai in mass X-ray surveys of the chest. *Sci. Rep. Res. Inst. Tohoku Univ. Ser. C..,* 12, 99–122.

Nilsson, B.S., Hanngren, A., Lins, L.E., Ripe, E., Ivemark, B., Askergren, J. and Sundblad, R. (1978) Acute phase of sarcoidosis with splenomegaly and hypercalcaemia. *Scand. J. Respir. Dis.,* 59, 199–209.

Nissen, A.W. and Berte, J.B. (1964) Cardiac arrhythmias in sarcoidosis. *Arch. Intern. Med.,* 113, 167–74.

Nitter, L. (1953) Changes in the chest roentgenogram in Boeck's sarcoid of the lungs. *Acta Radiol.,* Suppl. 105.

Nobechi, K. (1961) Epidemiology of sarcoidosis in Japan: preliminary report. *Am. Rev. Respir. Dis.,* 84, 148–52.

Nolan, J.P. and Klatskin, G. (1964) The fever of sarcoidosis. *Ann. Intern. Med.,* 61, 455–61.

Nora, J.R., Levitsky, J.M. and Zimmerman, H.J. (1959) Sarcoidosis with panhypopituitarism and diabetes insipidus. *Ann. Intern. Med.,* 51, 1400–9.

Norberg, R. (1964) Studies in sarcoidosis, I. Serum proteins. *Acta Med. Scand.,* 175, 359–72.

Norberg, R. (1967) Studies in sarcoidosis, IV Serum immunoglobin levels. *Acta Med. Scand.,* 175, 497–504.

Nordentoft, V., and Møller, P.M. (1970) Mediastinoscopy with lymph-node biopsy carried out in patients with endogenous uveitis of unknown etiology. *Acta Ophthalmol.,* 48, 331–44.

Nordland, M., Ylvisaker, R.S., Larson, P. and Reiff, P. (1946) Pregnancy complicated by idiopathic thrombocytopenic purpura and sarcoidosis of the spleen. *Minn. Med.,* 29, 166–70.

Nordstedt, (1936) Lymphogranulomatosis benigna in the light of prolonged clinical observations and autopsy findings. *Br. J. Dermatol.,* 48, 309–446.

North, A.F., Jr., Fink, C.W., Gibson, W.M., Levinson, J.E., Schuchter, S.L., Howard, W.K., Johnson, N. H. and Harris, C. (1970) Sarcoid arthritis in children. *Am. J. Med.* **48**, 449–55.

Norwood, C.W. and Kelly, D.L. (1974) Intracerebral sarcoidosis acting as a mass lesion. *Surg. Neurol.*, **2**, 367–72.

Nosal, A., Schleissner, L.A., Michkin, F.S. and Lieberman, J. (1979) Angiotension-I converting enzyme and gallium scan in noninvasive evaluation of sarcoidosis. *Ann. Intern. Med.*, **90**, 328–31.

Nottebart, H.C., McGehee, R. F., and Utz, J.P. (1973) Cryptococcosis complicating sarcoidosis. *Am. Rev. Respir. Dis.*, **107**, 1060–3.

Nou, E. (1965) Sarcoidosis with skull lesions. *Acta Tuberc. Scand.*, **47**, 147–52.

Novy, F.G., Jr. (1936) Sarcoid. *Calif. West Med.*, **45**, 41–5.

Numao, Y., Sekiguchi, M., Fruic, T., Matsui, Y., Izumi, T., Mikami, R. (1980) A study of cardiac involvement in 963 cases of sarcoidosis by ECG and endomyocardial biopsy. In *Proc. 8th International conference on Sarcoidosis, Cardiff 1978.* (eds. W. Jones-Williams and B.H. Davies), Alpha Omega, Cardiff, pp. 607–14.

Nurick, S., Blackwood, W., Mair, W.C.P. (1972) Giant-cell granulomatous angiitis of the central nervous system. *Brain*, **95**, 133–42.

Obel, A.L. and Löfgren, S. (1964) Pathogenesis of hyaline formation in sarcoidotic lymph-nodes. *Acta Med. Scand.*, Suppl. **425**, 27–32.

Obenauf, C.D., Shaw, H.E., Sydnor, C.F. and Klintworth, G.K. (1978) Sarcoidosis and its ocular manifestations. *Am. J. Ophthalmol.*, **86**, 648–55.

Obermayer, M.E. and Hassen, M. (1955) Sarcoidosis with sarcoidal reaction in tattoo. *Arch. Dermatol.*, **71**, 766–7.

Obitisch-Mayer, I. (1958) Ueber Sarcoidosis Boeck des Magens. *Wien. Klin. Wochenschr.*, **70**, 312–5.

Oelbaum, M.H. and Wainwright, J. (1950) Hypopituitarism in a male due to giant-cell granuloma of the anterior pituitary. *J. Clin. Pathol.*, **3**, 122–9.

Ogilvie, R.I., Kaye, M. and Moore, S. (1964) Granulomatous sarcoid disease of the kidney. *Ann. Intern. Med.*, **61**, 711–5.

Ogunlesi, T.O. and Rankin, T.B. (1961) Sarcoidosis in West Africa. *J. Trop. Med. Hyg.*, **64**, 318–20.

Oh, S.J. (1979) Sarcoid polyneuropathy: a histologically proved case. *Ann. Neurol.*, **7**, 178–81.

Oille, W.A., Ritchie, R.C. and Barrie, H.J. (1953) The age of the lesions in a case of cardiac sarcoidosis. *Can. Med. Assoc. J.*, **68**, 277–8.

Oldberg, S. (1943) Morbus Schaumann–Morbus Basedow. *Acta Med. Scand.*, **115**, 163–76.

Oldershaw, P.J. and Edmondson, R.P.S. (1978) Renal tuberculosis presenting with accelerated hypertension. *Tubercle*, **59**, 197–9.

O'Leary, J.A. (1962) Ten-year study of sarcoidosis and pregnancy. *Am. J. Obstet. Gynecol.*, **84**, 462–6.

Olsen, T.G. (1963) Sarcoidosis of the skull. *Radiology*, **80**, 232–5.

Olson, J.A., Steffenson, E.H., Margolis, R.R., Smith, R.W. and Whitney, R.L. (1950) Effect of ACTH on certain inflammatory diseases of the eye. *J. Am. Med. Assoc.*, **142**, 1276–8.

Olsson, T., Björmstad-Pettersen, H. and Sternberg, N.L. (1979) Bronchostenosis due to sarcoidosis. *Chest*, **75**, 663–6.

O'Neill, R.P. and Penman, R.W.B. (1969) 'Sarcoidosis' complicated with Nocardiosis. *J. Ir. Med. Assoc.*, **62**, 287–90.

Opal, S.M., Pittman, D.L. and Hofeldt, F.D. (1979) Testicular sarcoidosis. *Am. J. Med.*, **67**, 147–50.

Oppenheim, A. and Pollack, R.S. (1947) Boeck's Sarcoid (sarcoidosis) *Am. J. Roentgenol.*, **57**, 28–35.

Oreskes, I. and Siltzbach, L.E. (1968) Changes in rheumatoid factor activity during the course of sarcoidosis. *Am. J. Med.*, **44**, 60–7.

Orie, N.G.M., Rijssel, T.G. Van and Zwaag, G.L. Van der (1950) Pyloric stenosis in sarcoidosis. *Acta Med. Scand.*, **138**, 139–43.

Oswald, N.C. and Parkinson, T. (1949) Honeycomb lungs. *Q. J. Med.*, **18**, 1–20.

Otero, O.G., Tano-Assini, M.T. and Cassino, E. (1967) Sarcoidosis generalizada: presentación de un caso que evo con purpura thrombocitopenica. *Rev. Clin. Esp.* **105**, 140–5.

Oudet, P. and Roegel, E. (1962) Adénopathies médiastinales bénignes dans les suites de la vaccination par le B.C.G. *Poumon Coeur*, **18**, 927–35.

Owen, T.K. and Henneman, J. (1953) Diffuse sarcoidosis associated with hypopituitarism and terminal renal failure. *Br. Med. J.* **2**, 1141–3.

Ozer, F.L., Johnson, W.A. and Waggener, J.D. (1961) Muscular sarcoidosis: a case with 'tumour' formation. *Lancet*, **1**, 22–4.

Pacheco, Y., Cordier, G., Perrin-Fayolle, M. and Revillard, J.P. (1981) Flow-cytometry analysis of activated T-cells from bronchoalveolar lavage fluids in sarcoidosis. *Bull. Eur. Pathophys. Resp.*, **17**, 56P.

Padilla, A.J. and Sparberg, M. (1972) Regional enteritis and sarcoidosis in one patient. *Gastroenterology*, **63**, 153–60.

Pagaltsos, A.S., Kumar, P., Willoughby, J.M.T. and Dawson, A.M. (1971) *In vitro* inhibition of leucocyte migration in Crohn's disease by a sarcoid spleen suspension. *Br. Med. J.*, **2**, 155–6.

Page, J.R. and Seth, S.M. (1969) Sarcoidosis of the upper respiratory tract. *J. Laryngol. Otol.* **83**, 1005–11.

Palazzo, E., Oberling, F., North, M.L., Lang, J.M., Mayer, S. and Waitz, R. (1972) Sarcoidosis in a patient with cold haemagglutinin disease. *Acta Haematol.*, **48**, 331–6.

Palestro, G., Mazzucco, G. and Code, R. (1975) Glomerulonephritis and sarcoidosis: report of a case. *Panminerva. Med.*, **17**, 127–31.

Palmer, E.D. (1958) A note on silent sarcoidosis of the gastric mucosa. *J. Lab. Clin. Med.*, **52**, 231–4.

Panitz, F. and Shinaberger, J.H. (1965) Nephrogenic diabetes insipidus due to sarcoidosis without hypercalcaemia. *Ann. Intern. Med.*, **62**, 113–20.

Panosetti, E. and Lehmann, W. (1979) Sarcoidose isolée de l'oesophage cervical. *Praxis*, **68**, 349–53.

Paola, D. de (1958) Erythematodes disseminatus mit Sarkoidgranulomen. *Frankf. Z. Pathol.*, **69**, 363–73.

Papadimitriou, J.M. (1976) The influence of the thymus on multinucleate giant-cell formation. *J. Pathol.*, **118**, 153–6.

Papadimitriou, J.M. and Spector, W.G. (1971) The origin, properties and fate of epithelioid cells. *J. Pathol.*, **105**, 187–203.

Papadimitriou, J.M. and Spector, W.G. (1972) The ultrastructure of high- and low-turnover inflammatory granulomata. *J. Pathol.*, **196**, 37–43.

Papapoulos, S.E., Fraher, L.J., Sandler, L.M., Clemens, T.L., Lewin, I.G. and O'Riordan, J.L.H. (1979) 1, 25-dihydroxycholecalcoferol in the pathogenesis of hypercalcaemia of sarcoidosis. *Lancet*, **1**, 627–30.

Papowitz, A.J. and Li, J.K.H. (1971) Abdominal sarcoidosis with ascites. *Chest*, 59, 692–5.

Parkinson, T. (1949) Eosinophilic xanthomatous granuloma with honeycomb lungs. *Br. Med. J.*, 1, 1029–30.

Parsons, V. (1960) Awareness of family and contact history of tuberculosis in generalized sarcoidosis. *Br. Med. J.*, 2, 1756–8.

Partenheimer, R.C., and Meredith, H.C. (1950) Splenomegaly with hypersplenism due to sarcoidosis, *N. Engl. J. Med.*, 243, 810–2.

Pascoe, H.R., (1964) Myocardial sarcoidosis. *Arch. Pathol.*, 77, 299–304.

Pascual, R.S., Gee, J.B.L. and Finch, S.C. (1973) Usefulness of serum lysozyme measurement in diagnosis of sarcoidosis. *N. Engl. J. Med.*, 289, 1074–6.

Patnode, R.A., Allin, R.C. and Carpenter, R.L. (1966) Serum immunoglobulin levels in sarcoidosis. *Am. J. Clin. Pathol.*, 45, 398–401.

Pauli, G., Bessot, J.C., Peterschmidt, J. and Isch, F. (1969) Sarcoidose d'expression myopathique avec localitisation thoracique. *Rev. Tuberc. Pneumol.* 33, 1111–7.

Pautrier, L.M. (1934) Leprome à histologie de sarcoide dermique. *Bull. Soc. Fr. Dermatol. Syphiligr.*, 41, 1284–91.

Pautrier, L.M. (1937) Syndrome de Heerfordt et maladie de Besnier–Boeck–Schaumann. *Bull. Soc. Med. Hôp., Paris*, 53, 1608–20.

Pautrier, L.M. (1940) *Une Nouvelle Grande Reticulo-endothéliose, maladie de Besnier–Boeck–Schaumann*, Paris.

Pautrier, L.M. and Glasser, R. (1936) Inoculation positive probable au lapin au point d'inoculation, de lesions cutanées de maladie de Besnier–Boeck–Schaumann. (Probable positive inoculation in a rabbit, at inoculation site of skin lesions from Besnier–Boeck–Schaumann disease). *Bull. Soc. Fr. Dermatol. Syphiligr.* 43, 505 –6.

Pearce, J. and Ehrlich, A. (1955) Gastric sarcoidosis. *Ann. Surg.*, 141, 115–9.

Pearson, J.M.M. Pettit, J.H.S., Siltzbach, L.E., Ridley, D.S., Hart, P.D'A. and Rees, R.J.W. (1969) The Kveim test in lepromatous and tuberculoid leprosy. *Int, J. Lepr.*, 37, 372–81.

Pederson, K.O. (1967) Coexistent sarcoidosis and hyperparathyroidism. *Acta Med. Scand.*, 182, 781–6.

Pennell, W.H. (1951) Boeck's sarcoid with involvement of the central nervous system. *Arch. Neurol. Psychiatry*, 66, 728–35.

Pepys, J. (1955) The relationship of non-specific and specific factors in the tuberculin reaction. *Am. Rev. Tuberc.*, 71, 49–73.

Pepys, J. (1977) Clinical and therapeutic significance of patterns of allergic reactions of the lungs to extrinsic agents. *Am. Rev. Respir. Dis.*, 116, 573–88.

Pepys, J., Jenkins, P.A., Festenstein, G.N., Gregorg, P.H., Lacey, M.E. and Skinner, F.A. (1963) Farmer's lung: thermophilic ackinomycetes as a source of 'farmer's lung hay' antigen. *Lancet*, 2, 607–11.

Pepys, J., Jenkins, P.A., Lachmann, P.J. and Mahon, W.E. (1966) An iatrogenic auto-antibody: immunological response to 'pituitary snuff' in patients with diabetes insipidus. *Clin, Exp. Immunol.*, 1, 377–89.

Pepys, J., Riddell, R.W., Citron, K.M. and Clayton, Y.M. (1962) Precipitins against extracts of hay and moulds in the serum of patients with farmer's lung, aspergillosis, asthma and sarcoidosis. *Thorax*, 17, 366–76.

Perkins, E.S. (1958) The aetiology and treatment of uveitis. *Trans. Ophthalmol. Soc. UK*, 78, 511.

Perkins, E.S. (1968) Uveitis survey at the Institute of Ophthalmology, London. In *Clinical Methods in Uveitis* (eds. S.B. Aronson, C.N. Gamble, E.K. Goodner, and G.R. O'Connor.) Mosby, St Louis, pp. 58–65.

Perrin-Fayolle, M., Bouvier, M., Queneau, P. and Deplante, J.P. (1971) Lacunes craiennes au cours d'une sarcoidose gangliopulmonaire. *Lyon Med.*, 225, 945–53.

Perrin-Fayolle, M., Pacheco, Y., Harf, R., Montagon, B. and Biot, N. (1981) Angiotensin converting enzume in bronchoalveolar lavage fluid in pulmonary sarcoidosis. *Thorax*, 36, 790–2.

Perry, C.B. The aetiology of erythema nodosum. *Br. Med. J.*, 1944, 2, 843–7.

Persellin, R.H., Baum, J. and Ziff, N.Y. (1966) Serum antibody response in sarcoidosis. *Proc. Soc. Exp. Biol.*, 121, 638–42.

Persson, I., Ryder, L.P., Nielsen, L.S. and Svejgaard, A. (1975) The HLA A7 histocompatibility antigen in sarcoidosis in relation to tuberculous sensitivity. *Tissue Antigens*, 6, 50–3.

Pfisterer, R., Wespi, H. and Herzog, H. (1954) Report of some cases of Boeck's disease after B.C.G. inoculation. *Helv. Med. Acta*, 21, 439–44.

Phear, D.N. (1958) The relation between regional ileitis and sarcoidosis. *Lancet*, 2, 1250–1.

Philips, A.K. and Luchette, A.A. (1952) Rupture of the spleen due to sarcoidosis. *Ohio Med. J.*, 48, 617–9.

Phillips, R.W. (1953) Hypercalcemia of sarcoid corrected with cortisone. *N. Engl. J. Med.*, 248, 934–6.

Phillips, R.W. and Phillips, A.M. (1956) The diagnosis of Boeck's sarcoid by skeletal muscle biopsy. *Arch. Intern. Med.*, 98, 732–6.

Pierson, D.J. and Willett, E.S. (1978) Sarcoidosis presenting with finger pain. *J. Am. Med. Assoc.*, 239, 2023–4.

Pinkerton, H. and Iverson, L. (1952) Histoplasmosis: three fatal cases with disseminated sarcoid-like lesions. *Arch. Intern. Med.*, 90, 456–67.

Pinkston, P., Bitterman, P.B. and Crystal, R.G. (1983) Spontaneous release of interleukin-2 by lung lymphocytes in active pulmonary sarcoidosis. *N. Engl. J. Med.*, 308, 793–800.

Pinner, M. (1938) Non-caseating tuberculosis. *Am. Rev. Tuberc.* 36, 690–728.

Pinner, M., Weiss, M. and Cohen, A.C. (1943) 'Procutins' and 'anticutins' *Yale J. Biol. Med.*, 15, 459–63.

Plair, C.M. and Perry, S. (1962) Hypothalamic-pituitary sarcoidosis: a clinical and pathological entity: report of a case. *Arch. Pathol.*, 76, 527–35.

Plimpton, C.H. and Gellhorn, A. (1956) Hypercalcemia in malignant disease without evidence of bone destruction. *Am. J. Med.*, 21, 750–9.

Plummer, N.S., Symmer, W.St.C. and Winner, H.I. (1957) Sarcoidosis in identical twins, with torulosis as a complication in one case. *Br. Med. J.*, 2, 599–603.

Poe, D.L. (1940a) Sarcoidosis of the larynx. *Arch. Otalaryngol.*, 32, 315–20.

Poe, D.L. (1940b) Sarcoidosis of the external ear. *Ann. Otol. St. Louis*, 49, 771–5.

Poe, D.L. (1942) Multiple benign sarcoid of the upper respiratory tract. *Ann. Otol. Rhinol. Laryngol.*, 51, 430–44.

Poe, D.L. and Seager, P.S. (1950) Sarcoidosis (Boeck's sarcoid) of the upper respiratory tract: report of a case with 10 years' clinical observation. *Arch. Otalryngol.*, 51, 414–9.

Poe, R.H. (1978) Middle-lobe atelectasis due to sarcoidosis with pleural effusion. *NY State J. Med.*, 79, 2095–7.

Poe, R.H., Israel, R.H., Utell, M.J. and Hall, W.J. (1979) Probability of a positive transbronchial lung biopsy result in sarcoidosis. *Arch. Intern. Med.*, 139, 761–3.

Polachek, A.A. and Matre, W.J. (1964) Gastrointestinal sarcoidosis: report of a case involving the oesophagus. *Am. J. Dig. Dis.*, **9**, 429–33.

Pongor, F. and Viragh, Z. (1959) Pulmonary histocytosis X with diabetes insipidus. *Am. Rev. Tuberc.*, **79**, 652–8.

Poon, T.P. and Forbus, W.D. (1959) Sudden death due to myocardial sarcoidosis with a comment on the aetiology of sarcoid. *Arch. Intern. Med.*, **104**, 771–8.

Popper, J.S., Bingham, W.G. and Armstrong, F.S. (1960) Sarcoid granuloma of the cerebellum. *Neurology*, **10**, 942–6.

Porter, G.H. (1960) Sarcoid heart disease. *N. Engl. J. Med.*, **263**, 1350–7.

Porter, G.H. (1961) Hepatic sarcoidosis: a cause of portal hypertension and liver failure. *Arch. Intern. Med.*, **103**, 483–95.

Posner, I. (1942) Sarcoidosis: case report. *J. Pediatr.*, **20**, 486–95.

Powell, L.W., Jr. (1953) Sarcoidosis of skeletal muscle: report of 6 cases. *Am. J. Clin. Pathol.*, **23**, 881–9.

Powell, L.W., Jr. (1954) Sarcoidosis of the myocardium. *N. C. Med. J.*, **15**, 28–33.

Powell, R.F. and Smith, E.B. (1976) Pruritic cutaneous sarcoidosis *Arch. Dermatol.*, **112**, 1465–6.

Powell-Jackson, J.D., Roberts, C.I. and Scott, G.W. (1971) Some unusual presentations of sarcoidosis. *Guy's Hosp. Rep.*, **120**, 277–94.

Present, D.H., Lindner, A.E. and Janowitz, H.D. (1966) Granulomatous diseases of the gastro-intestinal tract. *Ann. Rev. Med.*, **17**, 243–56.

Present, D.H. and Siltzbach, L.E. (1967) Sarcoidosis among the Chinese and review of the worldwide epidemiology of sarcoidosis. *Am. Rev. Respir. Dis.*, **95**, 285–91.

Press, P. and Wacker, T. (1962) Images ganglio-pulmonaires d'aspect sarcoidosique chez les vaccinés au B.C.G. *Poumon Coeur*, **18**, 937–49.

Preuss, O.P., Deodhar, S.D. and van Ordstrand, H.S. (1980) Lymphoblast transformation in beryllium workers. In *Proc. 8th International Conference on Sarcoidosis, Cardiff, 1978* (eds. W. Jones-Williams and B.H. Davies), Alpha Omega, Cardiff, pp. 711–4.

Pringle, J.J. (ed.) (1897) *A Pictorial Atlas of Skin Diseases and Syphilitic Affections*, Rebman, London and Saunders, Philadelphia. (English edition of Besnier, E. (1895–1897). Le Musée de l'Hôpital Saint-Louis, Rueff, Paris.).

Pruvost, P., Hautefeuille, E., Canetti, G. and Mabileau, J. (1941) Etude anatomo-clinique d'un cas de maladie de Besnier–Boeck–Schaumann terminée par une tuberculose disséminée. *Bull. Soc. Med. Hôp. Paris*, **57**, 481–90.

Pryse-Davies, J. (1964) Gastro-duodenal Crohn's disease. *J. Clin. Pathol.*, **17**, 90–94.

Pulaski, E.J. and White, T.T. (1948) Streptomycin: report of its clinical effects in 44 patients treated for various infections of the respiratory tract. *Arch. Intern. Med.*, **82**, 217–28.

Purriel, P. and Navarrete, E. (1961) Epidemiology of sarcoidosis in Uruguay and other countries of Latin America. Report of International Conference on Sarcoidosis, Washington, 1960. *Am. Rev. Respir. Dis.*, **84**, 155–61.

Putkonen, T. (1943) Über die Intrakutanreaktion von Kveim bei lymphogranulomatosis benigna. *Acta Derm.-Venereol.*, **23**, Suppl. 10.

Putkonen, T. (1945) Uber die Kveim reaktion bei lymphogranulomatosis benigna. *Acta Derm.-Venereol.*, **25**, 393–410.

Putkonen, T. (1952) A case of skin tuberculosis with a positive Kveim reaction as late as 5 years after injection of antigen. *Acta Derm.-Venereol.*, **32**, Suppl. 29, 294–6.

Putkonen, T. (1964) Source of potent Kveim antigen *Acta Med. Scand.*, Suppl. 425, 83–5.

Putkonen, T. (1967) Influence of prednisone on the Kveim potency of sarcoid lymph-nodes. In *Proc. 4th International Conference on Sarcoidosis, Paris*, pp. 189–93.

Putkonen, T., Hannuksela, M. and Halme, H. (1965a) Calcium and phosphorus metabolism in sarcoidosis. *Acta Med. Scand.*, 177, 327–35.

Putkonen, T., Virkkunen, M. and Wager, O. (1965b) Joint involvement in sarcoidosis with special reference to the co-existence of sarcoidosis and rheumatoid arthritis. *Acta Rheum. Scand.*, 11, 53–61.

Putnam, C.E., Rothman, S.L., Littner, M.R., Allen, W.A., Schachter, E.N., McLoud, T.C., Bein, M.E. and Gee, J.B. (1977) Computerized tomography in pulmonary sarcoidosis. *J. Computer Ass. Tomography*, 1, 1126–28.

Pyke, D.A. and Scadding, J.G. (1952) Effect of cortisone upon skin sensitivity to tuberculin in sarcoidosis. *Br. Med. J.*, 2, 1126–8.

Quinn, E.L., Bunch, O.C. and Yagle, E.M. (1955) The mumps skin test and comple-ment-fixation test as a diagnostic aid in sarcoidosis. *J. Invest. Dermatol.*, 24, 595–8.

Quismorio, F.P., Sharma, O.P. and Chandor, S. (1977) Immunopathological studies on the cutaneous lesions in sarcoidosis. *Br. J. Dermatol.*, 97, 635–642.

Quock, C.P. and Donohoe, R.F. (1967) Flame-shaped retinal haemorrhages in sarcoidosis. *J. Am. Med. Assoc.*, 202, 239–341.

Rab, S.M., Choudhury, G.M. and Choudhury, A.R. (1963) Giant-cell myocarditis. *Lancet*, 2, 172–3.

Rabello, F.E., Jr. (1936) Données nouvelles pour l'interprétation de l'affection de Besnier–Boeck; rôle de la lèpre. *Ann. Dermatol. Syphiligr.* 7, 571–97.

Raben, A.S., Bogdanovich, N.K. and Golochevskaya, V.S. (1961) Transformation of sarcoidosis into reticulosarcomatosis. *Probl. Hematol. Blood Transfus. (USSR)*, 6, 33–8.

Rabinowitz, J.G., Ulreich, S. and Soriano, C. (1974) The usual and unusual man-ifestations of sarcoidosis and the 'hilar haze'; a new diagnostic aid. *Am. J. Roentgenol.*, 120, 821–31.

Radewill, F.H. (1943) Malakoplakia of the urinary bladder and generalised sar-coidosis. *J. Urol.*, 49, 401–7.

Raftery, E.B., Oakley, C.M. and Goodwin, J.F. (1966) Acute subvalvar mitral incompetance. *Lancet*, 2, 360–5.

Rakov, H.L. and Taylor, J.S. (1942) Sarcoidosis: consideration of clinical and histologic criteria differentiating sarcoidosis from tuberculosis. *J. Lab. Clin. Med.*, 27, 1284 –93.

Rakower, J. (1963) Sarcoidal bilateral lymphoma syndrome (Löfgren's syndrome): a review of 31 cases. *Am. Rev. Respir. Dis.*, 87, 518–24.

Ramachandar, K., Douglas, S.d., Siltzbach, L.E. and Taub, R.N. (1975) Peripheral blood lymphocyte subpopulations in sarcoidosis. *Cell. Immunol.*, 16, 422–6.

Ramanujam, K. (1982) Tuberculoid leprosy or sarcoidosis? *Lepr. India*, 54, 318–23.

Ramasoota, T., Johnson, W.C. and Graham, J.H. (1967) Cutaneous sarcoidosis and tuberculoid leprosy. *Arch. Dermatol.*, 96, 259–68.

Ramel, M.E. (1934) Syndrome de Besnier–Boeck, à nodules miliaire, associé à une anétodermie maculeuse. Inoculation positive des lésions cutanées et du sédiment urinaire au cobaye. *Bull. Soc. Fr. Dermatol.*, 41, 1122–34.

Ramirez, J.J., Ponka, J.L. and Haubrich, W.S. (1964) Massive haemorrhage from sarcoid ulcers in the stomach. *Henry Ford Hosp. Med. Bull.,* 12, 15–21.

Rankin, J.A., Naegel, G.P., Schrader, C.E., Matthay, R.A. and Reynolds, H.Y. (1983) Air-space immunoglobulin production and levels in bronchoalveolar lavage fluid of normal subjects and patients with sarcoidosis. *Am. Rev. Respir. Dis.,* 127, 442–8.

Ravaut, P., Valtis, J. and Nellis, P. (1929) Résultats de l'inoculation au cobaye d'une sarcoïde et d'une tuberculide papulo-necrotique. *C. R. Soc. Biol., Paris,* 101, 444–5.

Raven, R.W. (1949) Surgical manifestations of sarcoidosis. *Ann. R. Coll. Surg.,* 5, 3–28.

Raymond, L.A., Spaulding, A.G. and Vilter, R.W. (1978) Peripheral retinal neovascularization in sarcoidosis with thalassaemia. *Ann. Ophthalmol.,* 10, 745–8.

Rebuck, J.W. and Crowley, J.H.A. (1955) A method of studing leucocyte functions *in vivo. Ann. NY Acad. Sci.,* 59, 757–805.

Rechardt, L. and Mustakallio, K.K. (1965) Macrophage response to dermal abrasion in sarcoidosis. *Acta Pathol. Microbiol. Scand.,* 65, 521–7.

Reenstierna, J. (1937) The possible role of leprosy in the etiology of the Besnier–Boeck syndrome and Schaumann's syndrome. *Int. J. Lepr.,* 5, 433–6.

Reenstierna, J. (1940) the possible role of leprosy in the etiology of the Besnier–Boeck sarcoid and Schaumann's syndrome. *Acta Med. Scand.,* 103, 118–22.

Rees, R.J.W. and Weddell, A.G.M. (1968) Experimental models for studying leprosy. *Ann. NY Acad. Sci.,* 154, 214–36.

Reeves, A.L. (1980) Delayed hypersensitivity in experimental pulmonary berylliosis. In *Proc. 8th International Conference on Sarcoidosis, Cardiff, 1978* (eds. W. Jones-Williams and B.H. Davies), Alpha Omega, Cardiff, pp. 715–21.

Refvem, O. (1954) The pathogenesis of Boeck's disease (sarcoidosis) *Acta Med. Scand.,* Suppl. 294, 1–146.

Refvem, O. (1974) Long-term corticosteroid treatment of pulmonary sarcoidosis. In *Proc. 6th International Conference on Sarcoidosis* (eds. K. Iwai and Y. Hosoda), University of Tokyo Press, 547.

Refvem, O. and Refvem, O.K. (1980) Long-term cortiocsteroid treatment of pulmonary sarcoidosis. In *Proc. 8th International Conference on Sarcoidosis, Cardiff,* pp. 648–51.

Regan, G.M., Tagg, B. and Thomson, M.P. (1967) Subjective assessment and objective measurement of finger clubbing. *Lancet,* 1, 529–32.

Reid, J.D. (1964) The nature and significance of the Kveim test. *Acta Med. Scand.,* Suppl. 425, 86–7.

Reid, J.D. and Gebbie, T. (1958) Kveim tests in cases of sarcoidosis and in family contacts. *NZ Med. J.,* 57, 588–92.

Reid, L. and Lorriman, G. (1960) Lung biopsy in sarcoidosis, with special reference to bacteriological and microscopic features. *Br. J. Dis. Chest,* 54, 321–34.

Reimann, H.A. and Price, A.H. (1949a) Histoplasmosis resembling sarcoidosis. *Trans. Assoc. Am. Physicians,* 62, 112–5.

Reimann, H.A. and Price, A.H. (1949b) Histoplasmosis in Pennsylvania: confusion with sarcoidosis and experimental therapy with bacillomycin. *P. Med. J.,* 52, 367–71.

Reiner, M., Sigurdsson, G., Nunziata, V., Malik, M.A., Poole, G.W. and Joplin, G.F. (1976) Abnormal calcium metabolism in normocalcaemic sarcoidosis.*Br. Med. J.,* 2, 1473–6.

Reinherz, E.L., Kung, P.C., Goldstein, G. and Schlossman, S.F. (1979) Further characterization of the human inducer T-cell subset by monoclonal antibody. *J. Immunol.*, **123**, 2894–6.

Reinherz, E.L. and Schlossman, S.F. (1980) Regulation of the immune response: inducer and suppressor T-lymphocytes subsets in human beings. *N. Engl. J. Med.*, **303**, 370–3.

Reis, W. and Rothfeld, J. (1931) Tuberkulide des Sehnerven als Komplication von Hautsarkoiden vom Typus Darier-Roussy. *Graefes Arch. Ophthalmol.*, **126**, 352–66.

Reisfield, D.R. (1958) Boeck's sarcoid and pregnancy. *Am. J. Obstet. Gynecol.*, **75**, 795–801.

Reisner, D. (1944) Boeck's sarcoid and systemic sarcoidosis: a study of 35 cases. *Am. Rev. Tuberc.*, **49**, 289–307; 437–62.

Reisner, D. (1967) Observations on the course and prognosis of sarcoidosis, with special consideration of its intrathoracic manifestations. *Am. Rev. Respir. Dis.*, **96**, 361–80.

Rennard, S.I., Hunnighake, G.W., Bitterman, P.B. and Crystal, R.G. (1981) Production of fibronectin by the human alveolar macrophage. *Proc. Nat. Acad. Sci. USA.*, **78**, 7147–51.

Renner, R.R., Lahiri, M. and Bragoli, A.J. (1977) Sarcoidosis in husband and wife. *NY State J. Med.*, **77**, 118–9.

Reske-Nielsen, E. and Harmsen, A. (1962) Periangiitis and panangiitis as a manifestation of sarcoidosis of the brain. *J. Nerv. Ment. Dis.*, **135**, 399–412.

Resnick, H., Roche, M. and Morgan, W.K.C. (1970) Immunoglobulin concentrations in berylliosis. *Am. Rev. Respir. Dis.*, **101**, 504–10.

Rey, J.C., Canepa, E. and Vivoli, D. (1947) Enfermedad de Besnier–Boeck–Schaumann con manifestaciones cutaneas, ganglionares, oseas y pulmonares; diabetes insípida y silicosis pulmonar asociadas – evolucíon fatal por tuberculosis. *An. Cátedra Patol. Clin. Tuberc. Univ. Buenos Aires*, **8**, 129–43.

Rey, J.C., Montaner, L.J.G. and Valli, E.F. (1967) Experience in sarcoidosis in Buenos Aires (Argentina). In *Proc. 4th International Conference on Sarcoidosis, Paris* (eds. J. Turiaf and J. Chabot), Masson, Paris, pp. 382–4.

Reynolds, H.Y. (1978) The importance of lymphocytes in pulmonary health and disease. *Lung*, **115**, 225–42.

Reynolds, H.Y., Fulmer, J.D., Kazmirowski, J.A., Roberts, W.C., Frank, M.M. and Crystal, R.G. (1977) Analysis of cellular and protein content of broncho-alveolar lavage fluid from patients with idiopathic pulmonary fibrosis and chronic hypersensitivity pneumonitis. *J. Clin. Invest.*, **59**, 165–75.

Reynolds, H.Y. and Newball, H.H. (1974) Analysis of proteins and respiratory cells obtained from human lung by bronchial lavage. *J. Lab. Clin. Med.*, **84**, 559–73.

Ribaudo, C.A., Gilligan, T.J. and Rotting, A. (1949) Purpura hemorrhagica associated with sarcoidosis. *Arch. Intern. Med.*, **83**, 322–30.

Rice-Oxley, J.M. and Truelove, S. (1950) Complications of ulcerative colitis. *Lancet*, **1**, 607–11.

Rich, A.R. (1951) *The Pathogenesis of Tuberculosis*, 2nd edn., Charles C. Springfield, Illinois.

Richards, L.D. and Steingold, L. (1952) Enlarged hilar and paratracheal glands following B.C.G. vaccination. *Br. J. Tuberc.*, **46**, 163–5.

Richardson, E.P. (1961) Progressive multifocal leucoencephalopathy. *N. Engl. J. Med.*, **265**, 815–23.

Richman, A., Zeifer, H.D., Winkelstein, A., Kirschner, P.A. and Steinhardt, R.D. (1955) Chronic non-specific granulomatous inflammation of the stomach, duodenum and intestine. *Gastroenterology*, 29, 358–69.

Rickards, A.G. and Barrett, G.M. (1954) Non-tuberculous Addison's disease and its relationship to 'giant-cell granuloma' and multiple glandular disease. *Q. J. Med.*, 23, 403–23.

Rickards, A.G. and Harvey, P.W. (1954) 'Giant-cell granuloma' and other pituitary granulomata. *Q. J. Med.*, 23, 425–35.

Ricker, W. and Clark, M. (1949) Sarcoidosis: a clinico-pathologic review of 300 cases, including 22 autopsies. *Am. J. Clin. Pathol.*, 19, 725–49.

Ridderwold, L. (1964) Sarcoidosis in Norway. *Acta Med. Scand.*, suppl., 425, 111.

Rider, J.A. and Dodson, J.W. (1950) Sarcoidosis: report of a case manifested by retrobulbar mass, destruction of orbit, and infiltration of paranasal sinuses. *Am. J. Ophthalmol.*, 33, 117–20.

Ridley, C.M. (1957) Sarcoidosis with unusual arthritis. *Proc. R. Soc. Med.*, 59, 609–10.

Ridley, M., Turk, J.L. and Badenoch-Jones, P. (1979) *In vitro* modification of membrane receptors on cells of the mononuclear phagocyte system. *J. Pathol.*, 127, 173–84.

Rieder, H. (1910) Über Kombination von chronishcher Osteomyelitis (spina ventosa) mit Lupus pernio. *Fortschr. Rötgenstr.*, 15, 125–35.

Rigden, B. (1978) Sarcoid lesion in breast after probable sarcoidosis in lung. *Br. Med. J.*, 2, 1533–4.

Rijssel, T.G. Van (1947) Die ziekte van Besnier–Boeck, en bacteriëel-allergische onstekingsprocessen, Utrecht.

Riley, E.A. (1950) Boeck's sarcoid: a review based upon a clinical study of 52 cases. *Am. Rev. Tuberc.*, 62, 231–285.

Riley, R.L., Riley, M.C. and Hill, H.M. (1952) Diffuse pulmonary sarcoidosis: diffusing capacity during exercise and other lung function studies in relation to ACTH therapy. *Bull. Johns Hopkins Hosp.*, 91, 345–70.

Ripe, E., Nilsson, B.S., Hanngren, Å., Lins, L.-E., Ivemark, B., Askergren, J. and Sundblad, R. (1980) Comparison of Kveim antigen from spleen and mediastinal lymph-nodes. In *Proc. 8th International Conference on Sarcoidosis, Cardiff* (eds. W. Jones-Williams and B.H. Davies), Alpha Omega, Cardiff, pp. 668–89.

Rizzato, G., Brambilla, I., Bertoli, L., Conti, F., Merlini, R. and Montero, O. (1980) Impaired airway function and pulmonary haemolynamics in sarcoidosis. In *Proc. 8th International conference on Sarcoidosis, Cardiff* (eds. W. Jones-Williams and B.H. Davies), Alpha Omega, Cardiff, pp. 349–59.

Robert, F. (1944) Les manifestations osseuses de la maladie de Besnier–Boeck–Schaumann (la maladie de Perthes-Jüngling). *Sém. Hôp. Paris*, 25, 2327–30.

Robert, F. (1962) Sarcoidosis of the central nervous system. *Arch. Neurol.*, 7, 442–9.

Roberts, W.C., and Rang, M.C. (1958) Sarcoidosis of the liver and spleen. *Lancet*, 2, 296–9.

Roberts, W.C. (1981) in N.I.H. Conference: Pulmonary Sarcoidosis. *Ann. Intern. Med.*, 94, 73–94.

Roberts, W.C., McAllister, H.A., Ferrans, V.J. (1977) Sarcoidosis of the heart. *Am. J. Med.*, 63, 86–108.

Robertson, R.F. (1948) Vitamin D in treatment of Boeck's sarcoidosis. *Br. Med. J.*, 2, 1059–61.

Robinson, B. and Pound, A.W. (1950) Sarcoidosis: a survey with report of 30 cases. *Med. J. Aust.*, 2, 568–82.

Robinson, E.K. and Ernst, R.W. (1954) Boeck's sarcoid of the peritoneal cavity. *Surgery*, 36, 986–91.

Robinson, R.C.V. and Hahn, R.D. (1947) Sarcoidosis in siblings. *Arch. Intern. Med.*, 80, 249–56.

Robinson, R.G., Kerwin, D.M. and Tsou, E. (1980) Parathyroid adenoma with coexistent sarcoid granulomas. *Arch. Intern. Med.*, 140, 1547–8.

Rodman, T., Funderburk, E.E., Jr. and Myerson, R.M. (1959) Sarcoidosis with vertebral involvement. *Ann. Intern. Med.*, 50, 213–8.

Roelsen, E., Paulsen, L. (1964) Hypercalcaemia treated with sodium phytate. *Acta Med. Scand.*, 175, 751–62.

Roethe, R.A., Fuller, P.B., Byrd, R.B. and Hafermann, D.R. (1980) Transbronchoscopic lung biopsy in sarcoidosis: optimal number and sites for diagnosis. *Chest*, 77, 400–2.

Rogers, F.J. and Haserick, J.R. (1954) Sarcoidosis and the Kveim reaction. *J. Invest. Dermatol.*, 23, 389–406.

Rogers, W.N. (1957) Chronic beryllium poisoning treated with corticotrophin. *Br. Med. J.*, 2, 267.

Rohatgi, P.K. (1980) Radioisotope scanning in osseous sarcoidosis. *Am. J. Radiol.*, 134, 189–91.

Rømer, F.K. (1967) Sarcoidosis with large nodular lesions simulating pulmonary metastases. *Scand. J. Respir. Dis.*, 58, 11–6.

Rømer, F.K. (1977) Notification of sarcoidosis in Denmark – the 'true' incidence. *Z. Erkr. Atmungsorgane*, 149, 59–64.

Rømer, F.K. (1980a) Renal manifestations and abnormal calcium metabolism in sarcoidosis. *Q. J. Med.*, 49, 233–47.

Rømer, F.K. (1980b) Sarcoidosis and cancer – a critical view. In *Proc. 8th International Conference on Sarcoidosis, Cardiff*, (eds. W. Jones-Williams and B.H. Davies), Alpha Omega, Cardiff, pp. 567–71.

Rømer, F.K. (1980c) Angiotensin converting enzyme in newly detected sarcoidosis. *Acta Med. Scand.*, 208, 437–43.

Ronchese, F. (1942) Sarcoid and tuberculosis: report of a case with autopsy. *Arch. Dermatol. Syphilol. NY* 46, 860–71.

Roos, B. (1937) Neurologische Symptome bei der Schaumannschen benigner lymphogranulomatose. *Z. Kinderheilkd.*, 59, 280–302.

Roos, B. (1937) Über das Vorkommen der Schaumannschen benignen Lymphogranulomatose (des Boeckschen benignen Miliarlupoids) bel Kindern. *Z. Kinderheilkd.* 59, 280–302

Rosedale, R.S. (1945) Boeck's sarcoid involving the face and larynx. *Arch. Otalaryngol.*, *Chicago*. 42, 281–3.

Rosen, F.S. and Janeway, C.A. (1966) The gamma globulins. III: The antibody deficiency syndromes. *N. Engl. J. Med.*, 275, 709–15.

Rosen, J.A. and Wang, Y. (1965) CNS sarcoid granuloma monitored by brain scanning. *Arch. Intern. Med.*, 115, 336–8.

Rosen, Y., Amorosa, J.K., Moon, S., Cohen, J. and Lyons, H.A. (1977a) Occurrence of lung granulomas in patients with stage I sarcoidosis. *Am. J. Roentgenol.*, 129, 1083–5.

Rosen, Y., Moon, S., Huang, C., Gourin, A. and Lyons, H.A. (1977b) Granulomatous pulmonary angiitis in sarcoidosis. *Arch. Pathol. Lab. Med.*, 101, 170–4.

Rosen, Y., Athanassides, T.J., Moon, S. and Lyons, H.A. (1978) Non-granulomatous interstitial pneumonitis in sarcoidosis: relationship to development of epithelioid granulomas. *Chest*, 74, 122–5.

Rosen, Y., Vuletin, J.C., Pertschuk, L.P. and Silverstein, E. (1979) Sarcoidosis from the pathologist's vantage point. *Pathobiol. Ann.*, 14, 405–9.

Rosenbaum, J. (1941) Boeck's sarcoid of the lacrimal gland. *Arch. ophthalmol.*, 25, 477–82.

Rosenberg, J.C. (1971) Portal hypertension complicating hepatic sarcoidosis. *Surgery*, 69, 294–9.

Rosenthal, M., Trabert, U., Müller, W., Müller, S. and Wurm, K. (1976) Levamisole in sarcoidosis. *N. Engl. J. Med.*, 294, 112–3.

Rosenthal, S.R. (1949) Pathological and experimental studies of Boeck's sarcoid. *Am. Rev. Tuberc.*, 60, 236–48.

Rösgen, M. and Heigl, W. (1952) Bemerkungen zum Morbus Besnier–Boeck–Schaumann. *Med. Monatsschr.* 6, 636–41.

Ross, J.A. (1955) Uveoparotid sarcoidosis with cerebral involvement. *Br. Med. J.*, 2, 593–6.

Ross, J.K., Mikhail, J.R., Drury, R.A.B. and Mitchell, D.N. (1970) Mediastinoscopy. *Thorax*, 25, 312–6.

Ross, R.J.M. and Empey, D.W. (1983) Bilateral spontaneous pneumothorax in sarcoidosis. *Postgrad. Med. J.*, 59, 106–7.

Rossman, M.D., Dauber, J.H. and Daniele, R.P. (1981) Nodular endobronchial sarcoidosis: a study comparing blood and lung lymphocytes. *Chest*, 79, 427–31.

Rossman, M.D., Dauber, J.H., Cardillo, and M.E. Daniele, R.P. (1982) Pulmonary sarcoidosis: correlation of serum angiotensin-converting enzyme with blood and broncho-alveolar lymphocytes. *Am. Rev. Respir. Dis.*, 125, 366–9.

Rossman, M.D., Dauber, J.H. and Daniele, R.P. (1978) Identification of activated T-cells in sarcoidosis. *Am. Rev. Respir. Dis.*, 117, 713–20.

Rostenberg, A., Jr., Szymanski, F.J., Brebis, G.J., Haeberlin, J.B. and Senear, F.E. (1953) Experimental studies on sarcoidosis: persistence and survival of inoculated micro-organisms. *Arch. Dermatol. Syphilol., NY*, 67, 306–14.

Rothfeld, E. and Folk, E. (1962) Sarcoid myopathy. *J. Am. Med. Assoc.*, 179, 903–5.

Rothfeld, J. (1930) Ein Fall von Lupus pernio mit schweren Gehirnerscheinungen. *Klin. Wochenschr.*, 9, 1030–2.

Roughton, F.J.W. and Forster, R.E. (1957) Relative importance of diffusion and chemical reaction rates in determining rate of exchange of gases in the human lung. *J. Appl. Physiol.*, 11, 290–302.

Rubin, E.H. and Pinner, M. (1944) Sarcoidosis: one case report and literature review of autopsied cases. *Am. Rev. Tuber.*, 49, 146–69.

Rubin, H.J. and Kling, D.H. (1948) Boeck's sarcoid of nasal vault. *Ann. Otol., Rhinol., Laryngol.*, 57, 1083–7.

Rudberg-Roos, I. and Roos, B.E. (1958) Pulmonary function in sarcoidosis before and after ACTH and cortisone therapy. *Acta Tuber. Scand.*, 35, 49–66.

Rudin, L., Megalli,. M., and Mesa-Tejada, R. (1974) Genital sarcoidosis. *Urology*, 111, 750–3.

Rudzki, J., Ishak, K.G. and Zimmerman, H.J. (1975) Chronic intrahepatic cholestasis of sarcoidosis. *Am. J. Med.*, 59, 373–87.

Ruete, A. (1922) Zur Aetiologie der Boeckschen Erkrankung. *Dermatol. Z.* 37, 129.

Rukavina, J.G., Oakin, M. and Lynch, F.W. (1958) The effect of an intravenous chelating agent, edathamil sodium (Na 2 EDTA) in 3 cases of sarcoidosis. *J. Invest. Dermatol.*, 31, 259–62.

Runyon, E.H. (1965) Pathogenic mycobacteria. *Adv. Tuberc. Res.*, 14, 235–87.

Rutishauser, E. and Rywlin, A. (1950) Besnier–Boeck rénal. *J. Urol. Med. Chir.*, 56, 277–85.

Ryrie, D.R. (1954) Sarcoidosis with obstructive jaundice. *Proc. R. Soc. Med.*, 47, 879.

Rywlin, A. (1952) Le Besnier–Boeck de la glande thyroide. *Pr. Med.* 60, 1278–80.

Saari, M., Miettinen, R., Alenko, H. (1975) Uveitis: report of a 20–year survey in northern Finland. *Can. J. Ophthalmol.*, 10, 356–60.

Sahetya, G.K., Cobb, W.B., Facen, H.T., Hassan, S.N., Kumar, B., Young, R.C. (1980) Pulmonary sarcoidosis: a significant cause of chronic airways obstruction. In *Proc. 8th International Conference on Sarcoidosis, Cardiff*, (eds. W. Jones–Williams and B.H. Davies), Alpha Omega, Cardiff, pp. 361–7.

Sahn, S.A., Schwarz, M.I., Lakshminarayan, S. (1974) Sarcoidosis: the significance of an acinar pattern on chest roentgenogram. *Chest.* 65, 684–7.

Saint-Remy, J-M.R., Mitchell, D.N., Cole, P.J. (1983) Variation in immunoglobulin levels and circulating immune complexes in sarcoidosis. *Am. Rev. Respir. Dis.*, 127, 23–7.

Sakula, A. (1963) Bronchial carcinoma and sarcoidosis. *Br. J., Cancer*, 17, 206–12.

Saldana, M.J., Patchewsky, A.S., Israel, H.L., Atkinson, G.W. (1977) Pulmonary angiitis and granulomatosis. *Hum. Pathol.*, 8, 391–409.

Sales, L.M. (1953) Sarcoidosis of myocardium: report of a case. *J. Fl. Med. Assoc.*, 40, 27–31.

Salm, R. (1969) Familial sarcoidosis terminating as neurosarcoidosis. *Postgrad. Med. J.*, 45, 668–74.

Salo, O.P., Hannuksela, M. (1972) Immunohistology of the Kveim reaction. *Ann. Clin. Res.*, 4, 169–72.

Salomon, M.I., Poon, T.P., Hsu, K.C., King, E.J. and Tchertkoff, V. (1975) Membranous glomerulopathy in a patient with sarcoidosis. *Arch. Pathol.*, 99, 479–83.

Saltzman, G.-F. (1958) Roentgenologic changes in cerebral sarcoidosis. *Acta Radiol.*, 50, 235–41.

Salvesen, H.A. (1935) The sarcoid of Boeck, a disease of importance to internal medicine. *Acta Med. Scand.*, 86, 127–51.

Sanders, M.A. and Shilling, J.S. (1976) Retinal, choroidal and optic disc involvement in sarcoidosis. *Trans. Ophthalmol. Soc. UK*, 96, 140–4.

Sandors, F. (1958) Development of sarcoid tubercles at the site of tuberculin injections. *Tubercle, Lond.*, 39, 372–9.

Sands, J.H., Palmer, P.P., Mayock, R.L. and Creger, W.P. (1955) Evidence for serologic hyper-reactivity in sarcoidosis. *Am. J. Med.*, 19, 401–9.

Sanner, T. and Seljelid, K. (1975) Macrophate cytolytic factor. *Exp. Cell. Res.*, 94, 221–6.

Santoianni, G. (1938) La malattia di Besnier–boeck–Schaumann (transmissione sperimentale negli animali. *Arch. Ital. Dermatol. Sifilogr. Venereol.*, 15, 78–90.

Santoianni, G. and Ayala, L. (1949) Ricerche sperimentali sulla etiologia della malattia di Besnier–Boeck–Schaumann. Risultati della prova biologica negli animali. *Ann. Ital. Dermatol. Sifilogr.*, 4, 9–16.

Sarkar, T.K. (1970) Anaplastic carcinoma of the lung and sarcoidosis. *Br. J. Clin. Pract.*, **24**, 297–9.

Sarner, M. and Wilson, R.J. (1965) Erythema nodosum and psittacosis: report of 5 cases. *Br. Med. J.*, **2**, 1469–70.

Sartwell, P.E. and Edwards, L.B. (1974) Epidemiology of sarcoidosis in the US Navy. *Am. J. Epidemiol.*, **99**, 250–7.

Saslaw, S. and Beman, F.M. (1959) Erythema nodosum as a manifestation of histoplasmosis. *J. Am. Med. Assoc.*, **170**, 1178–9.

Saumon, G., Georges, R., Loiseau, A. and Turiaf, J. (1976) Membrane diffusing capacity and pulmonary capillary blood volume in pulmonary sarcoidosis. *Ann. NY Acad. Sci.*, **278**, 284–91.

Savin, L.H. (1934) An analysis of the signs and symptoms of 66 published cases of the uveoparotid Syndrome with details of an additional case. *Trans. Ophthal. Soc. UK*, **54**, 549–66.

Scadding, J.G. (1950) Sarcoidosis with special reference to lung changes, *Br. Med. J.*, **1**, 745–53.

Scadding, J.G. (1956) Insensitivity to tuberculin in pulmonary tuberculosis. *Tubercle*, **37**, 371–80.

Scadding, J.G. (1959) Principles of definition in Medicine. *Lancet*, **1**, 323–5.

Scadding, J.G. (1960a) Chronic diffuse interstitial fibrosis of the lungs. *Br. Med. J.*, **1**, 443–50.

Scadding, J.G. (1960b) *Mycobacterium tuberculosis* in the aetiology of sarcoidosis. *Br. Med. J.*, **2**, 1617–23.

Scadding, J.G. (1961a) Calcification in sarcoidosis. *Tubercle*, **42**, 121–35.

Scadding, J.G. (1961b) Prognosis of intrathoracic sarcoidosis in England. *Br. Med. J.*, **2**, 1165–72.

Scadding, J.G. (1963) The meaning of diagnostic terms in bronchopulmonary disease. *Br. Med. J.*, **2**, 1425–30.

Scadding, J.G. (1964) Fibrosing alveolitis. *Br. Med. J.*, **2**, 686.

Scadding, J.G. (1967) *Sarcoidosis*, Eyre and Spottiswoode, London, pp. 46, 229, 244, 253, 266, 330, 408.

Scadding, J.G. (1968) Further observations on calcification in sarcoidosis. *Scand. J. Respir. Dis.*, Suppl. **65**, 235–42.

Scadding, J.G. (1968) A 'burnt-out' case of sarcoidosis. *Postgrad. Med. J.*, **44**, 105–8.

Scadding, J.G. (1971a) Further observations on sarcoidosis associated with M. *tuberculosis* infection. In *Proc. 5th International Conference on Sarcdoidosis, Prague, 1969* (eds. L. Levinsky and F. Macholda), Universita Karlova, Prague, pp 89–92.

Scadding, J.G. (1971b) Tuberculin sensitivity in tuberculosis. *Postgrad. Med. J.*, **47**, 694–7.

Scadding, J.G. (1972) Skin infiltrations in 500 cases of sarcoidosis. *Praxis*, **61**, 133–6.

Scadding, J.G. (1972) The semantics of medical diagnosis. *Int. J. Bio.-Med. Comput.*, **3**, 83–90.

Scadding, J.G. (1981a) The eponymy of sarcoidosis. *J. R. Soc. Med.*, **74**, 147–57.

Scadding, J.G. (1981b) Talking clearly about bronchopulmonary diseases. In *Scientific Foundations of Respiratory Medicine*, (eds. J.G. Scadding and G. Cumming), Heinemann Medical, London: W.B. Saunders, Philadelphia, Chapter 58.

Scadding, J.G. and Hinson, K.F.W. (1967) Diffuse fibrosing alveolitis (diffuse interstitial fibrosis of the lungs). *Thorax*, **22**, 291–304.

Scadding, J.G. and Sherlock, S. (1948) Liver biopsy in sarcoidosis. *Thorax*, 3, 79–87.

Schabel, S.I., Forte, G.A. and McKee, K.A. (1978) Posterior lymphadenopathy in sarcoidosis. *Radiology*, 129, 591–3.

Schaefer, M., Lapras, C., Thomalske, G., Grau, H. and Schober, R. (1977) Sarcoidosis of the pineal gland. *J. Neurosurg.*, 47, 630–2.

Scharkoff, T. (1977) Sarkoidose und Beruf. *Z. Erkr. Atmungsorgane*, 149, 50–8.

Schattenburg, H.J. and Harris, W.H., Jr. (1946) Malignant granulosa–cell tumour with pseudo-tubercles. *Am. J. Pathol.*, 22, 539–49.

Schaumann, J. (1917) Étude sur le lupus pernio et ses rapports avec les sarcoïdes et la tuberculose. *Ann. Dermatol. Syphiligr.*, 6, 357–73.

Schaumann, J. (1919) Études histologiques et bactériologiques sur les manifestations médullaires du lymphogranulome bénin. *Ann. Dermatol. Syphiligr.*, 7, 385–98.

Schaumann, J. (1924) Benign lymphogranuloma and its cutaneous manifestations. *Br. J. Dermatol. Syph.*, 36, 515–44.

Schaumann, J. (1926) Notes on the histology of the medullary and osseous lesions in benign lymphogranuloma and especially on their relationship to the radiographic picture. *Acta Radiol.*, 7, 358–64.

Schaumann, J. (1933) Etude anatomo-pathologique et histologique sur les localisations viscerales de la lymphogranulomatose benigne. *Bull. Soc. Fr. Dermatol. Syphiligr.*, 40, 1167–8.

Schaumann, J. (1934a) Observations cliniques, bactériologiques et sérologiques pour servir à l'étiologie de la lymphogranulomatose bénigne. *Bull. Soc. Fr. Dermatol. Syphiligr.* 41, 1296–322.

Schaumann, J. (1934b) Sur le lupus pernio. Mémoire présenté en Novembre 1914 à la Société française de Dermatologie et de Syphiligraphie pour le Prix Zambaco, Stockholm.

Schaumann, J. (1936) Lymphogranulomatosis benigna in the light of prolonged clinical observations and autopsy findings. *Br. J. Dermatol.*, 48, 399–446.

Schaumann, J. (1941) On the nature of certain peculiar corpuscles present in the tissue of lymphogranulomatosis benigna. *Acta Med. Scand.*, 106, 239–53.

Schaumann, J. and Seeberg, G. (1948) On cutaneous reactions in cases of lymphogranulomatosis benigna. *Acta Derm.-Venereol.*, 28, 158–68.

Schiessle, W., Konn, G., Wurm, K., and Reindell, H. (1963) Considérations radiologiques bronchoscopiques et biopsiques dans la sarcoïdose endothoracique (302 cas): éléments pathogéniques. *J. Fr. Med. Chir. thorac.*, 17, 465–80.

Schiff, A.D., Blatt, C.J. and Colp. C. (1969) Recurrent pericardial effusion secondary to sarcoidosis of the pericardium. *N. Engl. J. Med.*, 281, 141–3.

Schiffner, J. and Sharma, O.P. (1977) Ulcerative sarcoidosis. *Arch. Dermatol.*, 113, 676–7.

Schmidt, M.E. and Douglas, S.D. (1977) Monocyte IgG receptor activity dynamics, and modulation: normal individuals and patients with granulomatous diseases. *J. Lab. Clin. Med.*, 89, 332–40.

Schoenberger, C.I., Line, B.R., Keogh, B.A., Hunninghake, G.W. and Crystal, R.G. (1982) Lung inflammation in sarcoidosis: comparison of serum angiotensin-converting enzyme levels with bronchoalveolar lavage and gallium–67 scanning assessment of the T-lymphocyte alveolitis. *Thorax*, 37, 19–25.

Schoenfield, Y., Avidor, E., Eldar, M., Vidne, B., Levy, M. and Pinkhas, J. (1978) Squamous cell carcinoma assoicated with sarcoidosis in the lung. *Oncology*, 35, 112–3.

Scholz, D.A. and Keating, F.R., Jr. (1956) Renal insufficiency, renal calculi and nephrocalcinosis in sarcoidosis: report of 8 cases. *Am. J. Med.*, **21**, 75–84.

Schönholzer, G. (1947) Morbus Besnier–Boeck–Schaumann und Armeedurchleuchtung. *Schweiz. Med. Wschr.*, **77**, 585–8.

Schoonhoven van Beurden, A.J.R.E. Van (1942) Bijdrage tot de pathogenese van de ziekte van Besnier–Boeck. *Ned. Tijdschr. Geneeskd.*, **89**, 2280.

Schrijver, H. and Schillings, P.H.M. (1952) Thrombocytopenic purpura with sarcoidosis, cured after splenectomy. *Acta Med. Scand.*, **144**, 213–6.

Schubothe, H. (1952) Antikorperbedingte hämolytische Anämien. *Verh. Dtsch. Ges. Inn. Med.*, **58**, 679–94.

Schubotz, R., Goebel, K.M., and Hausmann, L. (1980) Kveim–induced migration inhibition in sarcoidosis. In *Proc. 8th International Conference on Sarcoidosis, Cardiff*, (eds. W. Jones-Williams and B.H. Davies), Alpha Omega, Cardiff, pp. 191–4.

Schultz, A. (1945) Boeck's sarcoid with uveoparotitis and dacryoadenitis. *Am. J. Ophthalmol.*, **28**, 1010–4.

Schumacher, H. (1909) Fall von beiderseitiger Iridocyclitis chronica bei Boeckschem multiplen benignem Sarkoid. *Muench. Med. Wochenschr.*, **56**, 2664.

Schüpbach, A. and Wernly, M. (1943) Hyperkalzaemic und Organverkalkungen bei Boeckscher Krankheit. *Acta Med. Scand.*, **115**, 401–22.

Schuyler, M.R., Thigpen, T.P. and Salvaggio, J.E. (1978) Local pulmonary immunity in pigeon breeder's disease. *Ann. Intern. Med.*, **88**, 355–8.

Schwartz, S.O. (1945) The prognostic value of marrow eosinophils in thrombocytopenic purpura. *Am. J. Med. Sci.*, **209**, 579–87.

Schwartz, E.L., and Baum, S. (1968) Radioisotope brain scanning in cerebral sarcoidosis. *J. Am. Med. Assoc.*, **203**, 365–6.

Schwarzschild, W. and Myerson, R.M. (1968) Venous insufficiency of the small intestine secondary to sarcoidosis of mesenteric lymph nodes. *Am. J. Gastroenterol.*, **50**, 69–72.

Schweitzer, V.G., Thompson, N.W., Clark, K.A., Nishiyama, R.H., and Bigos, S.T. (1981) Sarcoidosis hypercalcaemia and primary hyperparathyroidism. *Am. J. Surg.*, **142**, 499–503.

Schweizer, A.T. and Kanaar, P. (1967) Sarcoidosis with polyarthritis in a child. *Arch. Dis. Child.*, **42**, 671–4.

Scott, N.M., Smith, V.M. Cox, P.A. and Palmer, E.D. (1953) Sarcoid and sarcoid-like granulomas of the stomach: a clinical evaluation. *Arch. Intern. Med.*, **92**, 741–9.

Scott, R.B. (1938) The sarcoidosis of Boeck. *Br. Med. J.*, **2**, 777–8.

Seal, R.M.E., Hapke, E.J., Thomas, G.O., Meek, J.C. and Hayes, M. (1968) The pathology of the acute and chronic stages of farmer's lung. *Thorax*, **23**, 469–89.

Seeberg, G. (1951) Tuberculin sensitivity in lymphogranulomatosis benigna studied with depot tuberculin. *Acta Derm.-Venereol.*, **31**, 427–34.

Segal, A.W. and Loewi, G. (1976) Neutrophil dysfunction in Crohn's disease. *Lancet*, **2**, 219–21.

Seibert, F.B. and Nelson, J.W. (1943) Electrophoresis of serum proteins in tuberculosis and other chronic diseases. *Am. Rev. Tuberc.*, **47**, 66–77.

Seibert, F.B., Seibert, M.V., Atno, A.J. and Campbell, H.W. (1947) Variation in protein and polysaccharide content of sera in the chronic diseases, tuberculosis, sarcoidosis and carcinoma. *J. Clin. Invest.* **26**, 90–102.

Seifert, O. (1939) Über benignes miliar lupoid (Typus Boeck) der oberen Luftwege. *Z. Hals-, Nasen-Ohrenheilkd.*, **46**, 69.

678 Sarcoidosis

Sekiguchi, M., Konno, S., Kondo, M. and Hirasawa, K. (1967) A case of myocardial sarcoidosis proved while living. *J. Circ. J.*, 311, 987.

Selenkow, H. A., Tyler, H.R., Matson, D.D. and Nelson, D.H. (1959) Hypopituitarism due to hypothalamic sarcoidosis. *Am. J. Med. Sci.*, 238, 456–63.

Selroos, O. (1966) Exudative pleurisy and sarcoidosis. *Br. J. Dis. Chest*, 60, 191–6.

Selroos, O. (1969) The frequency, clinical picture and prognosis of pulmonary sarcoidosis in Finland. *Acta Med. Scand.*, Suppl. 503.

Selroos, O. (1974) The frequency of sarcoidosis in Finland. In *Proc. 6th International Conference on Sarcoidosis, Tokyo*, (eds. K. Iwai and Y. Hosoda), University of Tokyo Press, Tokyo, p. 319–21.

Selroos, O. (1976a) Sarcoidosis of the spleen. *Acta Med. Scand.*, 200, 337–40.

Selroos, O. (1976b) Fine-needle aspiration biopsy of spleen in diagnosis of sarcoidosis. *Ann. NY Acad., Sci.*, 278, 511–20.

Selroos, O. (1977) Fine-needle aspiration biopsy of spleen in diagnosis of sarcoidosis. *Z. Erkr. Atmungsorgane*, 149, 109–11.

Selroos, O., Brander, L. and Virolainen, M. (1974) Sarcoidosis and myeloma of lambda-type IgG. *Acta Med. Scand.*, 195, 59–63.

Selroos, O. and Klockars, M. (1977) Serum lysozyme in sarcoidosis. *Scand. J. Respir. Dis.*, 58, 110–6.

Selroos, O. and Koivunen, E. (1979) Prognostic significance of lymphopenia in sarcoidosis. *Acta Med. Scand.*, 206, 259–62.

Selroos, O. and Kuhlbäck, B. (1972) Renal involvement in sarcoidosis. In *La Sarcoïdose particulièrement dans ses localisations extrathoraciques*. Rapport du symposium européen, Sept. 1971, (ed. Y. Gallopin), Hallwag, Geneva (Re-printed from *Praxis*), 158–163.

Selroos, O. and Liewendahl, K. (1972) Clinical manifestations of thyroid sarcoidosis. In *La Sarcoïdose particulièrement dans ses localisations extrathoraciques*. Rapport du symposium européen, Sept. 1971, (ed. Y. Gallopin), Hallwag, Geneva (Reprinted from *Praxis*, 151–7.

Selroos, O. and Niemistö, M. (1977) Sarcoidosis of the nose. *Scand. J. Respir. Dis.*, 58, 57–62.

Selroos, O., and Sellergren, T.L. (1979) Corticosteroid therapy of pulmonary sarcoidosis: a prospective evlauation of alternate day and daily dosage in stage II disease. *Scand. J. Respir. Dis.*, 60, 215–21.

Selroos, O., Sellergren, T-L., Vuorio, M. and Virolainen, M. (1973) Sarcoidosis in identical twins. *Am. Rev. Respir. Dis.*, 108, 1401–6.

Semins, H., Nugent, G.R. and Chou, S.M. (1972) Intramedullary spinal cord sarcoidosis. *J. Neurosurg.*, 37, 233–6.

Semple, A.B. and Hughes, T.L. (1959) *Report on Liverpool's X-ray Campaign*, Liverpool Health Dept and Liverpool Hospital Board, p. 77.

Semple, P. d'A. (1975) Thrombocytopenia, haemolytic anaemia and sarcoidosis. *Br. Med. J.*, 2, 440–1.

Serwer, G.A., Edwards, S.B., Benson, D.W., Anderson, P.A.W. and Spach, M. (1978) Ventricular tachyarrhythmia due to cardiac sarcoidosis in a child. *Pediatrics*, 62, 322–5.

Seshul, R., Grubb, D.J. (1960) Transition from tuberculosis to sarcoidosis. *Dis. Chest*, 38, 462–4.

Shaffer, B., Cahn, M.M., and Levy, E.J. (1953) Sarcoidosis apparently cured by quinacrine (Atabrine) hydrochloride. *Arch. Dermatol. Syphilol. NY*, 67, 640–1.

Sharma, O.P. (1967) Splenic rupture in sarcoidosis. *Am. Rev. Respir. Dis.*, 96, 101–2.

Sharma, O.P. (1980) Unusual manifestations of pulmonary sarcoidosis. In *Proc. 8th International Conference on Sarcoidosis Cardiff, 1978* (eds. W. Jones-Williams and B.H. Davies), Alpha Omega, Cardiff, pp. 378–85.

Sharma, O.P., Colp, C. and Williams, M.H. (1966a) Pulmonary function studies in patients with bilateral sarcoidosis of hilar lymph-nodes. *Arch. Intern. Med.*, 177, 436–9.

Sharma, O.P., Colp, C. and Williams, M.H. (1966b) Course of pulmonary sarcoidosis with and without corticosteroid therapy as determined by pulmonary function studies. *Am. J. Med.*, 41, 541–51.

Sharma, O.P. and Chandor, S.R. (1972) IgA deficiency in sarcoidosis. *Am. Rev. Respir. Dis.*, 106, 600–3.

Sharma, O.P. and Gordonson, J. (1975) Pleural effusion in sarcoidosis: a report of 6 cases. *Thorax*, 30, 95–101.

Sharma, O.P., Hewlett, R. and Gordonson, J. (1973) Nodular sarcoidosis: an unusual radiographic appearance. *Chest*, 64, 189–92.

Sharma, O., Hughes, D.T.D., James, D.G. and Naish, P. (1971a) Immunosuppressive therapy with azathioprine in sarcoidosis. In *Proc. 5th International Conference on Sarcoidosis, Prague*, (eds. L. Levinsky and F. Macholda), Universita Karlova, Prague, pp. 635–7.

Sharma, O.P. and James, D.G. (1971) Hypogammaglobulinaemia, depressed delayed-type hypersensitivity and granuloma formation. *Am. Rev. Respir. Dis.*, 104, 228–31.

Sharma, O.P., James, D.G. and Fox, R.A. (1971b) A correlation of *in vitro* delayed-type hypersensitivity and *in vitro* lymphocyte transformation in sarcoidosis. *Chest*, 60, 35–7.

Sharma, O.P., Neville, E., Walker, A.N. and James, D.G. (1976) Familial sarcoidosis: a possible genetic influence. *Ann. NY Acad. Sci.*, 278, 386–400.

Sharma, O.P., Peters, R.L., Ashcavai, M. and Balchum, O.J. (1970) Australia (hepatitis) antigen in sarcoidosis. *Lancet*, 2, 928.

Shay, H., Berk, J.E., Sones, M., Aegerter, E.E., Weston, J.K. and Adams, A.B. (1951) The liver in sarcoidosis. *Gastroenterology*, 19, 441–61.

Shealy, C.N., Kahama, L., Engel, F.L. and McPherson, H.T. (1961) Hypothalamic-pituitary sarcoidosis: a report on 4 patients, one with prolonged remission of diabetes insipidus following steroid therapy. *Am. J. Med.*, 30, 46–55.

Sheehan, H.L. and Summers, V.K. (1949) The syndrome of hypopituitarism. *Q. J. Med.*, 18, 319–78.

Sheffer, A.L., Ruddy, S. and Israel, H.L. (1971) Serum complement levels in sarcoidosis. In *Proc. 5th International Conference on Sarcoidosis, Prague*, (eds. L. Levinsky and F. Macholda), Universita Karlova, Prague, pp. 195–7.

Sheinfield, W.I. and Rubinov, M. (1964) Noncaseating epithelioid granuloma of the appendix. (localized sarcoid disease?). *J. Int. Coll. Surg.*, 1, 1–4.

Shelley, W.B. and Hurley, H.J. (1958a) Experimental evidence for an allergic basis for granuloma formation in man. *Nature (London)*, 180, 1060.

Shelley, W.B. and Hurley, H.L. (1958b) The allergic origin of zirconium deodorant granulomas. *Br. J. Dermatol.*, 70, 75–101.

Shepard, C.C. (1960) Acid-fast bacilli in nasal secretions in leprosy, and results of inoculation of mice. *Am. J. Hyg.*, 71, 147–57.

Sherlock, S. (1958) Diseases of the liver and biliary system. Blackwell, Oxford, p. 495.

Sherman, F.E. and Moran, T.J. (1954) Granulomas of stomach. *Am. J. Clin. Pathol.*, 24, 415–21.

Shields, L.H. (1959) Disseminated cryptococcosis producing a sarcoid type reaction. *Arch. Intern. Med.,* 104, 763–70.

Shigematsu, M., Kitamura, K., Norbechi, K. and Hosada, Y. (1967) Epidemiologic features of sarcoidosis in Japan basing upon 700 case studies. In *Proc. 4th International Conference on Sarcoidosis, Paris* (eds. J. Turiaf and J. Chabot), Masson, Paris, pp. 365–8.

Shigemitsu, N., Emuri, K., Matsuba, K., Harada, S. and Takahashi, T. (1978) Clinicopathologic characteristics of pulmonary acinar sarcoidosis. *Chest,* 73, 186–8.

Shmuhes, E., Lantis, L.R. and Hurley, H.J. (1970) Verrucose sarcoidosis. *Arch. Dermatol.,* 102, 665–9.

Shulman, L.E., Schoenrich, E.H. and Harvey, A.M. (1952) The effects of adrenocorticotrophic hormone (ACTH) and cortisone on sarcoidosis. *Bull. Johns Hopkins Hosp.,* 912, 371–415.

Siegel, C.J., Honda, M., Salik, J. and Mendeloff, A.I. (1961) Dysphagia due to granulomatous myositis of the cricopharyngeus muscle. *Trans. Assoc. Am. Physicians,* 74, 342–52.

Siegler, D. (1978) Sarcoidosis and selective IgA deficiency. *Br. J. Dis. Chest,* 72, 143–6.

Siemsen, J.K., Grebe, S.F., Sargent, E.N. and Wentz, D. (1976) Gallium–67 scintigraphy of pulmonary diseases as a complement to radiography. *Radiology,* 118, 371–5.

Sieracki, J.C. and Fisher, E.R. (1973) Ceroid nature of so-called Hamazaki-Wesenberg bodies. *Am. J. Clin. Pathl.,* 59, 248–53.

Siltzbach, L.E. (1952) Effects of cortisone on sarcoidosis: a study of 13 patients. *Am. J. Med.,* 12, 139–60.

Siltzbach, L.E. (1958) Clinical conference on sarcoidosis. *J. Mt Sinai Hosp.,* 25, 548.

Siltzbach, L.E. (1961a) Current status of the Nickerson–Kveim reaction. *Am. Rev. Respir. Dis.,* 84, 89–93;

Siltzbach, L.E. (1961b) The Kveim test in sarcoidosis: a study of 750 patients. *J. Am. Med. Ass.,* 178, 476–82.

Siltzbach, L.E. (1964a) Significance and specificity of the Kveim test. *Acta Med. Scand.,* Suppl. 425, 74–8.

Siltzbach, L.E. (1964b) An international Kveim test study. *Acta Med. Scand.,* Suppl. 425, 178–86.

Siltzbach, L.E. (1964c) Schema for course of sarcoidosis. *Acta Med. Scand.,* Suppl. 425, 273–4.

Siltzbach, L.E. (1967) An international Kveim test study 1960–1966. In *Proc. 4th International Conference on Sarcoidosis, Paris* (eds. J. Turiaf and J. Chabot), Masson, Paris, pp. 201–13.

Siltzbach, L.E. (1976) Qualities and behaviour of satisfactory Kveim suspensions. *Ann. NY Acad. Sci.,* 278, 665–8.

Siltzbach, L.E. and Blaugrund, S.M. (1963) Sarcoidosis of the mucosa of the respiratory tract. *Trans. 43rd Ann. Meet. Am. Broncho-esophagol. Assoc.,* 25.

Siltzbach, L.E. and Duberstein, J.L. (1968) Arthritis in sarcoidosis. *Clin. Orthop.* 57, 31–50.

Siltzbach, L.E. and Ehrlich, J.C. (1954) The Nickerson-Kveim reaction in sarcoidosis. *Am. J. Med.,* 16, 790–803.

Siltzbach, L.E., Glade, R.R., Hirshaut, Y., Vieira, L.O.B.D., Celikoglu, I.S. and Hirschhorn, K. (1971) *In vitro* stimulation of peripheral lymphocytes in sarcoidosis. In *Proc. 5th International Conference on Sarcoidosis, Prague, 1969* (eds. L. Levinsky and F. Macholda), Universita Karlova, Prague, pp. 217–20.

Siltzbach, L.E., Greenberg, G.M. (1968) Childhood sarcoidosis: a study of 18 patients. *N. Engl. J. Med.,* **279**, 1239–45.

Siltzbach, L.E., James, D.G., Neville, E., Turiaf, J., Battesti, J.P., Sharma, O.P., Hosoda, Y., Mikami, R., Odaka, M. (1974) Course and prognosis of sarcoidosis around the world. *Am. J. Med.,* **57**, 847–52.

Siltzbach, L.E., Posner, A. and Medine, M.M. (1951) Cortisone therapy in sarcoidosis. *J. Am. Med. Assoc.,* **147**, 927–9.

Siltzbach, L.E. and Ruttemberg, M.A. (1971a) Chemical and physical characteristics of the active principle in Kveim suspensions. In *Proc. 5th International conference on Sarcoidosis, Prague, 1969* (eds. L. Levinsky and F. Macholda), Universita Karlova, Prague, pp. 371–4

Siltzbach, L. and Som, M.L. (1952) Sarcoidosis with bronchial involvement: 2 cases with bronchoscopic biopsies. *J. Mt Sinai Hosp.,* **19**, 473–80.

Siltzbach, L.E. and Teirstein, A.S. (1964) Chloroquine therapy in 43 patients with intrathoracic and cutaneous sarcoidosis. *Acta Med. Scand.,* Suppl. **425**, 302–6.

Siltzbach, L.E., Vieira, L.O.B., Topilsky, M. and Yanowitz, H.D. (1971c) Is there Kveim responsiveness in Crohn's disease? *Lancet,* **2**, 634–6.

Siltzbach, L.E., Vieira, L.O.B.D. and Waraich, B.A. (1971b) Effects of oral corticosteroids on Kveim reactivity in 30 Kveim-positive subjects with sarcoidosis. In *Proc. 5th International Conference on Sarcoidosis. Prague, 1969* (eds. L. Levinsky and F. Macholda), Universita Karlova, Prague, pp. 365–6.

Silver, H.M., Shirkhoda, A. and Simon, D.B. (1978) Symptomatic osseous sarcoidosis with findings on bone scan. *Chest,* **73**, 238–41.

Silverman, K.J., Hutchins, G.M. and Bulkley, B.M. (1978) Cardiac saracoid: a clinicopathological study of 84 unselected patients with systemic sarcoidosis. *Circulation,* **58**, 1204–11.

Silverstein, A., Feuer, M.M. and Siltzbach, L.E. (1965) Neurologic sarcoidosis: study of 18 cases. **28**, 23–9.

Silverstein, A., Siltzbach, L.E. (1969) Muscle involvement in sarcoidosis. *Arch. Neurol.,* **21**, 235–41.

Silverstein, E. (1976) Pathogenesis of sarcoidosis: an hypothetical model. *Med. Hypotheses,* **2**, 75–8.

Silverstein, E. and Friedland, J. (1979) Serum angiotensin-converting enzyme in sarcoidosis and other diseases. *Lancet,* **1**, 382–3.

Silverstein, E., Friedland, J., Lyons, H. and Gourin, A. (1976) Elevation of angiotesin–converting enzyme in granulomatous lymph-nodes and serum in sarcoidosis: clinical and possible pathogenic significance. *Ann. NY Acad. Sci.,* **278**, 498–513.

Silverstein, E., Friedland, J., Stanek, A.E., Smith, P.R., Dearson, D.R. and Lyons, H.A. (1983) Pathogenesis of sarcoidosis. Mechanism of angiotensin converting enzyme elevation: T-lymphocyte modulation of enzyme induction in mononuclear phagocytes, enzyme properties. In *Proc. 9th International Conference Sarcoidosis and other granulomatous disorders.* Pergamon Press, Oxford, pp. 319–325.

Silverstein, E., Pertschuk, L.P. and Friedland, J. (1979) Immunofluorescent localisation of angiotensin-converting enzyme in epithelioid and giant-cells of sarcoidosis granulomas. *Proc. Nat. Acad. Sci. USA,* **76**, 6646–8.

Šimeček, C. (1970) Nachweis der Tuberkelbazillen bei der sarkoidose mittels der Tierimpfung. *Prax. Pneumol.,* **24**, 494–7.

Simkins, S. (1951) Boeck's sarcoid with complete heart block mimicking carotid sinus syndrome. *J. Am. Med. Assoc.* **146**, 794–7.

Simmonds, M. (1917) Über das Vorkommen von Riesenzellen in der Hypophyse. *Virchows Arch. Pathol. Anat. Physiol.,* 223, 281.

Simon, H.B. and Wolfe, S. (1973) Granulomatous hepatitis and prolonged fever of unknown origin. *Medicine Baltimore,* 52, 1–21.

Simpson, J.A. (1960) Myasthenia gravis: a new hypothesis. *Scott. Med. J.* 5, 419–36.

Simpson, J.R. (1963) Sarcoidosis with erythrodermia and ulceration. *Br. J. Dermatol.,* 75, 193–8.

Simpson, R.G. (1950) Erythema nodosum: the provocation problem with special reference to lymphogranuloma venereum. *Dermatologica,* 101, 94–107.

Singer, E.P., Hensler, N.M. and Flynn, P.F. (1959) Sarcoidosis: an analysis of 45 cases in a large military hospital. *Am. J. Med.* 26, 364–75.

Singh, M.D. and Fitzpatrick, M.J. (1964) Cranial neuropathy associated with sarcoidosis. Case report. *Dis. Chest,* 45, 431–5.

Singh, R., Kaur, D. and Parameswaran, M. (1971) Sarcoidal reaction of the skin in syphilis. *Br. J. Vener. Dis.,* 47, 209–11.

Sirak, H.D. (1954) Boeck's sarcoid of the stomach simulating linitis plastica. *Arch. Surg.,* 69, 769–76.

Skillicorn, S.A. and Garity, R.W. (1955) Intra-cranial Boeck's sarcoid resembling meningioma. *J. Neurosurg.,* 12, 407–13.

Slavin, P. (1949) Diffuse pulmonary granulomatosis in young women following exposure to beryllium compounds in the manufacture of radio tubes. *Am. Rev. Tuberc.,* 60, 755–72.

Small, M.J. (1951) Favourable response of sarcoidosis to cortisone treatment. *J. Am. Med. Assoc.,* 147, 932–7.

Smellie, H.C. (1956) Rhesus (D) factor in sarcoidosis. *Lancet,* 1, 863.

Smellie, H. and Hoyle, C. (1960) The natural history of pulmonary sarcoidosis. *Q. J. Med.,* 29, 539–58.

Smellie, H.C., Apthorp, G.H. and Marshall, R. (1961) The effect of corticosteroid treatment on pulmonary function in sarcoidosis. *Thorax,* 16, 87-90.

Smith, C.E. (1940) Epidemiology of coccidioidomycosis with erythema nodosum (San Joaquin or Valley fever) *Am. J. Public Health,* 30, 600–11.

Smith, J.G., Harris, J.S., Conant, N.F. and Smith, D.T. (1955) An epidemic of North American blastomycosis. *J. Am. Med. Assoc.,* 158, 641–6.

Smith, M.J., Turton, C.W.G., Mitchell, D.N., Turner-Warwick, M., Morris, L.M. and Lawler, S.D. (1981) Association of HLA B8 with spontaneous resolution in sarcoidosis. *Thorax,* 36, 296–8.

Snapper, I. and Pompen, A.W.N. (1938) *Pseudotuberculosis in man.* Bohn, Haarlem, pp. 23 and 71.

Snapper, I., Yarvis, J.J., Freud, H.R. and Goldberg, A.F. (1958) Hyperparathyroidism in identical twins, one of whom suffered concomitantly from Boeck's sarcoidosis. *Metab. Clin. Exp.,* 7, 671–80.

Sneddon, I.E. (1955) Berylliosis: a case report. *Br. Med. J.,* 1, 1448–50.

Sneddon, I.E. (1958) Beryllium disease. *Postgrad. Med. J.,* 34, 262–8.

Snell, N.J.C. and Karlish, A.J. (1975) Heerfordt's syndrome in two sisters. *Br. Med. J.,* 4, 731–2.

Snider, G.E. (1948) The treatment of Boeck's sarcoid with nitrogen mustard: a preliminary report. *South. Med. J.,* 41, 11–4.

Sniderman, H.R. (1941) Boeck's sarcoid of the lacrimal gland. *Am. J. Ophthalmol.,* 24, 676–80.

Snorasson, E. (1947) Myositis fibrosa progressiva – lymphogranulomatosis benigna Boeck. *Nord. Med.,* 36, 2424–5.

Snyder, R., Towfighi, J. and Gonatas, N.K. (1976) Sarcoidosis of the spinal cord. *J. Neurosurg.*, **44**, 740–3.

Söderstrom, N. (1960) Two cases of sarcoidosis treated with mepacrine. *Lancet*, **2**, 947–8.

Sokoloff, L. and Bunim, J.J. (1959) Clinical and pathological studies of joint involvement in sarcoidosis. *N. Engl. J. Med.*, **260**, 841–7.

Sokolowski, J.W., Schillaci, R.F. and Motley, T.E. (1969) Disseminated cryptococcosis complicating sarcoidosis. *Am. Rev. Respir. Dis.*, **100**, 717–22.

Solomon, A., Kreel, L., McNicol, M., Johnson, N. (1979) Computed tomography in pulmonary sarcoidosis. *J. Comput. Ass. Tomography*, **3**, 754–8.

Som, P.M. and Krespi, Y.P. (1979) Laryngeal sarcoid. *Radiology*, **133**, 341–2.

Sommer, E. (1977) Les calcifications endothoraciques dans la sarcoïdose. In *Sarcoïdose. Rapp. 4th International Conf., 1967.* Masson, Paris, pp. 667–73.

Søndergaard, G. (1951) Kveim's reaction anvendt ved diagnosen af den pulmonale form af lymfogranulomatosis benigna (Schaumann). *Ugeskr. Laeg.*, **113**, 1412–5.

Sones, M. and Israel, H.L. (1954) Altered immunologic reactions in sarcoidosis. *Ann. Intern Med.*, **40**, 260–8.

Sones, M. and Israel, H.L. (1960) Course and prognosis of sarcoidosis. *Am. J. Med.*, **29**, 84–93.

Sones, M., and Israel, H.L. (1961) Effects of potassium para-aminobenzoate in sarcoidosis. *Am. Rev. Respir. Dis.*, **83**, 907–8.

Sones, M., Israel, H.L., Dratman, M.B. and Frank, J.H. (1951) Effect of cortisone in sarcoidosis. *N. Engl. J. Med.*, **244**, 200–13.

Sones, M., Israel, H.L., Krain, R. and Beerman, H. (1955) Kveim test in sarcoidosis and tuberculosis. *J. Invest. Dermatol.*, **24**, 353–64.

Sorber, W.A., Leake, E.S. and Myrvik, B.N. (1974) Isolation and characterization of hydrolase containing granules from rabbit lung macrophages. *J. Reticuloendothelial Soc.*, **16**, 184–92.

Sørensen, S.F., Hardt, F., Veien, N.F. (1976) Estimation of lymphocyte subpopulations in the peripheral blood of patients with sarcoidosis. *Scand. J. Immunol.*, **5**, 1117–21.

Sorger, K. and Taylor, W.A. (1961) Generalized sarcoidosis: report of a case terminating in fatal nephropathy. *Arch. Pathol.*, **71**, 35–43.

Souter, W.C. (1929) A case of uveo-parotid fever with autopsy findings. *Trans. Ophthalmol. Soc. UK*, **49**, 113–27.

Spalton, D.J. (1979) Fundal changes in sarcoidosis. *Trans. Ophthalmol. Soc. UK*, **99**, 167–9.

Spector, W.G. (1969) The granulomatous inflammatory exudate. *Int. Rev. Exp. Pathol.*, **8**, 1–8.

Spector, W.G. (1975) The dynamics of granulomas and the significance of epithelioid cells. *Pathol. et Biol.*, **23**, 437–9.

Spencer, J. and Warren, S. (1938) Boeck's sarcoid: report of a case with clinical diagnosis confirmed at autopsy. *Arch. Intern. Med.*, **62**, 285–96.

Spilberg, I., Siltzbach, L.E. and McEwen, C. (1969) The arthritis of sarcoidosis. *Arthritis Rheum.*, **12**, 126–37.

Spillane, J.D. (1952) Four cases of diabetes insipidus and pulmonary disease. *Thorax*, **7**, 134–47.

Spink, W. (1937) Pathogenesis of erythema nodosum, with special reference to tuberculous and streptococcic infection and rheumatic fever. *Arch. Intern. Med.*, **59**, 65–81.

Spink, W.W., Hofbauer, F.W., Walker, W.W. and Green, R.A. (1949) Histopathology of the liver in human brucellosis. *J. Lab. Clin. Med.,* 34, 40–58.

Spivack, A.P., Nadel, J.A. and Eisenberg, G.M. (1957) Cryptococcus renal infection: report of a case. *Ann. Intern. Med.,* 47, 990–1002.

Sprince, N.L., Kazemi, H. and Fanburg, B.L. (1980) Serum angiotensin I converting enzyme in chronic beryllium disease. In *Proc 8th International Conference on Sarcoidosis, Cardiff, 1978* (eds. W. Jones-Williams and B.H. Davies), Alpha Omega, Cardiff, pp. 287–9.

Sprince, N.L. Kazemi, H. and Hardy, H.L. (1976) Current (1976) problem of differentiating between beryllium disease and sarcoidosis. *Ann. NY Acad. Sci.,* 278, 654–2.

Stableforth, D.E., Knight, R.K., Collins, J.W., Heard, B.E. and Clarke, S.W. (1978) Transbronchial lung biopsy through the fibreoptic bronchoscope. *Br. J. Dis. Chest,* 72, 108–14.

Stahl, D., Veien, N.K. and Brodthagen, H. (1980) Cutaneous manifestations of sarcoidosis. In *Proc. 8th International Coference of Sarcoidosis, Cardiff, 1978* (eds. W. Jones-Williams and B.H. Davies), Alpha Omega, Cardiff, pp. 551–7.

Ståhle, I. (1958) Sarcoidos och tuberculos. *Nord. Med.,* 59, 302–3.

Ståhle, I. (1963) Les bronches dans la sarcoïdose. *Bronches,* 13, 559–86.

Stallard, H.B. and Tait, C.B.V. (1939) Boeck's sarcoid: a case record. *Lancet,* 1, 440–2.

Stanley, N.N., Fox, R.A., Whimster, W.F., Sherlock, S. and James, D.G. (1972) Primary biliary cirrhosis or sarcoidosis – or both. *N. Engl. J. Med.,* 287, 1282–4.

Stark, J.E. (1963) Sarcoidosis and hyperthyroidism. *Proc. R. Soc. Med.* 56, 612–3.

Stats, D., Rosenthal, N. and Wasserman, L.R. (1947) Hemolytic anaemia associated with malignant diseases. *Am. J. Clin. Pathol.,* 17, 585–613.

Statton, R., Blodi, F.C. and Hanigan, J. (1964) Sarcoidosis of the optic nerve. *Arch. Ophthalmol.,* 71, 834–6.

Steigleder, G.K., Silvla, A., Jr. and Nelson, C.T. (1961) Histopathology of the Kveim test. *Arch. Dermatol. Syphilol. NY,* 84, 828–34.

Stein, E., Jackler, I., Stimmel, B., Stein, W. and Siltzbach, L.E. (1973) Asymptomatic electrocardiographic alterations in sarcoidosis. *Am. Heart J.,* 86, 474–7.

Stein, E., Stimmel, B. and Siltzbach, L.E. (1976) Clinical course of cardiac sarcoidosis. *Ann. NY Acad. Sci.,* 278, 470–4.

Stein, G.N., Israel, H.L. and Sones, M. (1956) A roentgenographic study of skeletal lesions in sarcoidosis. *Arch. Intern. Med.,* 97, 532–6.

Steinberg, I. (1958) Fatal fungus infections in sarcoidosis: report of 2 cases treated with antibiotics and cortisone. *Ann. Intern. Med.,* 48, 1359–72.

Stephen, J.D. (1954) Fatal myocardial sarcoidosis: a case of sudden death. *Circulation,* 9, 886–9.

Stephen, J., Braimbridge, M.V., Corrin, B., Wilkinson, S.P., Day, D. and Whimster, W.F. (1976) Necrotizing sarcoidal angiitis and granulomatosis of the lung. *Thorax,* 31, 356–60.

Steplewski, Z. and Israel, H.L. (1976) The search for viruses in sarcoidosis. *Ann. NY Acad. Sci.,* 276, 260–3.

Stirling, K. (1950) Erythema nodosum, with tuberculin neutralising serum. *Am. Rev. Tuberc.,* 62, 112–5.

Stjernberg, N., Truedson, H. and Björnstad-Petersen, H. (1980) Scalene node biopsy in sarcoidosis. *Acta Med. Scand.,* 207, 111–3.

Stjernberg, N., Wiman, L.-G. (1974) Uveo-parotid fever (Heerfordt's syndrome) or sarcoid affection of the eyes and parotid glands. In *Proc. 6th International Conference on Sarcoidosis, Tokyo* (eds. K. Iwai and Y. Hosoda), University of Tokyo Press, Tokyo, pp. 331–7.

Stoeckle, J.D., Hardy, H.L. and Weber, A.L. (1969) Chronic beryllium disease: long-term follow-up of 60 cases. *Am. J. Med.,* **46,** 545–61.

Stone, D.J. and Schwartz, A. (1966) A long-term study of sarcoid and its modification by steroid therapy. Lung function and other factors in prognosis. *Am. J. Med.,* **41,** 528–40.

Strickland, G.T. and Moser, K.M. (1967) Sarcoidosis with a Landry–Guillainé–Barré syndrome and clinical response to corticosteroids. *Am. J. Med.,* **43,** 131–5.

Stuart, B.M. (1944) Sarcoidosis of Boeck; metabolic studies of 3 cases. *Am. J. Med. Sci.,* **203,** 717–27.

Stuart, C.A., Neelon, F.A. and Lebovitz, H.E. (1978) Hypothalamic insufficiency: the cause of hypopituitarism in sarcoidosis. *Ann. Intern. Med.,* **88,** 589–94.

Stuart, C.A., Neelon, F.A. and Lebovitz, H.E. (1980) Disordered control of thirst in hypothalamic-pituitary sarcoidosis. *N. Engl. J. Med.,* **303,** 1078–82.

Studdert, T.C. (1953) Farmer's lung. *Br. Med. J.,* **1,** 1305–9.

Studdy, P., Bird, R., James,. G.D. and Sherlock, S. (1978) Serum angiotensin-converting enzyme (SACE) in sarcoidosis and other granulomatous disorders. *Lancet,* **2,** 1331–4.

Studdy, P.R., James, D.G. (1983) The specificity and sensitivity of serum angiotensin converting enzyme in sarcoidosis and other diseases. Experience in twelve centres in six different countries. In *Proc. 9th International Conference on Sarcoidosis, Paris,* Pergamon Press, Oxford, pp. 332–44.

Stump, D., Spock, A. and Grossman, H. (1976) Vertebral sarcoidosis in adolescents. *Radiology,* **121,** 153–5.

Sundelin, F. (1925) Tumeurs multiples disséminées dans les muscles des extrémités et rappelant la tuberculose par leur stucture histologique. *Acta Med. Scand.,* **62,** 442–60.

Sunderman, F.W. and Sunderman F.W., Jr. (1957) Clinical application of the fractionation of serum protein by paper electrophoresis. *Am. J. Clin. Pathol.* **27,** 125–58.

Sutherland, A.M. (1960) Genital tuberculosis in women. *Am. J. Obstet. Gynecol.,* **79,** 486–97.

Sutherland, I., Mitchell, D.N. and D'Arcy Hart, P. (1965) The incidence of pulmonary sarcoidosis among the participants in a trial of tuberculosis vaccines. *Br. Med. J.,* **2,** 497–500.

Sutton, J.S. and Weiss, L. (1966) Transformation of monocytes in tissue culture into macrophages, epithelioid cells, and multinucleated giant cells. *J. Cell. Biol.,* **28,** 303–32.

Svanborg, N. (1961) Studies on cardiopulmonary function in sarcoidosis. *Acta Med. Scand.,* Suppl. 366.

Swanton, R.H. (1971) Sarcoidosis and amyloidosis. *Proc. R. Soc. Med.* **64,** 44–5.

Sweeney, E.G. and McDonnell, L. (1979) Herpes simplex encephalitis and sarcoidosis. *Ir. J. Med. Sci.,* **148,** 54–7.

Sweet, L.C., Anderson, J.A., Callies, Q.C. and Coates, E.D. (1971) Hypersensitivity pneumonitis related to a home furnace humidifier. *J. Allergy Clin. Immunol.,* **48,** 171–8.

Sybert, A. and Butler, T.P. (1978) Sarcoidosis following adjuvant high-dose methotrexate therapy for osteosarcoma. *Arch. Intern. Med.*, 138, 488–9.

Symmers, W.St.C. (1951) Localised tuberculoid granulomas associated with carcinoma: their relationship to sarcoidosis. *Am. J. Pathol.*, 27, 493–521.

Symmers, W.St.C. (1956) Histoplasmosis contracted in Britain: a case of histoplasmic lymphadenitis following clinical recovery from sarcoidosis. *Br. Med. J.*, 2, 786–90.

Symmers, W.St.C. and Gillett, R. (1951) Polyarteritis nodosa, associated with malignant hypertension, disseminated platelet thrombosis, 'wire-loop' glomeruli, pulmonary silico-tuberculosis and sarcoidosis-like lymphadenopathy. *Arch. Pathol.*, 52, 489–504.

Taafe, A. and Feinman, L. (1977) Familial sarcoidosis: a report of three cases. *Br. J. Clin. Pract.*, 31, 225–6.

Tachibana, T., Aratake, K., Okada, S., Yamamoto, Y., Kato, S. and Naito, M. (1974) Sarcoidosis in childhood, In *Proc. 6th International conference on sarcoidosis, Tokyo.* (eds. K. Iwai and Y. Hosoda), University of Tokyo Press, Tokyo, pp. 503–6.

Talbot, F.J., Katz, S., Matthews, M.J. (1959) Broncho-pulmonary sarcoidosis. *Am. J. Med.*, 26, 340–55.

Talbot, P.S. (1967) Sarcoid myopathy. *Br. Med. J.*, 4, 465–6.

Tangen, M. (1954) Tissue immunity reactions in Boeck's sarcoid. *Acta Pathol. Microbiol. Scand.*, 34, 375–82.

Tannenbaum, H., Pinkus, G.S. and Schur, P.H. (1976a) Immunological characterisation of subpopulations of mononuclear cells in tissue and in peripheral blood from patients with sarcoidosis. *Clin. Immunol. Immunopathol.*, 5, 133–41.

Tannenbaum, H., Rocklin, R.E., Schur, P.H., and Sheffer, A.L. (1976b) Immune function in sarcoidosis. *Clin. Exp. Immunol.*, 26, 511–9.

Tanner, S.E. and McCurry, A.L. (1934) Uveo-parotid tuberculosis: a report of 3 cases. *Br. Med. J.*, 2, 1041–2.

Taub, R.N., Sachar, D., Siltzbach, L.E. and Janowitz, H. (1974) Transmission of ileitis and sarcoid granulomas to mice. *Trans. Assoc. Am. Physicians*, 87, 219–24.

Taussig, H.B. and Oppenheimer, E.H. (1936) Severe myocarditis of unknown etiology. *Bull. Johns Hopkins Hosp.*, 59, 155–70.

Taylor, A.B. (1960) Sarcoidosis of the uterus. *J. Obstet. Gynaecol. Br. Emp.*, 67, 32–5.

Taylor, A.J. (1958) The association of sarcoidosis, active pulmonary tuberculkosis and insensitivity to tuberculin. *Br. J. Tuber.*, 52, 70–3.

Taylor, G., Fisher, C. and Hoffbrand, B.I. (1982) Sarcoidosis and membramous glomerulonephritis: a significant association. *Br. Med. J.*, 1, 1297–8.

Taylor, R.L., Lynch, H.J. and Wysor, W.G. (1963) Seasonal influence of sunlight on the hypercalcaemia of sarcoidosis. *Am. J. Med.*, 34, 221–7.

Taylor, T.K., Senekjian, H.O., Knight, T.F., Györkey, F. and Weinman, E.J. (1979) Membranous nephropathy with epithelial crescents in a patient with pulmonary sarcoidosis. *Arch. Intern. Med.*, 139, 1183–5.

Taylor-Robinson, D., Canchola, J., Fox, H. and Chanock, R.M. (1964) A newly identified oral mycoplasma (*M. orale*) and its relationship to other human mycoplasmas. *Am. J. Hyg.*, 80, 135–48.

Teilum, G. (1948) Allergic hyperglobulmaemia and hyalinosis (paramyloidosis) in the reticulo-endothelial system in Boeck's sarcoid. *Am. J. Pathol.*, 24, 389–407.

Teilum, G. (1949) The nature of the double-contoured and stratified intracellular bodies in sarcoidosis (Boeck–Schaumann). *Am. J. Pathol.,* 25, 85–91.

Teilum, G. (1951) Glomerular lesions of kidneys in sarcoidosis (Boeck's sarcoid). *Acta Pathol. Microbiol. Scand.,* 28, 294–301.

Teirstein, A.S., Chuang, M., Miller, A. and Siltzbach, L.E. (1976a) Flexible bronchoscope biopsy of lung and bronchial wall for the diagnosis of sarcoidosis. *Ann. NY Acad. Sci.,* 278. 522–7.

Teirstein, A.S., Siltzbach, L.E. and Berger, H. (1976b) Patterns of sarcoidosis in three populations groups in New York City. *Ann. NY Acad. Sci.,* 278, 371–6.

Teirstein, A.S., Siltzbach, L.E. and Dorph, D. (1980) Report of international questionnaire regarding diagnostic procedures in sarcoidosis: the impact of fibreoptic brochoscopy. In *Proc. 8th International Conference on Sarcoidosis, Cardiff* (eds. W. Jones-Williams and B.H. Davies), Alpha Omega, Cardiff, pp. 233–7.

Teirstein, A.S., Wolf, B.S. and Siltzbach, L.E. (1961) Sarcodosis of the skull. *N. Engl. J. Med.,* 265, 65–8.

Tellis, C.J. and Putnam, J.S. (1977) Cavitation in large multinodular pulmonary disease: a rare manifestation of sarcoidosis. *Chest,* 71, 792–3.

Ten Have, H. (1958) *Morbus Besnier–Boeck–Schaumann,* Thesis, Gröningen.

Ten Have, H. and Orie, N.G.M. (1961) Tuberculosis and asthmatic bronchitis in sarcoidosis. *Dis. Chest,* 39, 42–9.

Tenneson, M. (1892) Lupus pernio. *Ann. Dermatol. Syphiligr. Paris,* 3, 1142–4.

Tepper, L.B., Hardy, H.L. and Chamberlin. R.I. (1961) *Toxicity of Beryllium Compounds,* Elsevier, Amsterdam.

Terpstra, J.J. (1944) Cerebrale stoornissen bij de ziekte van Besnier–Boeck. *Ned. Rev. Tijdschr. Geneeskd,* 88, 476–9.

Terris, M. and Chaves, A.D. (1966) An epidemiological study of sarcoidosis. *Am. Rev. Respir. Dis.,* 94, 50–5.

Tesluk, H. (1966) Giant-cell versus granulomatous myocarditis. *Am. J. Clin. Pathol.,* 261, 1326–33.

Thannhauser, S.J. (1950) *Lipidoses: Deseases of Cellular Lipid Metabolism,* Oxford Medical Publications, New York.

Theodoropoulos, G., Archimandritis, A., Davaris, P., Platarius, J. and Melissinos, K. (1981) Ulcerative colitis and sarcoidosis. *Dis. Colon Rectum,* 24, 308–10.

Thomas, G.O. (1969) Hypercalciuria in sarcoidosis treated with inorganic phosphates. *Br. Med. J.,* 2, 92–8.

Thomas, L.L.M., Alberts, C., Pegels, J.G., Balk, A.G. and von dem Borne, A.E. (1982) Sarcoidosis with auto-immune thrombocytopenia and selective IgA deficiency. *Scand. J. Haematol.,* 28, 357–9.

Thomas, T.V., Wiere, K.C., Heilbrunn, A. and Thio, R.T. (1972) Sarcoidosis of the stomach. *Ann. Surg.,* 38, 465–7.

Thomas, W.C. (1957) Diabetes insipidus. *J. Clin. Endocrineol. Metab.,* 17, 565–82.

Thomas, W.C., Morgan, H.G., Connor, T.B., Haddock, L., Bills, C.E., and Howard, J.E. (1959) Studies of antiricketic activity in sera from patients with disorders of calcium metabolism and preliminary observations on the mode of transport of vitamin D in human serum. *J. Clin. Invest.,* 38, 1078–85.

Thompson, J.R. (1961) Sarcoidosis of the central nervous system: report of a case simulating intracranial neoplasm. *Am. J. Med.,* 31, 977–80.

Thompson, J.R. (1966) Vascular changes in sarcoidosis. *Dis. Chest,* 50, 357–61.

Thompson, W.D., McGrouther, D.A. and Stockdill, G. (1973) Thyrotoxicosis with sarcoid-like granulomata. *J. Pathol.,* 111, 289–91.

Thomson, A.D. (1958) The pathology of sarcoidosis. *Postgrad. Med. J.,* 34, 248–53.

Thorbjarnarson, B. and Glenn, F. (1956) Sarcoidosis associated with sudden death during mitral valvulotomy. *Arch. Surg.,* **73**, 862–9.

Thorn, G., Forsham, P.H., Frawley, F.T., Hill, S.R., Roche, M., Staehelin, D. and Wilson, D.L. (1950) The clinical usefulness of ACTH and cortisone. *N. Eng. J. Med.,* **242**, 865–72.

Thudani, U., Aber, C.P. and Taylor, J.J. (1975) Massive splenomegaly, pancytopenia and haemolytic anaemia in sarcoidosis. *Acta Haematol.,* **53**, 230–40.

Tice, D.A., Cohen, R. and Rader, B. (1967) Myocardial sarcoidosis and complete repair of tetralogy of Fallot. *J. Thor. Cardiovasc. Surg.,* **54**, 573–8.

Tice, F. and Sweany, H.C. (1941) A fatal case of Besnier–Boeck–Schumann's disease with autopsy findings. *Ann. Intern. Med.,* **15**, 597–607.

Tillgren, J. (1935) Diabetes insipidus as a symptom of Schaumann's disease. *Br. J. Dermatol.,* **47**, 223–9.

Tobi, M., Kubrin, I. and Ariel, I. (1982) Rectal involvement in sarcoidosis. *Dis. Colon Rectum,* **47**, 491–3.

Todd, R.F. and Garnick, M.B. (1980) Prostatic adenocarcinoma, sarcoidosis and hypercalcemia. *J. Urol.,* **123**, 133–4.

Tolis, G., Goldstein, M. and Friesen, H.G. (1973) Functional evaluation of prolactin secretion in patients with hypothalamic-pituitary disorders. *J. Clin. Invest.,* **52**, 783–8.

Tonnel, A.B., Lahoute, C., Lebar, J., Rubin, H., Ramon, P., Aerts, C. and Voisin, C. (1979) Charactéristiques cellulaires et biochimiques du liquide de lavage bronchoalvéolaire au cours du poumon d'éléveur d'oiseaux. *Bull. Eur. Physiopath. Resp.,* **15**, 33P.

Toomey, F. and Bautista, A. (1970) Rare manifestations of sarcoidosis in children. *Radiology,* **94**, 569–73.

Topilsky, M., Siltzbach, L.E., Williams, M. and Glade, P.R. (1972) Lymphocyte response in sarcoidosis. *Lancet,* **1**, 117–20.

Toulant, P. and Morard, G. (1936) A propos d'un cas d'uvéo-parotidite (syndrome d'Heerfordt). *Arch. Ophthalmol.,* **53**, 321–45.

Transbøl, I.B. and Halver, B. (1967) Relation of renal glycosuria and parathyroid function in hypercalcaemic sarcoidosis. *J. Clin. Endocrinol Metab.,* **27**, 1193–6.

Trible, W.H. (1958) Sarcoidosis of the larynx. *Arch. Otalaryngol.,* **63**, 382–3.

Tripodi, D., Leon, C. and Brugmans, J. (1973) Drug-induced restoration of delayed hypersensitivity in anergic patients with cancer. *N. Engl. J. Med.,* **289**, 354–7.

Trujillo, N.J., Halstead, L.S. and Ticktin, H.E. (1967) Chronic ulcerative colitis, xanthomatous biliary cirrhosis and sarcoidosis. *Med. Ann. D. C.,* **36**, 170–4.

Tsega, E., Getahun, B. and Teklehaimanot, R. (1978) Sarcoidosis in Ethiopia. *Tubercle,* **59**, 261–8.

Turiaf, J. and Battesti, J.P. (1971) La sarcoïdose d'après l'étude de 350 cas. *Rev. Tuberc. Pneumol.,* **35**, 569–99.

Turiaf, J., Basset, G. and Georges, R. (1967) Indications, méthode et résultats du traitement de la sarcoidose médiastino-pulmonaire par les corticosteroides. In *Proc. 4th International Conference on Sarcoidosis, Paris* (eds. J. Turiaf and J. Chabot), Masson, Paris, pp. 722–34.

Turiaf, J., Battesti, J.P. and Minault, M. (1968) Anergie tuberculinique, test de Kveim et immunoglobulines sériques dans la sarcoïdose. *Le poumon et le coeur,* **24**, 625–45.

Turiaf, J., Battesti, J.P. and Menault, M. (1970) La sarcoïdosi des sujets natifs des Antilles françaises. *Presse Méd.,* **78**, 1003–8.

Turiaf, J., Basset, F., Menault, M. and Jeanjean, Y. (1980) The Kveim test: a personal experiment using an allergen obtained from a sarcoid spleen. In *Proc. 8th International conference on Sarcoidosis, Cardiff, 1978* (eds. W. Jones-Williams and B.H. Davies), Alpha Omega, Cardiff, p. 678.

Turiaf, J. and Brun, J. (1955) *La Sarcoidose Endothoracique de Besnier–Boeck–Schaumann*, Expansion Scientifique Française, Paris.

Turiaf, J., Carlotti, J., Blanchon, P. and Herrault, A. (1947) Maladie de Besnier–Boeck–Schaumann à localisations faciale, oculaire et gangliopulmonaire: méningite subaigue inauguarale: tuberculose pulmonaire terminale. *J. Fr. Med. Chir. Thorac.,* **1**, 195–200.

Turiaf, J., Marland, P. and Basset, F. (1969) La sarcoïdose du corps thyroide (à propos d'un cas de sarcoïdose kystique du corps thyroide). *Ann. Méd. Int.,* **120**, 837–45.

Turiaf, J., Marland, P., Rose, Y. and Sors, C. (1952) Le diagnostic bronchoscopique et bronchobiopsique des formes pulmonaires de la maladie de Besnier–Boeck–Schaumann. *Bull. Soc. Med. Hop. Paris,* **68**, 1089–15.

Turiaf, J., Menault, M., Basset, F., Jeanjean, Y. and Battesti, J.P. (1974) Absence of relation between Kveim test and adenopathies in sarcoidosis and other diseases with lymph localizations. In *Proc. 6th International Conference on Sarcoidosis, Tokyo* (eds. K. Iwai and Y. Hosoda), University of Tokyo Press, Tokyo, pp. 84–7.

Turiaf, J., Rose, Y. and Basset, F. (1963) La sarcoïdose bronchique. *Bronches,* **13**, 587–609.

Turiaf, J., Thibier, R. Basset, F., Roucou, Y. and Duroux, P. (1965) Les cavités nécrotiques intrafocales de la sarcoïdose pulmonaire. *J. Fr. Med. Chir. Thrac.,* **19**, 139–58.

Turek, S.L. (1953) Sarcoid disease of bone at ankle joint. *J. Bone J. Surg.,* **35**, 465–8.

Turkington, R.W., and Buckley, C.E. (1966) Macrocryoglobulinemia and sarcoidosis. *Am. J. Med.,* **40**, 156–64.

Turkington, R.W. and MacIndoe, J.H. (1972) Hyperprolactinemia in sarcoidosis. *Ann. Intern. Med.,* **76**, 545–9.

Turner, M.C., Shin, M.L. and Ruley, E.J. (1977) Renal failure as a presenting sign of diffuse sarcoidosis in an adolescent girl. *Am. J. Dis. child.,* **131**, 997–1000.

Turner, O.A. and Weiss, S.R. (1969) Sarcoidosis of the skull. *Am. J. Roentgenol.,* **105**, 322–5.

Turner, R.G., James, D.G., Friedman, A.I., Vijendram, M. and Davies, J.P.H. (1975) Neuro-ophthalmic sarcoidosis. *Br. J. Ophthalmol.,* **59**, 657–63.

Turner-Warwick, M. (1974) Autoantibodies in allergic respiratory disease. In *Progress in immunology II vol. 4. Clinical Aspects I.* (eds. L. Brent and J. Holborrow), North Holland, Amsterdam, p. 238.

Turner-Warwick, M. (1978) *Immunology of the Lung,* Edward Arnold, London, pp. 221–41.

Turton, C.M.G., Grundy, E., Firth, G., Mitchell, D.N., Rigden, B.G. and Turner-Warwick, M. (1979) Value of measuring serum angiotensin I converting enzyme and serum lysozyme in the management of sarcoidosis. *Thorax,* **34**, 57–62.

Turton, C.M.G., Morris, L., Lawler, S.D. and Turner-Warwick, M. (1980) HLA in familial sarcoidosis. In *Proc. 8th International conference on Sarcoidosis, Cardiff, 1978* (eds. W. Jones-Williams and B.H. Davies), Alpha Omega, Cardiff, pp. 195–200.

Uehlinger, E. (1945) Ueber Morbus Boeck mit Uebergang in Tuberkulosesepsis. *Schweiz. Med. Wochenschr.*, **75**, 474.

Uehlinger, E. (1955) Die pathologische Anatomie des Morbus Boeck. *Beitr. Klin. Tuberk. Spezifischen Tuberk.-Forsch.*, **114**, 17–45.

Uehlinger, E.A. (1961) Epidemiology of sarcoidosis in Switzerland. *Am. Rev. Respir. Dis.*, **84**, 153–4.

Uesaka, I., Izumi, T. and Tsuji, S. (1974) Nocardia-like organisms isolated from lesions of sarcoidosis. In *Proc. 6th International Conference on Sarcoidosis, Tokyo* (eds. K. Iwai and Y. Hosoda), University of Tokyo Press, Tokyo, p. 3.

Ulrich, K. (1918) Die Schleimhautveranderungen der oberen Luftwege beim 'Boeck-schen Sarkoid' und ihre Stellung zum lupus pernio. *Arch. Laryngol. Rhinol., Berl.*, **31**, 506–34.

Umbert, P., Belcher, R.W. and Winklemann, R.K. (1976) Lymphokines (MIF) in the serum of patients with sarcoidosis and cutaneous granuloma annulare. *Br. J. Dermatol.*, **95**, 481–5.

Umbert, P., Winkelmann, R.K. (1977) Granuloma annulare and sarcoidosis. *Br. J. Dermatol.*, **97**, 481–6.

Urbach, F., Sones, M. and Israel, H.L. (1952) Passive transfer of tuberculin sensitivity to patients with sarcoidosis. *N. Engl. J. Med.*, **247**, 794–7.

Urich, H. (1976) The optic pathway in sarcoidosis. *Ann. NY Acad. Sci.*, **278**, 406–15.

Urich, H. (1977) Neurosarcoidosis or granulomatous angiitis: a problem of definition. *Mt Sinai J. Med.*, **44**, 718–25.

Ustvedt, H.J. (1939) Nosography and diagnosis of Boeck's sarcoid. *Nord. Med.*, **2**, 1677–85.

Ustvedt, H.J. (1948) Autopsy findings in Boeck's sarcoid. *Tubercle.* **29**, 107–11.

Ustvedt, H.J. and Aanonsen, A. (1949) Diagnostic BCG test. *Acta Tuberc. Scand.*, **23**, 1–35.

Uyama, M. (1974) Sarcoid uveitis – clinical course and treatment. In *Proc. 6th International Conference on Sarcoidosis, Tokyo.* (eds. K. Iwai and Y. Hosoda), University of Tokyo Press, Tokyo, pp. 354–9.

Valdimarsson, H. and Gross, N.J. (1973) Human skin response to products of concanavalin A-activated lymphocytes. *J. Immunol.* **111**, 483–91.

Valenti, S., Scordamaglia, A., Crimi, P. and Meren, C. (1982) Bronchoalveolar lavage and transbronchial lung biopsy in sarcoidosis and extrinsic allergic alveolitis. *Eur. J. Respir. Dis.*, **63**, 564–9.

VA-Armed Forces Study of Chemotherapy of Tuberculosis (1963) *Transactions of 22nd Research Conference, Cincinnati, Ohio.* p. 31.

Van de Rhee, H.J., Hillebrands, W. and Daems, W.T. (1978) Are Langhans giant-cells precursors of foreign-body giant cells? *Arch. Dermatol. Res.*, **265**, 15–21.

Van Ditmars, M.J. (1967) A comparison between sarcoidosis in the Netherlands and Pennsylvania. In *Proc. 4th International Conference on Sarcoidosis, Paris* (eds. J. Turiaf and J. Chabot), Masson, Paris, pp. 353–9.

Vaněk, J. (1968) Acid-fast bacilli of mycobacterial nature in sarcoidosis. *Beitr. Pathol. Anat.*, **136**, 303–15.

Vaněk, J. and Schwarz, J. (1970) Demonstration of acid-fast rods in sarcoidosis. *Am. Rev. Respir. Dis.*, **101**, 395–400.

Van Epps, D.D., Palmer, D.L. and Williams, R.C. (1974) Characterisation of serum inhibitors associated with anergy. *J. Immunol*, **113**,189–200.

Van Furth, R. (1970) The origin and turnover of promonocytes, monocytes and macrophages in normal mice. *Mononuclear Phagocytes,* (ed. R. van Furth), Blackwell, Oxford, pp. 151–61.

Van Ganse, W.F., Oleffe, J., van Hove, W. and Grotenbriel, C. (1970) Contribution à l'étude des aspects immunologiques de la bérylliose chronique. *Lille Med.,* 16, 680–6.

Van Ganse, W.F., Oleffe, J., van Hove, W. and Grotenbriel, C. (1971) Lymphocyte transformation in chronic pulmonary berylliosis. *Lancet,* 1, 1023.

Vanhille, P., Dequiedt, P., Raviart, B., Leliève, G. and Tacquet, A. (1977) Insuffisance rénale par néphrite granulomateuse au cours d'une sarcoïdose. *Lille Med.,* 22, 778–82.

Veien, N.K. (1977) Cutaneous sarcoidosis treated with levamisole. *Dermatologica,* 154, 185–9.

Veien, N.K. and Brodthagen, H. (1977) Cutaneous sarcoidosis treated with methotrexate. *Br. J. Dermatol.,* 97, 213–6.

Veien, N.K. and Kobayasa, T. (1980) Ultrastructure of cutaneous granulomas and mononuclear cells from patients with sarcoidosis. *Acta Dermato.-Venereol.* 60, 13–9.

Venet, A., Wewers, M. and Crystal, R.G. (1982)Enhanced antigen presentation by alveolar macrophages of patients with sarcoidosis. *Clin. Res.,* 30, 360.

Verner, J.V.,Jr., Engel, F.L. and McPherson, H.T. (1958) Vitamin D intoxication: report of 2 cases treated with cortisone. *Ann. Intern. Med.,* 48, 765–73.

Verier-Jones, J. (1967) Development of sensitivity to dinitrochlorobenzene in patients with sarcoidosis. *Clin. Exp. Immunol.,* 2, 477–87.

Verrier-Jones, J., Cumming, R.H., Asplin, C.M., Laszlo, G. and White, R.J. (1976) Circulating immune complexes in erythema nodosum and early sarcoidosis. *Lancet,* 1, 153.

Verstraeten, J.M. and Bekaert, J. (1951) Association de spondylite ankylosante et de sarcoïdose. *Acta Tuberc. Belg.,* 42, 149–51.

Vesely, D.L., Maldonodo, A. and Levey, G.S. (1977) Partial hypopituitarism and possible hypothalamic involvement in sarcoidosis. *Am. J. Med.,* 62, 425–31.

Vesey, C.M.R. and Wilkinson, D.S. (1959) Erythema nodosum: a study of 70 cases. *Br. J. Dermatol.,* 71, 139–55.

Vezendi, S. and Mandi, L. (1977) Family occurrence of sarcoidosis. *Z. Erkr. Atmungsorgane,* 149, 274–5.

Vico, J.J. and Larsen, C.R. (1979) Sarcoidosis of the larynx. *Radiology,* 131, 636–8.

Vilinskas, T., Joyeuse, R. and Serlin, O. (1970) Hepatic sarcoidosis with portal hypertension. *Am. J. Surg.,* 120, 393–6.

Virmani, R., Bures, J.C. and Roberts, W.C. (1980) Cardiac sarcoidosis: a major cause of sudden death in young individuals. *Chest,* 77, 423–8.

Vitenson, J.H. and Wilson, J.M. (1972) Sarcoid of the glans penis. *J. Urol.,* 108, 284–6.

Vitye, B., Ostiguy, G. and LeBel, E. (1969) Abnormal $99^{m}Tc$ brain scan in cerebral sarcoidosis. *Can. Med. Assoc. J.,* 101, 169–70.

Vogt, J.H. (1939) Erythema nodosum – ligende eksantem og protrahert hilusadenitt hos en tuberkulinnegativ patient. *Nord. Med.,* 3, 2341–2.

Vogt, H. (1949) Morbus Besnier–Boeck–Schaumann: klinische und pathologische anatomische Studie. *Helv. Med. Acta,* 16, Suppl. 25.

Voigt-Richter, R. (1965) Über doppelseitigne Spontanpneumothorax und über die sogenannte Pleurabeteiligung bei Sarkoidose Boeck. *Prax. Pneumol.,* 19, 747–50.

Voog, R., Marchal, A., Couderc, P. and Cabanel, G. (1969) La pleurésie sarcoïdosique. (A propos d'une observation personelle avec revue de la littérature). *J. Fr. Med. Chir. Thorac.*, **23**, 15–29.

Voog, R., Schaever, R. and Sarrazin, R. (1969) Contribution des techniques cytologiques au diagnostic des processus pathologiques médiastinaux. Poumon Coeur, **25**, 47–58.

Vorwald, A.J., Bowditch, M., Durkan, T.M. and Waters, T.C. (1950) *Pneumoconiosis*: Leroy U. Gardner Memorial Volume, Hoeber, New York.

Vuletin, J.C. and Rosen, Y. (1977) Nature of pseudo-fungal budding structures (Hamazaki-Wessenberg bodies) and asteroid bodies in sarcoidosis. *Am. J. Clin. Path.*, **68**, 99.

Wade, H.W. (1951) Leprosy and sarcoid. The Kveim test in leprosy patients and contacts. *J. Invest. Dermatol.*, **17**, 337–47.

Wadina, G.S. and Melamed, A. (1966) Gastric granuloma (? sarcoid) *Am. J. Gastroenterol.*, **45**, 11–21.

Wagoner, G.P., Freiman, D.G. and Schiff, L. (1953) An unusual case of jaundice in a patient with sarcoidosis. *Gastroenterology*, **25**, 574–81.

Wahlgren, F. (1936) In discussion on 'So-called chronic miliary tuberculosis'. *Acta Pathol. Scand.*, Suppl. 26, 168.

Wahren, B., Carlens, E., Espmark, A., Lundbeck, H., Löfgren, H., Madar, E., Henle, G. and Henle, W. (1971) Antibodies to various herpes viruses in sera from patients with sarcoidosis. *J. Natl. Cancer Inst.*, **47**, 747–55.

Waksman, B.H. (1959) The diagnosis of beryllium disease, with special reference to the patch test. *Arch. Ind. Health*, **19**, 190.

Waldek, S., Agius-Ferrante, A.M. and Lawler, W. (1978) Renal failure due to glomerulonephritis in sarcoidosis. *Br. Med. J.*, **1**, 1110–1.

Waldman, D.J. and Stiehm, E.R. (1977) Cutaneous sarcoidosis of childhood. *J. Pediatr.*, **91**, 271–3.

Walker, A.G. (1961) Sarcoidosis of the brain and spinal cord. *Postgrad. Med. J.*, **37**, 431–6.

Walker, A.N. and James, G.G. (1972) The course, prognosis and management of sarcoidosis. In *Proc. European Conference on Sarcoidosis, Geneva*, Hallwag, Geneva (reprinted from *Praxis*), pp. 200–7.

Wall, A.J. and Peters, T.J. (1972) Change in structure and peptidase activity of rat small intestine induced by prednisolone. *Gut*, **12**, 445–8.

Wallace, S.L., Lattes, R., Malia, J.P. and Ragan, C. (1958) Muscle involvement in Boeck's sarcoid. *Ann. Intern. Med.*, **48**, 497–511.

Wallgren, A. (1930) A new argument in favour of the tuberculous nature of erythema nodosum. *Acta Paediatr.*, **11**, 590–1.

Walsh, F.B. (1939) Ocular importance of sarcoid: its relation to uveo-parotid fever. *Arch. Opthalmol.*, **21**, 421–38.

Walsh, M.J. (1978) Systemic sarcoidosis with refractory ventricular tachycardia and heart failure. *Br. Heart J.*, **40**, 931–3.

Wambergne, F.P., Duchatelle, P., Riberi, P., Routier, G., Palliez, T.M., Dequiedt, P. and Lelièvre, G. (1978) Localisation rénale spécifique de la sarcoïdose. *J. Urol. Nephrol.*, **84**, 859–65.

Wanstrup, J. and Elling, P. (1968) Immunochemistry of sarcoidosis. *Acta Pathol. Microbiol. Scand.*, **73**, 37–48.

Wanstrup, J. and Christensen, H.E. (1966) Sarcoidosis. I Ultrastructural investigations on epithelioid cell granulomas. *Acta Path. Microbiol. Scand.*, **67**, 433–50.

Warburg, M. (1955) A case of symmetrical muscular contractures due to sarcoidosis. *J. Neuropathol.*, **14**, 313–6.

Ward, P.A., Goralnick, S. and Bullock, W.D. (1976) Defective leukotaxis in patients with lepromatous lepro. *J. Lab. Clin. Med.*, **87**, 1025–32.

Warfel, A.H. (1978) Macrophage fusion and multinucleated giant cell formation, surface morphology. *Exp. Mol. Pathol.*, **28**, 163–76.

Warfvinge, L.E. (1943) Boeck's sarcoid, experimentally produced by virulent human tubercle bacilli in a case of Schaumann's disease. *Acta Med. Scand.*, **114**, 259–70.

Warfvinge, L.E. (1945) Lymphogranulomatosis benigna und Tuberkulose. *Acta Tuberc. Scand.*, **19**, 195–210.

Warfvinge, L.E. (1945) Über eine von abgetoten tuberkelbazillin hervorgerufene Haut Reaktion bei Lymphogranulomatosis benigna. *Acta Tuberc. Scand.*, **19**, 126–41.

Waring, W.W., Wilkinson, R.W., Wiebe, R.A., Faul, C. and Hilman, B.C. (1971) Quantitation of digital clubbing in children. *Am. Rev. Respir. Dis*, **104**, 166–74.

Warr, G.A., Martin, R.R., Holleman, C.L. and Criswell, B.S. (1976) Classification of bronchial lymphocytes from smokers and non–smokers. *Am. Rev. Respir. Dis.*, **113**, 96–100.

Watson, C.J., Rigler, L.G., Wangensteen, O.H. and McCartney, J.S. (1945) Isolated sarcoidosis of the small intestines simulating non-specific ileo-jejunitis. *Gastroenterology*, **4**, 30–52.

Watson, D.W., Friedman, H.M. and Quigley, A. (1971) Immunological studies in a patient with ulcerative colitis and sarcoidosis. *Gut*, **12**, 541–5.

Watson, R.C. and Cahen, I. (1973) Pathological fracture in long bone sarcoidosis. *J. Bone J. Surg.*, **55**, 613–7.

Webb, A.K., Mitchell, D.N., Bradstreet, C.N.P. and Salsbury, A.J. (1980) Splenomegaly and splenectomy in sarcoidosis. *J. Clin. Pathol.*, **32**, 1050–3.

Weber, A.L., Stoeckle, J.D. and Hardy, H.L. (1965) Roentgenologic patterns in long-standing beryllium disease. *Am. J. Roentgenol.*, **93**, 879–90.

Weeks, K.D. and Smith, D.T. (1945) Lepromin skin tests in Boeck's sarcoid. *Am. J. Trop. Med.*, **25**, 519–21.

Wegener, F. (1939) Über eine eigenartige rhinogene Granulomatose mit besonderer Beteiligung des Arteriensystems und der Nieren. *Beitr. Pathol. Anat. allg. Pathol.*, **102**, 36–68.

Weidman, A.I., Andrade, R. and Franks, A.G. (1966) Sarcoidosis: report of a case of sarcoidal lesions in a tattoo and subsequent discovery of pulmonary sarcoidosis. *Arch. Dermatol.*, **94**, 320–5.

Weinberg, R.S. and Tessler, H.H. (1976) Serum lysozyme in sarcoid uveitis. *Am. J. Ophthalmol.*, **82**, 105–8.

Weinberger, M. (1933) Über eine chronisch verlaufene Polymyositis mit Ausgang in progressive Muskelatrophie. *Wien. Med. Wochenschr.*, **83**, 100, 137, 162.

Weinberger, S.E., Kelman, J.A., Elson, N.A., Young, R.C., Reynolds, H.Y., Fulmer, J.D. and Crystal, R.G. (1978) Broncho-alveolar lavage in interstitial lung disease. *Ann. Intern. Med.*, **89**, 459–66.

Weinreb, R.N. and Kimura, S.J. (1980) Uveitis associated with sarcoidosis and angiotensin converting enzyme. *Am. J. Ophthalmol.*, **89**, 180–5.

Weisman, R.A., Canalis, R.F. and Powell, W.J. (1980) Laryngeal sarcoidosis with airway obstruction. *Ann. Otol.*, **80**, 58–61.

Weiss, J.A. (1960) Sarcoidosis in otalaryngology: report of 11 cases. *Laryngoscope*, **70**, 1351–98.

Wells, A.Q., and Robb-Smith, A.H.T. (1946) *The Murine Type of Tubercle Bacillus*, Medical Research Council Special Report Series No. 259, London.

Wells, A.Q. and Wylklie, J.A.H. (1949) Tuberculin neutralising factor in serum of patients with sarcoidosis. *Lancet*, 1, 439–41.

Wells, C.E.C. (1967) The natural history of neurosarcoidosis. *Proc. R. Soc. Med.*, 60, 1172–4.

Wells, R.S. and Smith, M.A. (1963) The natural history of granuloma annulare. *Br. J. Dermatol.*, 75, 199–205.

Welsh, L.W. and Welsh, J.J. (1977) Problems of diagnosis in the evaluation of mediastinal sarcoidosis. *Laryngoscope*, 87, 1635–44.

Wemambu, S.N.C., Turk, J.L., Waters, M.F.R. and Rees, R.J.W. (1969) *Erythema nodosum leprosum*: a clinical manifestation of the Arthus phenomenon. *Lancet*, 2, 933–5.

Werb, Z. and Gordon, S. (1975a) Secretion of a specific collagenase by stimulated macrophages. *J. Exp. Med.*, 142, 346–60.

Werb, Z. and Gordon, S. (1975b) Elastase secretion by stimulated macrophages. *J. Exp. Med.*, 142, 361–71.

Werner, E. (1962) Übergang einer ansteckenden Lungentuberkulose in einer atypische Form (Morbus Boeck). *Beitr. Klin. Tuberk. Spezifischen Tuberk-Forsch.*, 126, 42–50.

Wessenberg, W. (1966) Tönsheide: über säurefeste 'Spindelkorper Hamazaki' bei Sarkoidose der Lymphknoten und über doppellicht brechende Zelleinschlüsse bei Sarkoidose der Lungen. *Arch. Klin. Exp. Dermatol.*, 227, 101–7.

West, S.G., Gilbraith, R.E. and Lawless, O.J. (1981) Painful clubbing and sarcoidosis. *J. Am. Med. Assoc.*, 246, 1338–9.

West, W.O. (1959) Acquired hemolytic anaemia secondary to Boeck's sarcoid *N. Engl. J. Med.*, 261, 688–90.

Westcott, J.L. and de Graff, C. (1973) Sarcoidosis, hilar adenopathy and pulmonary artery narrowing. *Radiology*, 585–6.

Westerhof, L., van Ditmars, M.J., der Kinderen, P.J., Thijssen, J.H.H. and Schwarz, F. (1970) Recovery of adrenocortical function during long-term treatment with corticosteroids. *Br. Med. J.*, 4, 534–7.

Westra, S.A. and Visser, J.F. (1949) Hypercalcamie bij de Ziekte van Besnier–Boeck. *Ned. Tijdschr. Geneeskd.*, 93, 18–25.

Widstrom, A. and Schnurer, L.B. (1978) The value of mediastinoscopy: experience in 374 cases. *J. Otolaryngol.*, 7, 103–9.

Wiederholt, W.C. and Sickert, R.G. (1965) Neurological manifestations of sarcoidosis. *Neurology*, 15, 1147–54.

Wilen, S.B., Rabinowitz, J.G., Ulreich, S. and Lyons, H.A. (1974) Pleural involvement in sarcoidosis. *Am. J. Med.*, 57, 200–9.

Wigley, J.E.M. and Musso, L.A. (1951) A case of sarcoidosis with erythrodermic lesions. *Br. J. Derm.*, 63, 398–407.

Willan, R. (1808) *On Cutaneous Diseases*, J. Johnson, London, vol. 1, p. 483.

Wille, C. (1946) Boeck's disease of the mucosa. *Acta Oto-Laryngol.*, 34, 182–91.

Williams, E. (1974) The Kveim test in brucellosis. In *Proc. 6th International Conference on Sarcoidosis, Tokyo* (eds. K. Iwai and Y. Hosoda), University of Tokyo Press, Tokyo, pp. 96–8.

Williams, G.T. and Williams, W.Jones (1983) Granulomatous inflammation – a review. *J. Clin. Pathol.*, 36, 723–33.

Williams, J.D., Smith, M.D. and Davies, B.H. (1982) Interaction of immune complexes and T-suppressor cells in sarcoidosis. *Thorax*, 37, 602–6.

Williams, M.J. (1961) Sarcoidosis presenting with polyarthritis. *Ann. Rheum. Dis.,* **20,** 138–43.

Williams, R.H. and Nickerson, D.A. (1935) Skin reactions in sarcoid. *Proc. Soc. Exp. Biol., NY,* **33,** 403–5.

Willoughby, J.M.T. and Mitchell, D.N. (1971) In vitro inhibition of leucocyte migration in Crohn's disease by a sarcoid spleen suspension. *Br. Med. J.,* **2,** 155–7.

Willoughby, J.M.T., Mitchell, D.N. and Wilson, J.D. (1971) Sarcoidosis and Crohn's disease in siblings. *Am. Rev. Respir. Dis.,* **104,** 249–54.

Wiman, L.G., Beskow, R. (1970) Familiäres Auftreten von sarkoidose. *Z. Erkr. Atmungsorgane,* **133,** 481–5.

Wiman, L.G. (1972) Familial occurrence of sarcoidosis. *Scand. J. Respir. Dis., Suppl.* **80,** 115–9.

Wiman, L.G. (1974) Familial occurrence of sarcoidosis. In *Proc. 6th International Conference on Sarcoidosis, Tokyo* (eds. K. Iwai and Y. Hosoda), University of Tokyo Press, Tokyo, pp. 22–6.

Winblad, S. (1969) Erythema nodosum associated with infection with Yersinia enterocolitica. *Scand. J. Infect. Dis.,* **1,** 12–6.

Winkler, M. (1905) Beitrag zur Frage der 'Sarkoide' (Boeck) resp der subkutanenen nodulären Tuberkulide (Darier). *Arch. Dermatol. Syph. Wien,* **77,** 1–23.

Winkler, M. (1948) Über zwei tödlich verlaufene Fälle von Sarkoid Boeck, *Dermatologica,* **97,** Suppl. 125.

Winnacker, J.L., Becker, K.L., Friedlander, M., Higgins, P.A. and Moore, C.F. (1969) Sarcoidosis and hyperparathyroidism. *Am. J. Med.,* **46,** 305–11.

Winnacker, J.L., Becker, K.L. and Katz, S. (1968) Endocrine aspects of sarcoidosis. *N. Engl. J. Med.,* **278,** 483–92.

Winnacker, J.L., Becker, K.L., Katz, S. and Matthews, M.J. (1967) Recurrent epididymitis in sarcoidosis. Report of a patient treated with corticosteroids. *Ann. Intern. Med.,* **66,** 743–8.

Winslow, R.C. and Funkhouser, J.W. (1968) Sarcoidosis of the female reproductive organs. *Obstet. Gynecol.,* **32,** 285–9.

Winter, M. (1976) Thrombocytopenia, haemolytic anaemia and sarcoidosis. *Br. Med. J.,* **1,** 44.

Winterbauer, R.H., Belic, N. and Moores, K.D. (1973) A clinical interpretation of bilateral hilar adenopathy. *Ann. Intern. Med.,* **78,** 65–71.

Winterbauer, R.H. and Hutchinson, J.F. (1980) Use of pulmonary function tests in the management of sarcoidosis. *Chest,* **78,** 640–7.

With, T.K. and Helweg-Larsen, P. (1938) A case of benign lymphogranulomatosis (Sarcoid–Boeck–Schaumann) of the lymph glands, tonsils and salivary glands: complication with pulmonary tuberculosis. *Acta Med. Scand.,* **95,** 92–109.

Witmer, R. (1948) Über eine Periphlebitis retinae vom Typus Boeck. *Ophthalmologica,* **116,** 288–90.

Wolbach, S.B. (1911) A new type of cell inclusion, not parasitic, associated with disseminated granulomatous lesions. *J. Med. Res.,* **24,** 243.

Wolf, J. (1946) Lichenoid sarcoid. *Arch. Dermatol. Syphilol.,* **54,** 765.

Wolf, S.M., Rowland, L.P., Schotland, D.L., McKinney, A.S., Hoefer, P.F.A. and Aranow, H. (1966) Myasthenia as an auto-immune disease: clinical aspects. *Ann. NY Acad. Sci.,* **135,** 517–35.

Wong, M. and Rosen, S.W. (1962) Ascites in sarcoidosis due to peritoneal involvement. *Ann. Intern. Med.,* **57,** 277–80.

Wood (1964) Sarcoidosis complicated by Battey infection (?). *Q. Progr. Rep. Vet Admin.,* **19,** 29.

Wood, E.H. and Bream, C.A. (1959) Spinal sarcoidosis. *Radiology*, 73, 226–33.

Wright, C.S., Doan, C.A., Bouroncle, B.A. and Zollinger, R.M. (1951) Direct splenic arterial and venous blood studues in the hypersplenic syndromes before and after epinephrine. *Blood*, 6, 195–212.

Wright, R.E., Clairmont, A.A., Pev-Lee, J.H. and Butz, W.C. (1974) Intranasal sarcoidosis. *Laryngoscope*, 84, 2058–64.

Wurm, K., Reindell, H. and Heilmeyer, L. (1958) *Der Lungenboeck im Röntgenbild*, Georg Thieme, Stuttgart.

Wurm, K., Kehler, E. and Reichelt, H. (1962) Zur pathogenese der Sarkoidose (Morbus Boeck): gehäuftes Sarkoidosevorkommen in tuberculosen Sippen. *Med. Klin.*, 57, 1760–4.

Wurm, K. (1963) Unterschunjen über das Tuberculin-verhalten bei Sarkoiodose. *Beitr. Klin. Tuberc.*, 127, 195–201.

Wurm, (1974) Prognosis of sarcoidosis. In *Proc 6th International Conference on Sarcoidosis, Tokyo* (eds. K. Iwai and Y. Hosoda), University of Tokyo Press Tokyo, pp. 485–7.

Wurm, K. and Rosner, R. (1976) Prognosis of chronic sarcoidosis. *Ann. NY Acad. Sci.*, 278, 732–35.

Wynn-Williams, N. (1961) On erythema nodosum, bilateral hilar lymphadenopathy and sarcoidosis. *Tubercle*, 42, 57–63.

Wyss, S. and Maier, C. (1967) Hämolytische Anämie bei Sarkoidose der Milz. *Acta Haemat.*, 37, 126–36.

Yagura, T., Shimiza, M., Yamamura, Y. and Tachibanu, T. (1975) Serum IgE levels and reaginic-type skin reactions in sarcoidosis. *Clin. Exp. Immunol.*, 21, 289–97.

Yamamoto, M., Saito, N., Tachibana, T., Hirago, Y., Horikawa, M., Osada, H., Shigematsu, N. and Mikami, R. (1983) Effects of an 18–month corticosteroid therapy on stage I and stage II sarcoidosis patients (a control trial). In *Proc. 9th International Conference on Sarcoidosis, Paris*, Pergamon Press, Oxford, pp. 470–4

Yamamato, M., Muramatsu, M. and Suzuki, T. (1980) Successful corticosteroid treatment of 7 cases of probable myocardial sarcoidosis. In *Proc. 8th International Conference on Sarcoidosis, Cardiff, 1978* (eds. W. Jones-Williams and B.H. Davies), Alpha Omega, Cardiff, pp. 615–23.

Yamazaki, J. and Harada, G. (1941) Zwel Fälle von Boeckschen Sarcoid mit positiven Tuberkelbazillenbelfund im Herde. *Jpn J. Med. Sci. 13*, 2, 177–81.

Yancey, J., Luxford, W. and Sharma, O.P. (1972) Clubbing of the fingers in sarcoidosis. *J. Am. Med. Assoc.*, 222, 582.

Yang, S.P., Wu, M.C. (1974) Sarcoidosis in Taiwan. In *Proc. 6th International Conference on Sarcoidosis, Tokyo* (eds. K. Iwai and Y. Hosoda), University of Tokyo Press, Tokyo, p. 309.

Yansson, E., Hannuksela, M., Eklung, H., Halme, H. and Tuari, S. (1972) Isolation of a mycoplasma from sarcoid tissue. *J. Clin. Pathol.* 25, 837–42.

Yeager, H., Lussier, L. and Prashad, J. (1979) Alveolar macrophage-lymphocyte interaction: alterations in smokers and in sarcoidosis. *Chest*, 75, 289.

Yeager, H., Lussier, L.M., Prashad, J. and Katz, S. (1980) Sarcoidosis: differing effects of recall antigens and Kveim–Siltzbach suspension on alveolar macrophage–lymphocyte binding. N.I.H. Conference, USDHEW, Bethesda, pp. 442–6.

Yeager, H., Williams, M.C., Beekman, J.F., Beaman, B.L. and Hawley R.J. (1977) Sarcoidosis: analysis of cells obtained by bronchial lavage. *Am. Rev. Respir. Dis.*, 116, 951–4.

Yesner, R. and Silver, M. (1951) Fatal myocardial sarcoidosis. *Am. Heart J.*, **41**, 777–85.

Yotsomoto, H., Hachiya, J., Furnie, T. and Mikami, R. (1980) An estimation of computed tomography in detecting the intrathoracic changes of sarcoidosis. In *Proc. 8th International Conference on Sarcoidosis, Cardiff, 1978* (eds. W. Jones-Williams and B.H. Davies), Alpha Omega, Cardiff, pp. 386–7.

Young, D.A. and Laman, M.L. (1972) Radiodense skeletal lesions in Boeck's sarcoid. *Am. J. Roentgenal*, **114**, 533–8.

Young, H.B. and Mouney, R.A.H. (1968) Giant splenomegaly in sarcoidosis. *Br. J. Surg.*, **55**, 554–7.

Young, R.C.,Jr., Carr, C., Shelton, T.G., Mann, M., Ferrin, A., Laurey, J.R. and Harden, K. (1967) Sarcoidosis: relationship between changes in lung structure and functions. In *Proc. 4th International Conference on Sarcoidosis, Paris* (eds. J. Turiaf and J. Chabot), Masson, Paris, pp. 453–64.

Young, R.L., Harkleroad, L.E., Lordon, R.E. and Weg, J.G. (1970) Pulmonary sarcoidosis: a prospective evaluation of glucocorticoid therapy. *Ann. Intern. Med.*, **73**, 207–12.

Young, R.L., Krumholz, R.A. and Harkleroad, L.E. (1966) A physiologic roentgenographic disparity in sarcoidosis. *Dis. Chest*, **50**, 81–6.

Young, R.L., Lordon, R.E., Krumholz, R.A., Harkleroad, L.E., Branam, G.E. and Weg, J.G. (1968) Pulmonary sarcoidosis. I. Pathophysiologic correlations. *Am. Rev. Respir. Dis.*, **97**, 997–1008.

Yunis, E.J., Estevez, J.M., Pinzon, C.J. and Moran, T.J. (1967) Malacoplakia. *Arch. Pathol.*, **83**, 180–7.

Zachwiej., E., Hatys-Skirzynska, H., and Szamborski, J. (1956) Sarkoioza macicy. *Ginekol. Pol.*, **28**, 655–62.

Zaki, M.H., Addrizzo, J.R., Patton, J.M., Murphy, J.J. (1971) Further exploratory studies in sarcoidosis. *Am. Rev. Respir. Dis.*, **103**, 539–45.

Zaki, P. (1964) Contribution to the origin development and experimental production of laminated calcinosiderotic Schaumann bodies. *Acta Med. Scand.*, Suppl. **425**, 21–4.

Zapatero, J. (1970) Sarcoidosis en España. *Hosp. Gen.*, **10**, 141–4.

Zeman, W. (1951) Über neuro-psychiatrische Syndrome beim Morbus Besnier–Boeck–Schaumann. *Dsch. Med. Wochenschr.*, **76**, 1621–2.

Zenen, J.C., Meyer, A. and Klainer, L.M. (1963) Vertebral sarcoidosis. *Arch. Intern. Med.*, **111**, 696–702.

Zettergren, L. (1954) Lymphogranulomatosis benigna: a clinical and histopathological study of its relation to tuberculosis. *Acta Soc. Med. Ups.*, Suppl. 5, **59**, 1–180.

Zimmer, J.G. and Demis, D.J. (1966) Associations between gout, psoriasis and sarcoidosis with considerations of their pathogenic significance. *Ann. Intern. Med.*, **64**, 786–96.

Zimmerman, L.E., Maumenee, A.E. (1961) Ocular aspects of sarcoidosis. *Am. Rev. Respir. Dis.*, **54**, 42–4.

Zimmerman, L.E., Leeds, N.E. (1976) Calvarial and vertebral sarcoidosis. *Radiology*, **119**, 384.

Zimmerman, J., Holick, M.F. and Silver, J. (1983) Normocalcemia in a hypoparathyroid patient with sarcoidosis: evidence for parathyroid-hormone-independent synthesis of 1,25 dihydroxyvitamin D. *Ann. Intern. Med.*, **98**, 338.

Zinneman, H.H., Hall, H.W. and Heller, B.I. (1954) Acquired agammaglobulinaemia: report of 3 cases. *J. Am. Med. Assoc.*, **156**, 1390–3.

Ziskind, M.M., Weill, H., Payzant, A.R. (1963) The recognition and significance of acinus-filling processes of the lung. *Am. Rev. Respir. Dis.,* 87, 551–9.

Zollinger, H.V. (1941) Groszellig-granulomatöse Lymphangitis cerebri (Morbus Boeck) unter dem Bilde einer multiplen Sklerose verlaufend. *Virchows Arch.,* 307, 597–615.

Zoneraich, S., Gupta, M.P., Mehta, J., Zoneraich, O. and Wessely, Z. (1974) Myocardial sarcoidosis presenting as acute mitral insufficiency. *Chest,* 66, 452–6.

Zweifel, E. (1946) Gleichzeitiges Vorkommen, eines Boeckschen Sarkoids mit einer primären chronischen Polyarthritis (beginnendes Sjögren-Syndrom). *Helv. Paediatr. Acta,* 1, 475–84.

Zweiman, B. and Israel, H.L. (1976) Comparative *in vitro* reactivities of leucocytes from sarcoids and normals to different Kveim preparations. *Ann. NY Acad. Sci.,* 278, 700–8.

Index